Vascular and Endovascular Challenges Update

BIBA Publishing, BIBA Medical Limited, 526 Fulham Road, Fulham, London, SW6 5NR.
www.bibamedical.com
First published in 2016 by BIBA Publishing.
ISBN: 978-0-9570419-4-3

Limit of Liability/Disclaimer Warranty

Head of Publishing: Marcio Brito; Managing editor: Dawn Elizabeth Powell. Subediting team: David Brennan, Susan Couch, Angela Gonzalez, Katherine Hignett, Urmila Kerslake and Amanda Nieves

Typeset by Naomi Amorra

Printed in the UK by Henry Ling Printers.

Published by BIBA Publishing, 2016

I

TEVAR follow-up

Radiation damage to the pioneer operators

Aortic transection challenges and a conundrum

Juxtarenal challenges

Challenging and short infrarenal neck

Abdominal aortic aneurysm challenges

Lifestyle and aneurysm growth

Population screening challenges

The threshold for elective intervention for abdominal aortic and iliac aneurysm

Venous challenges

Contributors

A

Alback A, MD, PhD
Department of Vascular Surgery
University of Helsinki
Helsinki University Hospital
Helsinki, Finland

Allen L
Imperial Vascular Unit
Imperial College Healthcare Trust
London, UK

Andersson T, MD, PhD
AZ Groeninge
Department of Medical Imaging
Department of Neuroradiology
Karolinska University Hospital
Stockholm, Sweden

Ansel GM, MD, FACC
System Medical Chief: Vascular
OhioHealth/ Riverside Methodist Hospital
Columbus, USA

Ante M
University Hospital Heidelberg
Heidelberg, Germany

Antonello M, MD, PhD
Vascular and Endovascular Surgery Clinic
Padova University School of Medicine
Padova, Italy

Arnoldussen CWKP, MD
Department of Radiology and Nuclear
Medicine
VieCuri Medical Centre
Venlo, The Netherlands
Department of Radiology
Maastricht University Medical Centre
Maastricht, The Netherlands

Ashley S, MS, FRCS, BM
Consultant Vascular Surgeon
Plymouth Hospitals NHS Trust
Plymouth, UK

Azizzadeh A, MD, FACS
Professor and Chief
Division of Vascular and Endovascular
Surgery
University of Texas Medical School at
Houston
Houston, USA

Azzaoui R, MD
Aortic Centre
Vascular Surgery
Hôpital Cardiologique
CHU Lille
Lille, France

B

Ball S, MBChB, MRCS
Academic Surgery Unit
University of Manchester
Manchester, UK

Barakat T, MB, BS, FRCS
Northern Vascular Unit
Freeman Hospital
Newcastle upon Tyne, UK

Beard JD
Sheffield Vascular Institute
Northern General Hospital
Sheffield Teaching Hospital NHS
Foundation Trust
Sheffield, UK

Beck AW, MD
University of Florida College of Medicine,
Division of Vascular Surgery
Gainesville, USA

Behrendt CA, MD
University Heart Center Hamburg
University Medical Center
Hamburg-Eppendorf
Hamburg, Germany

Benson R, BSc, MBChB, MRCS
Department of Vascular Surgery
University Hospital of North Staffordshire
Stoke-on-Trent, UK

Beschorner U, MD
Clinic for Cardiology and Angiology II
University Heart Center Freiburg – Bad
Krozingen
Bad Krozingen, Germany

Bhattacharya V, MB, MD, FRCS
Queen Elizabeth Hospital
Gateshead, UK

Bicknell C, MBBS, MD, FRCS
Academic Division of Surgery (Imperial
College London)
Imperial Vascular Unit (Imperial College
Healthcare Trust)
London, UK

Bischoff MS, MD
University Hospital Heidelberg
Heidelberg, Germany

Björck M, MD, PhD
Department of Surgical Sciences, Section
of Vascular Surgery,
Uppsala University
Uppsala, Sweden

Black S, MD FRCS FEBVS
Vascular Surgery
St Thomas' Hospital
London, UK

Blankensteijn JD, MD, PhD
VU Medical Centre
Amsterdam, The Netherlands

Böckler D, MD, PhD, MBA
University Hospital Heidelberg
Heidelberg, Germany

Boersma HH, PharmD, PhD
Department of Clinical Pharmacy and
Pharmacology, University Medical Center
Groningen, University of Groningen,
Groningen, The Netherlands

**Bown M, MBBCh, MD, FRCS, PGCert
(Bioinformatics)**
Department of Cardiovascular Sciences
University of Leicester, Leicester Royal
Infirmary
Leicester, UK

Buijs R, Bsc
Department of Surgery, Division of
Vascular Surgery,
University Medical Center Groningen
University of Groningen
Groningen, The Netherlands

C

Cannavale A, MD
East Kent Hospitals University NHS
Foundation Trust
Kent and Canterbury Hospital
Canterbury , UK

Cao P, MD, Prof
Vascular and Endovascular Surgery,
Hospital S M Misericordia
University of Perugia
Perugia, Italy

Capoccia L, MD , PhD
Vascular and Endovascular Surgery
Division
Department of Surgery "Paride Stefanini"
Policlinico Umberto I
"Sapienza" University of Rome
Rome, Italy

Caradu C, MD
Unit of Vascular Surgery
Hopital Pellegrin
University Hospital of Bordeaux
Bordeaux, France

Castellano R, MD
Department of Vascular Surgery
San Raffaele Scientific Institute
Vita-Salute University School of Medicine
Milano, Italy

Chakfe N, MD, PhD, FEBVS
Vascular Surgery and Kidney
Transplantation Department
Novel Hopital Civil
Strasbourg, France

Cheshire N, MD, FRCS
Academic Division of Surgery
Imperial College London
London, UK

Chiesa R, MD, Full Professor
Department of Vascular Surgery, San
Raffaele Scientific Institute,
Vita-Salute University School of Medicine
Milano, Italy

**Cleveland TJ, BMedSci, BM, BS, FRCS,
FRCR**
Sheffield Vascular Institute
Sheffield Teaching Hospitals
Northern General Hospital
Sheffield, UK

Clough RE, PhD
Aortic Centre
Vascular Surgery
Hôpital Cardiologique
CHU Lille
Lille, France

Criado FJ, MD, FACS, FSVM
Vascular Surgeon – Endovascular
Specialist
MedStar Union Memorial Hospital
Baltimore, USA

D

**Davies AH, MA, DM, DSc, FRCS, FHEA,
FEBVS, FACPh**
Section of Vascular Surgery
Imperial College London
London, UK

**Darzi A, OM, KBE, PC, FRS, FMedSci,
FRCSI, FRCS, FRCSE, FRCPGlas, FACS,
FRCP**
Academic Division of Surgery
Imperial College London
London, UK

De Beaufort HWL, MD
Department of Vascular Surgery
University Medical Center Utrecht
Utrecht, The Netherlands

De Boer SA, MD
Department of Internal Medicine, Division
of Vascular Medicine,
University Medical Center Groningen,
University of Groningen,
Groningen, The Netherlands

**Debus ES, Prof, MD, FEBS, FEBVS
Professor and chair**
German Aortic Centre
Department for Vascular Medicine -
University Heart Centre Hamburg
University Clinics of Hamburg-Eppendorf
Hamburg, Germany

De Rango P, MD
Vascular and Endovascular Surgery
Hospital S M Misericordia
University of Perugia
Perugia, Italy

De Vries JPPM, MD, PhD
Head of Department of Vascular Surgery
St Antonius Hospital
Nieuwegein, The Netherlands

Donas KP, Assistant Professor
St Franziskus Hospital
Münster, Germany

Dovell G, MBBCh, MRCS
CT1, Vascular Surgery
Plymouth Hospitals NHS Trust
Plymouth, UK

Ducasse E, MD PhD
Unit of vascular surgery
Hopital Pellegrin
University Hospital of Bordeaux,
Bordeaux, France

Durham C, MD
Assistant professor
Division of Vascular and Endovascular
Surgery
University of Texas Medical School at
Houston
Houston, USA

E

Earnshaw JJ, DM, FRCS
Gloucestershire Hospitals NHS
Foundation Trust
Cheltenham General Hospital
Cheltenham, UK

Eriksson J, MD
Department of Surgical Sciences
Section of Vascular Surgery
Uppsala University
Uppsala, Sweden

F

Fanelli F, MD, EBIR
"SAPIENZA" – University of Rome
Rome, Italy

Ferrer C, MD
Vascular and Endovascular Surgery
Hospital S M Misericordia
University of Perugia
Perugia, Italy

Forsythe RO, MBChB, MRCS
Centre for Cardiovascular Science
University of Edinburgh
Edinburgh, UK

Francois O, MD
AZ Groeninge
Department of Medical Imaging
Department of Neuroradiology
Stockholm, Sweden

G

Gable DR, MD
Chief of Vascular and Endovascular
Surgery
Professor of Vascular Surgery
The Heart Hospital Baylor Plano
Plano, USA

Gaines P, MD Chb, FRCP, FRCR
Sheffield Hallam University
Sheffield, UK

Gibbs R, MD, FRCS
Imperial Vascular Unit
Imperial College Healthcare Trust
London, UK

Gohel M, MD FRCS FEBVS
Cambridge University Hospitals
Cambridge, UK &
Imperial College London
London, UK

Goodyear SJ, MD, FRCS
Worcestershire Royal Hospital
Worcester, UK

Grant SW, MRCS, PhD
Academic Surgery Unit
Institute of Cardiovascular Sciences
University of Manchester
Manchester, UK

Grego F, MD
Vascular and Endovascular Surgery Clinic
Padova University School of Medicine
Padova, Italy

H

Harnish P, MD
Department of Internal Medicine
OhioHealth/Riverside Methodist Hospital
Columbus, USA

Haulon S, MD, PhD
Aortic Centre
Vascular Surgery
Hôpital Cardiologique
CHU Lille
Lille, France

Hazenberg CEVB, MD, PhD
Department of Vascular Surgery
University Medical Centre Utrecht
Utrecht, The Netherlands

Heidemann F, MD
University Heart Center Hamburg
University Medical Center
Hamburg-Eppendorf
Hamburg, Germany

Hellgren T, MD
Department of Surgical Sciences
Section of Vascular Surgery
Uppsala University
Uppsala, Sweden

Hertault A, MD
Aortic Centre
Vascular Surgery
Hôpital Cardiologique
CHU Lille
Lille, France

Hinchliffe RJ, MD, FRCS
St George's Vascular Institute
St George's Hospital
London, UK

Holden A, MBChb, FRANZCR, EBIR
Director of Interventional Radiology
Auckland Hospital
Auckland, New Zealand

J

Jenkins M, MBBS, BSc, MS, FRCS
Imperial Vascular Unit, Imperial College
Healthcare Trust
London, UK

Jordan WD Jr, MD
Emory University School of Medicine
Atlanta, USA

K

Kabnick LS, MD, RPhS, FACS, FACVLM
New York University Vein Center
New York, USA

Kahlberg A, MD, Assistant professor
Department of Vascular Surgery, San
Raffaele Scientific Institute, Vita-Salute
University School of Medicine
Milano, Italy

Kamman AV, MD
Thoracic Aortic Research Center
Policlinico San Donato I.R.C.C.S
University of Milan
Milan, Italy

Karmeli R, MD
Carmel Medical Centre Haifa
Haifa, Israel

Karthikesalingam A, PhD, MRCS MA(Cantab)
St George's Vascular Institute
St George's Hospital
London, UK

Katsargyris A, MD,
Department of Vascular and Endovascular
Surgery
Paracelsus Medical University
Nuremberg, Germany

Kauhanen P, MD PhD
Department of Vascular Surgery
University of Helsinki
Helsinki University Hospital
Helsinki, Finland

Kölbel T, MD, Professor
German Aortic Centre
Department for Vascular Medicine
University Heart Centre Hamburg
University Clinics of Hamburg-Eppendorf
Hamburg, Germany

Kolvenbach R, MD, PhD
Catholic Hospital Group Duesseldorf
Augusta Hospital
Duesseldorf, Germany

Konge L, MD, PhD
Copenhagen Academy for Medical
Education and Simulation
University of Copenhagen,
Rigshospitalet,
Copenhagen, Denmark

Kouvelos G, MD
Department of Vascular and
Endovascular Surgery
Paracelsus Medical University
Nuremberg, Germany

Kwasnicki R, MBBS, BSc, PhD
Academic Division of Surgery
Imperial College London
London, UK

L

Laine M, MD
Helsinki University Hospital
Helsinki University
Helsinki, Finland

Lane TRA, MBBS, BSc, MRCS, PhD
Section of Vascular Surgery
Imperial College London
London, UK

Lardenoije JW, PhD, MD
Department of Surgery,
Rijnstate Hospital
Arnhem, The Netherlands

Lejay A, MD, PhD
Vascular Surgery and Kidney
Transplantation Department
Nouvel Hopital Civil
Strasbourg, France

Leopardi M, MD
Division of Vascular Surgery
San Raffaele Scientific Institute
"Vita-Salute" University
Milan, Italy

Lichtenberg M, MD, FESC
Vascular Centre
Arnsberg Clinic
Arnsberg, Germany

L'Hoest H
Barmer GEK
Berlin, Germany

Loftus I, MD, FRCS
St George's Vascular Institute
St George's Hospital
London, UK

Lönn LB, MD, Ph D
Department of Radiology
Department of Vascular Surgery,
Rigshospitalet
Copenhagen, Denmark

Lyons OT, MRCS, PhD
Vascular Surgery, St Thomas' Hospital
Cardiovascular Division, King's College
London
London, UK

M

Macharzina R, MD
Clinic for Cardiology and Angiology II
University Heart Center Freiburg – Bad
Krozingen
Bad Krozingen, Germany

Mani K, MD, PhD, FEBVS
Department of Surgical Sciences
Section of Vascualr Surgery
Uppsala University
Uppsala, Sweden

Martin T, BSc, MBBS, FRANZCR
Interventional Radiology Fellow
Auckland Hospital
Auckland, New Zealand

Martin-Gonzalez T, MD, PhD
Aortic Centre
Vascular Surgery
Hôpital Cardiologique
CHU Lille
Lille, France

Marschall U, MD
Barmer GEK
Berlin, Germany

Mascia D, MD
Department of Vascular Surgery, San
Raffaele Scientific Institute,
Vita-Salute University School of Medicine
Milano, Italy

Mayer KS, MD
Goethe-University Hospital
Department of Vascular and Endovascular
Surgery
Frankfurt, Germany

McCollum CN, FRCS, MD
Academic Surgery Unit
Institute of Cardiovascular Sciences
University of Manchester
Manchester, UK

Melissano G, MD, Associate Professor
Department of Vascular Surgery, San
Raffaele Scientific Institute, Vita-Salute
University School of Medicine
Milano, Italy

Menegolo M, MD, PHD
Vascular and Endovascular Surgery Clinic
Padova University School of Medicine
Padova, Italy

Meteyer V, MD
Vascular Surgery and Kidney
Transplantation Department
Novel Hopital Civil
Strasbourg, France

Midy D, MD, PhD
Unit of Vascular Surgery
Hopital Pellegrin
University Hospital of Bordeaux
Bordeaux, France

Miller A, MD
President, Amsel Medical
Cambridge, USA

Miyake K, MD, PhD
President of the International Meeting on
Aesthetic Phlebology
Clinica Miyake and Centro De Estudos
Hiroshi Miyake
Sao Paulo, Brazil

Moll FL, MD, PhD
Department of Vascular Surgery
University Medical Center Utrecht
Utrecht, The Netherlands

Mossop PJ, MBBS
Department of Medical Imaging
University of Melbourne School of
Medicine
St Vincent's Australia
Melbourne, Australia

Mulder DJ, MD, PhD
Department of Internal Medicine,
Division of Vascular Medicine, University
Medical Center Groningen, University of
Groningen, Groningen, The Netherlands

Murphy KE, MBChB, MRCS
Registrar in Vascular Surgery,
Sheffield Vascular Institute, Northern
General Hospital
Sheffield Teaching Hospital NHS
Foundation Trust
Sheffield, UK

N

Noory E, MD
Clinic for Cardiology and Angiology II
University Heart Center Freiburg – Bad
Krozingen
Bad Krozingen, Germany

**Normahani P, MBBS, BSc (Hons), MSc,
MRCS (Eng)**
Academic Division of Surgery
Imperial College London
London, UK

Nyamekye IK, MD, FRCS
Worcestershire Royal Hospital
Worcester, UK

O

Oakley C, Senior Physiotherapist
STEPS Physiotherapy
Sheffield UK

P

Paraskevas K, MD
St Georges' Vascular Institute
St George's Hospital
London, UK

Patterson BO, MRCS
NIHR Academic Clinical Lecturer in
Vascular Surgery
St Georges' Vascular Institute
St George's Hospital
London, UK

Piazza M, MD
Vascular and Endovascular Surgery Clinic
Padova University School of Medicine
Padova, Italy

Price BA, MD MS FRCS FCPhleb
The Whiteley Clinic
Guildford, UK

R

Rabin A, MD
Carmel Medical Centre Haifa
Haifa, Israel

Rastan A, MD
Clinic for Cardiology and Angiology II
University Heart Center Freiburg - Bad
Krozingen,
Bad Krozingen, Germany

Reijnen MPJ, MD, PhD
Department of Surgery,
Rijnstate Hospital
Arnhem, The Netherlands

Resch T, MD, PhD
Vascular Center
Department of Vascular and Thoracic
Surgery
Skane University Hospital
Malmö, Sweden

Rhee R, MD
Maimonides Medical Center
Brooklyn, USA

Riambau V, MD, PhD
Professor and chief of Vascular Surgery
Vascular Surgery Division
Cardiovascular Institute
Hospital Clinic
University of Barcelona

Richards CR, MPH, MS, MD
Tripler Army Medical Center
Honolulu, USA

Riga C, MBBS, BSc, MD, FRCS
Academic Division of Surgery (Imperial
College London)
Imperial Vascular Unit (Imperial College
Healthcare Trust)
London, UK

Rohlffs F, MD
German Aortic Centre
Department for Vascular Medicine -
University Heart Centre Hamburg
University Clinics of Hamburg-Eppendorf
Hamburg, Germany

S

Saarinen E, MD, PhD
Department of Vascular Surgery
University of Helsinki
Helsinki University Hospital
Helsinki, Finland

Sabbagh C, MB, BS
Cambridge University Hospitals
Cambridge, UK

Sakhinia F, MB, ChB, FRCR
Sheffield Vascular Institute
Northern General Hospital
Herries Road
Sheffield, UK

Saratzis A, MBBS, MRCS, PhD
Department of Cardiovascular Sciences
University of Leicester, Leicester Royal
Infirmary
Leicester, UK

Sayed S, MBChB, MD, FRCS
Department of Vascular Surgery
King's College Hospital London
London, UK

Sayers R, MBChB, (Hons), FRCS (Ed),
FRCS (Eng), MD
Department of Cardiovascular Sciences
University of Leicester, Leicester Royal
Infirmary
Leicester, UK

Schmitz-Rixen T, MD, Professor for
Vascular Surgery
Goethe-University Hospital
Department of Vascular and Endovascular
Surgery
Frankfurt, Germany

Schneider PA, MD
Kaiser Permanente Moanalua Medical
Center
Honolulu, USA

Schroeder TV, MD, DMSc
Copenhagen Academy for Medical
Education and Simulation
University of Copenhagen, DENMARK
Copenhagen, Denmark

Schuurmann RC, MD
Department of Vascular Surgery
St Antonius Hospital
Nieuwegein, The Netherlands

Settembre N, MD PhD
Department of Vascular Surgery
University of Helsinki
Helsinki University Hospital
Helsinki, Finland

Shames M, MD
Professor of Surgery and Radiology
Division of Vascular and Cardiac Surgery
USF Health Morsani School of Medicine
Tampa, USA

Shih M, MD
Maimonides Medical Center
Brooklyn, USA

Shutze W, MD
Professor of Vascular Surgery
The Heart Hospital Baylor Plano
Plano, USA

Sidloff D, MD, MRCS, BSc (Hons)
Department of Cardiovascular Sciences
University of Leicester, Leicester Royal
Infirmary
Leicester, UK

Sim E, MB BS
Alfred Health
Prahran, Australia

Slart, RHJA
Department of Nuclear Medicine
and Molecular ImagingUniversity
Medical Center Groningen, University
of Groningen, Groningen & University
of Twente, Department of Biomedical
Photonic Imaging, Enschede, The
Netherlands

Smith RS, MD
University of Alabama at Birmingham
Birmingham, AL, USA

Sobocinski J, MD, PhD
Aortic Centre
Vascular Surgery
Hôpital Cardiologique
CHU Lille
Lille, France

Spafford C, Senior physiotherapist
STEPS Physiotherapy
Sheffield UK

Spear R, MD, PhD
Aortic Centre
Vascular Surgery
Hôpital Cardiologique
CHU Lille
Lille, France

Spillerova K, MD
Department of Vascular Surgery
University of Helsinki
Helsinki University Hospital
Helsinki, Finland

Stackelberg O, MD
Unit of Nutritional Epidemiology, Institute
of Environmental Medicine,
Karolinska Institutet
Stockholm, Sweden

Stansby G, MB, MChir, FRCS
Northern Vascular Unit
Freeman Hospital
Newcastle upon Tyne, UK

Stavroulakis K, MD
St Franziskus Hospital
Münster, Germany

Stenson K, MA, MBBS, MRCS
St George's Vascular Institute
St George's Hospital
London, UK

Strijkers RHW, MD
Department of Vascular Surgery
Maastricht University Medical Centre
Maastricht, The Netherlands

Strøm M, MD
Copenhagen Academy for Medical
Education and Simulation
Department of Vascular Surgery
Rigshospitalet
Copenhagen, Denmark

T

Tanious A, MD
Integrated Vascular Surgery Resident
Division of Vascular and Cardiac Surgery
USF Health Morsani School of Medicine
Tampa, USA

Thaveau F, MD, PhD, FEBVS
Vascular Surgery and Kidney
Transplantation Department
Novel Hopital Civil
Strasbourg, France

Thompson MM, MD FRCS
St George's Vascular Institute
St George's Hospital
London, UK

Thorbjørnsen K, MD
Department of Surgical Sciences
Section of Vascular Surgery
Uppsala University
Uppsala, Sweden

Torsello G, University Professor
Münster University Hospital
St. Franziskus Hospital
Münster, Germany

Trimarchi S, MD PhD
Thoracic Aortic Research Center
Policlinico San Donato I.R.C.C.S
University of Milan
Milan, Italy

Truijers M, PhD, MD
VU Medical Centre
Amsterdam, The Netherlands

Tshomba Y, MD
Department of Vascular Surgery
San Raffaele Scientific Institute
Vita-Salute University School of Medicine
Milano, Italy

Tsilimparis N, MD, PhD
German Aortic Centre
Department for Vascular Medicine -
University Heart Centre Hamburg
University Clinics of Hamburg-Eppendorf
Hamburg, Germany

V

**Valenti D, DMChir, PhD, FRCS (Eng),
FRCS (Ed), FEBVS**
Department of Vascular Surgery
King's College Hospital London
London, UK

Van Baal JG, MD, PhD
Department of Surgery
Ziekenhuisgroep Twente
Almelo, The Netherlands

Van den berg JC, MD, PhD
Service of Interventional Radiology
Ospedale Regionale di Lugano
Lugano, Switzerland

Van den Ham LH, MD
Department of Surgery,
Rijnstate Hospital
Arnhem, The Netherlands

van Herwaarden JA, MD PhD
Department of Vascular Surgery
University Medical Center Utrecht
Utrecht, The Netherlands

Van Netten JJ, PhD
Department of Surgery
Ziekenhuisgroep Twente
Almelo, The Netherlands

Van Sterkenberg SMM, MD
Department of Surgery,
Rijnstate Hospital
Arnhem, The Netherlands

Venermo M, MD, PhD
Department of Vascular Surgery
University of Helsinki
Helsinki University Hospital
Helsinki, Finland

Verhoeven ELG, MD, PhD
Department of Vascular and
Endovascular Surgery
Paracelsus Medical University
Nuremberg, Germany

Vermeulen CFW, MD, PhD
German Aortic Centre
Department for Vascular Medicine -
University Heart Centre Hamburg
University Clinics of Hamburg-Eppendorf
Hamburg, Germany

Verzini F, MD, Prof
Vascular and Endovascular Surgery
Hospital S M Misericordia
University of Perugia
Perugia, Italy

W

Wanhainen A, MD, PhD
Department of Surgical Sciences
Section of Vascular Surgery
Uppsala University
Uppsala, Sweden

Waltenburg HN, Cand.scient, PhD
The Danish Health Authority
Radiation Protection
Copenhagen, Denmark

Wooster M, MD
Integrated Vascular Surgery Resident
Division of Vascular and Cardiac Surgery
USF Health Morsani School of Medicine
Tampa, USA

Z

Zeebregts, CJAM, MD, PhD
Department of Surgery, Division of
Vascular Surgery, University   Medical
Center Groningen, University of
Groningen, Groningen, The Netherlands

Zeller T, MD
Clinic for Cardiology and Angiology II
University Heart Center Freiburg – Bad
Krozingen
Bad Krozingen, Germany

CONTROVERSIES, CHALLENGES, CONSENSUS

This year we have challenges in the three-yearly cycle of controversies, challenges, consensus: **controversies** that enable a world-class Faculty and an expert audience to **challenge** the available evidence to reach a **consensus** after discussion. At last year's Charing Cross, we started the new cycle with **controversies**. This was to explore those uncertainties about which there was not **consensus** at the end of the last cycle.

Now we approach **challenges** and there are many. We will see a new section on **Acute Stroke Challenges**. This replaces the former carotid section. This new section draws attention to the need for a multidisciplinary approach to the pathways of care required when a patient suffers a cerebral embolism after, for example, endovascular manipulation of the arch of the aorta. It is now possible to retrieve such emboli from the brain. As long as this is done rapidly, the outcome of stroke is enormously better and this is a major breakthrough. The advance is currently the domain of neuroradiologists. They have been provided with very fine technology to retrieve emboli from the brain and this has had remarkable results.

In the **aortic** section of this book, particularly the **thoracic** portion, we are reminded that we live in an era to be able to replace segments of the aorta over the whole length by an endovascular method. Inevitably, there are some unwanted emboli passing via the great vessels to the brain. It would seem irresponsible not to have a complete understanding of the pathways of care so that such an unfortunate patient can have intracranial retrieval as soon as possible.

There are also new ways of using mesh devices in the arch of the aorta to discourage embolisation to the brain. All of these will be discussed at the Charing Cross Symposium in 2016. A key challenge is to agree on the optimal treatment for dissection of the aorta. This depends upon a knowledge of the natural history of the disease and the effect of any proposed intervention. It has been noticed that, when a dissecting aneurysm has a thrombus in the false lumen, the prognosis is better. This has led some to embolise the false lumen therapeutically in the hope of conveying an improved prognosis by this activity. This has proven to be a most challenging area and is disputed. There are those who would embolise all types of materials into the false lumen to thrombose it and others who would prefer to use an endovascular device to establish one single true lumen rather than meddle with the false lumen, and after various trials there is still an argument whether any intervention is beneficial at all! Open repair remains an option.

The **abdominal** session will be dominated on the day by new data that will be presented to the Charing Cross audience. There will be two aspects of the new data. The first will be a merging of the Individual Patient Data as a meta-analysis of the EVAR (Endovascular aneurysm repair) 1, DREAM (Dutch randomized endovascular aneurysm management), OVER (Open *versus* endovascular repair) and ACE (Anevrysme de l'aorte abdominale: chirurgie *versus* endoprothese) trials. These will be merged into a new form and analysed at Cambridge University. The first to hear the results will be the audience at Charing Cross in 2016. As these new data will be a first in a journal, sadly, they do not appear in a chapter in this book this year. These randomised controlled trials now are reaching the point of having long-term data. The 15-year results of the EVAR 1 trial will also be presented to the audience of Charing Cross. The average age of the patients was 74 years and after 15 years, they are a ripe old age! The audience will learn about the outcomes of the patients randomised to endovascular repair on the one hand or open repair on the other.

This year we recognise the debt of gratitude we owe to pioneers of endovascular surgery such as Dr Edward (Ted) Diethrich. Ted has suffered a brain tumour which is associated with exposure to radiation whilst he performed so many pioneering endovascular procedures leading the way in our specialty. Dr Roy Greenberg died after an extensive abdominal tumour and Lindsay Machan and Krassi Ivancev suffered cataracts in the eyes. These pioneers paid the price of the advance of our subject. Chapters in the book relate to aims to reduce radiation and reduce the amount of contrast, which are challenges at the moment. We honour our pioneers.

The **peripheral arterial** section focuses around challenges posed in the superficial femoral artery segment. This is particularly so for the longer lesions. There is a wide consensus of opinion that symptomatic lesions of a fairly short length can be treated by balloon angioplasty with successful results but the challenge is how long the benefit lasts. The concept of a drug-coated balloon is to achieve a longer durability and patency of this target lesion. We live in an era when there is an attempt to establish the length of lesion that can be conquered by the drug-coated balloon. The challenge is also the durability beyond two years. We anxiously await three- to five-year substantial long-term data with the use of drug-coated balloon to see how durable this is compared with, for example, open surgery, vein bypass or other forms of vascular reconstruction. The opinion is divided on whether, for example, a 25cm superficial femoral artery lesion should be treated by extensive drug-coated balloon use or whether there should be use of stent or stents in series in the first instance, with or without pre-treatment. The value of pre-treatment has escalated. This usually takes place in a form of atherectomy and an attempt to reduce the calcification before using drug-coated balloon or a stent in the hope of maintaining long-term patency. The extremely long lesions are chosen to be treated by a stent graft system in some cases.

In the background, the BASIL (Bypass *versus* angioplasty in severe ischaemia of the leg) 2 and 3 trials and the BEST (Best endovascular *versus* best surgical therapy) trial are progress, comparing endovascular reconstruction to the below-the-knee vessels against open bypass at five years.

The **venous** section divides comfortably into superficial venous challenges but what is new and has gained much ground over the last year is the increase in the performance of deep venous interventions. We are now seeing the use of venous stents for post-thrombotic syndrome. Clinical trials are emerging with the use of venous stents and prove their efficacy. Trials are taking place comparing modes of imaging before such interventions and the place of intravascular ultrasound against venography is of great importance.

We cannot remember so many of the Faculty at Charing Cross offering chapters for this book. I am pleased to say that the BIBA Publishing Team has been able to manage this increased load and occasionally been able to smile about it! Dawn Elizabeth Powell coordinated the management of the book in the publishing department headed by Marcio Brito and colleagues David Brennan, Susan Couch, Angela Gonzalez, Katherine Hignett, Urmila Kerslake, and Amanda Nieves, and I wish to thank them all.

Roger M Greenhalgh

Acute stroke challenges

Selection for intervention challenges

Specialised imaging to identify high-risk plaque

SA de Boer, HH Boersma, RHJA Slart, DJ Mulder and CJAM Zeebregts

Introduction

The development of an atherosclerotic plaque is a complex and dynamic process involving various pathological events such as endothelial cell dysfunction, inflammation, proteolysis, apoptosis, lipid accumulation, angiogenesis, thrombosis, and calcification.[1] A high-risk plaque is usually characterised by a thin vulnerable fibrous cap. If the fibrous cap degenerates, the plaque ruptures and dispels its thrombogenic lipid core into the vessel lumen, potentially leading to an acute vascular event. Several endothelial, inflammatory, and smooth muscle cells have the ability to excrete proteases such as matrix-metalloproteinases (MMPs) and cathepsin cysteine proteases (CCPs). These proteases degenerate extracellular matrix and collagen inside the fibrous cap, resulting in a lesion more prone to rupture.[2,3]

The identification of plaques in patients who are at high risk for an acute vascular event potentially allows early preventative interventions. It has become clear that the pathological property of an atherosclerotic plaque, rather than its size or the degree of stenosis, is important to identify a high-risk plaque.[1] Conventional anatomic imaging modalities, such as duplex ultrasound imaging, identify stenotic plaques and allow assessment of the degree of stenosis, but they do not provide any information on its pathological state. To allow better clinical risk stratification and to identify a high-risk plaque, there is a clear need for advanced imaging techniques. With targeted, specialised imaging, molecular pathophysiological processes can be visualised and as a consequence, the number of irreversible ischaemic events may be reduced (Figure 1).[4,5]

Nuclear imaging: PET and SPECT

Positron emission tomography (PET) and single-photon emission computed tomography (SPECT) imaging allow assessment of several *in vivo* pathological processes within the atherosclerotic plaque. These nuclear medicine techniques are based on the use of radioactive imaging agents. PET has the advantage over SPECT by allowing a more precise quantification of signals as well as localisation of the plaque activity due to a two-to-three times better spatial resolution. Since PET and SPECT imaging are limited in spatial resolution, co-registration with computed tomography (CT) scanning or magnetic resonance imaging (MRI) is necessary for accurate anatomic localisation of the radioactive signal. CT imaging is very effective for detailed vascular imaging because of its high spatial resolution, accompanied by a short acquisition time. Combining cameras such as hybrid PET/ CT is a reliable method to visualise and quantify atherosclerosis and inflammation. However, co-registration with MRI has some additional advantages. MRI is superior to CT in that it provides better soft tissue contrast and a precise analysis of the arterial wall without exposure to radiation.

Bio-optical imaging

Bio-optical imaging is a technique based on visible, ultraviolet, and infrared light to obtain molecular imaging without the need of radiation. An additional advantage of bio-optical imaging is visualising and measuring different properties of tissue at the same time due to use of various wavelengths of light. In the field of bio-optical imaging, bioluminescence and fluorescence are the most commonly used techniques. Use of bio-optical imaging is hampered by limitations such as the short penetration depth of the fluorescent signal, high costs, and the complexity of the tracers and camera equipment. However, despite all disadvantages, intra-operative use of these techniques is currently under development in oncology,[6] and we expect clinical cardiovascular application of optical imaging agents to follow in the near future.

Bioluminescence

Bioluminescence imaging is based on the capacity of several organisms to produce light by an enzyme-catalysed reaction. The pigment luciferin is administered and oxidised by an enzyme called luciferase, resulting in the emission of light without the use of an external light source. This process can be used to non-invasively visualise biological processes. However, until now, bioluminescence imaging was restricted to experimental approaches, as cells or whole organisms always need to be transfected with the luciferase gene before luciferase can be expressed.

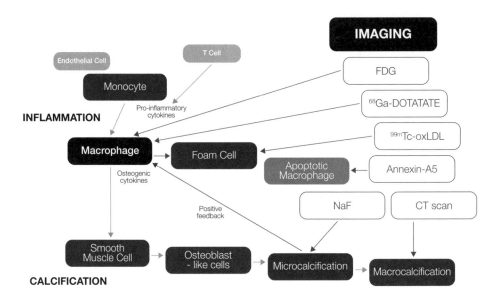

Figure 1: Scheme of inflammation and related pathogenic processes occurring of the high-risk plaque and targeted *in vivo* imaging. Adapted from Chen *et al.*[5]

Fluorescence imaging

In fluorescence imaging, an external light of a certain wavelength is used to excite a fluorescent molecule. The excited molecule will almost immediately release a longer wavelength, lower-energy light to enable imaging. Fluorescence, especially the use of light in the near-infrared fluorescence (NIRF) spectrum, contributes to a highly versatile platform for *in vivo* molecular imaging. The sensitivity for detection of certain processes with NIRF imaging exceeds that which can be detected with other molecular imaging modalities. Pathological processes that can be measured include endothelial cell dysfunction, inflammation, proteolysis, apoptosis, and thrombosis. For direct fluorescence imaging of these processes, probes targeting a specific receptor or an enzyme are necessary. The use of fluorescent imaging probes to identify the high-risk plaque is a promising modality, but clinical proof-of-concept studies are necessary.

Multispectral optoacoustic tomography

The problem with NIRF is that penetration of light is limited by tissue scattering. This scattering degrades the spatial resolution and overall accuracy, especially at increased penetration depths. Besides, the previous Bio-optical imaging techniques result in two-dimensional images. Using multispectral optoacoustic tomography (MSOT),[7] it is possible to generate a three-dimensional image (Figure 2). Optoacoustic imaging is based on the generation of the optoacoustic effect, in which pulses of laser-light that are absorbed in tissue giving rise to hyperthermia followed by broadband ultrasound waves, which can be easily non-invasively detected.

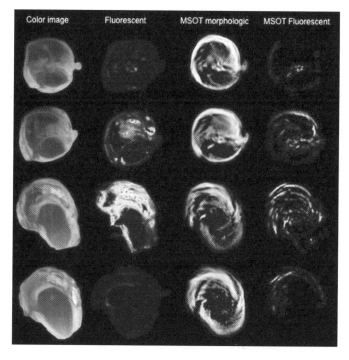

Figure 2: Imaging results from intact plaques made with MSOT. The colour images were taken in a cryo slicer system. The fluorescent images were taken from 50 micron cryo section. MSOT morphologic reconstruction and the reconstruction from the MMPSense 680 signal. Obtained from experiments performed at our department.

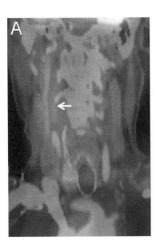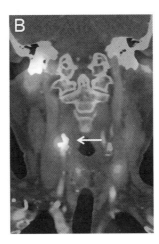

Figure 3: Examples of *in vivo* imaging of a symptomatic carotid plaque ,(A) Clinical PET/CT image with coronal plane slice of a patient showing FDG uptake in the affected right carotid artery. Obtained from previously published research.[8] (B) Clinical SPECT/CT image with coronal plane slice of a patient showing IL-2 uptake at the location of the near-occlusion symptomatic plaque in the affected right carotid artery.

Imaging agents for the high-risk plaque

In molecular imaging, imaging agents are labelled with radioactivity or fluorescence (or other suitable dyes) to visualise different pathological processes.

Inflammation

Inflammation of the arterial wall plays a key role in the development of a high-risk atherosclerotic plaque. The most commonly used imaging agent is the radioactively labelled glucose molecule [^{18}F]-2-fluoro-2-deoxy-D-glucose (FDG). FDG is especially consumed by cells with a high metabolic rate. The FDG signal has been shown to be significantly associated with macrophage infiltration and levels of inflammatory activity in carotid plaques in *ex vivo* studies.[8] Previous *in vivo* studies have demonstrated that the vascular FDG signal was associated with inflammatory biomarkers,[9] early recurrent stroke,[10] and even predicted cardiovascular events independent of traditional risk factors in asymptomatic adults.[4] In clinical trials, FDG uptake has also been used successfully as a monitoring tool for evaluating anti-atherosclerotic therapies.

Another PET tracer that has been studied in humans for evaluating atherosclerotic plaques and inflammation is ^{68}Ga-DOTATATE. This tracer binds to somatostatin receptor 2, which is expressed on activated macrophages. Previous studies have shown that the vascular ^{68}Ga-DOTATATE uptake correlated with cardiovascular risk factors.[11]

In addition to macrophages, lymphocytes play a significant role in development of a high-risk plaque. If lymphocytes are activated, they stimulate macrophages to produce MMPs. IL-2 is a pro-inflammatory cytokine, which is produced by T lymphocytes and associated with an increased carotid artery intima media thickness (a predictor of stroke).[12] The IL-2 receptor is over expressed on activated T lymphocytes during inflammation. IL-2 can be radiolabelled as its regular drug derivative, aldesleukin. However, the labelling procedure is complex and long, mainly due to aldesleukin instability during the labelling procedure.[13] Several groups have demonstrated that ^{99m}Tc-IL-2 accumulated in symptomatic carotid plaques and correlated with the amount of IL-2R+ cells, and T lymphocytes within the plaque.[14,15]

Proteolysis

An important process in plaque progression is the metabolic activation of the fibrous cap. Metabolic activation will be triggered from the release of proteolytic enzymes such as MMPs and CCPs.[3] For example, ^{99m}Tc-labeled MMP inhibitors showed a higher uptake in carotid artery stenosis compared with normal arteries in mice.[16] Furthermore, in another *ex vivo* study in which MMP-9 was visualised with NIRF imaging, MMP-9 was also shown to have an important role in the pathogenesis of plaque rupture.[2] Nevertheless, the relation between MMP expression and stroke needs to be further established and imaging agents should be validated in humans instead of animals.

Apoptosis

Carotid plaques with an increased necrotic core due to extensive apoptosis of macrophages appear to be closely associated with higher likelihood of plaque rupture.[17] Apoptotic cells start to express phosphatidylserine on the outside of the membrane. Annexin-A5 has a high affinity for phosphatidylserine and can be labelled with either ^{99m}Tc or ^{18}F to serve as an imaging agent. In a proof of concept study of four patients with a history of a transient ischaemic attack as a result of carotid artery stenosis, *in vivo* Annexin-A5 uptake corresponded with histopathological analysis of the high-risk plaque.[18] Unstable plaques showed higher uptake of Annexin-A5. There are also other imaging agents that bind to phosphatidylserine to detect apoptosis. Synaptotagmin C2A is a peptide that has been conjugated to magnetic nanoparticles for MRI as well as ^{99m}Tc for nuclear imaging.[19] However, more research is needed to validate this peptide in humans.

Lipid accumulation

The extent of the lipid core is critical to the stability of the high-risk plaque. High-risk plaques were shown to have a much larger central lipid pool.[20] There are several imaging agents available to image lipid accumulation such as ^{99m}Tc-LDL, ^{99m}Tc-oxLDL, and ^{99m}Tc-LOX-1, but most of those agents are evaluated in dated studies. However, high lipid accumulation can also be measured by MRI.[21]

Angiogenesis

Intraplaque angiogenesis is associated with plaque destabilisation. Neoangiogenesis causes plaque growth and is a source of intraplaque haemorrhage.[22] The intraplaque release of several angiogenic cytokines, such as vascular endothelium growth factor (VEGF), and the local hypoxic environment stimulates angiogenesis. As such, VEGF is a target for imaging. For example, [89]Zr-bevacizumab PET for targeting of VEGF-A has been shown to correlate with immunohistochemistry scores related to plaque instability in human carotid plaque in an *ex vivo* study.[23] Although it has been suggested that VEGF may have a protective role in atherosclerosis due to regeneration of endothelium, the overall evidence underlines a substantial role in plaque rupture, due to the formation of immature capillary vessels. To explain this discrepancy, further evaluation is needed. However, the use of radioactive [89]Zr-bevacizumab in a clinical setting has a high radiation burden. The latter can be drastically reduced by using ^{18}F-labelled, labelled to smaller VEGF proteins, such as fab-fragments.[23]

Calcification

Microcalcification is another feature of high-risk plaques that develops in response to inflammation. While macrocalcification is considered a characteristic of plaque stability, microcalcifications may be related to plaque rupture. Microcalcifications are associated with plaque inflammation and necrosis.[24] Detection of microcalcification is not possible with a CT scan since it only identifies macrocalcification (Figure 4). The feasibility of [18]F -sodium fluoride (NaF) PET to visualise microcalcification in the atherosclerotic plaque was recently demonstrated.[25] Currently, NaF is the only available clinical imaging agent that can non-invasively detect microcalcification in vascular plaque activity. Additional clinical trials are required to evaluate the value of NaF PET-for the prediction of cardiovascular events.

Conclusion

Specialised molecular imaging techniques to identify a high-risk plaque are available, but further evaluation is required to validate imaging agents. Clinical studies are needed to establish the predictive value of these imaging agents and to evaluate their applicability as a surrogate endpoint in clinical trials. Until now, only FDG is more or less clinically established to be used as a radiopharmaceutical for imaging of inflammation in atherosclerosis.

Hybrid imaging systems such as PET/CT and PET/MRI can play a pivotal role in this, including the use of whole body vascular imaging. Most promising tracers are FDG and NaF for hybrid imaging in the near future. Bio-optical imaging without using potentially harmful radiation is a technique with clinical potential but needs to be further developed and validated in humans.

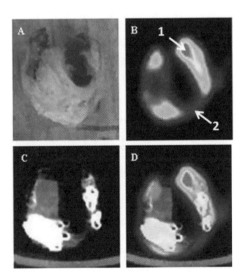

Figure 4: Transverse view of a heavily calcified carotid artery endarterectomy specimen. (A) Photograph of cut segment after scanning procedure. (B) µPET image of CEA specimen incubated with 18F-NaF; arrow 1 corresponds with low uptake and arrow 2 is correlated with high uptake. (C) CT-image of the same CEA specimen. (D) Fused µPET and CT image. Obtained from previously unpublished experiments performed at our department.

Summary

- Various imaging modalities such as nuclear molecular imaging, including PET and SPECT, and Bio-optical imaging can be used to identify the high-risk carotid plaque but need to be further validated and developed.

- Of all imaging agents, FDG is currently the most validated and clinical potential imaging agent to identify the high-risk plaque. In addition to FDG, NaF is also a promising imaging agent.

- Imaging agents to visualise and quantify proteolytic enzymes, especially matrix metallo-proteinases-9, can be of great potential to identify the high-risk plaque, but validation of imaging agents in humans is complicated and needs to be further developed.

- There is a clear need for large population-based studies for more accurate plaque assessment, as a good selection policy for intervention is important.

References

1. Naghavi M, Libby P, Falk E, *et al*. From vulnerable plaque to vulnerable patient: a call for new definitions and risk assessment strategies: Part I. *Circulation* 2003; **108** (14): 1664–72.
2. Jager NA, Wallis de Vries BM, *et al*. Distribution of matrix metalloproteinases in human atherosclerotic carotid plaques and their production by smooth muscle cells and macrophage subsets. *Mol Imaging Biol* 2015; Epub.
3. Morgan AR, Rerkasem K, Gallagher PJ, *et al*. Differences in matrix metalloproteinase-1 and matrix metalloproteinase-12 transcript levels among carotid atherosclerotic plaques with different histopathological characteristics. *Stroke* 2004; **35** (6): 1310–15.
4. Moon SH, Cho YS, Noh TS, *et al*. Carotid FDG uptake improves prediction of future cardiovascular events in asymptomatic individuals. *JACC Cardiovasc Imaging* 2015; **8** (8): 949–56.
5. Chen W, Dilsizian V. Targeted PET/CT imaging of vulnerable atherosclerotic plaques: microcalcification with sodium fluoride and inflammation with fluorodeoxyglucose. *Curr Cardiol Rep* 2013; **15** (6): 364: 1–6.
6. van Dam GM, Themelis G, Crane LM, *et al*. Intraoperative tumor-specific fluorescence imaging in ovarian cancer by folate receptor-alpha targeting: first in-human results. *Nat Med* 2011; **17** (10): 1315–19.
7. Razansky D, Harlaar NJ, Hillebrands JL, *et al*. Multispectral optoacoustic tomography of matrix metalloproteinase activity in vulnerable human carotid plaques. *Mol Imaging Biol* 2012; **14** (3): 277–85.
8. Masteling MG, Zeebregts CJ, Tio RA, *et al*. High-resolution imaging of human atherosclerotic carotid plaques with micro 18F-FDG PET scanning exploring plaque vulnerability. *J Nucl Cardiol* 2011; **18** (6): 1066–75.
9. Rudd JH, Myers KS, Bansilal S, *et al*. Relationships among regional arterial inflammation, calcification, risk factors, and biomarkers: a prospective fluorodeoxyglucose positron-emission tomography/ computed tomography imaging study. *Circ Cardiovasc Imaging* 2009; **2** (2): 107–15.
10. Marnane M, Merwick A, Sheehan OC, *et al*. Carotid plaque inflammation on 18F-fluorodeoxyglucose positron emission tomography predicts early stroke recurrence. *Ann Neurol* 2012; **71** (5): 709–18.
11. Mojtahedi A, Alavi A, Thamake S, *et al*. Assessment of vulnerable atherosclerotic and fibrotic plaques in coronary arteries using (68)Ga-DOTATATE PET/CT. *Am J Nucl Med Mol Imaging* 2014; **5** (1): 65–71.
12. Elkind MS, Rundek T, Sciacca RR, *et al*. Interleukin-2 levels are associated with carotid artery intima-media thickness. *Atherosclerosis* 2005; **180** (1): 181–87.
13. Signore A, Capriotti G, Scopinaro F, *et al*. Radiolabelled lymphokines and growth factors for in vivo imaging of inflammation, infection and cancer. *Trends Immunol* 2003; **24** (7): 395–02.
14. Annovazzi A, Bonanno E, Arca M, *et al*. 99mTc-interleukin-2 scintigraphy for the in vivo imaging of vulnerable atherosclerotic plaques. *Eur J Nucl Med Mol Imaging* 2006; **33** (2): 117–26.
15. Glaudemans AW, Bonanno E, Galli F, *et al*. In vivo and in vitro evidence that (99)mTc-HYNIC-interleukin-2 is able to detect T lymphocytes in vulnerable atherosclerotic plaques of the carotid artery. *Eur J Nucl Med Mol Imaging* 2014; **41** (9): 1710–19.

16. Schafers M, Riemann B, Kopka K, *et al.* Scintigraphic imaging of matrix metalloproteinase activity in the arterial wall in vivo. *Circulation* 2004; 1; **109** (21): 2554–59.

17. Leist M, Jaattela M. Four deaths and a funeral: from caspases to alternative mechanisms. *Nat Rev Mol Cell Biol* 2001; **2** (8): 589–98.

18. Kietselaer BL, Reutelingsperger CP, Heidendal GA, *et al.* Noninvasive detection of plaque instability with use of radiolabeled annexin A5 in patients with carotid-artery atherosclerosis. *N Engl J Med* 2004; **350** (14): 1472–73.

19. Korngold EC, Jaffer FA, Weissleder R, Sosnovik DE. Noninvasive imaging of apoptosis in cardiovascular disease. *Heart Fail Rev* 2008; **v13** (2): 163-73.

20. Davies MJ, Richardson PD, Woolf N, *et al.* Risk of thrombosis in human atherosclerotic plaques: role of extracellular lipid, macrophage, and smooth muscle cell content. Br Heart J 1993; **69** (5): 377–81.

21. Hatsukami TS, Ross R, Polissar NL, Yuan C. Visualization of fibrous cap thickness and rupture in human atherosclerotic carotid plaque in vivo with high-resolution magnetic resonance imaging. *Circulation* 2000; **102** (9): 959–64.

22. Takaya N, Yuan C, Chu B, *et al.* Presence of intraplaque hemorrhage stimulates progression of carotid atherosclerotic plaques: a high-resolution magnetic resonance imaging study. *Circulation* 2005; **111** (21): 2768–75.

23. Golestani R, Zeebregts CJ, Terwisscha van Scheltinga AG, *et al.* Feasibility of vascular endothelial growth factor imaging in human atherosclerotic plaque using (89)Zr-bevacizumab positron emission tomography. Mol Imaging 2013; **12** (4): 235–43.

24. Joshi NV, Vesey AT, Williams MC, *et al.* 18F-fluoride positron emission tomography for identification of ruptured and high-risk coronary atherosclerotic plaques: a prospective clinical trial. *Lancet* 2014; **383** (9918): 705–13.

25. Irkle A, Vesey AT, Lewis DY, *et al.* Identifying active vascular microcalcification by (18)F-sodium fluoride positron emission tomography. *Nat Commun* 2015; **6**: 7495.

Microemboli and the cause of dementia

S Ball and CN McCollum

Introduction

Dementia is a progressive, neurodegenerative disorder causing severe cognitive impairment, behavioural changes and dependence on others for activities of daily living. Sufferers lose weight and ultimately become bed bound and incontinent. In the UK, 850,000 people suffer from dementia with one in 14 aged over 65 affected. By 2025 an estimated one million people will be living with dementia; an increase of 40% compared with current numbers. The overall prevalence of dementia at death increases from 6% for those aged 65–69 to 58% for those aged over 95. Delaying the onset of dementia by five years would half the number of people dying with dementia. Early onset dementia affects more than 44,000 UK people a year and follows a more aggressive course. The overall cost of dementia to the UK is an estimated £26 billion/year.[1]

Alzheimer's disease and vascular dementia account for over 80% of all the dementias; there is considerable overlap between the two based on clinical, epidemiological and histopathological evidence. Vascular risk factors are associated with an increased risk of both Alzheimer's disease and vascular dementia. The exact pathophysiology remains unknown; it is suggested that arterial disease or cerebral emboli trigger neurodegeneration or reduce the amount of neurofibrillary tangles and senile plaques needed for the clinical manifestation of dementia.[2] However, regardless of the pathology, treatment of vascular risk factors forms an important part of management.[3-6]

The notion that cerebral emboli that are too small to cause acute symptoms may be involved in the development of dementia was based on evidence that patients with prosthetic heart valves and those undergoing carotid or open heart surgery suffered cognitive deficits.[2] Cognitive impairment persists in some 10–30% of patients following cardiac surgery and autopsy studies on such patients are consistent with widespread microembolism to the brain.[7,8] This led to the hypothesis that widespread microembolism to the brain over a period of time leads to cognitive impairment.[8]

Paradoxical cerebral embolisation is recognised to be important in cryptogenic stroke, post-operative confusion following hip replacement, migraine, decompression sickness in scuba divers and transient global amnesia.[9-12] Paradoxical emboli may pass through a patent foramen ovale or other atrial/ventricular septal defect to enter the cerebral circulation. As paradoxical embolisation may also occur through pulmonary arteriovenous fistulae, we use the term "venous to arterial circulation shunt". Paradoxical embolisation may

13

conceivably occur over many years, producing a gradual deterioration in cerebral function typical of dementia.

These works led us to study the association of cerebral emboli and dementia in a series of studies.[3,8,13–16] The middle cerebral artery supplies blood to the frontal, parietal and temporal areas of the brain, which are considered critical in dementia.[3] By insonating the middle cerebral artery through the transtemporal window, cerebral emboli can be detected and their frequency counted. In all studies, patients underwent one hour of continuous transcranial Doppler insonation of the middle cerebral artery using a 2MHz pulsed-wave Doppler probe. Patients were observed for any movement or potential artefacts and the data analysed by two vascular scientists, blinded to each other's results. The international consensus criteria[17] for emboli detection was used, including: embolic signals should be transient (lasting <300 milliseconds), at least 3dB higher than the background blood flow, unidirectional, within the Doppler spectrum, and accompanied by an audible "snap", "chirp", or "moan" (Figure 1).

The presence of a venous to arterial circulation shunt was investigated using an emulsion of air microbubbles in saline as an ultrasound contrast medium following the completion of one-hour transcranial Doppler. The bubble suspension was rapidly injected intravenously under three conditions, each separated by one minute: resting quietly; coughing repeatedly during injection and for a further 10 seconds; and performing a standardised Valsalva manoeuvre with five-second release after injection. The presence of a venous to arterial circulation shunt equivalent to a patent foramen ovale was defined as 15 or more embolic signals with the first within 12 cardiac cycles of contrast administration.

Frequency of spontaneous cerebral emboli in dementia

Our first investigation was a pilot study exploring the role of cerebral and paradoxical embolisation in dementia.[2] Cerebral emboli were detected in 27.5% of dementia patients compared with 7% of controls (p=0.15) with emboli being most frequent in both Alzheimer's disease and vascular dementia compared with controls (Odds ratio [OR] 10.5, p=0.04). A significant venous to arterial circulation shunt, equivalent to patent foramen ovale, was detected in 61% of dementia patients and 44% of controls (p=0.24). In dementia patients with cerebral emboli, moderate-to -severe carotid stenosis was present in three (p=0.41). It was, therefore, concluded that cerebral emboli were more frequent in patients with both Alzheimer's disease and vascular dementia, but these emboli were not due to carotid disease or a venous to arterial circulation shunt.

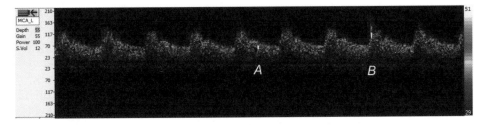

Figure 1: Transcranial Doppler recording showing a solid emboli (A) and a gaseous emboli (B).

This formed the basis of a case control study comparing the occurrence of spontaneous cerebral emboli and venous to arterial circulation shunt in patients with Alzheimer's disease and vascular dementia to controls.[13] A total of 320 patients were involved; 170 dementia patients and 150 controls. Cerebral emboli were detected in 32 (40%) patients with Alzheimer's disease and 31 (37%) with vascular dementia compared with only 12 (15%) and 12 (14%) of their respective controls. Two or more spontaneous cerebral emboli were detected in 17 (21%) patients with Alzheimer's disease and 18 (21%) with vascular dementia, and in nine (11%) and eight (9%) of their respective controls. The odds ratio (OR) for cerebral emboli was 3.22 (1.52 to 6.81; p=0.002) in Alzheimer's disease and 4.80 (1.83 to 12.58, p=0.001) in vascular dementia. The OR for spontaneous cerebral emboli remained similar and highly significant at 2.7 (1.18 to 6.21; p=0.019) for Alzheimer's disease and 5.36 (1.24 to 23.18; p=0.025) for vascular dementia after adjustment for cardiovascular risk factors.

We detected a significant venous to arterial circulation shunt (equivalent to patent foramen ovale) in 27 (32%) patients with Alzheimer's disease and 25 (29%) with vascular dementia compared with respectively 19 (22%) and 17 (20%) controls. The OR for Alzheimer's was 1.57 and for vascular dementia 1.67. This study was the first to show an association between spontaneous cerebral emboli and dementia, leading us to conduct further studies on the effects that spontaneous cerebral emboli have on cognitive decline in dementia patients.[3,14]

Cerebral emboli and progression of dementia

We compared cognitive decline in dementia patients who were positive for cerebral emboli with those who were negative, concluding that spontaneous cerebral emboli are associated with an accelerated decline in cognition and function in Alzheimer's dementia and vascular dementia. A total of 132 patients, 74 with Alzheimer's and 58 with vascular dementia, underwent baseline transcranial Doppler to detect cerebral emboli and various neuropsychological tests for cognition and function; Alzheimer's Disease Assessment Scale-Cognitive (ADAS-cog) score, Mini-Mental State Examination (MMSE) and Interview for Deterioration in Daily Living Activities in Dementia (IDDD). These tests were repeated at six months.

All patients, regardless of their cerebral emboli status, showed significant deterioration in cognition and function over the six months (Figure 2).

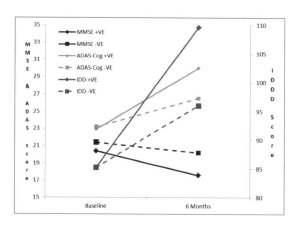

Figure 2: The rate of decline in cognitive functioning over six months between those positive for cerebral emboli and those without.

This was the first study to document that spontaneous cerebral emboli are related to cognitive decline in dementia and led us to further evaluate if the numbers of emboli had an influence on cognitive decline. A total of 99 patients completed the study, undergoing both cognitive function testing at baseline and every six months for two years, along with detection of cerebral emboli at baseline and every six months for 18 months.

The results again showed a significantly more rapid decline in cognition and function as measured by ADAS-Cog, MMSE and IDDD (p=0.009; 0.01; 0.008, respectively) over the two years. In this study, Neuropsychiatric Inventory (NPI) was also measured and showed a mean increase in score of 12 in cerebral emboli positive patients, compared with a mean decrease in score of 3.8 in those with no cerebral emboli (p<0.001).

For cerebral emboli-positive patients, the percentage of patients with >40% decline in cognitive function at six, 12, 18, and 24 months were 31%, 45%, 53%, and 57%, respectively, compared with 21%, 30%, 23%, and 30%, respectively, in cerebral emboli-negative patients (p=0.003).

The ranking based on the number of emboli detected per Doppler session was significantly correlated with cognitive deterioration over two years, as indicated by scores on the ADAS-Cog (rs=0.28; p=0.008), Interview for Deterioration in Daily Living Activities in Dementia (rs =0.36; p<0.001), and Neuropsychiatric Inventory (rs=0.42, p<0.001). However, when this correlation was repeated in only patients who were emboli positive, no statistical significance was achieved.

Cerebral emboli and cerebral white matter

Deep white matter hyperintensities are associated with a more rapid decline in patients with dementia and older people without dementia.[15,18-20] The exact mechanisms of white matter hyperintensities are not fully known but are thought to be related to hypertension and small vessel arteriosclerosis. Some studies have found an association between white matter hyperintensities and cerebral infarctions while others excluded patients with cerebral infarction.

We studied the relationship between spontaneous cerebral emboli, patent foramen ovale, deep white matter hyperintensities and periventricular hyperintensities on cerebral magnetic resonance imaging (MRI) in patients with Alzheimer's disease and vascular dementia.

In patients with Alzheimer's disease, a significant venous to arterial circulation shunt was associated with more severe deep white matter hyperintensities (p=0.005) and periventricular hyperintensities (p=0.038), which persisted following adjustment for age, MMSE score, hypertension, carotid disease and presence of cerebral infarcts (p=0.030). Alzheimer's disease patients with a significant venous to arterial circulation shunt had an OR of 3.9 (p=0.021) for severe periventricular hyperintensities which when adjusted as above, rose to 8.7 (p=0.011). This association remained after exclusion of cerebral infarcts. There was no relationship between the presence of a significant venous to arterial circulation shunt and deep white matter hyperintensities or periventricular hyperintensities in vascular dementia.

When compared with Alzheimer patients, vascular dementia patients had more severe deep white matter hyperintensities and periventricular hyperintensities.

There was a negative correlation between cerebral emboli and severity deep white matter hyperintensities.

In Alzheimer's disease patients, there was no relationship between cerebral emboli and deep white matter hyperintensities, but the presence of a significant venous to arterial circulation shunt was associated with a significant increase in both deep white matter hyperintensities and periventricular hyperintensities.

Carotid artery disease and dementia

The Rotterdam study was the first to report an association between carotid artery disease and dementia.[21] The pathophysiology being that cerebral hypoperfusion causes cell death and cerebral atrophy, which we know is related to dementia.[22]

Balucani et al evaluated the extent of cognitive impairment in bilateral asymptomatic carotid stenosis, unilateral asymptomatic carotid stenosis and no carotid stenosis.[23] Cerebral haemodynamics were measured by cerebral vasomotor reactivity and neuropsychological assessments evaluating cognitive function specific to each hemisphere were undertaken. A significant difference was found in cognitive function in those with carotid stenosis (bilateral or unilateral). This was also true for patients with impaired cerebral vasomotor reactivity and was observed in relation to the performance of each hemisphere. Impaired cerebral vasomotor reactivity was found ipsilateral to the side of stenosis. There was no significant difference between those with no carotid stenosis and those with preserved cerebral vasomotor reactivity. The fact that the observed difference was ipsilateral to the stenosis supports the theory of hypoperfusion.

Balestrini et al evaluated the relationship between severe carotid stenosis, haemodynamic impairment and cognitive decline.[24] Patients with carotid artery stenosis had an increased probability of developing cognitive impairment (OR 4.16, $p<0.001$) and the risk increased significantly if there was associated haemodynamic impairment (OR 14.66, $p<0.001$).

Saleh et al's systematic review on carotid artery intima media thickness and cognitive impairment included 20 studies of which 14 found a significant association. The investigators suggested that the lack of a strong relationship between intima-media thickness and cognitive impairment was in part due to a lack of a definition of cognitive impairment and inconsistent intima-media thickness measurement techniques.[25]

Conclusion

Since publication of the above studies, there has been little further research in the area; only a few review articles reinforcing our knowledge on cardiac disease as a risk factor for dementia.

It is clear from our published works that cerebral emboli have a role in the pathophysiology of Alzheimer's disease and vascular dementia. The frequency of cerebral emboli was similar in Alzheimer's disease and vascular dementia, suggesting that the causation of both may be the same with larger emboli causing the cerebral infarcts that lead to the classification of dementia as "vascular".

The most plausible mechanism is cerebral microemboli-induced repetitive low-grade ischaemia in the cerebral microcirculation, potentially triggering microglial activation and inflammatory brain injury leading to dementia without causing symptomatic neurological events. The occurrence of cerebral emboli and their effect on the rate of progression of dementia were also similar in both Alzheimer's disease and vascular dementia. The cognitive decline observed in our dementia patients was similar to that observed in other clinical trials on Alzheimer's disease. These studies also report considerable variability in the progression of dementia between individuals; cerebral emboli may explain at least some of this variability. The difference in the cognitive decline over two years between dementia patients with and without cerebral emboli is similar to the annual decline in Alzheimer's disease, which suggests a meaningful effect of emboli and one which could be inhibited.

None of the above studies explored the aetiology of cerebral emboli but they are common in patients with atrial fibrillation, prosthetic heart valves, carotid artery disease, patent foramen ovale and those undergoing cardiac surgery.

Cerebral emboli fall into the basket of vascular risk factors where there is good evidence of an important influence on the causation and progression of dementia to suggest that further work needs to be done. This should include randomised controlled trials on therapies to reduce vascular risk, especially cerebral emboli in the prevention or treatment of dementia.

Summary

- Alzheimer's disease and vascular dementia have common vascular risk factors.

- Cerebral microemboli have an important role in dementia and progression of dementia.

- Further work should focus on therapies to reduce vascular risk, especially cerebral emboli in the prevention of dementia.

References

1. Alzheimer's Society. Dementia UK: Update 2014 (second edition). http://bit.ly/1ROKMKW (date accessed 28 January 2016).
2. Purandare N, Welsh S, Hutchinson S, *et al*. Cerebral emboli and paradoxical embolisation in dementia: a pilot study. *Int J Geriatr Psychiatry* 2005; **20** (1): 12–16.
3. Purandare N, Burns A, Morris J *et al*. Association of cerebral emboli with accelerated cognitive deterioration in Alzheimer's disease and vascular dementia. *Am J Psychiatry* 2012; **169** (3): 300–08
4. Kivipelto M, Ngandu T, Laatikainen T, *et al*. Risk score for the prediction of dementia risk in 20 years among middle aged people: a longitudinal, population-based study. *Lancet Neurol* 2006; **5** (9): 735–41
5. Kalaria RN. The role of cerebral ischemia in Alzheimer's disease. *Neurobiol Aging* 2000; **21** (2): 321–30.
6. Launer LJ, Petrovitch H, Ross GW, *et al*. AD brain pathology: vascular origins? Results from the HAAS autopsy study. *Neurobiol Aging* 2008; **29** (10):1587–90.
7. Moody DM, Bell MA, Challa VR, Johnston WE, Prough DS. Brain microemboli during cardiac surgery or aortography. *Ann Neurol* 1990; **28** (4): 477–86
8. Voshaar RC, Purandare N, Hardicre J, *et al*. Asymptomatic spontaneous cerebral emboli and cognitive decline in a cohort of older people: a prospective study. *Int J Geriatr Psychiatry* 2007; **22**(8): 794–800.
9. Lechat P, Mas JL, Lascault G, *et al*. Prevalence of patent foramen ovale in patients with stroke. *N Engl J Med* 1988; **318** (18): 1148–52.
10. Webster MW, Chancellor AM, Smith HJ *et al*. Patent foramen ovale in young stroke patients. *Lancet* 1988; **2** (8601): 11–12.
11. Riding G, Rao S, Hutchinson S, *et al*. Cerebral emboli during hip and knee replacement: the role of venous to arterial shunting. *Brit J Surg* 2001; **88** (5): 745.
12. Anzola GP. Clinical impact of patent foramen ovale diagnosis with transcranial Doppler. European *Ultraschall Med* 2002; **16** (1-2): 11–20.

13. Purandare N, Burns A, Daly KJ, *et al.* Cerebral emboli as a potential cause of Alzheimer's disease and vascular dementia: case-control study. *BMJ* 2006; **332** (7550): 1119–24.

14. Purandare N, Voshaar RC, Morris J, *et al.* Asymptomatic spontaneous cerebral emboli predict cognitive and functional decline in dementia. *Biol Psychiatry* 2007; **62** (4): 339–44.

15. Purandare N, Oude Voshaar RC, McCollum C, *et al.* Paradoxical embolisation and cerebral white matter lesions in dementia. *Br J Radiol* 2008; **81** (961): 30–34.

16. Oude Voshaar RC, Purandare N, Hardicre J, *et al.* Asymptomatic spontaneous cerebral emboli and mood in a cohort of older people: a prospective study. *Am J Geriatr Psychiatry* 2007; **15** (12): 1057–60.

17. Basic identification criteria of Doppler microembolic signals. Consensus Committee of the Ninth International Cerebral Hemodynamic Symposium. *Stroke* 1995; **26** (6): 1123.

18. De Groot JC, De Leeuw FE, Oudkerk M, *et al.* Periventricular cerebral white matter lesions predict rate of cognitive decline. *Ann Neurol* 2002; **52** (3): 335-41.

19. Vermeer SE, Prins ND, den Heijer T, *et al.* Silent brain infarcts and the risk of dementia and cognitive decline. *N Engl J Med* 2003; **348** (13): 1215–22.

20. Prins ND, van Dijk EJ, den Heijer T, *et al.* Cerebral white matter lesions and the risk of dementia. Archives of *Neurology* 2004; **61**(10): 1531–34.

21. Hofman A, Ott A, Breteler MM, *et al.* Atherosclerosis, apolipoprotein E, and prevalence of dementia and Alzheimer's disease in the Rotterdam Study. *Lancet* 1997; **349** (9046): 151–54.

22. Romero JR, Beiser A, Seshadri S, *et al.* Carotid artery atherosclerosis, MRI indices of brain ischemia, aging, and cognitive impairment: the Framingham study. *Stroke* 2009; **40** (5): 1590–96.

23. Balucani C, Viticchi G, Falsetti L, Silvestrini M. Cerebral hemodynamics and cognitive performance in bilateral asymptomatic carotid stenosis. *Neurology* 2012; **79** (17): 1788–95.

24. Balestrini S, Perozzi C, Altamura C, *et al.* Severe carotid stenosis and impaired cerebral hemodynamics can influence cognitive deterioration. *Neurology* 2013; **80** (23): 2145–50.

25. Saleh C. Carotid artery intima media thickness: a predictor of cognitive impairment? Frontiers in bioscience (Elite edition) 2009; **2**: 980–90.

Carotid stenting and endarterectomy

A modern stroke service must have timely access to carotid stenting if it is to offer optimal outcomes

F Sakhinia and TJ Cleveland

Introduction

A stroke is when a focal—and sometimes global—neurological deficit develops acutely with a vascular cause.[1] It lasts longer than 24 hours and can be ischaemic (87%) or haemorrhagic (13%).[1] Furthermore, stroke is a major worldwide cause of morbidity and mortality, with approximately 150,000 people in the UK having their first stroke each year.[2] On the other hand, a transient ischaemic attack has the same initial symptoms as a stroke but these resolve completely within 24 hours; the most important aspect of a transient ischaemic attack is that it is associated with a very high (albeit short-term) risk of a further event, which may be a complete or even fatal stroke.

The prevalence of ischaemic stroke increases with increasing age and varies by race and ethnicity. Risk factors for stroke include smoking, hypertension, ischaemic heart disease, transient ischaemic attack, peripheral vascular disease, diabetes, hyperfibrinogenaemia, and hypercholesterolaemia.[2]

Atherosclerotic plaque in the carotid artery contributes to a major portion of ischaemic strokes though thromboembolism (which occurs due to rupture of the fibrous cap within the plaque, resulting in platelet activation and emboli) and hypoperfusion. Additionally, there is a strong association between the severity of the carotid artery stenosis and the development of subsequent stroke in symptomatic patients.[1]

The need for timely treatment

Patients who present with clinical symptoms of stroke or transient ischaemic attack need timely assessment and treatment. Overall outcomes are improved if a patient is managed in a dedicated stroke unit, with treatment instigated promptly; the highest risk for recurrent stroke is in the first few days or weeks after a primary event.[3]

This knowledge has precipitated healthcare systems to invest significant amounts of money and resources into the development of services that deliver timely treatments.[4,5] Integral to these pathways is the identification and treatment of carotid artery stenoses, which can be responsible for recurrent neurological events.

Carotid endarterectomy is a recognised treatment for stroke prevention, and its role is recognised in the treatment pathways in stroke strategies. While it is a treatment for the prevention of future stroke (and thus, its place is late in the pathway), endarterectomy provides the most benefit if performed in the acute phase (preferably within a week of symptom onset). Any other potential treatments for carotid bifurcation stenoses (such as stenting) need to be available in a similarly timely fashion or much of their potential benefit will be lost.

The role of carotid artery stenting

Carotid endarterectomy is an effective method of stroke prevention by treating high-grade carotid bifurcation stenosis. For example, NASCET (North American symptomatic carotid endarterectomy trial) and ESCT (European carotid surgery trial)[6,7] provided conclusive evidence that it gave additional benefit over optimal medical treatment alone when the risk of recurrent stroke (tight carotid stenosis) was high and when the operation could be performed with a low risk of complications.

There was reticence to consider angioplasty as a viable alternative (or even in addition) to endarterectomy because the risk of embolisation was thought to be too high. However, Mathias et al[8,9] and Kerber et al[10] reported successful results for angioplasty using the technology of that time (late 70s/early 80s). Balloon-expandable stents were used initially, but then self-expanding stents were introduced and used.[1] The balloon-expandable stents were prone to extrinsic compression and, therefore, self-expanding stents became the standard of care. However, the risk of embolic stroke at the time of carotid artery stenting was still a major concern, leading to the development of embolic protection devices in the 1990s.[11]

Compared with endarterectomy, the simplicity, short hospital stay, and comfort of stenting attracted a lot of support from both patients and endovascular operators. Stenting has undergone tremendous scrutiny and criticism over the last 15 years, and 13 randomised clinical trials have compared endarterectomy and stenting in both symptomatic and asymptomatic patients.[12] Multiple meta-analyses, large registries and clinical studies have also been published.[1]

The result of some of the early trials were not favourable towards stenting and several were abandoned due to high procedural risks observed with the procedure.[13] One of the largest earlier trials was CAVATAS (Carotid and vertebral artery transluminal angioplasty study),[14] which showed no significant difference in procedural risk between endarterectomy and stenting. However, it found that stenting was associated with a higher rate of 30-day death/any stroke (13%) than was endarterectomy (10%). These results were heavily criticised at the time by the vascular community.[13]

The evidence base in detail

The results of stenting from the trials can be divided into two periods: the early period from 1979 to 1999, and the modern endovascular period from 2000 onwards.[1] The transition from the early to modern period has been slow because of a reluctance to embrace new technologies and because of the poor outcomes with stenting seen in the early studies; however, the results of these studies may have been effected by poor operator skills and non-standardised criteria that contributed to suboptimal patient selection.

The introduction of several changes—including routine use of stents, embolic protection devices, dedicated devices, and modern antiplatelet drugs—has meant that stenting is now considered to be an effective technique for selected patients.[15] Overall, the randomised controlled trials (since 1999) for stenting include:

- SAPPHIRE (Stenting and angioplasty with protection in patients at high risk for endarterectomy) trial[16,17]
- EVA-3S (Endarterectomy *versus* angioplasty in patients with symptomatic severe carotid stenosis) study[18,19]
- SPACE (Stent-protected angioplasty *versus* carotid endarterectomy)[20–22]
- ICSS (International carotid stenting study)[23]
- CREST (Carotid revascularisation endarterectomy *versus* stenting trial)[24–26]
- ACT-1 (Asymptomatic carotid surgery trial)[27]
- ACST-2 (Asymptomatic carotid surgery trial)[28]
- ECST-2 (European carotid surgery trial 2)[29]
- SPACE-2 (Stent-protected angioplasty in asymptomatic carotid artery stenosis *versus* endarterectomy).[30]

The four studies EVA-3S, SPACE, ICSS and CREST randomised a total of 5,932 patients[13] (comprising 80% of the total randomised patients in the 13 trials) and these have had the greatest impact on current opinions.

The evidence[13,31,32] from these studies suggests that stenting is associated with an increased risk of procedural death/all stroke (the differences being so-called "minor strokes") compared with endarterectomy. However, longer term data confirm the suspicion that patients recover from these minor strokes and that at six to 12 months after the procedure, the functional outcomes for stenting and carotid endarterectomy are equivalent.

These data also indicate that when "chemical myocardial infarction" is studied (asymptomatic increase in cardiac enzyme levels and no ECG changes), endarterectomy is associated with a two-fold excess risk of myocardial infarction. In time, this translates into a higher risk of clinical myocardial infarction. But if chemical myocardial infarction is included within an endpoint of 30-day death/stroke/myocardial infarction, outcomes are similar between the two procedures. Other findings include:

- The 30-day rates of death/all stroke after stenting in patients under 70 are similar to those after endarterectomy. However, the rate of death/all stroke is higher after stenting in patients aged older than 70
- Randomised controlled trials reporting mid- to long-term outcomes show that endarterectomy and stenting are equally durable at preventing stroke.
- Restenosis rates are higher after stenting, but this does not seem to translate into an increased risk of late ipsilateral stroke.
- Endarterectomy can cause cranial nerve injury (the clinical significance of which is debatable).
- Stenting is associated with an increased number of both new and persisting lesions seen on magnetic resonance imaging (MRI) compared with endarterectomy (clinical significance unknown).

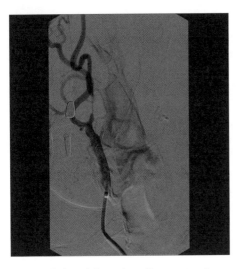

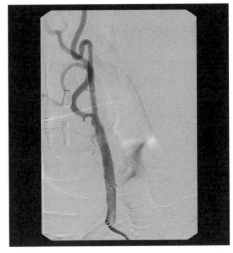

Figure 1: High-grade internal carotid artery stenosis following carotid endarterectomy.

Figure 2: Appearance following carotid artery stenting.

Summarising the evidence base

The published evidence, therefore, suggests that: there remains debate about the efficacy of stenting *versus* endarterectomy; patients at high risk of stroke and endarterectomy may be better served with stenting (if morphologically suitable); patients should expect a higher risk of periprocedural minor stroke in stenting, which will even out by six to 12 months; and the risk of significant cardiac events is higher with carotid endarterectomy.

It also indicates that: younger patients are more suited to stenting, which probably reflects the adverse aortic arch disease in elderly patients (good quality imaging may mitigate this issue); both endarterectomy and stenting need to be performed by experienced teams; case selection for both treatments is key; and that timing is important as delays will result in loss of benefit from intervention.

Patients excluded from studies

Some subgroups have been considered at high risk for endarterectomy and, therefore, do not appear in the randomised trials that compare endarterectomy with stenting. It has been suggested that stenting better serves these patients, if symptomatic, even when endarterectomy is readily available. These patients include those with restenosis from a previous endarterectomy (Figure 1 and Figure 2), those who have received neck radiotherapy, those with a high carotid bifurcation, and patients with previous endarterectomy with recurrent laryngeal nerve injury.

Guidelines for stenting

There is no international consensus, based on the latest guidelines, regarding the choice of treatment for stroke. The American Heart Association (AHA) and the North American Inter-Society guidelines released their recommendations in 2011, recognising the role of stenting in "average" risk symptomatic and asymptomatic patients.[13] These guidelines were heavily influenced by CREST (Carotid revascularization endarterectomy *versus* stenting trial), without making reference to some European trials.

In contrast, a multidisciplinary Australasian group concluded that stenting was appropriate in recently symptomatic patients aged less than 70 years and in symptomatic patients who are deemed "high risk" for endarterectomy. They did not recommend stenting in average risk asymptomatic patients.[33]

The National Institute for Health and Care Excellence (NICE) recommends the use of stenting in symptomatic patients, provided that procedural risk is kept within the same thresholds as those for endarterectomy. It also recommends that stenting is only offered to asymptomatic patients as part of a trial or by special arrangement.[13]

Therefore, while there remains debate, there is agreement that stenting has a significant role in stroke prevention, and like endarterectomy, this should be available within the timescale indicated in guidelines such as the UK's National Stroke Strategy.

Patient access to stenting

Stenting is a procedure that requires technical skill, training and practice. This requirement may be pronounced because the complications are obvious and significant and because the parameters for delivering benefit are tight.

The benefits of a multidisciplinary team approach to stroke management have been established. It is also clear that case selection for both endarterectomy and stenting is key, and that access to clinicians trained in both procedures is important for appropriate intervention.

In the UK, a small number of centres deliver regular stenting, with good results. The National Vascular Registry reviews the small number of centres reporting their stenting results. The majority of stroke multidisciplinary teams are not able to provide rapid assessment of those who may benefit from stenting. This results in: patients undergoing high-risk endarterectomy; delays in referral for stenting; patients being inappropriately referred for stenting, and patients not being offered a stroke prevention pathway that is best suited to them.

As in many areas, networking and centralisation may be the answer to these shortcomings.

Conclusion

Patients presenting with stroke or transient ischaemic attack require timely assessment of their symptoms and treatment by skilled operators to prevent future strokes. NICE guidance and the National Stroke Strategy mandate timely access to interventions.

Randomised controlled trial data show that stenting is a minimally invasive alternative to endarterectomy, which fulfils the criteria of preventing long-term stroke with good results in well-selected cases. This is, however, only achieved if performed by experienced and well-trained operators.

Summary

- Centralisation of stenting services and efficient networking across the regions would allow patient access to expert assessment and consideration of stenting in patients who would otherwise be considered high risk for endarterectomy.

- Stroke is a major cause of morbidity and mortality, which requires timely assessment and treatment to minimise the risk of recurrence.

- Evidence shows stenting to be an effective treatment, particularly in the younger population and patients who are deemed high risk for endarterectomy.

- Stenting may cause a higher number of peri-procedural minor strokes, but this evens out in the long term, with similar stroke disability in six to 12 months when compared with endarterectomy.

- Stenting is an elective procedure in which patients should be transferred to an expert or a centre with the necessary facilities.

- Results of stenting are closely related to training, technical skills, appropriate patient selection, and availability of adequate equipment.

- Better patient subgroup selection is associated with notably fewer complications associated with stenting.

- Efficient networked and centralised services are the key to allowing patients timely access to both treatments, performed by experienced operators to aid short- as well as long-term benefit and survival.

References

1. Cao P, De Rango P. Carotid Artery: Stenting. In: Cronenwett JL, Johnston KW. (eds.) Rutherford's Vascular Surgery. 8th edition. Philadelphia. Elsevier Saunders; 2014. p.1544-1567.
2. Naylor AR. Carotid artery disease, clinical features and management. *Surgery* (United Kingdom) 2012; **30** (8): 415–19.
3. Coull AJ, Silver LE, Rothwell PM. Implications of rates of non-fatal acute cerebrovascular events *versus* acute coronary events for provision of acute clinical services: Oxford Vascular Study. *Cerebrovasc Dis* 2003; **16** (suppl 4): 1–125.
4. National Institute for Health and Clinical Excellence: Stroke: Diagnosis and initial management of acute stroke and transient ischaemic attack (TIA). www.nice.org.uk/guidance/cg68 (accessed: 12 January 2016).
5. Department of Health National Stroke Strategy. Published December 2007.
6. North American Symptomatic Carotid Endarterectomy Trial Collaborators. Beneficial effect of carotid endarterectomy in symptomatic patients with high-grade stenosis. *N Engl J Med* 1991; **325**: 445–53.
7. European Carotid Surgery Trialists' Collaborative Group. Randomised trial of endarterectomy for recently symptomatic carotid stenosis: final results of the MRC European Carotid Surgery Trial (ECST). *Lancet* 1998; **351**: 1379–87.
8. Mathias K. A new catheter system for percutaneous transluminal angioplasty (PTA) of carotid artery stenoses. *Fortschr Med* 1977; **95**: 1007–11.
9. Mathias K, Mittermayer C, Ensinger H, Neff W. Percutaneous catheter dilatation of carotid stenoses. *Rofo* 1980; **133**: 258–61.
10. Kerber CW, Cromwell LD, Loehden OL. Catheter dilatation of proximal carotid stenosis during distal bifurcation endarterectomy. *Am J Neuroradiol* 1980; **1**: 348–49.
11. Theron J, Courtheoux P, Alachkar F, *et al.* New triple coaxial catheter system for carotid angioplasty with cerebral protection. *Am J Neuroradiol* 1990; **11**: 869–74.

12. Economoupoulos KP, Sergentanis TN, Tsivgoulis G, *et al.* Carotid artery stenting *versus* carotid endarterectomy: comprehensive meta-analysis of short and long- term outcomes. *Stroke* 2011; **42**: 687–92.

13. Naylor AR. A surgeon's view on endarterectomy and stenting in 2011: lest we forget, it's all about preventing stroke. *Cardiovasc Intervent Radiol* 2012; **35** (2): 225–33.

14. Ederle J, Dobson J, Featherstone RL, *et al.* On behalf of the CAVATAS Investigators (2009) Endovascular treatment with angioplasty or stenting *versus* end- arterectomy in patients with carotid artery stenosis in the Carotid and Vertebral Artery Transluminal Angioplasty Study (CAVA- TAS): long term follow-up of a randomised trial. *Lancet Neurol* 2009; **8**: 898–907.

15. Randall MS, McKevitt FM, Kumar S, *et al.* Long-Term Results of Carotid Artery Stents to Manage Symptomatic Carotid Artery Stenosis and Factors That Affect Outcome. *Circ Cardiovasc Interv* 2010; **3**: 50–56.

16. Yadav JS, Wholey MH, Kuntz RE, *et al.* Protected carotid-artery stenting *versus* endarterectomy in high-risk patients. Stenting and angioplasty with protection in patients at high risk for endarterectomy investigators. *N Engl J Med* 2004; **351**: 1493–1501.

17. Gurm HS, Yadav JS, Fayad P, *et al.* Long-term results of carotid stenting *versus* endarterectomy in high-risk patients. SAPPHIRE Investigators. *N Engl J Med* 2008; **358**: 1572–79.

18. Mas JL, Chatellier G, Beyssen B, *et al.* Endarterectomy *versus* stenting in patients with symptomatic severe carotid stenosis. EVA-3S Investigators. *N Engl J Med* 2006; **355**: 1660–71.

19. Mas JL, Trinquart L, Leys D, *et al.* Endarterectomy Versus Angioplasty in Patients with Symptomatic Severe Carotid Stenosis (EVA-3S) trial: results up to 4 years from a randomised, multicentre trial. EVA-3S Investigators. *Lancet Neurol* 2008; **7**: 885–92.

20. Ringleb PA, *et al.* SPACE Collaborative Group. 30 day results from the SPACE trial of stent-protected angioplasty *versus* carotid endarterectomy in symptomatic patients: a randomised non-inferiority trial. *Lancet* 2006; **368**:1239–47.

21. Stingele R, Berger J, Alfke K, *et al.* Clinical and angiographic risk factors for stroke and death within 30 days after carotid endarterectomy and stent-protected angioplasty: a subanalysis of the SPACE study. *Lancet Neurol* 2008; **7**: 216–22.

22. Eckstein HH, Ringleb P, Allenberg JR, *et al.* Results of the Stent-Protected Angioplasty *versus* Carotid Endarterectomy (SPACE) study to treat symptomatic stenoses at 2 years: a multinational, prospective, randomised trial. *Lancet Neurol* 2008; **7**: 893–902.

23. Ederle J, Dobson J, Featherstone RL, *et al.* International Carotid Stenting Study investigators. Carotid artery stenting compared with endarterectomy in patients with symptomatic carotid stenosis (International Carotid Stenting Study): an interim analysis of a randomised controlled trial. *Lancet* 2010; **375**: 985–97.

24. Brott TG , Hobson RW 2nd, Howard G, *et al.* Stenting *versus* endarterectomy for treatment of carotid-artery stenosis. CREST Investigators *N Engl J Med* 2010; **363**: 11–23.

25. Hopkins LN, *et al.* The Carotid Revascularization Endarterectomy *versus* Stenting Trial: credentialing of interventionalists and final results of lead-in phase. J Stroke *Cerebrovasc Dis* 2010; **19**: 153–62.

26. Voeks JH, Howard G, Roubin GS, *et al.* Age and outcomes after carotid stenting and endarterectomy: the carotid revascularization endarterectomy *versus* stenting trial. CREST Investigators. *Stroke* 2011; **42**: 3484–90.

27. Halliday A, Harrison M, Hayter E, *et al.* 10-year stroke prevention after successful carotid endarterectomy for asymptomatic stenosis (ACST-1): a multicentre randomised trial. Asymptomatic Carotid Surgery Trial (ACST) Collaborative Group *Lancet* 2010; **376**: 1074-1084

28. ACST Collaborators. MRC asymptomatic carotid surgery trial: carotid endarterectomy prevents disabling and fatal carotid territory strokes. *Lancet* 2004; **363**: 1491–1502.

29. European Carotid Surgery Trial 2 (ECST-2) Available at www.controlled-trials.com/ISRCTN97744893 (accessed 12 January 2016).

30. Reiff T, Stingele R, Eckstein HH, *et al.* Stent-protected angioplasty in asymptomatic carotid artery stenosis vs. endarterectomy: SPACE2—a three-arm randomised-controlled clinical trial. SPACE2 Study Group. *Int J Stroke* 2009; **4**: 294–99.

31. Brott TG, Hobson RW, Howard G, *et al.* Stenting *versus* endarterectomy for treatment of carotid-artery stenosis. *N Engl J Med* 2010; **363**: 11–23.

32. Carotid Stenting Trialists Collaboration. Short term out- come after stenting *versus* carotid endarterectomy for symptomatic carotid stenosis: preplanned meta-analysis of individual patient data. *Lancet* 2010; **376**: 1062–73.

33. Bladin C, Chambers B, Crimmins D, *et al.* Guidelines for patient selection and performance of carotid-artery-stenting: Inter-Collegiate Committee of the RACP/ RACS/RANZCR. *Intern Med J* 2011; **41**: 344–47.

Urgent carotid endarterectomy does not increase risk and will prevent more strokes

IM Loftus and KI Paraskevas

Introduction

In the last few years, the management of patients with symptomatic carotid artery stenosis has undergone considerable changes. Previously conceived concepts regarding delayed rather than urgent surgery have been proven wrong and international guidelines have been revised accordingly. Current evidence dictates that carotid endarterectomy should be performed within two weeks of an ischaemic cerebrovascular event (transient ischaemic or stroke episode). Emerging evidence suggests that the earlier endarterectomy is performed, the more strokes are prevented. Consequently, many advocate performing the procedure as early as within two days after the occurrence of a transient ischaemic attack/stroke episode. Despite the general assumption that urgent endarterectomy is associated with increased periprocedural stroke risk, several studies have demonstrated that this is not the case. This chapter will present the data proving that urgent carotid endarterectomy does not increase stroke risk, but actually prevents more strokes.

Evidence base

Two landmark randomised controlled trials, NASCET (North American symptomatic carotid endarterectomy trial)[1] and ECST (European carotid surgery),[2] demonstrated the relative benefit of carotid endarterectomy performed within six months of an ipsilateral cerebrovascular event (transient ischaemic attack or stroke episode) compared with medical treatment alone for patients with 70–99% carotid artery stenosis. Based on these findings, the 1998 American Heart Association (AHA) guidelines recommended endarterectomy for the management of patients with an ipsilateral 70–99% carotid artery stenosis and a recent (<6 months) non-disabling carotid artery ischaemic event (Grade A recommendation).[3]

The general belief at that time was that endarterectomy should be delayed for six to eight weeks after a transient ischaemic attack or an ischaemic stroke episode because: a) there was an increased risk of haemorrhagic transformation of the infarct; b) early surgery was thought to be associated with an increased rate of complications; and, c) the risk of suffering a stroke in the first few weeks after presentation was not considered to be high.[4] It was further thought that a slight delay would probably be beneficial for the patient (as it would allow time for the unstable carotid plaque to become more stable).[4]

A re-analysis of pooled data from NASCET and ECST (n=5,893 patients; 33,000 patient-years of follow-up), however, showed that the benefit of endarterectomy was greatest in patients randomised within two weeks of their last ischaemic event and that this benefit fell rapidly with increasing delay.[5] In male patients with ≥70% carotid stenosis, the five-year absolute risk reduction in ipsilateral ischaemic stroke with endarterectomy was 30.2% for men randomised within two weeks of their last event (number needed to treat [NNT] to prevent one ipsilateral stroke =3). However, this reduction in stroke risk was reduced by half for male patients randomised two to four weeks after their last event (NNT=6) and was even further reduced in men randomised after four weeks (NNT=9). For females, the benefit of endarterectomy for ≥70% stenosis was seen only if they underwent the procedure within two weeks of symptoms and not later. Importantly, these results were consistent across the individual trials.[5] Furthermore, there was no association between perioperative risk of stroke or death and time since the last ischaemic event.[5] These results verified and extended the results of an earlier NASCET subgroup analysis, which showed that stroke and death rates in symptomatic patients undergoing early (<30 days) endarterectomy did not differ from those of patients undergoing late (>30 days) endarterectomy (relative risk: 0.92; 95% confidence interval: 0.16-5.27; p=1.00).[6]

Revised recommendations

Following the publication of these results, both the 2009 European Society for Vascular Surgery[7] and the 2011 AHA/American Stroke Association (ASA)[8] guidelines provided revised recommendations regarding the timing of endarterectomy. Both guidelines indicated that in symptomatic patients, performing endarterectomy within two weeks is reasonable unless otherwise contraindicated.[7,8] This recommendation referred to patients having experienced a single recent neurologic event and who were at average or low surgical risk.

A subgroup of symptomatic patients who may be at higher stroke risk if operated on urgently are those patients with crescendo transient ischaemic attack and stroke-in-evolution. Three systematic reviews have demonstrated that patients with unstable neurologic presentations (crescendo transient ischaemic attack and stroke-in-evolution) are at higher risk of complications if operated on urgently compared with symptomatic patients with stable symptoms.[9-11] Nevertheless, urgent carotid endarterectomy may be justified even in these patients due to the high rate of recurrent events if they do not undergo carotid endarterectomy.

The recommendations of the UK National Stroke Strategy[12] are more aggressive than the other guidelines.[7,8] Intervention for symptomatic severe carotid stenosis is recommended within two days in neurologically stable patients.

In contrast, the benefit of very early endarterectomy was questioned by the Swedish Vascular Registry (Swedvasc).[13] This study analysed the outcomes of all symptomatic patients undergoing carotid endarterectomy between 12 May 2008 and 31 May 2011, and assessed outcomes according to time between the qualifying event and endarterectomy—zero to two days; three to seven days; eight to 14 days; and 15 to 180 days. The combined mortality and stroke rates for patients treated very urgently were considerably higher compared with those treated later. For example, the rate was 11.5% for patients undergoing endarterectomy zero to two days after the qualifying event *versus* 3.6%, 4.0%, and 5.4%, for patients undergoing endarterectomy at three to seven, eight to 14, and 15 to 180 days after the event. Also, patients treated very urgently had a more than four-fold higher stroke and death rates compared with patients operated on three to seven days after the event (odds ratio: 4.24; 95% confidence interval: 2.07–8.70; p<0.001).[13] A possible explanation for the higher stroke rates in the very urgent endarterectomy group may be because nearly 12% of the patients in this group presented with crescendo transient ischaemic attack.[14] As previously discussed, these patients are at higher risk of complications if operated on urgently.[9-11]

Recent data

An international multicentre study recently reported that the stroke risk associated with carotid endarterectomy in symptomatic patients does not differ when the procedure is performed within two days compared with within two weeks from symptom onset.[15] In the study, patients were divided into two groups: those who underwent urgent carotid endarterectomy (zero to two days after symptom onset; n=20) and those who underwent early carotid endarterectomy (three to 14 days after symptom onset; n=145). The 30-day stroke rate in patients who underwent urgent endarterectomy was similar to the stroke rates seen in patients who underwent early endarterectomy (10.0% vs. 4.1%, respectively; p=0.260).[15]

These results were verified in another recent, independent report presenting the outcomes of 761 symptomatic patients undergoing carotid endarterectomy within four different timing groups: a) within zero and two days; b) between three and seven days; c) between eight and 14 days; and d) thereafter.[16] The stroke and death rates for the four groups were, respectively: 4.4% (9/206), 1.8% (4/219), 4.4% (6/136), and 2.5% (5/200); p=0.25 for the difference between the groups. Furthermore, the timing of surgery did not influence the perioperative outcome in multivariate regression analysis (odds ratio: 0.93; 95% confidence interval: 0.63–1.36; p=0.71).[16]

An interesting finding is that urgent (rather than delayed) endarterectomy is more beneficial for patients even if intervening early is associated with a procedural risk as high as 10%. A re-analysis of pooled data from NASCET,[1] ECST[2] and the Veterans Affairs trial[17] suggests that a surgeon who operates within two weeks in patients with a 10% procedural stroke risk will actually prevent more strokes at five years than a surgeon who waits four weeks and who then operates in patients with a 0% procedural stroke risk.[18] This analysis provides proof that the increased stroke risk associated with urgent endarterectomy is considerably less when compared with the risk of suffering a recurrent stroke by delaying endarterectomy.[18]

Conclusion

Urgent carotid endarterectomy is not associated with an increased periprocedural stroke risk compared with delayed carotid endarterectomy. Furthermore, due to the high rates of early recurrent stroke after a recent cerebrovascular event, it prevents more strokes than does delaying the procedure. All members of the multidisciplinary team involved in the management of stroke patients should be aware of the benefits associated with urgent endarterectomy and should make sure that symptomatic carotid patients are referred and operated on as soon as possible following a transient ischaemic attack or minor stroke episode.

Summary

- Current evidence dictates that carotid endarterectomy should be performed within two weeks of an ischaemic cerebrovascular event.

- Despite the general assumption that urgent carotid endarterectomy is associated with increased periprocedural stroke risk, several large scale studies have demonstrated that this is not the case.

- All members of the multidisciplinary team should be aware of the benefits associated with urgent carotid endarterectomy and ensure that symptomatic carotid patients are referred, and operated upon, as soon as possible following a cerebral ischaemic event.

References

1. North American Symptomatic Carotid Endarterectomy Trial Collaborators. Beneficial effect of carotid endarterectomy in symptomatic patients with high-grade carotid stenosis. *N Engl J Med* 1991; **352** (7): 445–53.
2. MRC European Carotid Surgery Trial: interim results for symptomatic patients with severe (70-99%) or with mild (0-29%) carotid stenosis. European Carotid Surgery Trialists' Collaborative Group. *Lancet* 1991; **337** (8752): 1235–43.
3. Biller J, Feinberg WM, Castaldo JE, *et al.* Guidelines for carotid endarterectomy: a statement for healthcare professionals from a special writing group of the Stroke Council, American Heart Association. *Stroke* 1998; **29** (2): 554–62.
4. Naylor AR. Delay may reduce procedural risk, but at what price to the patient? *Eur J Vasc Endovasc Surg* 2008; **35** (4): 383–91.
5. Rothwell PM, Eliasziw M, Gutnikov SA, *et al*; Carotid Endarterectomy Trialists Collaboration. Endarterectomy for symptomatic carotid stenosis in relation to clinical subgroups and timing of surgery. *Lancet* 2004; **363** (9413): 915–24.
6. Gasecki AP, Ferguson GG, Eliasziw M, *et al.* Early endarterectomy for severe carotid artery stenosis after a nondisabling stroke: results from the North American Symptomatic Carotid Endarterectomy Trial. *J Vasc Surg* 1994; **20** (2): 288–95.
7. Liapis CD, Bell PF, Mikhailidis DP, *et al*; ESVS Guidelines Collaborators. ESVS guidelines. Invasive treatment for carotid stenosis: indications, techniques. *Eur J Vasc Endovasc Surg* 2009; **37** (4 Suppl): 1–19.
8. Furie KL, Kasner SE, Adams RJ, *et al*; American Heart Association Stroke Counciil, Council on Cardiovascular Nursing, Council on Clinical Cardiology, and Interdisciplinary Council on Quality of Care and Outcomes Research. Guidelines for the prevention of stroke in patients with stroke or transient ischemic attack: a guideline for healthcare professionals from the American Heart Association/ American Stroke Association. Stroke 2011; **42** (1): 227–76.
9. Karkos CD, Hernandez-Lahoz I, Naylor AR. Urgent carotid surgery in patients with crescendo transient ischaemic attacks and stroke-in-evolution: a systematic review. *Eur J Vasc Endovasc Surg* 2009; **37** (3): 279–88.
10. Rerkasem K, Rothwell PM. Systematic review of the operative risks of carotid endarterectomy for recently symptomatic stenosis in relation to the timing of surgery. *Stroke* 2009; **40** (10): e564–72.
11. Patterson BO, Holt PJ, Hinchliffe RJ, *et al.* Urgent carotid endarterectomy for patients with unstable symptoms: systematic review and meta-analysis of outcomes. *Vascular* 2009; **17** (5): 243–52.
12. Department of Health. National Stroke Strategy. http://bit.ly/1ZHau8L (accessed 18 January 2016).
13. Stromberg S, Gelin J, Osterberg T, *et al* K; Swedish Vascular Registry (Swedvasc) Steering Committee. Very urgent carotid endarterectomy confers increased procedural risk. Stroke 2012; **43** (5): 1331–35.
14. Naylor AR. Letter by Naylor regarding article, "Very urgent carotid endarterectomy confers increased procedural risk". *Stroke* 2012; **43** (9): e94.
15. Tsivgoulis G, Krogias C, Georgiadis GS, *et al.* Safety of early endarterectomy in patients with symptomatic carotid artery stenosis: an international multicenter study. *Eur J Neurol* 2014; **21** (10): 1251–57.

16. Rantner B, Schmidauer C, Knoflach M, Fraedrich G. Very urgent carotid endarterectomy does not increase the procedural risk. *Eur J Vasc Endovasc Surg* 2015; **49** (2): 129–36.
17. Mayberg MR, Wilson SE, Yatsu F, *et al.* Carotid endarterectomy and prevention of cerebral ischemia in symptomatic carotid stenosis. Veterans Affairs Cooperative Studies Program 309 Trialist Group. *JAMA* 1991; **266** (23): 3289–94.
18. Naylor AR. Time is brain! *Surgeon* 2007; **5** (1): 23–30.

Carotid bypass using hybrid as a rescue technique for on-table failed carotid endarterectomy

S Sayed and D Valenti

Introduction

Carotid endarterectomy traditionally involves removal of the intimal and inner medial layers of the vessel with either primary closure of the arteriotomy or patch angioplasty.[1,2] This surgery remains the gold standard for atherosclerotic lesions involving the carotid bifurcation. While this procedure is technically feasible for most lesions, it may prove to be difficult in select cases, such as in patients with extensive lesions extending distally into the internal carotid artery, radiation induced stenoses,[3] excessive endarterectomy and zone thinning, penetrating atheroma and severe internal carotid artery coiling above the endarterectomy zone. For such cases, carotid artery bypass grafting with or without re-implantation of the external carotid artery maybe indicated as a suitable alternative to endarterectomy. Our practice has been to use expanded polytetrafluoroethylene (ePTFE) vascular grafts in carotid artery bypass grafts, although the long saphenous vein may also be used.[4–7]

We are a high volume centre and have performed 590 carotid endarterectomy cases in the last seven years. Twenty four (4%) required carotid interposition grafts using PTFE and 67 (11%) needed eversion endarterectomies.

Endovascular technological advances have expanded our treatment options for these challenging patients. Intraoperative placement of intraluminal self-expanding stents for the management of unsatisfactory distal internal carotid artery endarterectomy endpoints has been reported previously with acceptable early 30 day and mid-term results.[8,9] The Gore Hybrid Vascular Graft (Gore) is a heparin-bonded ePTFE graft with a nitinol reinforced end.[10] It has been used in arteriovenous access grafts in dialysis, aortic[11,12] and cerebral debranching procedures[13] and peripheral vascular disease.[14]

We report our experience of using the Gore Hybrid Vascular Graft in nine patients as a rescue technique where standard endarterectomy was unsuccessful.

Deployment technique

The Gore Hybrid Vascular Graft is a combination graft consisting of a proximal 45cm thromboresistant flexible ePTFE heparin-coated graft and a 5cm heparin coated nitinol reinforced stent graft. The nitinol reinforced section is partially constrained to facilitate easy insertion and deployment into challenging target

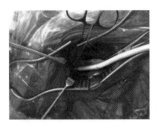

Figure 1: Intra-operative picture of the nitinol reinforced section once introduced and deployed into the vessel.

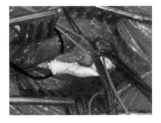

Figure 2: Implantation of external carotid artery once stent deployed distally and proximal anastomosis created.

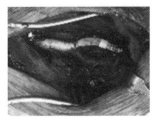

Figure 3: The Hybrid Vascular Graft fully deployed and in position.

vessels without the need for a sutured outflow anastamosis.[10] We use a standard approach to the carotid vessels with adequate exposure of the distal internal carotid artery. The common carotid artery is mobilised proximal to the carotid lesion and the dissection is continued distally to isolate the external carotid artery and internal carotid artery. Once the decision is made to use the Gore Hybrid Vascular Graft (6mm x 5cm), with the arteries clamped, the nitinol reinforced end of the hybrid graft is introduced into the internal carotid artery directly under vision for approximately 1.5cm with the deployment line facing upwards (Figure 1).

A purse string is subsequently placed in the distal internal carotid artery using a six polypropylene (Prolene, Ethicon) suture. Once in position, the internal carotid artery clamp is removed and the deployment line is pulled, keeping it parallel to the vascular prosthesis. The Gore Hybrid Vascular Graft is introduced a further 1cm. To ensure adequate anchoring, the purse string is pulled. The PTFE end of the graft is then trimmed to length and a proximal anastomosis is fashioned with the common carotid artery in an end-to-end fashion using a six Prolene (Figure 2).

The diameter of the nitinol section should be oversized by 5% to 20%. The nitinol reinforced segment of the graft is used to cover and re-line the suboptimal portion of the distal endpoint, reducing the risk of a dissection while creating a favourable laminar flow pattern. The primary determinant for a successful outcome is accurate measurement of the graft length, which is essential so that the distal anastomosis can be made without tension or kinking after clamp removal.

Case series

Between November 2014 and December 2015, 10 Gore Hybrid Vascular Grafts were used in patients undergoing carotid endarterectomy. All patients were scheduled to undergo routine endarterectomy with patch plasty. As per routine practice, preoperative detailed duplex imaging was undertaken to accurately measure the proximal and distal diameters of the internal carotid artery. Surgery was performed under local anaesthetic for all but two patients and none required a shunt. Carotid bypass grafting was not anticipated in any patient prior to surgery. The graft was used in four cases where the plaque extended beyond the surgical exposure resulting in an unacceptable distal endpoint. Two patients had penetrating atherosclerotic ulcers causing disruption of the posterior carotid wall, two had significant wall thinning after endarterectomy and one had a distal intimal dissection after endarterectomy. The total operative time and thus cerebral ischaemic time were reduced by using the Gore Hybrid Vascular Grafts due to the easy deployment technique and the avoidance of creating two sutured anastomosis.

Results

Procedural success was achieved in all cases. All patients made a good postoperative recovery with no perioperative strokes or deaths. All were discharged on day three on dual antiplatelets.

Patients were followed up at one, three, six and 12 months postimplantation with arterial duplex or computed tomography (CT) imaging (Figure 4).

There was 100% stent patency rate with no cases of in-stent restenosis or stenosis in the distal internal carotid artery at three months. At six-month follow-up, only one patient was found to have an occluded stent on duplex ultrasound. At the time of writing this chapter, only one patient had reached their 12-month follow-up duplex scan and this patient had an occluded stent. Clinically, all nine patients at the six-month follow-up remained asymptomatic.

Patients will be continually followed up every six months as there are a lack of data regarding the long-term patency of these grafts for this cohort of patients. All nine patients consented to publication of this report.

Discussion

The optimal flow surface after carotid endarterectomy should ideally not contain any embolic surface, should not be flow limiting and should be minimally thrombogenic. Standard endarterectomy with or without patch plasty and eversion endarterectomy remains the gold standard for significant carotid atherosclerotic disease. However, technically this may not always be possible due to the challenging pathologies as discussed earlier. Carotid interposition bypass grafting using either PTFE or long saphenous vein is a safe and durable alternative in these cases. We believe our centre is the first to use the sutureless Gore Hybrid Vascular Graft for carotid atherosclerotic disease as a rescue technique for failed carotid endarterectomy. We report our early experience of using the graft in 10 patients where standard carotid endarterectomy failed.

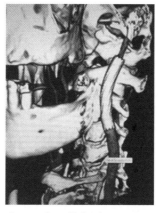

Figure 4: CT angiogram of carotid showing patent stent graft.

When the plaque extends distally into the internal carotid artery, one option is to tack the distal atheromatous plaque. This may prove to be suboptimal in some cases as residual thrombogenic plaque remains, potentially resulting in restenosis, plaque fracture or dissection. Other rescue techniques include adequate exposure of the internal carotid artery beyond the distal extent of the plaque and patching beyond the distal end point. In our experience, PTFE carotid interposition grafts have been performed in patients with extensive lesions of the internal carotid artery or where a safe internal carotid artery distal endpoint could not be achieved. We have also used grafts in patients with carotid wall perforations because of technically difficult endarterectomies for transmural lesions or recurrent stenosis.[5,7]

The Gore Hybrid Vascular Graft is a heparin-bonded ePTFE graft with a nitinol reinforced end, which allows easy deployment into the target vessel without the need for a sutured anastomosis.[10] The sutureless hybrid graft was primarily developed for use in arteriovenous grafts for access in dialysis. The nitinol segment at the venous outflow end creates a haemodynamically favourable laminar flow, which potentially reduces the risk of thrombosis and increases the longevity of the graft, while the sutureless distal anastomosis decreases the anastomotic suture burden (which itself leads to scarring and intimal hyperplasia). The graft has also been used in de-branching procedures for aortic dissections[11] or aneurysmal disease, cerebral debranching[12] renal artery bypass procedures in hybrid cases[13] involving aortic endograft placements and lower limb arterial occlusive disease.[14]

Recently Nigaro et al[15] reported the use of the Gore Hybrid Vascular Graft for a high lying extra-cranial carotid aneurysm. Potential benefits for using this sutureless graft in carotid surgery include reduced intimal hyperplasia and reduced time with cerebral ischaemia for difficult or revision procedures and improved flow dynamics distally.[16] Additionally, it offers a treatment modality for hostile anatomy minimising vessel manipulation, risk of dissection and nerve injuries.

The sutureless Gore Hybrid Vascular Graft is a viable option in such challenging patients. Sutureless techniques have been described previously. The Viabahn Open Revascularisation Technique (VORTEC) was first used for renal artery revascularisation.[17] Here the Viabahn stent graft (Also from Gore) is introduced via a direct puncture in the anterior wall of the target artery. The other end of the stent graft is then sutured in an end-to-end fashion to an ePTFE graft that is used for the extra anatomic bypass during aortic debranching. Another composite graft is the Viabahn Padova Sutureless. Here, the system is prepared preoperatively by suturing a Viabahn stent to an ePTFE graft prior to deployment thus creating a sutureless anastomosis for lower limb bypass surgery.[18] The advantage of Viabahn Padova Sutureless over VORTEC is that the modified graft may be implanted on the inside of the transected artery under direct vision with minimal risk of damaging the vessel. The technique we used for implantation of the Gore Hybrid Vascular Graft is similar to the Viabahn Padova Sutureless system in that the stent graft is introduced and deployed under direct vision. Our initial experience with this graft has been for complex re-do arteriovenous access and revision procedures in dialysis patients (n=5). Additionally, we have used the Gore Hybrid Vascular Graft in two infrainguinal bypasses (femoropopliteal) and two cases where the renal artery was re-implanted in aortic aneurysmal surgery.

Summary

- The Gore Hybrid Vascular Graft is a promising new technology in patients with extensive carotid atherosclerotic disease where conventional on-table endarterectomy has failed.

- We are the first group to report the use of the graft for carotid atherosclerotic disease.[19]

- Our experience suggests a potential role for the use of this graft in challenging carotid pathologies.

- Long-term follow-up is necessary to evaluate which patients would benefit from the use of this graft and in particular to assess the patency and durability of this graft.

References

1. Randomised trial of endarterectomy for recently symptomatic carotid stenosis: final results of the MRC European Carotid Surgery Trial (ECST). *The Lancet* 1998; **351** (9113): 1379–87.
2. North American Symptomatic Carotid Endarterectomy Trial Collaborators. Beneficial effect of carotid endarterectomy in symptomatic patients with high-grade carotid stenosis. *N Engl J Med* 1999; **325** (7): 445–53.
3. Cormier JM, Brisset D, Speir Y, *et al.* Fifty-three atherosclerotic carotid stenoses in an irradiated environment. *J Mal Vasc* 1993; **18** (3): 269–74.
4. Camiade C, Maher A, Ricco JB, *et al.* Carotid bypass with polytetrafluoroethylene grafts: a study of 110 consecutive patients. *J Vasc Surg* 2003; **38** (5): 1031–37.
5. Branchereau A, Pietri P, Magnan PE, Rosset E. Saphenous vein bypass: an alternative to internal carotid reconstruction. *Eur J Vasc Endovasc Surg* 1996; **12** (1): 26–30.
6. Ward AS, Operative techniques in arterial surgery. ISBN 0852003900 1986; 1: 236-Lancaster; MTP press.
7. Cormier JM, Cormier F, Laurian C, *et al.* Polytetrafluoroethylene bypass for revascularization of the atherosclerotic internal carotid artery: late results. *Ann Vasc Surg* 1987; **1** (5): 564–71.
8. Ross CB, Ranval TJ. Intraoperative use of stents for the management of unacceptable distal internal carotid artery end points during carotid endarterectomy: short-term and midterm results. *J Vasc Surg* 2000; **32** (3): 420–27.
9. Tameo MN, Dougherty MJ, Calligaro KD. Carotid endarterectomy with adjunctive cephalad carotid stenting: Complementary, not competitive, techniques. *J Vasc Surg* 2008; **48** (2): 351–54.
10. WL Gore & Associates. Instructions for use of hybrid vascular graft: http://www.goremedical.com/resources/dam/assets/AP3350ML3.HYVG.US_IFU.pdf (date accessed 28 January 2016).
11. Levack MM, Bavaria JE, Gorman RC, *et al.* Rapid aortic arch debranching using the Gore hybrid vascular graft. *Ann Thorac Surg* 2013; **95** (6): e163–65.
12. Wipper S, Ahlbrecht O, Kolbel T, *et al.* First implantation of Gore Hybrid Vascular Graft in the right vertebral artery for cerebral debranching in a patient with Loeys-Dietz syndrome. *J Vasc Surg* 2015; **61** (3): 793–95.
13. Chiesa R, Kahlberg A, Mascia D, *et al.* Use of a novel hybrid vascular graft for sutureless revascularization of the renal arteries during open thoracoabdominal aortic aneurysm repair. *J Vasc Surg* 2014; **60** (3): 622–30.
14. Brant W, Ullery M, Ben M, *et al.* Applicability of heparin-bonded hybrid vascular grafts; *Endovascular Today* 2012.
15. Nigro G, Gatta E, Pagliariccio G, *et al.* Use of the Gore Hybrid Vascular Graft in a challenging high-lying extracranial carotid artery aneurysm. *J Vasc Surg* 2014; **59** (3): 817–20.
16. W.L Gore & Associates. Gore Hybrid Vascular Graft: http://www.goremedical.com/hybrid/ (date accessed 28 January 2016).
17. Lachat M, Mayer D, Criado FJ, *et al.* New technique to facilitate renal revascularization with use of telescoping self-expanding stent grafts: VORTEC. *Vascular* 2008; **16** (2): 69–72.
18. Bonvini S, Ricotta JJ, Piazza M, *et al.* ViPS technique as a novel concept for a sutureless vascular anastomosis. *J Vasc Surg* 2011; **54** (3): 889–92.
19. Valenti D, Sayed S, Mistry H, *et al.* Carotid bypass using the Gore Hybrid Vascular Graft as a rescue technique for on table failed carotid endarterectomy. *J Vasc Surg* 2015 in press.

Intracranial clot retrieval

Clot properties and technique may impact technical result and patient outcome

T Andersson and O Francois

Introduction

Over the past two years, five randomised controlled trials have reported the superiority of intra-arterial treatment and intravenous thrombolysis (IVT) of large artery stroke in the anterior circulation compared with standalone IVT.[1–5] These results were obviously welcomed by the neurointerventional community, but they also clearly showed that challenges remain. The revascularisation percentage was far from 100% in all of the studies, and the percentage of patients with a good outcome was much less than that of patients achieving revascularisation (Figure 1). Such futile revascularisation may, in some instances, be because of a prolonged procedure time in which the patient develops a stroke while being on the angiography table. So, when is achieving revascularisation impossible? Or when the revascularisation does take too long, is this related to the clot properties and/or technique? What are the crucial technical points and should the technique differ for different clot types? And, do certain clot properties beside the obvious ratio between red blood cells and fibrin as well as reperfusion-related pathophysiological incidents lead to a bad outcome for the patients? These are the questions that will be addressed in this chapter.

Clot properties that may influence the revascularisation rate

One factor that seems to be very important for determining the properties of thromboemboli is the relative content of fibrin.[6–7] From our research and clinical experience, it is clear that the proportion of fibrin compared with the proportion of red blood cells in a clot substantially alters the clot's physical properties and, subsequently, the possibility to extract it (Figure 2A and Figure 2B). A mature, fibrin-rich clot is firm, tough and sticky and, therefore, much less likely to deform. With this comes the obvious risk of it being difficult to remove with conventional stent retrievers or with aspiration alone. In contrast, clots rich in red blood cells are soft, friable and slippery—which means that they may be easier to remove but are more prone to embolisation into the same or a previously unaffected territory.

Importance of a proper technique

To avoid a prolonged procedure and the associated risk that the patient develops an infarct on the angiography table, procedures need to be fast and efficient but still

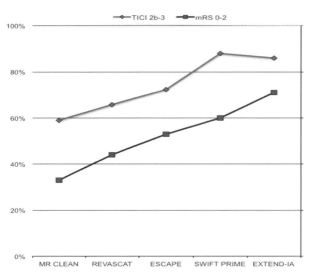

Figure 1: Revascularisation and good patient outcome after mechanical thrombectomy in five recently published randomised controlled trials. *Used TICI scale vs. modified TICI.

safe. Therefore, interventionalists should aim for a thrombectomy procedure to last no longer than 15–20 minutes from groin puncture to final results, and never more than 30 minutes. By using a proper technique and having access to a trained team, this is absolutely achievable. Another reason to strive for fast procedures is that a clot changes during the occlusion process. The longer a clot remains in place, the stickier and the more difficult it becomes to remove. When the clot is compressed by the water-hammer effect of the systemic blood pressure, it changes its properties to become more compacted and difficult to remove. Further, clot properties are altered by each of our attempts to remove them. For every failed thrombectomy attempt, the clot becomes more difficult to remove.

Therefore, what is the optimal technique? As this is a microsurgical procedure, different operators, as always, will have different views. But, from our experience, some points are crucial, taking into account that the properties of the clots vary

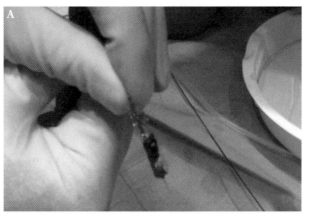
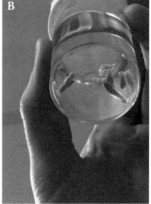

Figure 2: Clots rich of red blood cells (A) and fibrin (B), respectively, retrieved from patients treated at AZ Groeninge, Kortrijk, Belgium.

quite substantially. If the clot is very rich in fibrin, our laboratory studies have shown that it is almost impossible to aspirate it into a small-sized catheter. It is also very challenging for a standard stent retriever to penetrate the clot sufficiently to grip it. All of the most commonly used stent retrievers rely on their radial force to be strong enough to allow the retriever to move into the clot from the side (the microcatheter always passes between the vessel wall and the clot; never through the clot) and hold it. In this scenario, a stent retriever with high radial force or one based on a different principle (more capturing than penetrating the clot) becomes vital. It is also very important that the guide catheter is large enough to be able to accept the clot without losing it; 8Fr or 9Fr are usually the optimal sizes.

If the clot contains a high proportion or red blood cells, the risk is instead that it will fragment and send smaller emboli into more peripheral arteries. In this context, it is crucial to arrest flow—something that can only be achieved with a catheter with a balloon (ballon-guide catheter). A so-called "intermediate" or "aspiration" catheter alone can never achieve flow arrest as it, by necessity, is smaller than the target artery and because it becomes obstructed when the first part of the clot enters, allowing free flow on the sides. Pure aspiration in this setting, therefore, inherits a risk of clot stripping and fragmentation.

For the reasons mentioned above, we advocate to always use a 8–9Fr balloon-guide catheter, regardless if an intermediate catheter is added or not. Furthermore, we advocate positioning the stent retriever carefully with the proximal part just proximal to the foot of the thrombus (Figure 3) and finally to exert a slow and steady pull under flow arrest with staged aspiration, only full when the clot actually enters the guide.

Other clot properties and reperfusion injury

Clots contain many other substances beside fibrin and red blood cells. In our research collaboration with KU Leuven Campus Kulak in Kortrijk, Belgium, the group at the Laboratory for Thrombosis Research showed that clots collected from our thrombectomised patients (Figure 4) contain various levels also of von Willebrand factor (Figure 5). This is a large multimeric plasma glycoprotein that, together with fibrin, links platelets together and may thereby make the clot more organised and tough. Destabilising the clot by counteracting the creation of large and more active multimers may prove to be beneficial both for intravenous thrombolysis and for thrombectomy.[8–9]

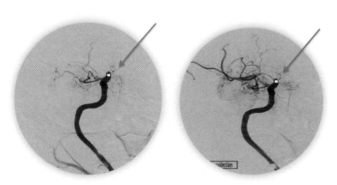

Figure 3: Optimal device positioning: align the proximal marker of the device approximately 5mm proximal to the proximal part of the clot. There is no need for distal microcatheter contrast injection.

In this context, another, perhaps not yet fully appreciated, reason for futile revascularisation (i.e. bad clinical outcome in spite of technical success) is injury caused by the reperfusion itself. Reperfusion into an ischaemic territory may indeed also activate von Willebrand factor, which in turn leads to thrombus formation in small arteries downstream. Blocking the function of von Willebrand factor has been shown to significantly reduce stroke reperfusion injury in mice.[9–10] In clinical cases where everything seemingly goes very quickly and smoothly yet there is futile revascularisation, we tend to blame our selection process for the bad outcome. But perhaps this kind of secondary injury deprives us, and especially the patient, of a good outcome.

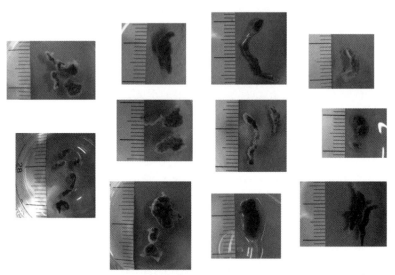

Figure 4: Thromboemboli collected from patients treated with thrombectomy at AZ Groeninge, Kortrijk, Belgium (courtesy of Frederik Denorme, Simon De Meyer *et al*, Laboratory for Thrombosis Research, KULAK, Kortrijk, Belgium).

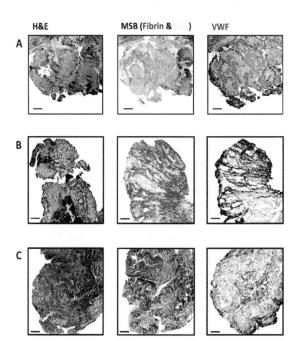

Figure 5: Staining for Hematoxylin & Eosin, Martius-Scarlet-Blue and anti-VWF antibodies, respectively, of thromboemboli collected from patients treated at AZ Groeninge, Kortrijk, Belgium (courtesy of Frederik Denorme, Simon De Meyer *et al*, Laboratory for Thrombosis Research, KULAK, Kortrijk, Belgium). Note the marked variability in VWF content.

Conclusion

We need to develop techniques and devices that make it possible to more safely and efficiently remove the clot. Ideally, this should be possible with one to two attempts and the total time of the procedure, from groin puncture to revascularisation, should not exceed 15–20 minutes—the final technical result is less important if the procedure takes 90 minutes!

In our clinical experience and in our laboratory investigations, the use of a balloon-guide catheter with concomitant flow arrest along with deliberate, optimal positioning of the devices have proved to be crucial in minimising the number of attempts required to revascularise the patient. Further, future thrombectomy devices should be designed to be able to manage all types of clots, or, there should be different devices specifically designed for a certain type of clot. We need to understand more the full spectrum of clot properties to try to find ways to more efficiently extract them. Finally, we need more research into the fascinating field of reperfusion injury to learn how to avoid and counteract this possible mechanism that results in bad outcomes.

Summary

- Mechanical thrombectomy is today a proven therapy for acute ischaemic stroke but failed or futile revascularisation diminishes the proportion of patients with a good outcome.

- Clot properties—content of red blood cells *versus* fibrin—and related technical shortcomings contribute to failed or futile revascularisation.

- With a trained team, adequate devices and proper technique including the use of a large size balloon-guide catheter, a thrombectomy procedure should ideally not last more than 15–20 minutes from groin puncture to revascularisation; never more than 30 minutes.

- The water-hammer effect of the systemic blood pressure and failed thrombectomy attempts cause an obstructive thromboembolus to change its properties and become more compacted and difficult to remove—time and the number of attempts (ideally never more than one or two) become crucial.

- Other factors such as the von Willebrand factor contribute to clot properties and may play an important role in reperfusion injury causing thrombus formation in microvessels downstream.

- To increase the proportion of patients with good outcome after intra-arterial stroke treatment, future thrombectomy devices should be designed to manage a variety of clot types and we need to optimise our technique accordingly and increase our understanding of secondary ischaemia caused by reperfusion injury.

References

1. Berkhemer OA, Fransen PS, Beumer D, *et al*, A randomized trial of intraarterial treatment for acute ischemic stroke. *N Engl J Med* 2015; **372**: 11–20.
2. Goyal M, Demchuk AM, Menon BK, *et al*, Randomized assessment of rapid endovascular treatment of ischemic stroke. *N Engl J Med* 2015; **372**: 1019–30.
3. Campbell BC, Mitchell PJ, Kleinig TJ, *et al*, Endovascular therapy for ischemic stroke with perfusion-imaging selection. *N Engl J Med* 2015; 372: 1009–18.
4. Saver JL, Goyal M, Bonafe A, *et al*. Stent-retriever thrombectomy after intravenous t-PA vs t-PA alone in stroke. *N Engl J Med* 2015; **372**: 2285–95.
5. Jovin TG, Chamorro A, Cobo E, *et al*, Thrombectomy within 8 hours after symptom onset in ischemic stroke. *N Eng J Med* 2015; **372**:2296–2306.
6. Liebeskind DS, Sanossian N, Yong WH, *et al*, CT and MRI early vessel signs reflect clot composition in acute stroke. *Stroke* 2011; **42**: 1237–43.
7. Cline B *et al*, O-027 Pathological analysis of extracted clots in embolectomy patients with acute ischaemic stroke. *J Neurointervent Surg* 2013; **5**: A15–A16.
8. Denorme F *et al*, ADAMTS13 destabilizes thrombi in a mouse model of thrombotic focal cerebral ischemia. *J Thromb Haemost* 2015;**13**(Suppl 2): 694–95.
9. De Meyer SF, Stoll G, Wagner DD, Kleinschnitz C. Von Willebrand factor: an emerging target in stroke therapy. *Stroke* 2012; **43**: 599–606.
10. De Meyer SF, Schwarz T, Deckmyn H, *et al*, Binding of von Willebrand factor to collagen and glycoprotein Ibalpha, but not to glycoprotein IIb/IIIa, contributes to ischemic stroke in mice--brief report. *Arteriosclerosis, Thrombosis, and Vascular Biology* 2010; **30**: 1949–51.

Thoracic aortic aneurysm challenges

Growth rate of small thoracic aortic aneurysm is not known but is relevant

M Truijers and JD Blankensteijn

Introduction

Management of asymptomatic thoracic aortic aneurysms is aimed primarily at preventing rupture. Patients are considered for prophylactic aneurysm repair when the risk of rupture exceeds the risk of surgery. Because of the well-established correlation between aneurysm size and rupture risk, patient selection is based upon aneurysm diameter and most patients with a large aneurysm are considered for elective repair.

Growth rate is suggested as a possible additional tool to identify patients at increased risk of rupture in spite of small thoracic aortic aneurysm size. To be able to use growth rate as a clinically relevant marker for aneurysm complications, the association between aneurysm growth and rupture needs to be quantified. Growth rate is also relevant as a possible marker to monitor the effect of medical interventions. Before it is possible to use growth rate as a marker for rupture or possible therapeutic target, it is essential to know aneurysm growth rate by measuring thoracic aortic size in a reliable and reproducible manner.

Aneurysm growth rate is known

The rate of thoracic aortic aneurysm growth depends upon aneurysm diameter, location and the presence of an underlying genetic or familial disorder.[1-4] Based upon observational data, idiopathic thoracic aortic aneurysms grow slowly; the average growth rate is estimated at 1mm/year, with small aneurysms growing even more slowly.[4-6] These small annual growth rates pose a significant challenge in medical imaging and there are some known pitfalls.

First, there is evidence for dynamic changes in aortic dimensions during the cardiac cycle. Most centres rely on non-electrocardiogram-gated computed tomography (CT) angiography for diameter measurement. This will provide images at random phases during the cardiac cycle. Recently, Parodi et al studied variations in thoracic aortic dimensions when using non-gated CT angiography and electrocardiogram-gated CT angiography. They found significant diameter differences between gated and non-gated scans. Specifically, during the cardiac cycle, diameter changed up to 5.4mm at the level of the descending thoracic aorta.[7] Consequently, electrocardiogram-gating is essential to determine aneurysm growth and changes in diameter over time should be studied in the same phase of the cardiac cycle.

To detect millimetres of aneurysm growth per year, accurate measurement and reproducibility are essential and a second possible pitfall for detecting thoracic aortic aneurysm growth is inter- and intraobserver variability. Reproducibility is especially poor for diameter measurements in orthogonal or multiplanar reconstructions. Techniques using automatic diameter measurements on reconstructions perpendicular to created centrelines show higher repeatability.[8,9] In a recent publication from Imperial College, London, both intraobserver and interobserver variation were less for perpendicular than for axial measurements. However, mean intraobserver and interobserver differences for the perpendicular images still approach or even exceed predicted annual CT angiography growth rate (5±3.8mm and 2.8±2.5mm respectively).[10]

Based upon these known pitfalls, most reports on rapid thoracic aortic expansion are reflective of measurement error.[11] To assess true aneurysm growth, accuracy has to be improved using electrocardiogram-gated CT angiography imaging, and aortic diameter has to be measured during the same phase of the cardiac cycle, at the exact same location, on reconstructions perpendicular to automatically generated centrelines.

Aneurysm growth rate and the risk of rupture

In 1978, McNamara et al described a possible relation between thoracic aortic aneurysm growth and rupture. In a series of 28 patients, 22 patients were not surgically repaired. Of these 22 patients, nine died of rupture. A recent increase in size preceded rupture in all patients for whom serial roentgenograms were available.[12]

Almost 40 years later, the literature is equivocal on the use of growth rate as a predictive marker for thoracic aortic aneurysm dissection or rupture risk. Current guidelines on thoracic aortic aneurysm disease, recommend that patients with a growth rate of >0.5cm/year in an aorta that is >5.5cm in diameter should be considered for operation. This recommendation results from case studies, standard of care or consensus opinion (Level of Evidence: C).[13] Based upon this level C recommendation, it is suggested that surgical intervention should be considered in rapidly growing aneurysms regardless of absolute diameter.[14] Part of these recommendations are based upon a single case series by Lobato et al, reporting on 31 patients with a thoracic aortic aneurysm.[15] All patients were considered unfit for repair or did not meet size criteria for elective repair. Patients were followed for a median period of 47 months. Nine patients suffered from aneurysm rupture and initial anteroposterior diameter (>5cm) and anteroposterior diameter growth rate were the major variables associated with rupture. Possible shortcomings of this study are a small sample size, diameter measurement on axial imaging and group heterogeneity (Crawford I to IV). In contrast to larger studies on the natural history of thoracic and thoracoabdominal aneurysms, median growth rates were large (3.4mm/year in the transverse and 2.8mm in the anterior-posterior direction) and irrespective of index aneurysm size. More recent studies on the natural history of thoracic aortic aneurysms do report on aneurysm growth rate but not on a possible correlation with the risk of rupture.[1,16]

In conclusion, aside from the study by Lobato *et al* and guidelines based upon consensus opinion, there are limited data on the association of growth rate and aortic rupture. This obviously does not mean there is no relationship. Based on common sense, all large aneurysms originate from small aneurysms, and, since there is a clear relationship between complication risk and aneurysm size, growth does matter. This alone justifies serial imaging and pre-emptive surgery when the aneurysm becomes too large or grows too fast. Consequently, many ruptures are prevented in these patients, which in turn leads to an underestimation of the value of growth rate to predict rupture. Additionally, large aneurysms grow faster and have a known higher risk of rupture. This collinearity of size and growth is an explanation for growth not being identified as an independent risk factor for rupture using multivariate analysis.

Aneurysm growth rate and risk management

The first step in the treatment of patients with aortic aneurysm disease aiming at reduction of aneurysm expansion rate, need for surgical repair, and rupture risk, is cardiovascular risk management.[17] Risk factor control includes medical therapy and lifestyle considerations.[14]

Smokers are more likely to develop aortic aneurysms, and current smoking accelerates aneurysm growth and increases dissection risk.[17] Smoking cessation is recommended for all patients, although there is limited evidence for the effect of cessation on returning complications risks and growth rates to normal.[13]

Based upon data from the Yale Center for Aortic Disease (a database including 3000 patients, 9,000 imaging studies and 9,000 patients-years of observation), Elefteriades *et al* report that acute exertion and emotion can precipitate the onset of acute aortic dissection. This observation has led to lifestyle alterations as part of the medical management of aortic aneurysms. The authors advise against heavy weight lifting and suggest sedative medication to prevent blood pressure spikes in emotional or stressful situations.[6] To prevent hypertensive spikes during training, some advocate a symptom limited stress test to ensure that the patient does not have a hypertensive response to exercise.[13] The beneficial effect of these lifestyle modifications on aneurysm growth is not known.

Aneurysm growth and medical therapy

Traditional endpoints in clinical studies on the effect of medical interventions in patients with a thoracic aortic aneurysm are dissection, rupture and mortality. Based upon multiple large studies on risk factor control in aneurysm patients, there is compelling evidence for a reduction in complication rate and mortality for patients on medical therapy. However, the effect of beta-blockers, statins, and angiotensin-converting-enzyme inhibitors etc., on thoracic aortic aneurysm growth is uncertain, and the use of aneurysm growth rate as a possible marker for the success of medical interventions is questionable.

The cornerstones of medical therapy in aneurysm disease are beta-blockers and statins. Beta-blockers have been suggested to reduce the rate of aortic dilatation by reducing blood pressure and subsequent aneurysm wall stress. This theoretical beneficial effect of beta-blockers on aneurysm growth has been studied in patients with chronic type B dissections and Marfan patients, showing reduced aortic dilatation in these patients.[13] To date, no studies on the effect of beta-blockers on growth rate in patients with an idiopathic thoracic aortic aneurysm have been published.[18] Moreover, randomised trials in abdominal aortic aneurysm patients showed no effect on aneurysm growth rate and low compliance rates because of an observed negative effect of beta-blockers on exercise tolerance and quality of life.[19–21] Unlike the suggested mechanical effect of beta-blockers, statins have a pleiotropic effect on inflammatory pathways involved in aneurysm formation and growth. Again, in spite of this theoretical effect on reducing aneurysm growth, large studies have failed to show reductions in growth rate in abdominal aortic aneurysms, and there is no clinical data for statin use and thoracic aortic aneurysm growth rate.[21,22]

Present and future research in aneurysm disease will focus on medical strategies to modify genetic and pathophysiological pathways involved in aneurysm disease. The effect of these strategies will most likely be monitored using traditional endpoints such as aneurysm-related complications and mortality as aneurysm growth is difficult to assess and because of the ill-defined relation between aneurysm growth and complication rate.

Summary

Growth rate is unknown

- Growth rate of small thoracic aortic aneurysm is low and difficult to measure.

- Imaging protocols will have to be improved to know thoracic aortic aneurysm growth rate.

Growth rate is relevant

- Because of the ill-defined relation between aneurysm growth rate and the risk of complications, the clinical relevance of aneurysm growth rate is limited.

- Little evidence for aneurysm growth rate as a surrogate marker for disease progression and limited evidence for the use of growth rate as tool to monitor the effect of medical interventions.

References

1. Elefteriades JA. Natural history of thoracic aortic aneurysms: indications for surgery, and surgical *versus* nonsurgical risks. *Ann Thorac Surg* 2002; **74** (5): S1877–S80.

2. Kuzmik GA, Sang AX, Elefteriades JA. Natural history of thoracic aortic aneurysms. *J Vasc Surg* 2012; **56** (2): 565–71.

3. Hansen PA, Richards JM, Tambyraja AL, *et al.* Natural history of thoraco-abdominal aneurysm in high-risk patients. *Eur J Vasc Endovasc Surg* 2010; **39** (3): 266–70.

4. Dudzinski DM, Isselbacher EM. Diagnosis and Management of Thoracic Aortic Disease. *Curr Cardiol Rep* 2015; **17** (12): 106.

5. Coady MA, Rizzo JA, Goldstein LJ, Elefteriades JA. Natural history, pathogenesis, and etiology of thoracic aortic aneurysms and dissections. *Cardiol Clin* 1999; **17** (4): 615–35.

6. Elefteriades JA, Farkas EA. Thoracic aortic aneurysm clinically pertinent controversies and uncertainties. *J Am Coll Cardiol* 2010; **55** (9): 841–57.

7. Parodi J, Berguer R, Carrascosa P, *et al.* Sources of error in the measurement of aortic diameter in computed tomography scans. *J Vasc Surg* 2014; **59** (1): 74–79.

8. Ahmed S, Zimmerman SL, Johnson PT, *et al.* MDCT interpretation of the ascending aorta with semiautomated measurement software: improved reproducibility compared with manual techniques. J Cardiovasc Comput Tomogr 2014; **8** (2): 108–14.

9. Rengier F, Weber TF, Partovi S, *et al.* Reliability of semiautomatic centerline analysis *versus* manual aortic measurement techniques for TEVAR among non-experts. *Eur J Vasc Endovasc Surg* 2011; **42** (3): 324–31.

10. Rudarakanchana N, Bicknell CD, Cheshire NJ, *et al.* Variation in maximum diameter measurements of descending thoracic aortic aneurysms using unformatted planes *versus* images corrected to aortic centerline. *Eur J Vasc Endovasc Surg* 2014; **47** (1): 19–26.

11. Elefteriades JA, Farkas EA. Thoracic aortic aneurysm clinically pertinent controversies and uncertainties. *J Am Coll Cardiol* 2010; **55** (9): 841–57.

12. McNamara JJ, Pressler VM. Natural history of arteriosclerotic thoracic aortic aneurysms. *Ann Thorac Surg* 1978; **26** (5): 468–73.

13. Hiratzka LF, Bakris GL, Beckman JA, *et al.* 2010 ACCF/AHA/AATS/ACR/ASA/SCA/SCAI/SIR/STS/SVM guidelines for the diagnosis and management of patients with thoracic aortic disease: executive summary. A report of the American College of Cardiology Foundation/American Heart Association Task Force on Practice Guidelines, American Association for Thoracic Surgery, American College of Radiology, American Stroke Association, Society of Cardiovascular Anesthesiologists, Society for Cardiovascular Angiography and Interventions, Society of Interventional Radiology, Society of Thoracic *Surgeons*, and Society for Vascular Medicine. *Catheter Cardiovasc Interv* 2010; **76** (2): E43–E86.

14. Boodhwani M, Andelfinger G, Leipsic J, *et al.* Canadian Cardiovascular Society position statement on the management of thoracic aortic disease. *Can J Cardiol* 2014; **30** (6): 577–89.

15. Lobato AC, Puech-Leao P. Predictive factors for rupture of thoracoabdominal aortic aneurysm. *J Vasc Surg* 1998; **27** (3): 446–53.

16. Davies RR, Goldstein LJ, Coady MA, *et al.* Yearly rupture or dissection rates for thoracic aortic aneurysms: simple prediction based on size. *Ann Thorac Surg* 2002; **73** (1): 17–27.

17. Goldfinger JZ, Halperin JL, Marin ML, *et al.* Thoracic aortic aneurysm and dissection. *J Am Coll Cardiol* 2014; **64** (16): 1725–39.

18. Danyi P, Elefteriades JA, Jovin IS. Medical therapy of thoracic aortic aneurysms: are we there yet? *Circulation* 2011; **124** (13): 1469–76.

19. Rughani G, Robertson L, Clarke M. Medical treatment for small abdominal aortic aneurysms. Cochrane Database Syst Rev 2012; **9**: CD009536.

20. Propanolol Aneurysm Trial Investigators. Propranolol for small abdominal aortic aneurysms: results of a randomized trial. *J Vasc Surg* 2002; **35** (1): 72–79.

21. Kokje VB, Hamming JF, Lindeman JH. Pharmaceutical Management of Small Abdominal Aortic Aneurysms: A Systematic Review of the Clinical Evidence. *Eur J Vasc Endovasc Surg* 2015; **50** (6): 702–13.

22. Castellano JM, Kovacic JC, Sanz J, Fuster V. Are we ignoring the dilated thoracic aorta? *Ann N Y Acad Sci* 2012; **1254**: 164–74.

Thoracic aneurysm challenges—risks of operative death and spinal cord ischaemia

The Uppsala algorithm to prevent spinal cord ischaemia during extensive aortic surgery

A Wanhainen, J Eriksson and K Mani

Introduction

Spinal cord ischaemia is a devastating complication after extensive open and endovascular aortic surgery, associated with significant mortality and morbidity as well as cost. The incidence of spinal cord ischaemia after thoracic and thoracoabdominal endovascular repair varies between 1% and 20%, depending on the extension and type of the aortic disease.[1–7]

The main risk factors for spinal cord ischaemia are: extensive aortic repair, including prior aortic surgery;[1,2,5,8] peri- or postoperative hypotension;[1,5,6] and compromised collaterals of the spinal circulation, including coverage of the left subclavian artery and hypogastric artery.[1,6,9] Additionally, general cardiovascular risk factors, such as age, chronic obstructive pulmonary disease, renal failure, and hypertension, have been associated with increased risk.[8]

The effectiveness of management algorithms, designed to detect spinal cord ischaemia and implement immediate therapeutic interventions to improve spinal cord perfusion, have been proven in several reports.[1,5–10] From Baltimore, USA, Arnaoutakis and colleagues showed that adjunctive use of cerebrospinal fluid drainage, left subclavian artery revascularisation and hypertensive therapy resulted in a permanent spinal cord ischaemia frequency of only 0.9% after thoracic endovascular aortic repair (TEVAR).[10] From Lille, France, Maurel and colleagues showed a significant reduction in spinal cord ischaemia rate following type I–III thoracoabdominal endovascular aortic repair after having introduced a dedicated management protocol (14% vs. 1.2%), including staged procedures, early restoration of arterial flow to the pelvis and lower limb, optimisation of oxygen delivery by means of blood transfusion, maintaining a middle artery pressure of >85mmHg, and cerebrospinal fluid drainage.[5] A similar finding was described by Rossi and colleagues where a strategy to reverse spinal cord ischaemia after thoracoabdominal endovascular aortic repair by rising middle artery pressure, cerebrospinal fluid drainage, angioplasty of stenosed hypogastric artery, and restoring perfusion to the aneurysm sac, reversed spinal cord ischaemia in two out of three patients developing neurological symptoms, leaving 6% with permanent paraplegia.[6]

Here, we describe the Uppsala algorithm to prevent spinal cord ischaemia during extensive aortic surgery, the scientific rationale behind it, and our clinical experience.

The Uppsala algorithm

Staged repair

Experimental pig studies showed return of spinal cord perfusion pressure five days after simulated thoracoabdominal aortic repair, by an increase in size of existing small arterioles within the collateral network and development of new small vessels within it.[11] This suggests a possible protective role for ischaemic preconditioning by means of staging the procedure, allowing the collateral circulation to adapt and stabilise. Further experimental studies later verified this hypothesis.[12]

Several clinical studies have confirmed the benefit of staged repair. From Cleveland, USA, O'Callaghan and colleagues reported an overall spinal cord ischaemia rate of 37% (12 of 32) in the non-staged group *versus* 11% (three of 27) in the staged group of type II endovascular repair (p=0.03). Furthermore, all neurological injuries in the staged group were temporary.[13] Harrison *et al* observed no cases of permanent paraplegia in 10 patients with type II thoracoabdominal aortic aneurysm with branched stent grafts in whom sac perfusion was maintained for seven to 10 days with an open side graft that was then closed.[14]

Our strategy is to stage not only the aortic stent graft procedure, but also all adjunct procedures, such as left subclavian artery bypasses and access conduit operations. Therefore, a thoracoabdominal endovascular aortic repair is typically staged in two to four separate procedures. The first step of the aorta stenting usually covers the descending portion of the aorta down to the level of the diaphragm, and the second procedure completes the repair.

Revascularisation of important collaterals

In experimental animal studies and clinical studies, segmental artery sacrifices were much better tolerated if the subclavian arteries and hypogastric artery were patent.[15] In a large European multicentre registry study, including 38 cases of spinal cord ischaemia among 2,235 TEVAR patients, simultaneous closure of at least two vascular territories supplying the spinal cord (i.e. left subclavian artery, intercostal arteries, lumbar arteries, and hypogastric arteries) was significantly associated with symptomatic spinal cord ischaemia, especially in combination with prolonged intraoperative hypotension. The authors emphasised the need to preserve the left subclavian artery during TEVAR.[16] We always try to preserve flow to both subclavian arteries and both hypogastric arteries whenever possible. Additionally, we try to minimise pelvic and lower extremity hypoperfusion during the procedure, either through shunts[16] and/or with early sheath removal.[5] In a few cases of high-risk patients, we have also preserved dominant intercostal arteries by designing a separate fenestration in the stent graft, with good clinical and imaging outcome.

Cerebrospinal fluid drainage

Cerebrospinal fluid drainage is an established technique to decrease the risk of spinal cord ischaemia after open thoracoabdominal aortic repair.[17] Reports also support the use of cerebrospinal fluid drainage for prevention and treatment of spinal cord ischaemia after endovascular repair.[1,18,19] In a prospective observational study by Hnath *et al* on 121 TEVAR patients, none in the cerebrospinal fluid drainage group developed spinal cord ischaemia, whereas 8% of those without cerebrospinal fluid drainage developed neurological deficit (p<0.05), despite more risk factors for spinal cord ischaemia in the cerebrospinal fluid drainage group.[18]

Three randomised controlled trials involving cerebrospinal fluid drainage during type I and II thoracoabdominal aortic aneurysm open surgery have been published. The largest study, including 145 thoracoabdominal aortic aneurysm repair, found an 80% reduction in relative risk of postoperative spinal cord ischaemia (12% vs. 3%).[17] A significant protective effect was also seen with a combination of cerebrospinal fluid drainage and intrathecal papaverine on 33 patients,[20] while a third trial with 98 randomised patients found no significant benefit of intraoperative cerebrospinal fluid drainage <50mL.[21] A recent Cochrane review recommends cerebrospinal fluid drainage as a component of a multimodality approach for prevention of neurological injury.[22]

The potential benefit of cerebrospinal fluid drainage must be balanced against the risks associated with its use. Intracranial haemorrhage is the most devastating of these complications. The incidence of symptomatic intracranial haemorrhage is about 1%[24] and the risk increases with large draining volumes.[23,24] Drainage volumes of ≤10ml per hour or <150ml per 24 hours (i.e. one third of the daily produced cerebrospinal fluid) has been recommended in asymptomatic patients.[25,26] Neuraxial haematoma can be a disastrous complication of cerebrospinal fluid drainage, which can resemble the signs of spinal cord ischaemia.[23] Systemic anticoagulation and platelet dysfunction increase the risk. The best imaging modality to differentiate between spinal cord ischaemia and haematoma is T2-weighted MRI.[27] Prompt neurosurgical treatment is essential to avoid permanent injury.

We use the Liquoguard-system, an automatic pressure controlled cerebrospinal fluid drainage system with continuous documentation of the drainage rate and volume that allows for reliable predefined drainage settings.[26] Our routine duration of drainage is 72 hours. We have no predefined upper limit of cerebrospinal fluid pressure, but guide the volume by estimated risk and symptoms of spinal cord ischaemia. To avoid excessive and uncontrolled cerebrospinal fluid drainage, which increases the risk of subdural haemorrhage, we typically drain small volumes (5mL) intraoperatively before the aorta has been completely excluded and postoperatively on asymptomatic patients when they are awake. The volume is increased to 10mL after the aorta has been excluded on anaesthetised patients, and even more on high-risk patients. In case of postoperative signs or symptoms of paraparesis, a drainage volume of 20mL or more is allowed.

In the emergency setting, we employ selective postoperative cerebrospinal fluid drainage in case of symptoms. This strategy is supported by a study from University of Alabama where 30% of post-TEVAR spinal cord ischaemia patients had complete resolution and 40% partial resolution when using selective postoperative cerebrospinal fluid drainage.[4]

Avoiding hypotension

Spinal cord perfusion is dependent on the net pressure of the middle artery pressure minus the mean intrathecal pressure. Several publications report spinal cord ischaemia recovery after hypertensive therapy with volume resuscitation and/or vasopressors.[1,3,10]

We aim to maintain a middle artery pressure of ≥85mmHg to ensure a spinal cord perfusion pressure (middle artery pressure minus lumbar cerebrospinal fluid pressure) of 70mmHg. Patients at risk are admitted to the intensive care unit for continuous haemodynamic monitoring for at least the first 24 postoperative hours. We aim for a haemoglobin level of >10g/dL and a central venous oxygen saturation of >75% with blood transfusion and oxygenation when necessary. Fresh frozen plasma and platelet transfusion are given according to massive transfusion protocol. Also, intra-abdominal pressure is monitored every four hours to avoid intra-abdominal hypertension/abdominal compartment syndrome.

For this reason, adjunctive procedures, such as left subclavian artery bypasses and access conduit operations are usually done as separate procedures, to avoid too excessive procedures in terms of complexity and time, with increased risk of bleeding and hypotension.

Neuromonitoring

Lower limb function cannot be evaluated in the anaesthetised patient. Experience suggests that intraoperative neuromonitoring by means of somatosensory evoked potentials and motor evoked potentials is an effective method to detect spinal cord ischaemia during complex endovascular aortic surgery.[18,29] However, neuromonitoring during aortic stent placement requires special considerations since the vascular access needed for endovascular repair may result in leg ischaemia eliminating cortical somatosensory evoked potentials and muscle motor evoked potentials monitoring from that leg.[30]

We have recently initiated a programme for neuromonitoring of high risk thoracoabdominal aortic aneurysm cases. We also try to avoid prolonged sedation and extubate the patients on the table as soon as feasible, to allow early neurological evaluation.

The Uppsala experience

The Uppsala experience of total thoracoabdominal endovascular aortic repair consists of 32 patients: 15 (47%) type II; 4 (12%) type III; and 13 (41%) type IV. Seven underwent urgent intervention for rupture. Thirty-day mortality was 3% (n=1). Four patients developed signs of spinal cord ischaemia, of whom two (6%) had permanent paraplegia. These included a 70-year old man operated on electively for a type II thoracoabdominal aortic aneurysm with a two-step procedure with a four-branched stent-graft. He received cerebrospinal fluid drainage according to protocol. Postoperatively, he developed sepsis with hypotension and subsequently developed symptoms of paraplegia. He deteriorated and developed multiorgan failure and died on day 69. Another patient who developed paraplegia was an 80-year old woman operated on electively for a type IV thoracoabdominal aortic aneurysm with a one-step procedure with a four-branched stent graft. She had significant bilateral hypogastric artery stenosis. Despite cerebrospinal fluid drainage, she developed signs of spinal cord ischaemia with left leg weakness that progressed to bilateral paraplegia. An attempt to improve flow in the hypogastric artery by angioplasty was complicated by rupture of the hypogastric artery with massive bleeding and hypotension and the development of abdominal compartment syndrome necessitating treatment with open abdomen. A deliberate excessive cerebrospinal fluid drainage was complicated by an intracranial haemorrhage, and she died on day 90. The third patient to develop signs of spinal cord ischaemia was a 71-year old man operated on emergently for a ruptured mycotic type IV thoracoabdominal aortic aneurysm with a one-step procedure with a four-branched stent graft. Perioperative cerebrospinal fluid drainage was not used. Postoperatively, he developed signs of spinal cord ischaemia with weakness in the legs. Cerebrospinal fluid drainage was initiated with complete reversion of the neurological symptoms. He is alive after two years. Another patient who developed signs of spinal cord ischaemia was a 78-year-old man with a chronic type B aortic dissection with type II thoracoabdominal aortic aneurysm formation. He had a history of open repair of the proximal descending aorta, TEVAR of the distal descending aorta, and endovascular aneurysm repair (EVAR) of the infrarenal abdominal aorta, with an episode of suspected spinal cord ischaemia with transient weakness of the legs. He was operated on electively for an aneurysm of the untreated remaining paravisceral aortic segments, with a fenestrated stent graft. A fifth fenestration was included for a dominating lumbar artery, and he had peri- and postoperative cerebrospinal fluid drainage. Postoperatively, he experienced a short episode of weakness in the left leg which went into complete regression. He is alive and still works as a physician after two years.

We conclude that the Uppsala experience conforms to what is presented in the literature. Spinal cord ischaemia is associated with extensive endovascular aortic surgery, impaired collateral circulation, bleeding and hypotension. Often these factors are present simultaneously, with an associated high mortality rate. Prevention and aggressive treatment algorithms is essential to improve outcome.

Summary

- Spinal cord ischaemia is a devastating complication after extensive open and endovascular aortic surgery.

- Management algorithms, designed to detect spinal cord ischaemia and implement immediate therapeutic interventions to improve spinal cord perfusion includes: Staging the procedure; preservation of left-subclavian and hypogastric artery flow; cerebrospinal fluid drainage; maintaining a high blood pressure and oxygenation, and perioperative neuromonitoring.

References

1. Cheung AT, Pchettina A, McGarvey L, Appoo JJ, et al. Strategies to manage paraplegia risk after endovascular stent repair of descending thoracic aortic aneurysms. Ann Thorac Surg 2005; 80: 1280–89.
2. Drinkwater SL, Goebells A, Haydar A, et al. The incidence of spinal cord ischaemia following thoracic and thoracoabdominal aortic endovascular intervention. Eur J Vasc Endovasc Surg 2010; 40: 729–35.
3. Etz CD, Weigang E, Hartert M, et al. Contemporary spinal cord protection during thoracic and thoracoabdominal aortic surgery and endovascular aortic repair: a position paper of the vascular domain of the European Association for Cardio-Thoracic Surgery. European Journal of Cardio-Thoracic Surgery 2015: 943–57.
4. Keith CJ, Passman MA, Carignan MJ, et al. Protocol implementation of selective postoperative lumbar spinal drainage after thoracic aortic endograft. J Vasc Surg 2012; 55: 1–9.
5. Maurel B, Delclaux N, Sobocinski J, Hertault A et al. The impact of early pelvic and lower limb reperfusion and attentive peri-operative management on the incidence of spinal cord ischemia during thoracoabdominal aortic aneurysm endovascular repair. Eur J Vasc Endovasc Surg 2015; 49: 248–54.
6. Rossi SH, Patel A, Saha P, et al. Neuroprotective strategies can prevent permanent paraplegia in the majority of patients who develop spinal cord ischaemia after endovascular repair of thoracoabdominal aortic aneurysms. Eur J Vasc Endovasc Surg 2015; 50: 599–607.
7. Ullery BW, Cheung AT, Fairman RM, et al. Risk factors, outcomes, and clinical manifestations of spinal cord ischemia following thoracic endovascular aortic repair. J Vasc Surg 2011; 54: 677–84.

8. Scali ST, Wang SK, Feezor RJ, *et al*. Preoperative prediction of spinal cord ischemia after thoracic endovascular aortic repair. *J Vasc Surg* 2014; **60**: 1481–90.

9. Czerny M, Eggebrecht H, Sodeck G, Verzini F, *et al*. Mechanisms of symptomatic spinal cord ischemia after TEVAR: insights from the European Registry of Endovascular Aortic Repair Complications (EuREC). *J Endovasc Ther* 2012; **19**: 37–43.

10. Arnaoutakis DJ, Arnaoutakis GJ, Beaulieu RJ *et al*. Results of adjunctive spinal drainage and/or left subclavian artery bypass in thoracic endovascular aortic repair. *Ann Vasc Surg* 2014; **28**: 65–73.

11. Etz CD, Kari FA, Mueller CS, *et al*. The collateral network concept: remodeling of the arterial collateral network after experimental segmental artery sacrifice. *J Thorac Cardiovasc Surg* 2011; **141**: 1029–36.

12. Bischoff MS, Scheumann J, Brenner RM, *et al*. Staged approach prevents spinal cord injury in hybrid surgical endovascular thoracoabdominal aortic aneurysm repair: an experimental model. *Ann Thorac Surg* 2011; **92**: 138–46.

13. O'Callaghan A, Mastracci TM, Eagleton MJ. Staged endovascular repair of thoracoabdominal aortic aneurysms limits incidence and severity of spinal cord ischemia. *J Vasc Surg* 2015; **61**: 347–54.

14. Harrison SC, Agu O, Harris PL, Ivancev K. Elective sac perfusion to reduce the risk of neurologic events following endovascular repair of thoracoabdominal aneurysms. *J Vasc Surg* 2012; **55**: 1202–05.

15. Strauch JT, Spielvogel D, Lauten A, *et al*. Importance of extrasegmental vessels for spinal cord blood supply in a chronic porcine model. *Rev Port Cir Cardiotorac Vasc* 2003; **10**: 185–91.

16. Österberg K, Falkenberg M, Resch T. Endovascular technique for arterial shunting to prevent intraoperative ischemia. *Eur J Vasc Endovasc Surg*. 2014; **48** (2): 126–30.

17. Coselli JS, Lemaire SA, Koksoy C, *et al*. Cerebrospinal fluid drainage reduces paraplegia after thoracoabdominal aortic aneurysm repair: results of a randomized clinical trial. *J Vasc Surg* 2002; **35**: 631–39.

18. Hnath JC, Mehta M, Taggert JB, *et al*. Strategies to improve spinal cord ischemia in endovascular thoracic aortic repair: outcomes of a prospective cerebrospinal fluid drainage protocol. *J Vasc Surg* 2008; **48**: 836–40.

19. Tiesenhausen K, Amann W, Koch G, *et al*. Cerebrospinal fluid drainage to reverse paraplegia after endovascular thoracic aortic aneurysm repair. *J Endovasc Ther* 2000; **7** (2): 132–35.

20. Svensson LG, Hess KR, D'Agostino RS, Entrup MH, Hreib K, Kimmel WA, *et al*. Reduction of neurologic injury after high-risk thoracoabdominal aortic operation. *Annals of Thoracic Surgery* 1998; **66** (1): 132–38.

21. Crawford ES, Svensson LG, Hess KR, *et al:* A prospective randomized study of cerebrospinal fluid drainage to prevent paraplegia after high risk surgery on the thoracoabdominal aorta. *J Vasc Surg* 1991; **13**: 36–45.

22. Khan SN, Stansby G. Cerebrospinal fluid drainage for thoracic and thoracoabdominal aortic aneurysm surgery. Cochrane Database of Systematic Reviews 2012, Issue 10. Art. No.: CD003635. DOI: 10.1002/14651858.CD003635.pub3

23. Fedorow CA, Moon MC, Mutch WA, *et al*. Lumbar cerebrospinal fluid drainage for thoracoabdominal aortic surgery: rationale and practical considerations for management. *Anesth Analg* 2010; **111**: 46–58.

24. Wynn MM, Mell MW, Tefera G, *et al*. Complications of spinal fluid drainage in thoracoabdominal aortic aneurysm repair: a report of 486 patients treated from 1987 to 2008. *J Vasc Surg* 2009; **49**: 29–35.

25. Estrera AL, Sheinbaum R, Miller CC, Azizzadeh A, *et al*. Cerebrospinal fluid drainage during thoracic aortic repair: safety and current management. *Ann Thorac Surg* 2009; **88** (1): 9–15.

26. Kotelis D, Bianchini C, Kovacs B, *et al*. Early experience with automatic pressure-controlled cerebrospinal fluid drainage during thoracic endovascular aortic repair. *J Endovasc Ther*apy 2015; 1–5

27. Weaver KD, Wiseman DB, Farber M, *et al*. Complications of lumbar drainage after thoracoabdominal aortic aneurysm repair. *J Vasc Surg* 2001; **34**: 623–27.

28. Weigang E, Hartert M, Siegenthaler MP, et. al. Perioperative management to improve neurologic outcome in thoracic or thoracoabdominal aortic stent-grafting. *Ann Thorac Surg* 2006; **82**: 1679–87.

29. Estrera AL, Sheinbaum R, Miller CC 3rd, *et al*. Neuromonitor-guided repair of thoracoabdominal aortic aneurysms. *J Thorac Cardiovasc Surg* 2010; **140** (6 Suppl): S131–35.

30. Sloan TB, Edmonds HL, Koht A. Intraoperative electrophysiologic monitoring in aortic surgery. *Journal of Cardiothoracic and Vascular Anesthesi*a 2013; **27**: 1364–73.

Low spinal cord ischaemia time with BEVAR and FEVAR is vital

A Katsargyris, G Kouvelos and ELG Verhoeven

Introduction

Spinal cord ischaemia represents a serious complication after both open and endovascular repair of thoracoabdominal aortic aneurysms, with frequently devastating outcomes such as persistent lower limb weakness or paraplegia. It also has a serious impact on perioperative mortality.[1]

Several factors have been associated with the occurrence of spinal cord ischaemia after open thoracoabdominal aortic aneurysm repair. For example, intercostal artery circulation interruption, intraoperative blood loss with prolonged hypotension, and aortic cross clamping.[2] Endovascular repair of thoracoabdominal aortic aneurysms with fenestrated and branched stent grafts eliminates the need for cross-clamping, potentially reduces the risks of haemodynamic instability, and could theoretically lower the incidence of spinal cord ischaemia.[3–6]

Published literature demonstrates an incidence of spinal cord ischaemia after endovascular thoracoabdominal aortic aneurysm repair of between 3.9% and 31%.[7,8] Several strategies have been proposed to reduce perioperative spinal cord ischaemia after the endovascular procedure, most of them extrapolated from the experience with open surgical thoracoabdominal aortic aneurysm repair.[2,9] Direct data for spinal cord ischaemia originating from endovascular thoracoabdominal aortic aneurysm repair are limited.[10-12]

The present chapter summarises current spinal cord protection strategies in endovascular thoracoabdominal aortic aneurysm repair. Particular emphasis is given on the role of minimising intraoperative spinal cord ischaemia time during fenestrated endovascular aneurysm repair (FEVAR) or branched endovascular aneurysm repair (BEVAR).

Vascular supply of the spinal cord

Understanding the anatomy of the blood supply of the spinal cord is essential for developing optimal strategies to prevent ischaemia during and after extensive thoracoabdominal aortic aneurysm repair.

The spinal cord is perfused by multiple aortic branches throughout its entire course. Traditionally, the anterior spinal artery represents the dominant blood supply to the motor region of the spinal cord, formed by branches of the vertebral arteries bilaterally. An additional network of intercostal and lumbar arteries supplements the blood supply of the spinal cord along its course.[13] A large intercostal artery, commonly referred to as the Artery of Adamkiewicz, arises from the confluence of a variable number of smaller tributaries in the lower thorax, and forms the greater radicular artery, a dominant supplier of the anterior spinal artery. The sensory areas of the spinal cord are supplied by two posterior spinal arteries, which originate from the subclavian arteries.

Lately, the anatomy of spinal cord perfusion has been reassessed and the "collateral network concept" has been introduced, at both an experimental and a clinical level. As investigated by Etz *et al,* the spinal cord is perfused by a collateral system, which involves an extensive axial arterial network in the spinal canal, the paravertebral tissues and the paraspinous muscles, in which vessels anastomose with one another and with the nutrient arteries of the spinal cord.[14] The configuration of the arterial network includes inputs not only from the segmental vessels (intercostal and lumbar), but also from the subclavian and the hypogastric arteries.[14] The presence of this extensive network allows for compensatory blood flow when part of the network is compromised, contributing to sufficient perfusion of the spinal cord after surgical or endovascular segmental artery occlusion.

Risk factors for spinal cord ischaemia after endovascular thoracoabdominal aortic aneurysm repair

A recent study from our group on a total of 218 patients with thoracoabdominal aortic aneurysm treated with fenestrated and branched stent-grafts identified baseline renal insufficiency (glomerular filtration rate<30 mL/minute), peripheral arterial disease, and long procedure duration as independent risk factors for spinal cord ischaemia.[12] Peripheral arterial disease, in particular, was shown to multiply the risk of spinal cord ischaemia by 6.6. This probably reflects a "defective" collateral network of spinal cord among patients with peripheral arterial disease. Long procedure duration (>300 minutes) also multiplied the spinal cord ischaemia risk by 7.4. This is probably related to longer intraoperative ischaemia times of the spinal cord, which can result in the compromise of the collateral circulation by large iliac sheaths. Additionally, longer duration of the procedure may indicate prolonged catheter and wire manipulations, with increased possibility of spinal cord embolisation. Other investigators have addressed the extent of aortic coverage as an independent risk factor for spinal cord ischaemia development.[15] Finally, peri- and postoperative hypotension, blood loss, and previous aortic surgery have also been associated with a significantly increased risk of spinal cord ischaemia.[16]

Spinal cord protection strategies in endovascular thoracoabdominal aortic aneurysm repair

Stent graft planning

When planning to use stent grafts, the aim should be to preserve the left subclavian artery, and one, or both, internal iliac arteries if possible, so as to maintain as much "spinal collateral circulation" as possible. Moreover, coverage of the aorta should be kept at the minimum possible length, without jeopardising a safe and durable proximal and distal landing zone in healthy aortic segments.

Cerebrospinal fluid drainage

Cerebrospinal fluid drainage is an established strategy to reduce spinal cord ischaemia in open thoracoabdominal aortic aneurysm repair.[2] Relevant data for the endovascular procedure are, however, lacking. Some groups use prophylactic cerebrospinal fluid drainage in patients with thoracoabdominal aortic aneurysm type I, II or III according to the modified Crawford classification, and in patients with previous abdominal aortic surgery.[7,16] Other authors advocate postoperative placement of cerebrospinal fluid drainage only upon spinal cord ischaemia symptoms, due to a significant incidence of related adverse events.[15] Our group favours prophylactic cerebrospinal fluid drainage in patients needing extensive aortic coverage.

Correction of blood pressure, haemoglobin, intravascular volume and oxygenation

Aggressive correction of haemoglobin, intravascular volume and arterial blood pressure is mandatory to aim for the best possible perfusion and oxygenation of the spinal cord.[1] A pre-emptive strategy of blood, plasma and platelet transfusion appears to be beneficial for several reasons.[7] First, endovascular exclusion of large aneurysms is associated with an acute reduction in coagulation factors and platelets, which leads to a postoperative coagulopathy with increased risk for postoperative bleeding. Second, an adequate intravascular volume with haemoglobin rich blood maximises oxygen delivery to the spinal cord tissue. Finally, a high cardiac output—as reflected by a high arterial blood pressure—increases perfusion of the spinal cord tissue.[7] The above parameters should be controlled and immediately corrected not only intraoperatively, but also during the first postoperative days, since many cases of spinal cord ischaemia can develop later (24–72 hours after the operation) partially due to postoperative ischaemia-reperfusion injury.[12]

Reduction of intraoperative spinal cord ischaemia time

The value of early re-establishment of hypogastric and lower-limb circulation, with the aim of restoring collateral circulation to the spinal cord as soon as possible, is in our opinion still underestimated and under used.

Prolonged ischaemia due to the obliterating sheaths has a negative impact on spinal cord ischaemia. Using the smallest possible sheaths and removing them as quickly as possible—in between separate steps of the procedure—lowers spinal cord ischaemia time. This should result in a direct positive effect to reduce spinal cord ischaemia. Additionally, lower spinal cord ischaemia time reduces the impact of ischaemia-reperfusion injury, which should further lower the risk of postoperative spinal cord ischaemia.[17]

Our strategy for quick hypogastric and lower limb reperfusion involves an open surgical access at both femoral arteries with the use of double purse string sutures (Prolene 4-0, Ethicon) fitted with a snugger.[18] These purse string sutures allow for complete removal of delivery sheaths between the steps of the procedure, while maintaining access with a stiff-wire in position to complete the later steps (e.g. introduction of a bifurcated graft, ballooning, angiography, etc.) (Figure 1). This manoeuvre serves to restore pelvic and lower limb perfusion as soon as possible between the different steps of the procedure.

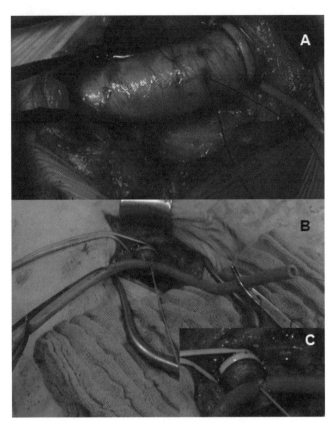

Figure 1: (A) Double purse string sutures (4-0 Prolene) at the common femoral artery before puncture. (B) Between the steps of the procedure, delivery sheaths can been removed to reperfuse the pelvis and lower limbs, while addressing the branches from an upper access. The purse sting sutures are pulled and clamped over snuggers, to achieve haemostasis over a stiff guidewire that will be used for the later steps of the procedure. (C) Close-up view.

In stent grafts with branches, only the branched graft can be deployed completely, and the delivery sheath can be removed before catheterisation of the branches and target vessels. These are subsequently addressed from an upper access, while the pelvis and lower limbs are being perfused without restriction. In grafts with fenestrations, the main stent graft can only be deployed, and the delivery sheath removed, after catheterisation of all target vessels.

Beyond the use of purse string sutures to allow quick removal of large sheaths as discussed above, additional measures to keep ischaemia time low during fenestrated endovascular aneurysm repair include:

- Use of a smaller 18F (instead of a 20F) sheath in the contralateral femoral artery during catheterisation of fenestrations. This allows some blood flow around the sheath to perfuse the hypogastric artery and the lower limb
- Introduction of guiding sheaths at the visceral vessels as late as possible (after catheterisation of all target vessels) to reduce visceral ischaemia time
- In 3-4x fenestrated endovascular aneurysm repair, placement of guiding sheaths initially only in the renal arteries. The superior mesenteric artery and coeliac are first secured with a stiff wire only to allow unrestricted perfusion during stenting of the renal arteries.

Achieving quick pelvic and lower limb reperfusion, along with the other above mentioned protection measures have resulted in low persistent spinal cord ischaemia rates (≈4%) after endovascular thoracoabdominal aortic aneurysm repair in our experience.[12] The value of quick re-establishment of hypogastric and lower limb circulation has been recently highlighted also by the group in Lille. The authors have noted a significant reduction of spinal cord ischaemia rates after modifying their deployment sequence to achieve quick pelvic and lower limb reperfusion.[7]

Procedure staging

Staging the procedure has emerged as an additional potentially useful strategy to reduce spinal cord ischaemia. The theoretical rationale behind staging is to provide some time for expansion of a pre-existing collateral network or formation of new vessels to maintain adequate perfusion to the spinal cord.[19] Also, splitting the procedure in to two stages could result in lower operative stress and lower ischaemia time of the spinal cord at each stage. Two different staging strategies have been more extensively tested in clinical cohorts:

- Temporary aneurysm sac perfusion with secondary stent graft side branch completion[10]
- Two step aortic coverage, with thoracic stent-graft deployment first followed by branch-fenestrated endovascular aneurysm repair/fenestrated endovascular aneurysm repair in a second stage[11]

Preliminary data from both techniques seem to result in lower spinal cord ischaemia rates. Quite recently, a third method of staging has been proposed. This consists of selective segmental artery endovascular coil embolisation initially, followed by open or endovascular thoracoabdominal aortic aneurysm repair a few weeks later.[20] Segmental artery coil embolisation uses the paraspinal arterial collateral network's ability to regenerate new arteries to secure sufficient spinal cord perfusion upon abrupt interruption of intercostal and lumbar arteries during open and endovascular thoracoabdominal aortic aneurysm repair. Clinical experience with this method is currently limited.

Disadvantages of staging include an ongoing risk of aneurysm rupture in the time between the two stages, and a risk of non-compliance, especially after a complicated first stage, should patients refuse to undergo the second stage of the procedure.[10,11]

Conclusion

Endovascular repair of thoracoabdominal aortic aneurysm cannot eliminate the risk for spinal cord ischaemia, despite its minimally invasive nature and the avoidance of cross-clamping. Several strategies are being applied with the aim to reduce the incidence of spinal cord ischaemia after endovascular thoracoabdominal aortic aneurysm repair. Most of them (cerebrospinal fluid drainage, aggressive correction of arterial blood pressure, intravascular volume, etc.) are based on evidence originating from open thoracoabdominal aortic aneurysm repair. Lately, a strategy to reduce spinal cord ischemia time by early reperfusion of the pelvis and lower limbs during branched EVAR and fenestrated EVAR has emerged as an important adjunct against spinal cord ischaemia. Adopting a deployment sequence that enables short and intermittent pelvic and lower limb ischaemia times during the procedure appears to be vital for preventing spinal cord ischaemia after thoracoabdominal aortic aneurysm endovascular repair.

Summary

- Spinal cord ischaemia continues to occur after endovascular thoracoabdominal aortic aneurysm repair with branched EVAR and fenestrated EVAR despite the minimally invasive nature of the technique.

- Low spinal cord ischaemia time appears to be vital in reducing the risk for spinal cord ischaemia during endovascular thoracoabdominal aortic aneurysm repair with branched EVAR and with fenestrated EVAR.

- Our strategy to keep ischaemia time low includes:

  - Use of purse string sutures to allow quick removal of large sheaths

  - Use of an 18Fr sheath in the contralateral femoral artery during catheterisation of fenestrations

  - Introduction of guiding sheaths at the visceral vessels as late as possible

  - In 3-4x fenestrated EVAR, placement of guiding sheaths initially only in the renal arteries. The superior mesenteric artery and coeliac are first secured with a stiff wire only.

References

1. Elefteriades JA. Natural history of thoracic aortic aneurysms: indications for surgery, and surgical *versus* nonsurgical risks. *Ann Thorac Surg* 2002; **74** (5): S1877–S80.
2. Kuzmik GA, Sang AX, Elefteriades JA. Natural history of thoracic aortic aneurysms. *J Vasc Surg* 2012; **56** (2): 565–71.
3. Hansen PA, Richards JM, Tambyraja AL, *et al*. Natural history of thoraco-abdominal aneurysm in high-risk patients. *Eur J Vasc Endovasc Surg* 2010; **39** (3): 266–70.
4. Dudzinski DM, Isselbacher EM. Diagnosis and management of thoracic aortic disease. *Curr Cardiol Rep* 2015; **17**(12): 106.
5. Coady MA, Rizzo JA, Goldstein LJ, Elefteriades JA. Natural history, pathogenesis, and etiology of thoracic aortic aneurysms and dissections. *Cardiol Clin* 1999; **17** (4): 615–35.
6. Elefteriades JA, Farkas EA. Thoracic aortic aneurysm clinically pertinent controversies and uncertainties. *J Am Coll Cardiol* 2010; **55** (9): 841–57.
7. Parodi J, Berguer R, Carrascosa P, *et al*. Sources of error in the measurement of aortic diameter in computed tomography scans. *J Vasc Surg* 2014; **59** (1): 74–79.
8. Ahmed S, Zimmerman SL, Johnson PT, *et al*. MDCT interpretation of the ascending aorta with semiautomated measurement software: improved reproducibility compared with manual techniques. *J Cardiovasc Comput Tomogr* 2014; **8** (2): 108–14.
9. Rengier F, Weber TF, Partovi S, *et al*. Reliability of semiautomatic centerline analysis *versus* manual aortic measurement techniques for TEVAR among non-experts. *Eur J Vasc Endovasc Surg* 2011; **42** (3): 324–31.
10. Rudarakanchana N, Bicknell CD, Cheshire NJ, *et al*. Variation in maximum diameter measurements of descending thoracic aortic aneurysms using unformatted planes *versus* images corrected to aortic centerline. *Eur J Vasc Endovasc Surg* 2014; **47** (1): 19–26.
11. Elefteriades JA, Farkas EA. Thoracic aortic aneurysm clinically pertinent controversies and uncertainties. *J Am Coll Cardiol* 2010; **55** (9): 841–57.
12. McNamara JJ, Pressler VM. Natural history of arteriosclerotic thoracic aortic aneurysms. *Ann Thorac Surg* 1978; **26** (5): 468–73.
13. Hiratzka LF, Bakris GL, Beckman JA, *et al*. 2010 ACCF/AHA/AATS/ACR/ASA/SCA/SCAI/SIR/STS/SVM guidelines for the diagnosis and management of patients with thoracic aortic disease: executive summary. A report of the American College of Cardiology Foundation/American Heart Association Task Force on Practice Guidelines, American Association for Thoracic Surgery, American College of Radiology, American Stroke Association, Society of Cardiovascular Anesthesiologists, Society for

Cardiovascular Angiography and Interventions, Society of Interventional Radiology, Society of Thoracic Surgeons, and Society for Vascular Medicine. *Catheter Cardiovasc Interv* 2010; **76** (2): E43–E86.

14. Boodhwani M, Andelfinger G, Leipsic J, *et al*. Canadian Cardiovascular Society position statement on the management of thoracic aortic disease. *Can J Cardiol* 2014; **30** (6): 577–89.

15. Lobato AC, Puech-Leao P. Predictive factors for rupture of thoracoabdominal aortic aneurysm. *J Vasc Surg* 1998; **27** (3): 446–53.

16. Davies RR, Goldstein LJ, Coady MA, *et al*. Yearly rupture or dissection rates for thoracic aortic aneurysms: simple prediction based on size. *Ann Thorac Surg* 2002; **73** (1): 17–27.

17. Goldfinger JZ, Halperin JL, Marin ML, *et al*. Thoracic aortic aneurysm and dissection. *J Am Coll Cardiol* 2014; **64** (16): 1725–39.

18. Danyi P, Elefteriades JA, Jovin IS. Medical therapy of thoracic aortic aneurysms: are we there yet? *Circulation* 2011; **124** (13): 1469–76.

19. Rughani G, Robertson L, Clarke M. Medical treatment for small abdominal aortic aneurysms. Cochrane Database Syst Rev 2012; **9**: CD009536.

20. Propanolol Aneurysm Trial Investigators. Propranolol for small abdominal aortic aneurysms: results of a randomized trial. *J Vasc Surg* 2002; **35** (1): 72–79.

21. Kokje VB, Hamming JF, Lindeman JH. Pharmaceutical Management of Small Abdominal Aortic Aneurysms: A Systematic Review of the Clinical Evidence. *Eur J Vasc Endovasc Surg* 2015; **50** (6): 702–13.

22. Castellano JM, Kovacic JC, Sanz J, Fuster V. Are we ignoring the dilated thoracic aorta? *Ann N Y Acad Sci* 2012; **1254**: 164–74.

Neurological consequences of endovascular aortic aneurysm surgery—EVAR and TEVAR

RA Benson and IM Loftus

Introduction

Postoperative cognitive decline is the formal research term used to describe cognitive difficulties noticed following a major surgical intervention. Unlike delirium or dementia, the term is not included in the Diagnostic and American Statistical Manual of medical Disorders or in the World Health Organisation-endorsed International Classification of Diseases, and there are no formal criteria for diagnosis. Despite this, postoperative cognitive decline is considered a distinct phenomenon within the broader remit of "mild cognitive impairment", lying within the spectrum of acute delirium, mild cognitive impairment and dementia.[1] Qualitatively, it can be described as a persistent deterioration after surgery, compared with levels demonstrated preoperatively, in one or more of: day-to-day memory, language skills, attention and learning.[2]

The majority of research related to postoperative cognitive decline and neurobehavioural outcomes has taken place within the field of cardiothoracic surgery, following the introduction of the concept by Bedford in 1955[3]. It has been suggested by some that postoperative cognitive decline be considered one of the most common significant neurological consequences of cardiac surgery, second only to stroke.[4] The condition is classified as a type II injury (type I injuries include brain death and stroke) and is often subdivided into short-term (up to six weeks post-surgery, reported in 20–50% of patients) and long-term (six weeks to six months following surgery reported in 10–30%).[5] Although postoperative cognitive decline has now been a topic of study for more than 50 years, there is still a notable lack of international consensus on diagnosis, pathophysiology of the disease, or possible preventative measures.

The burden of postoperative cognitive decline

Postoperative cognitive decline is a precursor for significant functional impairment in the months following major surgery, such as aortic procedures, and increased mortality at median follow-up periods of between one year and 8.5 years (1.11-2.38, p=0.01, 1.63 hazard ratio [HR}, 95% confidence interval [CI]).[6–8] Patients often experience increased lengths of stay due to delayed physical rehabilitation, and increased rates of discharge to nursing homes or other rehabilitation facilities.[9,10] The effects of poor short- and long-term cognitive impairment on functional status and quality of life raises potential medico-legal issues for the consenting surgeon, in terms of clear communication of all possible risks of surgery.

Patient-reported outcomes include poorer concentration and decreased ability to perform day-to-day activities such as reading, managing finances or household activities.[3] For those still in work at the time of surgery and wishing to return, awareness that insight may be affected by postoperative cognitive decline is vital for those working in hazardous environments. Results from the multicentre ISPOCD (International study of post-operative cognitive dysfunction) 1 and 2 trials into the effects of major non-cardiothoracic surgery (including, but not limited to, major aortic surgery) demonstrated a clear link between identification at one week and an increased and prolonged need for financial support (p=0.03) as well as a higher likelihood of requiring medical or voluntary early retirement (HR 2.26 [CI 1.24-4.12] p=0.01).[7]

The field of abdominal and thoracic aneurysm surgery has been slower to take on the challenges of postoperative cognitive decline, with only five small scale prospective observational studies published between 1989 and 2011, and only one containing an endovascular aneurysm repair (EVAR) cohort.[11–15] Following the use of a variety of test batteries and statistical analysis, two groups identified a cohort of patients reaching their defined threshold for postoperative cognitive decline in the period after open aortic surgery, with reported incidence of 50% and 44.8% linked to increasing age and fewer years in formal education. Other studies linked several variables to poorer mean cognitive scores such as age, smoking history and anaesthetic time.[13,15] However, all of these factors had already been identified in literature following other forms of specialist surgery, suggesting generic surgical and patient factors, rather than those specific to type or site of surgery.

As the published literature increasingly favours EVAR as an alternative to open repair in high-risk patients, aortic aneurysm surgery has become available to an older, more complex patient cohort. Based on the above, albeit flawed, studies, it suggests the incidence of postoperative cognitive decline will begin to rise.

Delirium and postoperative cognitive decline

Delirium is defined as an acute disturbance of consciousness or cognition developing over hours or days as a physiological consequence of patients' medical state. Recent evidence shows that its prevalence is higher in patients who have undergone open aortic surgery when compared with other major vascular surgery, and importantly, two of the aortic research groups found links between postoperative delirium and a decline in scores at discharge and three months after aortic surgery.[16,11,12]

Historically, delirium incidence has been reported to be as high as 46% following open aortic surgery. However, a recently published study by Visser *et al* identified delirium in only 15% of open abdominal aortic aneurysm patients and in only 2% of EVAR patients.[17] The most common risk factors following aortic surgery have been reported as pre-existing cognitive impairment, age >65 years and current alcohol excess.[18]

As with postoperative cognitive decline, delirium has been linked to higher inpatient mortality, increased length of stay, longer intensive care stays, higher rates of surgical complications, more frequent discharge to rehabilitation facilities and higher mortality at one year.[17,19]

Current avenues of research

There are several events that occur during aortic aneurysm repair that could be linked to risk of these forms of neurological injury, based on similar studies within related specialties. These include, but are not limited to, the significant haemodynamic shifts caused by aortic clamping or ballooning, the period of hypotension used to prevent "windsocking" during stent deployment around the aortic arch, and the incidence of microembolisation to the brain during manipulation of wires or deployment of thoracic grafts.

Perioperative microembolic damage

Cerebral microembolisation describes the passage of material (i.e. thrombus, atherosclerotic plaque, gas, medullary fat or synthetic material) into the cerebral circulation via the arterial blood supply. During aortic manipulation and aortic surgery, such as during EVAR, fragments from an atherosclerotic vessel wall are thought to be dislodged into the circulation and move with antegrade flow into the carotid or vertebral circulation.

Although this can result in symptomatic transient ischaemic attack or stroke, magnetic resonance imaging (MRI) studies have indicated that a proportion of patients demonstrate postoperative ischaemic changes without obvious neurological injury.

It has become increasingly important to differentiate between gas and solid microembolic signals due to the difference in cause (gaseous emboli are associated with open cardiothoracic procedures and valve implantation, whereas solid emboli are associated with atherosclerotic burden), and therefore potential therapeutic targets.[20] It appears that specific manoeuvres during surgery are also particularly high risk for microembolic signal volume. Bismuth *et al* published their findings from monitoring microembolic signal frequency during thoracic endovascular aortic repair (TEVAR) in 20 patients; the greatest frequency signals occurred during pigtail catheter insertion and manipulation, and device deployment, with the period during deployment showing a greater mean number of microembolic symbols overall (44 vs. 9 respectively).[21] Mean microembolic signal frequency was similar bilaterally, increasing relative to proximity of the graft's landing zone.

This suggests a role for arch thrombus and atherosclerotic burden on microembolic signal frequency. Various techniques have been used to quantify burden, such as computed tomography (CT) angiography and intravascular ultrasound (IVUS) scanning, but a universally accepted classification system remains elusive. There is some small scale evidence to suggest correlation between increased microembolic signal counts and worse confusion scores at day five.[22] Khalert *et al* quantified new MRI lesions against post-operative cognitive testing following endovascular repair.[23] New ischaemic lesions were identified on MRI in 12 patients, with zero incidence of new stroke or TIA in the immediate post-operative period. However, unlike earlier studies, they failed to link these findings to arch atheroma burden, and failed to find an association with cognitive decline within the seven days following surgery.

Prolonged hypotension and cerebral hypoxaemia

The impact of perioperative hypotension, iatrogenic or otherwise, should be reviewed in the context of the typical aneurysm patient with longstanding cardio and cerebrovascular disease, who is likely to be chronically hypertensive. A significant controversy in preoperative optimisation in recent times has involved introduction of a beta-blocker in patients undergoing non-cardiothoracic surgery. A recent meta-analysis of valid trial results confirmed that indiscriminate perioperative beta-blocker use led to higher than expected risk of symptomatic hypotension (relative risk 1.51) and ischaemic stroke at 30-days (relative risk 1.73).[24]

There is an ongoing case for maintaining optimal cerebral oxygenation during surgery and improved postoperative neurological outcomes. Casati *et al* observed the protective effects of making perioperative cerebral saturation monitoring available to anaesthetists, noting lower test scores in the control group at seven days, with a significant correlation with perioperative drop in cerebral saturations (p=0.01). Ballard *et al* also found that optimising cerebral oxygenation provided significant protection against mild and moderate postoperative cognitive decline up to 52 weeks after surgery.[25]

The effects of suboptimal cerebral perfusion are more relevant during TEVAR, during which many operators create a short period of induced hypotension to reduce the "windsocking" effect that can lead to unintended distal graft movement during deployment.[26] There are several methods reported in the literature, including rapid right ventricular pacing, controlled hypotension (systolic pressure ≤45mmHg) and intermittent induced cardiac arrest, although a study by Nienaber *et al* failed to find a difference in cognitive scores in the immediate postoperative period regardless of method used.[27]

Serum biomarkers related to neurological injury

Although the theory of neuroinflammation due to crossover of systemic pro-inflammatory cytokines in the cerebral circulation is well described, work on identifying downstream markers specific to neuronal inflammation is in its early stages. The potential advantages of finding such a marker include assessing the extent of injury, use as a prognostic marker, and to assess any protective effects of experimental interventions.

S-100B and neurone-specific enolase

S100B is a member of a larger S100, calcium-mediated protein family, constituting a major component of glial cells, the support cells within the central nervous system.[28] Neurone-specific enolase (NSE) is a soluble cytoplasmic enzyme found in neurons and neuroendocrine cells. It can also be found within cerebrospinal fluid and peripheral blood, but is also found within red cells and platelets, so specificity for evidence of neurological injury during procedures involving external bypass circuits and haemolysis is poor. These markers were commonly used historically, as cerebrospinal fluid levels of both were relatively easily available from spinal drains used to reduce the risk of paraplegia and paralysis during open thoracoabdominal aneurysm repair.[29] For surgery that does not require routine use of spinal drains such as EVAR, regular cerebrospinal fluid samples are impractical and carry significant risk of morbidity (including intracranial bleeding, spinal haematoma, and permanent neurological deficit) compared with a peripheral blood sample. Results from studies attempting to link elevated serum levels with postoperative cognitive outcomes are varied and inconclusive.[28]

Glial fibrillary protein

Glial fibrillary protein is an intermediate filament protein, upregulated in astrocytes following neuronal injury. It has demonstrated good experimental correlation with neurological damage in the setting of stroke and traumatic brain injury.[30] Murine models have been used to demonstrate astrocyte activation following orthopaedic trauma, mechanical ventilation, general anaesthetic (isoflurane), or various combinations of all three. Studies have demonstrated convincing links between IL-6 and TNF-a levels, and cognitive decline associated with increased ventilation time and astrocyte upregulation.[31]

Future challenges and controversies

Challenges faced by future studies include addressing the need for a core battery of tests that should be used by any study looking at postoperative cognitive decline following aneurysm repair, which would allow for more formal criteria for diagnosis to be published. These tests should also address the learning effects that are a result of repeated testing using the same format within a relatively short period of time, at least partially addressed with the next generation of cognitive tests such as the repeatable battery for the assessment of neuropsychological status.

The use of several tests in combination to study a variety of domains makes analysis of scores as a single overall result contentious. Therefore in future, the reporting of decline in scores for specific cognitive domains may be more appropriate. Neurological damage due to ischaemic change following microembolisation, watershed infarcts or haemorrhagic damage can occur in any part of the brain and have the potential to affect any number of cognitive functions alone or in combination. Finally, the search for an effective, low-risk preventative strategy remains the ultimate goal and, while the search continues, patients must be warned of the potential impact postoperative cognitive decline will have on their recovery. The demonstrable health and economic burden in the intermediate and longer term continues to drive research in the field, despite ongoing controversies.

Summary

- Postoperative cognitive decline is the persistent deterioration after surgery in one or more of: day-to-day memory, language skills, attention and learning, compared with levels demonstrated pre-operatively

- It has negative links with poorer functional status and quality of life, and increased mortality at one year and beyond

- It raises potential medico-legal issues for the consenting surgeon, in terms of clear communication of all possible risks of surgery

- Significant ongoing controversies regarding causality, measurement of outcomes, and protective strategies persist, driving the need for further research

References

1. The ICD-10 Classification of Mental and Behavioral Disorders: Diagnostic Criteria for Research. (World Health Organization, 1993).
2. Funder KS, Steinmetz, J. Post-operative cognitive dysfunction - Lessons from the ISPOCD studies. Trends Anaesth Crit Care 2012; **2**: 94–97.
3. Bedford PD. Adverse cerebral effects of anaesthesia on old people. Lancet 1995; **269**: 259–63.
4. Tan AMY, Amoako D. Postoperative cognitive dysfunction after cardiac surgery. Contin Educ Anaesthesia Crit Care Pain 2013; **13**: 218–23.
5. Newman M, Kirchner JL, Phillips-Bute B, et al. Longitudinal assessment of neurocognitive function after coronary artery bypass surgery. N Engl J Med 2001; **344**: 395–402.
6. Newman S, Stygall J, Hirani S, et al. Postoperative cognitive dysfunction after noncardiac surgery. Anesthesiology 2007; **106**: 572–90.
7. Steinmetz J, Christensen KB, Lund T, et al. Long term consequences of postoperative cognitive dysfunction. Anesthesiology 2009; **110**: 548–55.
8. Moller J, Cluitmans P, Rasmussen LS, et al. Long-term postoperative cognitive dysfunction in the elderly: ISPOCD1 study. Lancet 1998; **351**: 857–61.
9. Rosen SF, Clagett GP, Valentine RJ, et al. Transient advanced mental impairment: An underappreciated morbidity after aortic surgery. J Vasc Surg 2002; **35**: 376–4A.
10. Johnson T, Monk T, Rasmussen LS, et al. Postoperative cognitive dysfunction in middle-aged patients. Anesthesiology 2002; **96**: 1351–7.
11. Benoit AG, Campbell BI, Tanner JR, et al. Risk factors and prevalence of perioperative cognitive dysfunction in abdominal aneurysm patients. J Vasc Surg 2005; **42**: 884–90.
12. Wallbridge HR, Benoit AG, Staley D et al. Risk factors for postoperative cognitive and functional difficulties in abdominal aortic aneurysm patients: A three month follow-up. Int J Geriatr Psychiatry 2011; **26**: 818–24.
13. Treasure T, Smith PL, Newman S, et al. Impairment of cerebral function following cardiac and other major surgery. Eur J Cardiothorac Surg 1989; **3**: 216–21.
14. Lloyd AJ, Boyle J, Bell PR, et al. Comparison of cognitive function and quality of life after endovascular or conventional aortic aneurysm repair. BJS 2000; **87**: 443–7.
15. Grichnik KP, Ijsselmuiden AJ, D'Amico TA, et al. Cognitive decline after major noncardiac operations: A preliminary prospective study. Ann Thorac Surg 1999; **68**: 1786–91.
16. Schneider F, Böhner H, Habel U, et al. Risk factors for postoperative delirium in vascular surgery. Gen Hosp Psychiatry 2002; **24**: 28–34.
17. Visser L, Prent A, van der Laan MJ, et al. Predicting postoperative delirium after vascular surgical procedures. J Vasc Surg 2015; **62**: 183–189.
18. Böhner H, Hummel TC, Habel U, et al. Predicting delirium after vascular surgery: a model based on pre- and intraoperative data. Ann Surg 2003; **238**: 149–56.

19. Marcantonio ER, Flacker JM, Michaels M, *et al*. Delirium is independently associated with poor functional recovery after hip fracture. *J Am Geriatr Soc* 2000; **48**: 618–24.
20. Grosset DG, Georgiadis D, Kelman AW, *et al*. Detection of microemboli by transcranial Doppler ultrasound. *Tex Heart Inst J* 1996; **23**: 289–92.
21. Bismuth J, Garami Z, Anaya-Ayala JE, *et al*. Transcranial Doppler findings during thoracic endovascular aortic repair. *J Vasc Surg* 2011; **54**: 364–9.
22. Djaiani G, *et al*. Mild to moderate atheromatous disease of the thoracic aorta and new ischemic brain lesions after conventional coronary artery bypass graft surgery. *Stroke* 2004; **35**: e356–8.
23. Kahlert P, Eggebrecht H, Jánosi RA, *et al*. Silent cerebral ischemia after thoracic endovascular aortic repair: A neuroimaging study. *Ann Thorac Surg* 2014; **98**: 53–58.
24. Bouri S, Shun-Shin MJ, Cole GD, *et al*. Meta-analysis of secure randomised controlled trials of β-blockade to prevent perioperative death in non-cardiac surgery. *Heart* 2014; **100**: 456–64.
25. Ballard C, *et al*. Optimised anaesthesia to reduce postoperative cognitive decline (POCD) in older patients undergoing elective surgery, a randomised controlled trial. *PLoS One* 2012; **7**: 1–9.
26. von Knobelsdorff G, Höppner RM, Tonner PH, *et al*. Induced arterial hypotension for interventional thoracic aortic stent-graft placement: impact on intracranial haemodynamics and cognitive function. *Eur J Anaesthesiol* 2003; **20**: 134–40.
27. Nienaber CA, Kische S, Rehders TC, *et al*. Rapid pacing for better placing: Comparison of techniques for precise deployment of endografts in the thoracic aorta. *J Endovasc Ther* 2007; **14**: 506–12.
28. Cata JP, Abdelmalak B, Farag E. Neurological biomarkers in the perioperative period. *Br J Anaesth* 2011; **107**: 844–58.
29. Lases EC, Schepens MA, Haas FJ, *et al*. Clinical prospective study of biochemical markers and evoked potentials for identifying adverse neurological outcome after thoracic and thoracoabdominal aortic aneurysm surgery. *Br J Anaesth* 2005; **95**: 651–61.
30. Bembea M, Savage W, Strouse JJ, *et al*. Glial fibriallary acidic protein as a brain injury biomarker in children undergoing extracorporeal membrane oxygenation. *Pediatr Crit Med* 2011; **12**: 572–9.
31. Chen C, Zhang Z, Chen T, *et al*. Prolonged mechanical ventilation-induced neuroinflammation affects postoperative memory dysfunction in surgical mice. *Crit Care* 2015; **19**: 159.

Aortic arch hybrid debranching

CFW Vermeulen, N Tsilimparis, T Kölbel
and ES Debus

Introduction

Traditionally, aortic arch disease was repaired with an open surgical technique using cardiopulmonary bypass, which is associated with considerable morbidity and mortality.[1–6]

The first endovascular repair of a false thoracic aneurysm was performed in 1987 by Nicholay Volodos, followed by Juan Parodi in 1990 with the first successful endovascular repair of an abdominal aortic aneurysm.[7,8] A hybrid procedure of the aortic arch was first described in 1998 by Buth.[9] In the past decade, the gained expertise and further development of endovascular techniques have resulted in more complex endovascular procedures to repair the aortic arch and descending aorta disease. Depending on the anatomy and pathology, the aortic arch can be managed by several combinations of branched or fenestrated stent grafts and cervical debranching.[10–13]

In our institution, the number of thoracic endovascular aortic repair (TEVAR) procedures has increased with the ongoing growth of indications and technical options. The extensive indications are a result of the international shift of type B dissection treatment strategy in recent years from predominantly conservative to operative because of a better long-term remodelling and outcome.[14,15] Additionally, multimorbid patients with disease of the ascending aorta and the aortic arch, unfit for open repair, are nowadays considered for a complete endovascular or hybrid procedure.

Hybrid procedures are defined as procedures that require a surgical revascularisation of one or more supra-aortic vessels to extend the proximal landing zone of TEVAR in the aortic arch.

Aortic arch debranching has increased significantly over recent years, respective to the increase of TEVAR procedures. All types of aortic arch debranching are performed in our institution, whereby the carotid-subclavian bypass is the most commonly performed. Because the increase in aortic arch hybrid debranching is fairly recent, our knowledge of prognosis and complications is still developing. In the past few years we have performed more than 200 of these operations. We present our experience with 200 aortic arch hybrid debranching procedures for different aortic repair indications and address technical aspects and outcomes of the procedures.

Current approach of aortic arch hybrid debranching

The carotid-subclavian bypass is the most common aortic arch debranching surgery in our clinic. When covering the subclavian artery in combination with stenting a considerable part of the thoracic aorta, we impede an important part of spinal cord circulation and collateral circulation through the vertebral artery. The most important indications for the carotid-subclavian bypass are decreasing the risk of spinal cord ischaemia and the risk of posterior stroke. Another advantage is the prevention of upper extremity ischaemia. Recently, a retrospective single-centre study was published with outcomes of TEVAR and subclavian artery revascularisation.[16] The study shows an increased risk of stroke and upper extremity ischaemia if the left subclavian artery was covered without revascularisation. The results did not show a difference in spinal cord ischaemia. The authors (Zamar *et al)* do not elaborate on this topic. A possible explanation could be that the majority of their TEVAR indications (i.e. 64%) usually require fairly short stent coverage of the descending aorta and, therefore, the primary spinal circulation is mostly intact. As they share our clinic's opinion that hypoperfusion is the main reason for the important postoperative complications, an insight in their management of blood pressure and cerebrospinal fluid drainage would have been interesting. A large registry comprising data of several trials was published by Patterson *et al.* They concluded that prior revascularisation of the left subclavian artery protects against posterior stroke.[17] Maldonado *et al* conclude in their multicentre retrospective study that left subclavian artery coverage does not increase spinal cord ischaemia and posterior stroke.[18] They do, however, promote selective revascularisation of the left subclavian artery based on risk factors.

Traditionally, a carotid-subclavian bypass was performed mostly because of a symptomatic subclavian artery origin occlusion. Nowadays, a carotid-subclavian bypass is mainly performed in a one- or two-stage hybrid procedure with TEVAR. Because of the subsequent endovascular procedure, we have adjusted our surgical technique. We have altered the descent of the bypass from reasonably steep to a more horizontal course by placing the carotid anastomosis more proximally (Figure 1). This improves the introduction angle for guidewires and catheters via the subclavian artery. Additionally, we choose to insert a common carotid artery

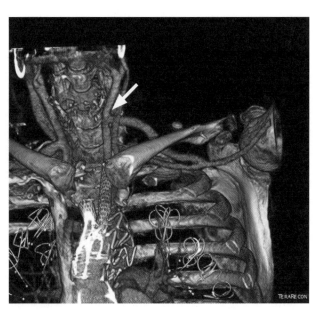

Figure 1: Horizontal course of the carotid-subclavian bypass with a favourable angle with the carotid artery for material introduction in subsequent TEVAR.

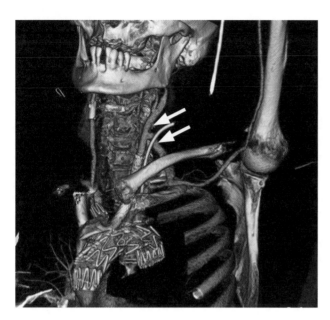

Figure 2: Common carotid artery interposition graft and carotid-subclavian bypass in a patient in whom the dissection extended into the carotid artery. Subsequently, the aortic arch prothesis and carotid stent could be inserted safely.

interposition graft in cases where the aorta dissection extends into the carotid artery for a safer endovascular approach (Figure 2). We always use a Dacron graft for the cervical bypasses.

We also perform subclavian transposition, carotid-carotid as well as subclavian-subclavian bypasses, but more rarely than carotid-subclavian bypasses. Our rapidly growing experience in branched and fenestrated aortic arch stenting results in fewer indications for these bypasses as a step in endovascular or hybrid procedures.

Outcomes in aortic arch hybrid debranching

In 2009, the University Heart Centre in Hamburg (Germany) expanded with the Clinic and Policlinic of Vascular Medicine and the Aorta Centre. Between 2009 and 2015, we operated on 219 cases of aortic arch debranching. The large majority were carotid-subclavian bypasses as aforementioned. The number of cervical debranching procedures increases every year with 63 procedures in 2015. This is a reflection of the recently changed treatment strategy of type B dissections and the common opinion in revascularising the left subclavian artery as well as our increased performance in aortic arch and ascending aorta stenting.[14,15,19,20]

Indications for a TEVAR were type B dissections, thoracoabdominal aneurysms, ascending aorta pathology in multimorbid patients unsuitable for open surgery and, rarely, traumatic aortic injury. We perform aortic arch debranching in a one- or two-stage procedure. In elective cases, a subclavian artery covering TEVAR is usually preceded by a carotid-subclavian bypass in a two-stage procedure. One-stage procedures are performed in (semi)acute situations.

Complications of the aortic arch debranching were relatively rare. Unfortunately, some of the complications that occurred were severe. No strokes were seen after aortic arch debranching procedures alone. In a few cases, a stroke did appear after the subsequent aortic arch TEVAR, which in three cases resulted in death. Stroke is a known risk of surgical procedures of the aortic arch.[21] The hypothesis is that the risk in endovascular procedures is less. However, endovascular procedures are often performed in severely ill patients who are too multimorbid for open surgery. Thus a selection bias occurs. Randomised trials are lacking and are difficult to design; therefore, a definite conclusion is complicated.

In less than 3% of paitents, postoperative bleeding led to reoperation. This was seen more often when the subsequent TEVAR was performed within two weeks of the cervical debranching. In one patient with Marfan syndrome and extensive anticoagulation because of mechanical heart valves, the postoperative bleeding resulted in brachial plexus damage with permanent severe neurological deficit of the left arm.

Patency of the aortic arch bypasses and transpositions was 100% in our institution, which is supported by literature on surgical subclavian revascularisation (carotid-subclavian bypass or subclavian transposition) in endovascular procedures.[16, 22] Previously published studies on surgical revascularisation of the subclavian artery in obstructive disease patients report a lower patency rate down to 73% after three years.[22–25]

We perform a surgical revascularisation of the subclavian artery in all our patients that are planned for an endovascular procedure where the aortic arch is involved to decrease the risk of spinal cord ischaemia. Spinal cord ischaemia is a devastating complication that occurs both in open and endovascular procedures of the thoracoabdominal aorta in up to 20%, depending on risk factors and the range of aorta that is repaired.[26–30] Because we perform a cervical debranching procedure in almost all aortic arch artery stent coverage, we could not conclude anything on spinal cord ischaemia. We can say that spinal cord ischaemia did occur in some of our high-risk cases, in spite of aortic arch debranching, cerebrospinal fluid drainage and mean arterial pressure management.

Conclusion

Aortic arch debranching and, in particular, surgical subclavian revascularisation by bypass or transposition is increasingly performed to extend the proximal landing zone for the thoracic endovascular repair of the aorta. We support aortic arch debranching in all of the cases in which the aortic arch is involved to reduce stroke rate and spinal cord ischaemia. We adjusted the surgical technique of the carotid-subclavian bypass to a more proximal carotid anastomosis to produce a more favourable angle for the introduction of material during the endovascular procedure. Patency is up to maximal, independent of the use of a synthetic graft. Aortic arch debranching can be performed in a one- or two-stage procedure, depending on the acuteness of the endovascular aorta repair. No differences in complications were seen between one- or two-stage procedures. The complication rate of aortic arch debranching alone was low.

Summary

- Technical advances and gained expertise have resulted in increased and more complicated thoracic endovascular procedures where the aortic arch is often involved.

- Aortic arch debranching, the large majority being surgical revascularisation of the (left) subclavian artery has simultaneously increased to extend the proximal landing zone of TEVAR in the aortic arch.

- An ever increasing number of aortic arch debranching procedures is performed in our aorta centre. Although all types of aortic arch debranching are performed, the large majority consists of the carotid-subclavian bypass.

- Complication rates of aortic arch debranching procedures are low, both in our institution as well as in reported studies.

- We have adjusted the surgical technique of the carotid-subclavian bypass to create a more favourable angle for material introduction in the endovascular procedure.

References

1. Okita Y, Ando M, Minatoya K, *et al*. Predictive factors for mortality and cerebral complications in arteriosclerotic aneurysm of the aortic arch. *Ann Thorac Surg* 1999; **67** (1): 72–78.

2. Jacobs MJ, De Mol BA, Veldman DJ. Aortic arch and proximal supraaortic arterial repair under continuous antegrade cerebral perfusion and moderate hypothermia. *Cardiovasc Surg* 2001; **9** (4): 396–402.

3. Matalanis G, Hata M, Buxton BF. A retrospective comparative study of deep hypothermic circulatory arrest, retrograde and antegrade cerebral perfusion in aortic arch surgery. *Cardiovasc Surg* 2003; **9** (3): 174–79.

4. Strauch JT, Spielvogel D, Lauten A, *et al*. Technical advances in total aortic arch replacement. *Ann Thorac Surg* 2004; **77** (2): 581–89.

5. Harrington DK, Walker AS, Kaukuntla H, *et al*. Selective antegrade cerebral perfusion attenuates brain metabolic deficit in aortic arch surgery: a prospective randomized trial. *Circulation* 2004; **110** (11 Suppl. 1): II 231–36.

6. Antoniou GA, El Sakka K, Hamady M, Wolfe JHN. Hybrid treatment of complex aortic arch disease with supra-aortic debranching and endovascular stent graft repair. *Eur J Vasc Endovasc Surg* 2010; **39**: 683–90.

7. Volodos NL, Karpovich IP, Shekhanin VE, *et al*. A case of distant transfemoral endoprosthesis of the thoracic artery using a self-fixing synthetic prosthesis in traumatic aneurysm (Russian). *Grudn Khir* 1988; **6**: 84–86.

8. Parodi JC, Palmaz JC, Barone HD. Transfemoral intraluminal graft implantation for abdominal aortic aneurysms. *Ann Vasc Surg* 1991; **5** (6): 491–99.

9. Buth J, Penn O, Tielbeek A, Mersman M. Combined approach to stent-graft treatment of an aortic arch aneurysm. *J Endovasc Surg* 1998; **5** (4): 329–32.

10. Eagleton MJ, Greenberg RK. Hybrid procedures for the treatment of aortic arch aneurysms. *J Cardiovasc Surg* (Torino) 2010; **51** (6): 807–19.

11. Ingrund JC, Nasser F, Jesus-Silva SG, *et al*. Hybrid procedures for complex thoracic aorta diseases. *Rev Bras Cir Cardiovasc* 2010; **25**: 303–10.

12. Antoniou GA, Mireskandari M, Bicknell CD, *et al*. Hybrid repair of the aortic arch in patients with extensive aortic disease. *Eur J Vasc Endovasc Surg* 2010; **40**: 715–21.

13. Cao P, De Rango P, Czerny M, *et al*. Systematic review of clinical outcomes in hybrid procedures for aortic arch dissections and other arch diseases. *J Thor Cardiovasc Surg* 2012; **144** (6): 1286–300; 1300.e1-2.

14. Fattori R, Montgomery D, Lovato L, *et al*. Survival after endovascular therapy in patients with type B aortic dissection: a report from the International Registry of Acute Aortic Dissection (IRAD). *JACC Cardiovasc Interv* 2013; **6** (8): 876–82.

15. Patel AY, Eagle KA, Vaishnava P. Acute type B aortic dissection: insights from the International Registry of Acute Aortic Dissection. Ann Cardiothor Surg 2014; **3** (4): 368–74.

16. Zamor KC, Eskandari MK, Rodriguez H, *et al*. Outcomes of thoracic endovascular aortic repair and subclavian revascularization techniques. J Am Coll Surg 2015; **221** (1): 93-101.

17. Patterson BO, Holt P, Nienaber C, *et al*. Management of the left subclavian artery and neurologic complications after thoracic endovascular aortic repair. *J Vasc Surg* 2014; **60** (6): 1491–98.e1.

18. Maldonado TS, Dexter D, Rockman CB, *et al*. Left subclavian artery coverage during thoracic endovascular aortic aneurysm repair does not mandate revascularization. *J Vasc Surg* 2013; **57** (1): 116–24.

19. Matsumura JS, Lee WA, Mitchell RS, *et al*. The Society for Vascular Surgery Practice Guidelines: management of the left subclavian artery with thoracic endovascular aortic repair. *J Vasc Surg* 2009; **50** (5): 1155–58.

20. Rolffs F, Tsilimparis N, Detter C, *et al*. New Advances in Endovascular Therapy: Endovascular Repair of a Chronic DeBakey Type II Aortic Dissection With a Scalloped Stent-Graft Designed for the Ascending Aorta. *J Endovasc Ther* 2016; **23** (1): 182–85.

21. Maurel B, Sobocinski J, Spear R, *et al*. Current and future perspectives in the repair of aneurysms involving the aortic arch. *J Cardiovasc Surg* (Torino). 2015; **56** (2): 197–215.

22. Scali ST, Chang CK, Pape SG, *et al*. Subclavian revascularization in the age of thoracic endovascular aortic repair and comparison of outcomes in patients with occlusive disease. *J Vasc Surg* 2013; **58** (4): 901–09.

23. Dietrich EB, Garrett HE, Ameriso J, *et al*. Occlusive disease of the common carotid and subclavian arteries treated by carotid-subclavian bypass. Analysis of 125 cases. Am J Surg 1967; **114**(5): 800–08.

24. Perler BA, Williams GM. Carotid-subclavian bypass – a decade of experience. *J Vasc Surg* 1990; **12**(6): 716–22.

25. Vitti MJ, Thompson BW, Read RC, *et al*. Carotid-subclavian bypass: a twenty-two-year experience. *J Vasc Surg* 1994; **20** (3): 411–17.

26. Cambria RP, Davison JK. Regional hypothermia with epidural cooling for spinal cord protection during thoracoabdominal aneurysm repair (Review). Semin Vasc Surg 2000; **13** (4): 315–24.

27. Safi HJ, Miller CC 3rd, Huynh TT, *et al*. Distal aortic perfusion and cerebrospinal fluid drainage for thoracoabdominal and descending thoracic aortic repair: ten years of organ protection. *Ann Surg* 2003; **238** (3): 372–80

28. Coselli JS, Bozinovski J, LeMaire SA. Open surgical repair of 2286 thoracoabdominal aortic aneurysms. *Ann Thorac Surg* 2007; **83** (2): S862–64; Discussion S890–92.

29. Greenberg RK, Lu Q, Roselli EE, *et al*. Contemporary analysis of descending thoracic and thoracoabdominal aneurysm repair: a comparison of endovascular and open techniques. *Circulation* 2008; **118** (8): 808–17.

30. Eagleton MJ, Shah S, Petkosevek D, *et al*. Hypogastric and subclavian artery patency affects onset and recovery of spinal cord ischemia associated with aortic endografting. *J Vasc Surg* 2014; **59** (1): 89–94.

The benefit of conformable design in treating challenging thoracic pathologies

RS Smith and WD Jordan

Introduction

Thoracic endovascular aortic repair (TEVAR) was first reported more than 20 years ago,[1] but the first thoracic endograft only received US Food and Drug Administration (FDA) approval in 2005 with the introduction to the US market of the TAG endograft (Gore).[2] TEVAR has evolved significantly over the last decade and has rapidly become the primary treatment modality for a wide variety of aortic pathology, including ruptured and elective aneurysms, acute and chronic dissections, and traumatic injuries,[3–7] largely due to reduced morbidity compared with open repair. The Conformable TAG (Gore) introduced several modifications of the original TAG device to increase conformability, increase resistance to compression, and expand the range of aortic diameters repairable with the device. The device is a nitinol wire frame stent covered with an expanded polytetrafluoroethylene and fluoroethylpropylene graft (Figure 1).

The endograft is constrained onto a delivery catheter which is introduced through an 18–24Fr sheath, and it is designed to be deployed in an aortic landing zone from 16–42mm diameter. The Conformable TAG device was FDA approved for endovascular repair of descending thoracic aortic aneurysms in 2011 and type B aortic dissections in 2013. Industry-sponsored clinical trials to evaluate the safety and efficacy of the device for aneurysms[8] and acute, complicated type B dissections[9] are currently underway, and two-year results of both trials were published in 2015. Follow-up for both trials will continue for five years. The primary safety and efficacy endpoints were completed at 30 days, and the two-year follow-up data addresses concerns of repair durability, endoleaks, and aortic remodelling that have been raised by advocates of open repair.[10,11] All computed tomography (CT) and magnetic resonance imaging (MRI) data were analysed by a core laboratory to reduce investigator bias. The two Conformable TAG studies provide a useful comparison of device performance in a relatively healthy, stable population (thoracic aneurysm repair) and also in an ill, physiologically compromised population (complicated type B dissection).

Four thoracic endografts are currently FDA approved in addition to the Conformable TAG: Talent (Medtronic), Valiant (Medtronic), Zenith (Cook), and Relay (Bolton). This review will focus on the two-year results of the Conformable TAG device. No direct head-to-head comparison studies have been performed,[12] and similar results have been reported with other devices.[13]

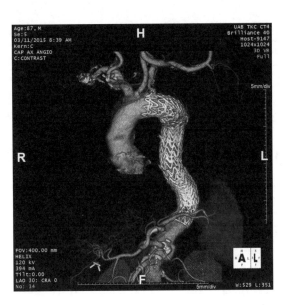

Figure 1: Gore Conformable TAG.

Descending thoracic aneurysm repair—two-year results

Risk of thoracic aneurysm rupture increases with size, and risk of aortic events within one year without treatment are reported to be 5.5% at 5cm and 9.3% at 6cm.[14] Successful TEVAR excludes the aneurysm from the systemic blood pressure and often results in its shrinkage. The Conformable TAG aneurysm study is an industry-sponsored, prospective, non-randomised, multicentre trial conducted to establish the safety and efficacy of the device. The total treatment group numbered 66 patients with descending thoracic aneurysms greater than 5cm and with anatomies meeting the instructions for use of the device. These instructions include a healthy proximal landing zone of at least 2cm beyond the left subclavian artery and distal landing zone at least 2cm above the coeliac artery. This patient population thus had favourable anatomy for TEVAR, and the device was successfully placed in 65 patients with an average aneurysm diameter of 60.1mm and aortic coverage length of 17cm.

Endoleaks are a prime concern after TEVAR and can lead to aneurysm enlargement and rupture. At two years, five out of 45 patients (11.1%) had an endoleak with two type II endoleaks and three endoleaks for which the origin could not be determined by the core lab. No patients required reintervention for an endoleak. Additionally, medium-term improvement in aneurysm diameter was seen after aneurysm exclusion with the Conformable TAG device. Of the 38 patients with imaging reviewed for aneurysm size at two years, only three (7.9%) had a 5mm or greater increase in aneurysm size, while 20 (52.6%) had a 5mm or greater decrease in size, and 15 (39.5%) had no change in size.

Overall survival at two years was 78% with two aneurysm-related deaths: rupture of an untreated ascending aortic aneurysm and an arterial access rupture during a secondary aortic intervention by a surgical team different from the original study team. There were no ruptures of the treated aneurysmal aortic segment. No other secondary interventions were required after aneurysm repair. Serious adverse events within 30 days occurred in 15 patients (22.7%), including one postoperative death. Thus, for the large majority of patients, TEVAR with the Conformable TAG device provided a successful and durable repair at two years.

Type B dissection—two-year results

TEVAR for acute, complicated type B dissection is accomplished by coverage of the aortic entry tear in the proximal descending thoracic aorta which re-establishes true lumen flow and improves the dynamic obstruction of aortic branches by the dissection flap, thereby stabilising distal malperfusion. An additional goal is to prevent rupture or aneurysm formation in the diseased segment. TEVAR has been shown to significantly improve survival in these patients compared to medical management.[15] The Conformable TAG type B dissection study is an industry-sponsored, prospective, non-randomised, multicentre trial. Patients had an acute dissection (<14 days from symptoms to diagnosis) and evidence of malperfusion treated with TEVAR less than 48 hours after diagnosis. Anatomic requirements included a dissection-free proximal landing zone of greater than 2cm distal to the left common carotid artery. Patients with renal failure, evidence of bowel ischaemia or shock were excluded. Fifty patients were enrolled and all had the device successfully placed with an average aortic coverage of 20.6cm. Twenty-six patients (52%) underwent an additional concurrent procedure, mostly to correct malperfusion. Mortality within 30 days occurred in four patients (8%), including one case of retrograde dissection and one case of type Ia endoleak with rupture.

The overall secondary intervention rate after TEVAR for type B dissection was 18%, including two ascending aorta replacements and one thoracoabdominal aneurysm repair for degeneration distal to the endograft. Additional aortic devices were implanted in 12% of the type B dissection patients, mostly due to persistent false lumen flow.

Thrombosis of the false lumen at two years was complete in 20 patients (74.1%) and partial in six patients (22.2%). Remodelling of the aorta was generally favourable with increases in true lumen and decreases in false lumen area. The overall aortic diameter in the treated segment was unchanged in 50%, increased in 11.5%, and decreased in 38.3% of patients. The type B dissection was therefore successfully treated in the majority of patients.

Retrograde dissection or *de novo* type A dissection remains a significant challenge for TEVAR.[16] Five patients (10%) had a proximal dissection noted on postoperative days 0, 6, 29, 89 and 183. Three were considered device-related, leading to one patient death. This complication is minimised by careful device delivery in a non-dissected proximal landing zone, although, in the setting of an acute dissection, the aorta at the area of the primary entry tear may be fragile and prone to propagate the dissection.

Overall survival at two years was 85%, which compares favourably to the pre-TEVAR era.[17]

Neurological complications and management

Stroke and spinal cord ischaemia are the dreaded complications of TEVAR related to manipulation of devices and wires in the arch and graft coverage of aortic branches. Stroke rates in the Conformable TAG aneurysm and acute, complicated type B dissection studies were 3% and 18%, respectively, and spinal cord ischaemia rates were 3% and 8%, respectively. These complication rates compare favourably with historic data of open repair and are comparable to other TEVAR device trials.[18]

TEVAR in the setting of stable, uncomplicated type B dissection has significantly lower rates of adverse events and improved two-year mortality, as would be expected from a more favourable patient population.[19]

The Conformable TAG study data reveal a wide variety of practice in regard to management of cerebrospinal fluid drain placement, intravascular ultrasound, and left subclavian artery coverage. Cerebrospinal fluid drain management was left to each treating surgeon and preoperative drains were placed in 30% (35 of 116) patients. Intravascular ultrasound was used in 58% of patients in the dissection study. The left subclavian artery was completely covered in 27 patients in the dissection study with eight patients undergoing revascularisation, while the left subclavian artery was completely covered in 15 patients in the aneurysm study with 11 undergoing revascularisation. No patients experienced left arm ischaemia, and there was no relationship between left subclavian coverage and spinal cord ischaemia. However, these groups are rather small to enable firm conclusions about optimal left subclavian artery management during TEVAR. Proper application of adjunctive techniques to prevent paraplegia remains an active area of ongoing research.[20,21]

Conclusion

Overall, the Conformable TAG device has been demonstrated to be safe and effective for the treatment of both descending thoracic aortic aneurysms and type B dissections in industry-sponsored studies at two years of follow-up. Favourable aortic remodelling, low rate of endoleak and low incidence of device related complications after implantation of the device provide additional evidence that TEVAR is the preferred treatment in patients with appropriate anatomy.

The engineering changes introduced in the Conformable TAG seem to have improved the applicability of the device. No adverse events due to endograft failure were noted during either study. Device collapse or compression—which had been rarely seen with the first generation endograft—were not observed. No wire fractures were noted, although one case of intercomponent migration associated with aneurysm remodelling was seen at 12 months. There were no resulting endoleaks, and no reintervention was required.

Future assessment of the Conformable TAG will include results of real-world use of the graft outside of industry-sponsored clinical trials. Durability of repair, aneurysm growth, endoleak rates and overall success might be less favourable for patients not meeting the rigorous anatomical criteria needed for inclusion in these early studies. Future work can better define which boundaries can be safely pushed and which require strict observation.

Summary

- TEVAR was FDA approved in 2005 and has become the treatment strategy of choice for descending thoracic aortic aneurysm and acute, complicated type B dissection.

- The Conformable TAG device is a second generation endograft for TEVAR, FDA approved in 2011 for treatment of descending thoracic aneurysm and in 2013 for treatment of type B dissection.

- Two-year results of concurrent industry sponsored studies of safety and efficacy of the Conformable TAG for the treatment of descending thoracic aneurysm and acute, complicated type B dissection were published in 2015.

- The Conformable TAG descending thoracic aneurysm trial demonstrated good results at two years with no device failures, low rate of endoleaks, and no ruptures of the treated aneurysm segment.

- The Conformable TAG acute, complicated type B dissection trial showed good results at two years with overall survival at 85% and favourable aortic remodelling.

- Follow-up data collection for both studies is planned for five years, and data of real world use of the device is necessary for a thorough evaluation of the performance of the device.

References

1. Dake MD, Miller DC, Semba CP, *et al.* Transluminal placement of endovascular stent grafts for the treatment of descending thoracic aortic aneurysms. *N Eng J Med* 1994; **331** (26): 1729–34.
2. Makaroun MS, Dillavou ED, Kee ST, *et al.* Endovascular treatment of thoracic aortic aneurysms: Results of the phase II multicenter trial of the GORE TAG thoracic endoprosthesis. *Journal of Vascular Surgery* 2005; **41** (1): 1–9.
3. Cambria RP, Crawford RS, Cho JS, *et al.* A multicenter clinical trial of endovascular stent graft repair of acute catastrophes of the descending thoracic aorta. *Journal of Vascular Surgery* 2009; **50**(6): 1255–64. e4.
4. Najibi S, Terramani TT, Weiss VJ, *et al.* Endoluminal *versus* open treatment of descending thoracic aortic aneurysms. *Journal of Vascular Surgery* 2002; **36** (4): 732–37.
5. Schaffer JM, Lingala B, Miller DC, *et al.* Midterm survival after thoracic endovascular aortic repair in more than 10,000 Medicare patients. *Journal of Thoracic and Cardiovascular Surgery* 2015; **149** (3): 808–23.
6. Mitchell ME, Rushton Jr FW, Boland AB, *et al.* Emergency procedures on the descending thoracic aorta in the endovascular era. *Journal of Vascular Surgery* 2011; **54** (5): 1298–302.
7. Jonker FHW, Trimarchi S, Verhagen HJM, *et al.* Meta-analysis of open *versus* endovascular repair for ruptured descending thoracic aortic aneurysm. *Journal of Vascular Surgery* 2010; **51** (4): 1026–32.e2.
8. Jordan Jr WD, Rovin J, Moainie S, *et al.* Results of a prospective multicenter trial of CTAG thoracic endograft. *Journal of Vascular Surgery* 2015; **61** (3): 589–95.
9. Cambria RP, Conrad MF, Matsumoto AH, *et al.* Multicenter clinical trial of the conformable stent graft for the treatment of acute, complicated type B dissection. *Journal of Vascular Surgery* 2015; **62** (2): 271–78.
10. Lee CJ, Rodriguez HE, Kibbe MR, *et al.* Secondary interventions after elective thoracic endovascular aortic repair for degenerative aneurysms. *Journal of Vascular Surgery* 2013; **57** (5): 1269–74.
11. LJ L, Harris PL, Buth J, Collaborators of the European collaborators registry (EUROSTAR). Secondary interventions after elective endovascular repair of degenerative thoracic aortic aneurysms: results of the European collaborators registry (EUROSTAR). *Journal of Vascular and Interventional Radiology* 2007; **18** (4): 491–5.

12. Rolph R, Duffy JM, Waltham M. Stent graft types for endovascular repair of thoracic aortic aneurysms. Cochrane Database of Systematic Reviews 2015 (9): CD008448.

13. Bavaria JE, Brinkman WT, Hughes GC, *et al.* . Outcomes of Thoracic Endovascular Aortic Repair in Acute Type B Aortic Dissection: Results From the Valiant United States Investigational Device Exemption Study. *The Annals of Thoracic Surgery* 2015; **100** (3): 802–09.

14. Kim JB, Kim K, Lindsay ME, *et al.* Risk of Rupture or Dissection in Descending Thoracic Aortic Aneurysm. *Circulation* 2015; **132** (17): 1620–29.

15. Durham CA, Cambria RP, Wang LJ, *et al.* The natural history of medically managed acute type B aortic dissection. *Journal of Vascular Surgery* 2015; **61** (5): 1192–99.

16. Canaud L, Ozdemir BA, Patterson BO, *et al.* Retrograde Aortic Dissection After Thoracic Endovascular Aortic Repair. *Annals of Surgery* 2014; **260** (2): 389–95.

17. Hagan PG, Nienaber CA, Isselbacher EM, *et al.* The international registry of acute aortic dissection (irad): New insights into an old disease. *JAMA* 2000; **283** (7): 897–903.

18. White RA, Miller DC, Criado FJ, *et al.* Report on the results of thoracic endovascular aortic repair for acute, complicated, type B aortic dissection at 30 days and 1 year from a multidisciplinary subcommittee of the Society for Vascular Surgery Outcomes Committee. *Journal of Vascular Surgery* 2011; **53** (4): 1082–90.

19. Nienaber CA, Rousseau H, Eggebrecht H, *et al.* Randomized Comparison of Strategies for Type B Aortic Dissection: The INvestigation of STEnt Grafts in Aortic Dissection (INSTEAD) Trial. *Circulation* 2009; **120** (25): 2519–28.

20. Cooper DG, Walsh SR, Sadat U, *et al.* . Neurological complications after left subclavian artery coverage during thoracic endovascular aortic repair: A systematic review and meta-analysis. *Journal of Vascular Surgery* 2009; **49** (6): 1594–601.

21. Buth J, Harris PL, Hobo R, Collaborators of the European collaborators registry (EUROSTAR). . Neurologic complications associated with endovascular repair of thoracic aortic pathology: Incidence and risk factors. A study from the European Collaborators on Stent/Graft Techniques for Aortic Aneurysm Repair (EUROSTAR) Registry. *Journal of Vascular Surgery* 2007; **46** (6): 1103–11.e2.

Acute and chronic type B dissection—false lumen challenges

Avoidance of retrograde type A dissection during intervention for acute complicated type B dissection

DR Gable and W Shutze

Introduction

Superior outcomes of thoracic endovascular aortic repair (TEVAR) compared with open repair have resulted in a shift in the treatment paradigm and recommendations for all thoracic aortic lesions including aortic dissection. Acute dissection of the ascending aorta is one of the more common aortic pathologies reported with an estimated incidence of 2.9 to 3.5 per 100,000 lives.[1,2] Although open surgical repair is still the recommended treatment for type A aortic dissection, there has been improved overall outcomes demonstrated for treatment of acute type B aortic dissection with endovascular stent grafts. It is generally agreed that uncomplicated acute type B aortic dissection treated conservatively with best medical therapy is associated with roughly 10% 30-day mortality and up to 25% need for intervention within four years of onset. Most recently, this has been demonstrated in comparison of TEVAR combined with best medical therapy *versus* best medical therapy alone at one year and at five years in the ADSORB[3] (Acute dissection: stent graft or best medical therapy) trial and INSTEAD (investigation of stent-grafts in aortic dissection)-XL[4] trial respectively. In the ADSORB trial, there was found to be incomplete thrombosis of the false lumen in 43% of the TEVAR and best medical therapy group *versus* 97% in the best medical therapy alone group. Additionally in the TEVAR and best medical therapy group, there was a reduction in size of the false lumen *versus* an increase in the best medical therapy alone group as well as an increase in the true lumen in the TEVAR and best medical therapy group *versus* no significant change in the best medical therapy alone group. In the INSTEAD trial (initially designed for two years and then expanded for five year follow-up), there was found to be complete false lumen thrombosis in 90% of the TEVAR and best medical therapy group *versus* 22% in the best medical therapy alone group as well as an overall 19% reduction of overall disease progression and 12% reduction of aortic specific mortality at five years in the TEVAR and best medical therapy group.

As this information has become evident, and treatment of acute and chronic type B aortic dissection with TEVAR has gained popularity, retrograde type A aortic dissection after TEVAR has become recognised as a new pathophysiologic entity and risk of treatment (Figure 1 and 2).

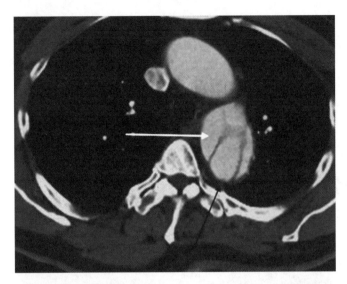

Figure 1: CT scan of an acute type B dissection. The black arrow demonstrates the true lumen and white arrow demonstrates the false lumen of the acute type B dissection prior to treatment.

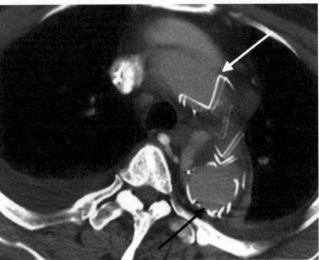

Figure 1: Intraoperative picture of the nitinol reinforced section once introduced and deployed into the vessel

Some early reports were published as early as 2002 but the incidence of this complication was felt to be rare.[5,6] Retrograde type A aortic dissection was identified more commonly in larger studies published in 2009, including 11 patients in a consecutive series of 443 patients undergoing TEVAR for acute type B dissection[6] and 63 in EuREC (European registry of endovascular complications).[7] These 63 cases (out of 3,714 total TEVAR cases aortic type B dissection) resulted in an incidence of 1.3%. The overall incidence of retrograde type A aortic dissection after TEVAR is reported to be between 1.3% and 24%.[8] Mortality of this feared complication has been documented to be 42.2% in the largest cohort reported[7] and has been reported as early as intra-procedurally and as late as several years after the initial repair. Avoidance of this dreaded complication must remain at the forefront of concern for all physicians who may consider repair of the acute or chronic type B dissection with an endovascular stent graft approach. Herein, we discuss common areas for consideration to assist in prevention of retrograde type A dissection after TEVAR.

Discussion

The complication of retrograde type A dissection after TEVAR can be broken down into three separate categories when considering potential causes. These categories are related to anatomical considerations, device related issues or procedure related issues. In regards to anatomic considerations, there have been shown to be several preoperative findings that may increase the risk for retrograde type A dissection and these must be considered when evaluating potential patients for treatment with TEVAR.

One of the most commonly accepted risk factors is an increased ascending aortic diameter of greater than or equal to 40mm.[9–11] The presence of an increased ascending aorta as described above has been shown to as much as double the risk in at least one study (15% vs. 33%).[12] This study also suggested aortic arch malformations were associated with an increased risk for retrograde type A dissection but an increase in the aortic root or the presence of a bicuspid valve did not appear to increase the risk. Additionally a bovine arch has been attributed to an increased risk of postoperative retrograde type A dissection.[13,14] Gandet et al suggested that loss of the sinotubular junction on preoperative imaging and female gender appeared to increase the overall risk for this complication as well. It is commonly held by many investigators that flow changes and alterations in haemodynamics related to debranching and/or transposition of the great vessels may cause an increase in the risk for retrograde type A dissection as well as a clamp injury during these procedures.[8,9,10,15] Use of a proximal stent graft landing zone in zones 0–2 may increase the risks for retrograde type A aortic dissection[8,10,11] and a recent study by Williams et al[13] demonstrated that all six out of 309 patients treated with TEVAR that developed retrograde type A dissection were patients that had these landing zones as the proximal target.

In terms of the type of device used for treatment, there are several concerns that have arisen as contributing to possible retrograde type A dissection. Along the lines of the prior discussion regarding an ascending aortic landing zone of over 40mm, the use a stent graft device of over 42mm has been shown to be associated with a higher risk for retrograde type A dissection.[12] In a similar fashion, oversizing the devices by more than 20% has been associated with a higher degree of risk[16,17] and Gandet et al suggested that oversizing by more than 10% was associated with a higher risk. The rigid structure of the devices that are currently available are felt to be a risk factor for retrograde type A dissection by several authors,[15,16] as is the potential compliance mismatch between the ascending aorta as a chosen landing zone compared to a more distal proximal landing zone.[15] This directly relates to the finding discussed previously regarding the higher incidence of retrograde type A dissection in procedures where the proximal landing zone is in zones 0–2.

A current ongoing debate is whether the presence of proximal bare metal springs on the stent graft device may contribute to the development of a retrograde type A dissection following TEVAR repair of a dissection. Many authors feel this is the case;[8,10,11,18] however, there are also some who feel that in their experience the presence of proximal bare metal springs makes no difference in the risk for this dreaded complication.[7,9,19,20] Many point to the results of the European Registry for Endovascular Complications in 2009, which demonstrated that 27 out of 29 patients (93%) suffering retrograde type A dissection had devices with proximal bare metal stents.[7] It is important to note, however, that more than 80% of the devices implanted in this registry were stents with bare metal proximal fixation. The abundant use of this type of device is attributable to the fact that they were the only type of device commercially available at the time of the study which offers a bias in the reported data for proximal bare metal springs as a concern for the cause of retrograde type A dissection. In a study reported by Idrees *et al,* with 766 patients, nearly half of the patients that developed retrograde type A dissection (seven out of 15) had devices used without bare metal proximal springs.[21]

In addition to the device and anatomical issues that increase the risk for retrograde type A dissection, the procedure itself also has areas and manoeuvres that may increase the risk for this complication. It is well accepted that the simple manipulation of the wires and catheters in the aortic arch may contribute to local intimal tears that may subsequently lead to retrograde type A dissection. Use of the injection catheter during the procedure, if left against the aortic wall, has also been implicated as a cause of increased risk.[12] Aortic wall injury may also occur following forward pressure on the device after initial device contact with the wall of the aorta. This may be especially true in acute aortic injury of the intimal wall following a dissection. Placement of the graft in a highly angulated neck has been shown to be associated with an increase in the risk for retrograde type A dissection by several authors especially if the angle is greater than 60 degrees.[18,22–24] Finally, a common consensus is that repetitive balloon remodelling is associated with increased risk for this disease process.[20,25]

Conclusion

There are multiple potential pitfalls associated with treatment of an aortic dissection with TEVAR as outlined above. Mortality of this disease process, even if diagnosed at the time of intervention, has been reported to be as high as 42–57%.[7,16] Avoidance of this complication begins with patient evaluation and selection for treatment pre-operatively. If an ascending aortic diameter of $\geq$40mm is noted, replacement of the ascending graft prior to TEVAR should be considered. Patients with the presence of an arch malformation, bovine configuration, presence of a connective tissue disorder or loss of the sinotubular junction must also be approached with caution if considering TEVAR as all of these factors will increase potential risk for retrograde type A dissection. The presence of a combination of these findings should give pause to the operator for TEVAR in this patient population, especially if it is planned that a debranching procedure with a proximal landing zone in zones 0-2 is required for treatment.

Once the decision is made for treatment, care must be taken during the procedure. Minimal wire and catheter manipulation in the arch must be done to decrease the risk for intimal injury. Care must be taken to avoid placement of the injection catheter immediately adjacent to the aortic wall if possible. Lowering the injection pressure, and potentially adding a 0.1 or 0.2 second rise on the injection may decrease the risks for intimal injury and therefore a subsequent retrograde type A dissection. Delivery of the device over a stiff wire and avoidance of multiple to-and-fro passes with the device through the arch may help decrease the risk for intimal injury. Selection of the type of device (presence or absence of bare proximal springs) remains controversial but has no increase risk for retrograde type A dissection in our own experience. The avoidance of post deployment balloon re-modelling, however, probably will help prevent possible intimal injury in an already fragile aortic wall after aortic dissection. Avoidance of post deployment balloon remodelling is of utmost importance in helping to prevent possible retrograde type A dissection.

The use of intra-operative rapid ventricular pacing to help reduce systolic pressure and aortic wall motion during deployment will also help reduce risks as well as avoidance of any attempt at graft movement or forward pressure after the first portion of the graft is deployed and has come in contact with the aortic wall. Additionally, it has become standard practice at our own institution to also use intravascular ultrasound (IVUS) during the TEVAR procedure, not only to evaluate true lumen placement of wires and devices, measurement of the aortic size and reduction of contrast usage, but also to evaluate for retrograde type A dissection after device placement. The use of intraoperative transoesophageal echo (TEE) will allow for help with monitoring for injury during treatment. TEE can be used to evaluate potential aortic valve injury from wire manipulation as well as the possible occurrence of intra-operative retrograde type A dissection that is otherwise asymptomatic. The finding of retrograde type A dissection has been reported as early as an intraoperative finding and as far out as seven years postoperative by several authors.[7,9,12,26] As many as 50% of retrograde type A dissection may be asymptomatic, seen only incidentally on follow-up computed tomography (CT) angiography.[12] Nonetheless, any postoperative complaints of chest or back pain should result in CT angiography evaluation. Additionally, many operators now recommend a follow-up CT on all patients if possible prior to discharge from hospital during the index procedure as part of routine practice.

Summary

- If possible, avoid TEVAR in treatment of acute type B aortic dissection in patients with ascending aortic diameter of ≥40mm, arch malformation, bovine arch configuration, connective tissue disorders or loss of the sinotubular junction on pre-operative CT angiography.

- If possible, avoid the proximal landing zones 0–2.

- Use care with aortic clamping in any debranching procedure but if possible, avoid debranching procedures in conjunction with TEVAR in acute type B dissection.

- Minimise wire and catheter manipulation in the aortic arch.

- Avoid excessive manipulation of the delivery device in the arch.

- Use intraoperative IVUS, TEE and rapid ventricular pacing to assist with device delivery.

- Avoid post-deployment balloon remodelling of the TEVAR device.

- Consider follow-up CT angiography evaluation in all patients prior to hospital discharge.

References

1. Clouse WD, Hallett JW Jr, Schaff HV, *et al.* Acute aortic dissection: population based incidence compared with degenerative aortic aneurysm rupture. *Mayo Clin Proc* 2004; **79** (2): 176–80.

2. Ramanth VS, Oh IK, Sundt TM III, *et al.* Acute aortic syndromes and thoracic aortic aneurysms and type B dissections. Cardiovasc Intervent Radiol 2009; **32** (5): 849–60.

3. J. Brunkwall P, Kasprzak, E. Verhoeven, *et al.* Endovascular repair of acute uncomplicated aortic type B dissection promotes aortic remodeling: 1 year results of the ADSORB trial. *Eur J Vasc Endovasc Surg.* 2014; **48** (3): 285–91.

4. Nienaber CA, Kisch S, Rousseau, H, *et al.* Endovascular repair of type B aortic dissection: long-term results of the randomized investigation of stent grafts in aortic dissection trial. *Circ Cardiovascular Inter* 2013; **6**: 407–16.

5. Grabenwoger M, Fleck T, Ehrich M, *et al.* Secondary surgical interventions after endovascular stent-grafting of the thoracic aorta. *Eur J Cardio-thorac Surg* 2004; **26**: 608–13.

6. Schwartz E, Langs G, Holfeld J *et al.* Quantifying the effects of stent-grafting in the thoracic aorta based on a motion manifold. *Med Image Anal* 2011.

7. ggebrecht H, Thompson M, Rousseau H, *et al.* Retrograde ascending aortic dissection during or after thoracic aortic stent graft placement: insight from the European registry on endovascular aortic repair complications. *Circulation* 2009; **120** (11): S276–81.

8. Cochennec F, Tresson P, Cross J, *et al.* Hybrid repair of aortic arch dissections. *J Vasc Surg* 2013; **57**: 1560–67.

9. Czerny M, Rieger M, Schmidli J. Incidence, risk factors, and outcome of retrograde type A aortic dissection after TEVAR. *Gefasschirurgie* 2015; **20**: S45–50.

10. Luehr M, Etz CD, Lehmkuhl L, *et al.* Surgical management of retrograde type A aortic dissection following complete supra-aortic debranching and stent-grafting of the transverse arch. *Eur J Cardiothorac Surg* 2013; **42**: 958–63.

11. Anderson ND, Williams JB, Hanna JM, *et al.* Results with an algorithmic approach to hybrid repair of the aortic arch. *J Vasc Surg* 2013; **57**: 655–67.

12. Gandet T, Canaud L, Ozdemir A, *et al.* Factors favoring retrograde aortic dissection after endovascular aortic arch repair. *J Thorac Cardiovasc Surg* 2015; **150** (1): 136–42.

13. Williams JB, Anderson ND, Bhattacharya SD, *et al.* Retrograde ascending aortic dissection as an early complication of thoracic endovascular aortic repair. *J Vasc Surg* 2012; **55** (5): 1255–62.

14. Neuhauser B, Czermak BV, Fish J, *et al.* Type A dissection following endovascular thoracic aortic stent-graft repair. *J Endovasc Ther* 2005; **12**: 74–81.

15. Czerny M, Weigang E, Gottfried S, *et al.* Targeting landing zone 0 by total arch rerouting and TEVAR: midterm results of a transcontinental registry. *Ann Thorac Surg* 2012: **94**: 84–89.

16. Piffaretti G, Mariscalco G, Tozzi M, *et al.* Acute iatrogenic type A aortic dissection following thoracic aortic endografting. *J Vasc Surg* 2010; **51** (4): 993–99.

17. Kpodonu J, Preventza O, Ramalah VG, *et al.* Retrograde type A dissection after endovascular stenting of the descending thoracic aorta. Is the risk real? *Eur J Cardiothoracic Surg* 2008; **33**: 1014–18.

18. Dong ZH, Fu WG, Wang YQ, *et al.* Retrograde type A aortic dissection after endovascular stent-graft placement for treatment of type B dissection. *Circulation* 2009; **119**: 735–41.

19. Canaud L, Ozdemir BA, Patterson BA, *et al.* Retrograde aortic dissection after thoracic endovascular aortic repair. *Ann Surg* 2014; **260**: 3889–95.

20. Neuhauser B, Greiner A, Jaschke W, *et al.* Serious complications following endovascular thoracic aortic stent-graft repair for type B dissection. *Eur J Cardiothoracic Surg* 2008; **33**: 58–3.

21. Idrees J, Arafat A, Johnston D, *et al.* Repair of retrograde ascending dissection after descending stent grafting. J Thoracic Cardiovasc Surg 2014; **147** (1): 151–54.

22. Girdauskas E, Falk V, Kuntze T, *et al.* Secondary surgical procedures after endovascular stent grafting of the thoracic aorta: successful approaches to a challenging clinical problem. *J Thorac Cardiovasc Surg* 2008; **136**: 1289–94.

23. Bethuyne N, Bove T, Vanden Brande P, *et al.* Acute retrograde aortic dissection during endovascular repair of a thoracic aortic aneurysm. *Ann Thorac Surg* 2003; **75**: 1967–69.

24. Fanelli F, Salvatore FM, Marcelli G, *et al.* Type A aortic dissection developing during endovascular repair of an acute type B dissection. *J Endovasc Ther* 2003; **10**: 254–59.

25. Steingruber IE, Chemelli A, Glodney B, *et al.* Endovascular repair of acute type B aortic dissection:midterm results. *J Endovasc Ther* 2008; **15**: 150–60.

26. Patterson B, Holt P, Nienaber C, Cambria R, *et al.* Aortic pathology determines mid-term outcome after endovascular repair of the thoracic aorta: report from the Medtronic Thoracic Endovascular Registry (MOTHER) database. *Circulation* 2013; **127**: 24–32.

Impact of TEVAR on late mortality in chronic type B dissection

BO Patterson and MM Thompson

Introduction

Aortic dissection occurs when the intima of the vessel separates from the media and blood flows between the two, creating an abnormal channel referred to as the false lumen.[1] This can present in a variety of ways, from mild back pain to sudden death due to rupture or malperfusion of organs. Stanford type B dissection occurs when the false aortic lumen arises from an entry tear distal to the left subclavian artery, and can present either in the acute or chronic phase. If the initial dissection event is not reported to a physician or if the correct diagnosis is not ascertained at the time of presentation, the condition will likely go undetected until it is discovered incidentally.

Once discovered, in the absence and significant dilatation, chronic uncomplicated type B aortic dissection is usually treated using pharmacological agents to reduce blood pressure. The goal of this is to reduce arterial wall stress and stop subsequent aneurysmal dilatation over time.[1,2] Patients then usually undergo annual imaging surveillance to monitor the status of the aorta. The main purpose of this is to determine if there is progressive expansion over time and if surgical intervention is warranted. Traditionally, only direct surgical replacement of the diseased aorta was possible, but in recent years thoracic endovascular aortic repair (TEVAR) has been increasingly offered based mainly on favourable short-term morbidity and mortality advantages. Corresponding long-term survival benefits have yet to be emphatically demonstrated.

Long-term death after TEVAR for chronic dissection

A systematic review of long-term outcomes following TEVAR for chronic dissection demonstrated that long-term all-cause survival varied between 60% and 100% in all studies that reported this, although the median follow-up was only 26 months when all studies were considered. Aortic-specific mortality was 4.2%, although it was not possible to determine pooled survival estimates.[3] Although this study represented a heterogeneous group with a strong possibility of reporting and publication bias, it suggested that TEVAR probably had some beneficial effect in preventing fatal aortic events when considering much of the published literature.

The MOTHER registry combined five clinical trials and one institutional case series, and included 195 patients with chronic dissection, in whom it is was possible to perform a detailed analysis of mid-term survival.[4] In this group, all-cause survival at five-year follow-up was 64%, whereas freedom from aortic-related death was 96%. If all deaths before 90 days were counted as "periprocedural" and discounted, then this equated to a mortality rate of 0.4 per 100 years of patient follow-up (Figure 1). This suggested that TEVAR was effective in preventing aortic-related deaths, with the caveat that some deaths may have been misclassified due to difficulties in the ascertainment of final cause of death in some patients. Aortic reintervention was relatively high in comparison with patients undergoing TEVAR for aneurysm, however, with only 71% remaining free from aortic reintervention at five years vs. 84% in aneurysm patients. Of the 34 reinterventions, 25 were recorded as being due to endoleak, aneurysmal expansion and continued perfusion of the false lumen. These could all be considered to be failures of primary treatment, specifically of TEVAR to achieve remodelling, either due to inadequate treatment or disease progression. In some cases, it is possible that TEVAR was the first treatment to be performed in the knowledge that distal segments would probably require treatment in the future. It is difficult to determine if this was the case without access to individual patient notes and information regarding preoperative planning. If it is assumed that all secondary interventions are performed due to a perceived threat of disease progression, it should be considered that they are necessary to prevent aortic-related death. This, therefore, may be the price to pay for reduced early morbidity and mortality in comparison with open repair and protection against late death compared with medical management alone.

A study of medically managed aortic dissections concluded that the event-free survival rate was sufficient to justify this strategy in many cases.[5] In this prospective study, an 82% freedom from aortic-related death was reported at five years. This study combined patients with classic aortic dissection and those with intramural haematoma, which is known to be a less lethal condition. In addition, all of the patients had an aortic diameter that was below threshold for surgery and were less at risk of aortic events by definition. In a direct comparison of medically managed dissection and those treated by endovascular means in the INSTEAD (Investigation of stent grafts in aortic dissection) XL study, it was suggested that medically-treated patients had a higher aortic-specific mortality rate than the interventional patient s(6.9% vs. 19.3%), and later disease progression was more frequent (27% vs. 46.1%). Furthermore, a total of 14 patients were crossed-over from best medical therapy to the intervention group, with five of these operations performed as an emergency and four requiring open repair,[6] presumably as the disease had become too complex to manage with an endovascular approach. It should be noted that many of the patients included in this study were treated within three months of initial presentation, which would classify them as being "subacute" dissections, which may mean that more patients demonstrated remodelling than would have been seen in a purely chronic dissection group. A further study from the International Registry of Aortic Dissection (IRAD) supported these findings by demonstrating that medically treated patients were more likely to develop aortic dilatation at follow-up and had a higher death rate at follow-up (29% vs. 15.5%).

These studies imply that achieving aortic remodelling is vital if TEVAR is to be efficacious in the long term, and as a consequence several different factors should be considered when planning and performing TEVAR for chronic dissection to promote long-term reintervention-free survival.

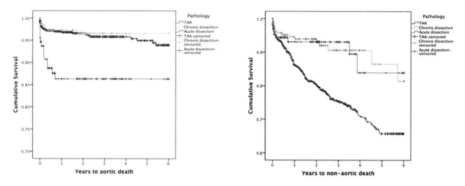

Figure 1: Low rate of aortic-related death in patients following TEVAR for chronic dissection who were included in the MOTHER registry in comparison with those undergoing surgery for other indications.[4]

Maximising aortic remodelling after TEVAR for chronic dissection

Remodelling can be defined as the restoration of the normal anatomy of the aorta by thrombosis and regression of the false lumen with expansion of the true lumen.[4,7] Endovascular treatment aims to induce false lumen thrombosis by depressurising the false lumen following coverage of the proximal entry tear and if possible the re-entry tear, thus inducing aortic remodelling. Several studies have agreed remodelling appears to occur more readily in those treated in the acute or subacute phase as opposed the chronic phase. A recent systematic review demonstrated that there was significantly greater variation in the tendency of chronic dissections to remodel in comparison with those treated in the acute phase. This is commonly ascribed to the more fixed, inflexible nature of the dissection flap in chronic disease, but various factors have been found to be associated with poor clinical outcomes.[8]

Failure to cover the main entry tear has not surprisingly been found to be associated with a poorer outcome.[9–11] If the proximal entry tear is inadequately covered, anterograde flow will likely persist in the false lumen and remodelling will be highly unlikely. A longer length of aortic coverage has been demonstrated to result in a greater tendency toward false lumen thrombosis at mid-term follow-up.[12] Aortic dissection with infrarenal extension displays less tendency to remodel, potentially because treating the segment of aorta above the diaphragm will often not address the main re-entry tear.[8] A study of purely extent IIIb chronic type B dissections suggested that longer coverage is necessary, as some reinterventions have been linked to patent fenestrations.[11] Other groups have subsequently found length of coverage to be less important,[10,13] and it could be that more extensive disease requiring longer coverage may be a confounding factor.

The number of aortic branches arising from the true aortic lumen and visible fenestrations in the dissection flap may determine the likelihood of false lumen thrombosis. Those with a greater number of patent distal fenestrations have been shown to require reintervention more frequently, although the solution to this problem is not clear.[9–11] Placing a fenestrated or branched endograft in all cases with distal extension would lead to dramatically increased morbidity and may be necessary. Attempting to individually recanalise individual branches from the true lumen is possible but is not well described.

The presence of stent graft induced new entry tears is also associated with reintervention.[14] This is most likely to be caused by oversizing of the stent graft at the distal extent of the treated area, with excessive radial force giving rise to trauma to the aortic wall and potentially perforation of the intimal flap.[15] This may be avoided by sizing the stent graft according to the dimensions of the distal true lumen, and may require the placement of tapered devices. The chronological definition of "chronic" dissection varies between different studies.[6,11] Some would group patients who are two weeks from presentation and those who were diagnosed five years previously together, which is perhaps not helpful.[10] The INSTEAD trial intervention arm recruited patients at a median of 3.5 weeks after the diagnosis and randomised patients to receive TEVAR or best medical therapy alone.[16] In those that were treated with TEVAR, there was a 92.6% for total false lumen thrombosis at one year, whereas in another study that treated patients at a mean of 100 weeks post diagnosis, false lumen thrombosis only occurred in 39% at three-year follow-up.[17] The difference noted between these two groups suggests that the classification of aortic dissection into simply "acute" and "chronic" may not adequate, and that the "subacute" classification described in the VIRTUE registry (14–92 days after the acute event) is probably more suitable.[18] This is borne out by the different rate of aortic remodelling seen in the three different groups in this study, which appears to translate into a difference in mid-term mortality.[19]

Conclusion

TEVAR for chronic aortic dissection may be performed with less perioperative morbidity and mortality than invasive open surgical techniques. There is emerging evidence from registries and trials that TEVAR is an effective method of preventing aortic-related death in the long term, but there is not enough to prove this conclusively.

It is assumed that the protection offered by TEVAR is linked to promoting aortic remodelling, or at least to preventing further degeneration. Often secondary interventions are necessary to ensure repair is ultimately durable. Improvements in long-term clinical outcomes may be achieved if predictors of poor outcomes can be identified either at the time of initial treatment or during follow-up surveillance.

Summary

- There are relatively few high-quality studies describing long-term mortality following TEVAR for chronic type B dissection.

- From existing data, it would appear that TEVAR is effective in protecting against aortic-related death in these patients.

- The caveat to this is that there may be a lack of ascertainment of the true cause of death in many causes given that this information is not always sought conclusively.

- Late mortality appears to be linked to a failure of treatment to achieve aortic remodelling, although this finding is not conclusive.

- Various strategies should be considered in order to maximise the chance of remodelling if TEVAR is to be successful:

  - Maximising coverage of the diseased aorta where possible

  - Coverage of distal false lumen fenestrations

  - Careful distal oversizing in order to avoid stent graft induced re-entry tears.

  - The number of aortic branches supplied by the false lumen predicts failure of remodelling after treatment, and treatment at time of the initial procedure may alleviate this.

- Ongoing imaging surveillance is vital to ensure that disease progression or treatment failure can be identified in good time and suitable treatment instigated.

References

1. Thrumurthy SG, Karthikesalingam A, Patterson BO, et al. The diagnosis and management of aortic dissection. BMJ. 2012; **344**: d8290.
2. Erbel R, Alfonso F, Boileau C, et al. Diagnosis and management of aortic dissection. European Heart Journal. 2001. pp. 1642–81.
3. Thrumurthy SG, Karthikesalingam A, Patterson BO, et al. A systematic review of mid-term outcomes of thoracic endovascular repair (TEVAR) of chronic type B aortic dissection. *Eur J Vasc Endovasc Surg* 2011; **42** (5): 632–47.
4. Patterson B, Holt P, Nienaber C, et al. Aortic Pathology Determines Midterm Outcome After Endovascular Repair of the Thoracic Aorta: Report From the Medtronic Thoracic Endovascular Registry (MOTHER) Database. *Circulation* 2013; **127** (1): 24–32.
5. Winnerkvist A, Lockowandt U, Rasmussen E, et al. A prospective study of medically treated acute type B aortic dissection. *European Journal of Vascular & Endovascular Surgery* 2006; **32** (4): 349–55.
6. Nienaber CA, Kische S, Rousseau H, et al. Endovascular repair of type B aortic dissection: long-term results of the randomized investigation of stent grafts in aortic dissection trial. *Circ Cardiovasc Interv* 2013; **6** (4): 407–16.
7. Resch TA, Delle M, Falkenberg M, et al. Remodeling of the thoracic aorta after stent grafting of type B dissection: a Swedish multicenter study. *J Cardiovasc Surg* (Torino) 2006; **47** (5): 503–8.
8. Patterson BO, Cobb RJ, Karthikesalingam A, et al. A Systematic Review of Aortic Remodeling After Endovascular Repair of Type B Aortic Dissection: Methods and Outcomes. *The Annals of Thoracic Surgery* 2014; **97** (2): 588–95.
9. Tolenaar JL, Kern JA, Jonker FHW, et al. Predictors of false lumen thrombosis in type B aortic dissection treated with TEVAR. *Ann Cardiothorac Surg* 2014; **3** (3): 255–63.

10. Kitamura T, Torii S, Oka N, Horai T, Nakashima K, Itatani K, *et al*. Key success factors for thoracic endovascular aortic repair for non-acute Stanford type B aortic dissection. *Eur J Cardiothorac Surg.* 2014; **46** (3): 432–37.

11. Hughes GC, Ganapathi AM, Keenan JE, *et al*. Thoracic Endovascular Aortic Repair for Chronic DeBakey IIIb Aortic Dissection. The Annals of Thoracic Surgery. 2014; **98** (6): 2092–98.

12. Qing K, Yiu W, Cheng SWK. A morphologic study of chronic type B aortic dissections and aneurysms after thoracic endovascular stent grafting. *J Vasc Surg* 2012; **55** (5): 1268–76.

13. Lee M, Lee DY, Kim MD, *et al*. Outcomes of endovascular management for complicated chronic type B aortic dissection: effect of the extent of stent graft coverage and anatomic properties of aortic dissection. *J Vasc Interv Radiol* 2013; **24** (10): 1451–60.

14. Weng S-H, Weng C-F, Chen W-Y, *et al*. Reintervention for distal stent graft-induced new entry after endovascular repair with a stainless steel-based device in aortic dissection. *J Vasc Surg* 2013; **57** (1): 64–71.

15. Zhang L, Zhou J, Lu Q, *et al*. Potential risk factors of re-intervention after endovascular repair for type B aortic dissections. *Cathet Cardiovasc Intervent* 2014; 86 (1): E1–E10.

16. Nienaber CA, Rousseau H, Eggebrecht H, *et al*. Randomized Comparison of Strategies for Type B Aortic Dissection: The INvestigation of STEnt Grafts in Aortic Dissection (INSTEAD) Trial. *Circulation* 2009; **120** (25): 2519–28.

17. Kang WC, Greenberg RK, Mastracci TM, *et al*. Endovascular repair of complicated chronic distal aortic dissections: Intermediate outcomes and complications. The Journal of Thoracic and Cardiovascular Surgery. *The American Association for Thoracic Surgery* 2011; **142** (5): 1074–83.

18. Investigators TVR. The VIRTUE Registry of type B thoracic dissections--study design and early results. *Eur J Vasc Endovasc Surg* 2011; **41** (2): 159–66.

19. Virtue Registry Investigators. Mid-term outcomes and aortic remodelling after thoracic endovascular repair for acute, subacute, and chronic aortic dissection: the VIRTUE Registry. *Eur J Vasc Endovasc Surg* 2014; **48** (4): 363–71.

Outcomes and predictors of intervention and mortality in patients with uncomplicated acute type B aortic dissection

CA Durham and A Azizzadeh

Introduction

Aortic dissection occurs in four to five persons per 100,000 annually, making it the most common aortic emergency. Furthermore, 20% to 30% of patients affected die prior to hospital admission.[1] Although substantial improvements have been made since Morris reported the first successful repair in 1963, immediate surgical correction has been a relatively static dogma for the treatment of acute type A aortic dissection.[2] However, consensus for the treatment of type B aortic dissection, where the entry tear originates distal to the left subclavian artery, has been more dynamic. Early attempts at repair of acute type B dissection included decompression of the false lumen via creation of distal reentry in the iliac artery, cellophane wrapping, and intimal tear excision and aortic replacement.[3–5] However, mortality with these strategies was markedly high, prompting Palmer and Wheat to introduce medical management focused on lowering systolic blood pressure and pulse as the standard of care.[6] Although this readily decreased in-hospital mortality for patients with acute uncomplicated type B dissection, the long-term consequences for such a strategy were not benign with as high as 40% progression to aneurysmal degeneration of the outer wall of the false lumen at a mean of 18 months.[7,8] Recent studies have shown favourable one-year survival with medical therapy alone over historical outcome of open repair; however, this focus on one-year survival has probably exaggerated the benefits of medical management as the primary late complication usually appears after this timeframe. The recent Food and Drug Administration (FDA) approval of thoracic stent grafting for the treatment of aortic dissection has opened a new era in the treatment of type B dissections. The FDA and the Society for Vascular Surgery have partnered to gather prospective data with five-year follow-up of thoracic endovascular aortic repair (TEVAR). This has led to re-evaluation of the natural history of the medically managed dissected aorta and recent updated and contemporary results regarding the outcomes of patients with uncomplicated acute type B aortic dissection.

Outcomes

Medical therapy aimed at lowering the systolic blood pressure and pulse has remained the standard of care for treatment of uncomplicated acute type B aortic

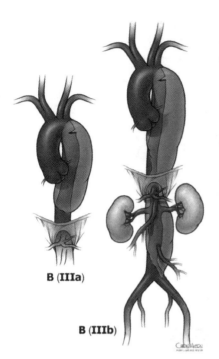

B (IIIa)

B (IIIb)

Figure 1: Aortic dissection distal to the left subclavian artery is classified as a Stanford B or Debakey III (a. limited to the thoracic aorta b. involving the thoracoabdominal aorta).

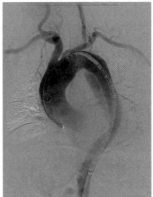

Figure 2a: Aortogram in a high-risk patient with uncomplicated type B (Debakey IIIb) aortic dissection who underwent TEVAR after failure of medical therapy. Note the proximal entry tear on the lesser curvature of the descending thoracic aorta with flow in the false lumen.

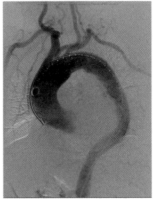

Figure 2b: Aortogram after deployment of the thoracic device distal to the left subclavian artery shows exclusion of the false lumen flow.

dissection, as the mortality of open surgery as primary management in patients with more complicated dissections has been known to be as high as 32%.[9] Indeed this strategy has demonstrated excellent historical short-term outcomes with 30-day mortality closer to 10% and favourable one-year survival with medical therapy alone ranging from 70% to 90%.[10–14] However, it is clear that the uncomplicated acute type B aortic dissection is not a benign disease process. Contemporary study has shown, however, that up to one eighth of patients will fail medical management in the first 30 days and require intervention, primarily due to the development of malperfusion syndrome. Five per cent will die in the first 30 days undergoing medical management alone.[15] Some studies have not identified this significant early morbidity and mortality by only including in the medical cohort those patients that were still being managed medically after 14 days; the subacute and chronic dissection.[11] However, the presentation of the malperfusion syndrome is variable, and many patients will have a waxing and waning course with regard to pulse deficits and clinical manifestations such as renal failure and mesenteric ischaemia.[16] There are a number of patients that do not neatly fit into a sophomoric triage algorithm, and patients who initially present as uncomplicated can rapidly deteriorate over the first 24–48 hours. This attests to the challenges inherent in managing acute aortic dissection, and further emphasises the importance of close follow-up and serial examination during the acute period.

The primary drawback of medical management is that it leaves the untreated wall of the false lumen susceptible to aneurysmal degeneration over time. DeBakey first demonstrated that 37% of patients develop this in 1982, and indeed the number of patients suffering this long-term complication does not appear to have changed over time.[7] Even with contemporary medical therapy, Juvonen showed 38% will develop late aneurysm formation and the International Registry of Acute Aortic Dissection (IRAD) investigators have reported the rate of aortic growth or aneurysm formation to be 34.5% at three years in patients undergoing medical therapy alone, both consistent with the original findings of the Baylor group.[17,18] The Massachusetts General Hospital reported similar findings with actuarial freedom from aortic growth to be 77.8% after two years and only 51.1% after five years.[19] The rate of aortic expansion or growth has been shown to be a strong predictor of imminent rupture in patients with degenerative abdominal aortic aneurysms. It is therefore intuitive that the same would be true for aneurysms of chronic aortic dissection.[20] However, there are little data regarding the expected rate of growth of the aorta in patients with medically managed type B dissections and only a few small series evaluate the rate of aortic enlargement in aortic dissections treated with medical therapy alone. The study from the Massachusetts General Hospital demonstrated an aortic growth rate of 12.3mm per year, driven by a rate of false lumen expansion of 8.6mm per year.[19] Although this was higher than some previous studies showing rates as low as 1.5mm per year, the latter studies were significantly smaller and included only those patients who had studies at least one year apart, minimising short-term changes but also potentially excluding patients demonstrating rapid aortic expansion in the first year.[21–23]

Furthermore, although the one-year mortality rates are significantly better with medical management as opposed to open surgical therapy, the effect of uncomplicated acute type B aortic dissection on long-term survival is also well documented. Debakey's review noted an overall survival only slightly higher than 50% after 50 years, and Massachusetts General Hospital's contemporary data are only slightly better—showing 58.4% survival after six years among patients with uncomplicated type B dissection who continued to be medically managed.[7,15] The intervention free survival was naturally even lower with the study group having an intervention free survival of 55.3% and 41.2% after three and six years, respectively. Interestingly this same study did, however, note a survival advantage among those ultimately failing medical management and requiring intervention. Those patients eventually undergoing an operation for their dissection demonstrated 76.4% survival after six years.[15] This is consistent with large registry data reviewing early intervention with TEVAR compared with medical management alone. The recent study from the IRAD group evaluated 1,100 patients, 75% of whom were treated with medical therapy alone and 25% were treated with an early aortic intervention. Although these cohorts had a similar early mortality, the five-year survival was superior in the cohort receiving an early intervention (84.5% vs. 71%).[18] Similarly, the INSTEAD (Investigation of stent grafts in aortic dissection) trial collaborators found improved long-term aorta-specific survival in the TEVAR cohort compared with the cohort treated with medical therapy alone.[24] The exact reasons for such a survival advantage are not yet entirely clear. However, it is clear that surgically altering the flow dynamics between the true and false lumens, either by sealing the entry tear or equalising pressure through fenestration, promotes aortic remodelling over blood pressure control alone. Indeed, there is an emerging consensus that late survival is better with intervention when compared with continued medical management.

Predictors

With the FDA approval for two thoracic stent grafts to be used in type B aortic dissection, it is clear that endovascular coverage of proximal aortic entry tear will become more common in the acute phase. Nonetheless, the utility of optimal medical therapy is not voided. The aim of much recent study has been identifying factors that predict mortality and intervention as a way of potentially determining who might derive benefit from early intervention.

The maximal diameter of the aorta has repeatedly been identified as a risk factor for morbidity and mortality in patients with uncomplicated acute type B aortic dissection. In a recent meta-analysis by van Bogerijen, 18 articles were reviewed for predictors of aortic growth in uncomplicated type B dissection. Nearly half of the studies included in the analysis identified a large maximum aortic diameter as predictive of future aortic growth, most showing that aortic diameter greater than 40mm correlates with aortic growth. However, one study has shown that an initial aortic diameter greater than 35mm correlates with growth.[19] Furthermore, our group has demonstrated that an initial aortic diameter greater than 44mm is an independent risk factor for mortality as well as decreased intervention free survival. We also found that false lumen diameter greater than 22mm predicts decreased intervention-free survival.[25]

Patency of the false lumen has also repeatedly been demonstrated to be a risk factor for aortic growth, although the majority of these evaluated patency of the false lumen based on the initial computed tomography (CT) scan.[22,26–28] But it has also been shown that a majority of false lumens are patent at the time of admission.[21] As such, it has also been demonstrated that thrombosis of the false lumen at discharge is protective against future growth and intervention, once hypertension has been able to be controlled with optimal medical management, and an initial opportunity for aortic remodelling has been provided. Yet, false lumen thrombosis occurs at a suboptimal rate with medical management alone.[19] TEVAR, however, has been shown to induce positive aortic remodelling in a large percentage of patients with acute type B aortic dissection. Nearly 90% of patients undergoing TEVAR for complicated type B dissections had thrombosis of the false lumen and a decrease in maximum aortic diameter at one year.[29] The prospective, multicentre STABLE (Study of thoracic aortic type B dissection using endoluminal repair) trial demonstrated a 100% rate of either partial or complete false lumen thrombosis in the initial post procedure imaging study compared with 0% at presentation, and 31% of patients had complete thrombosis of the false lumen at one year.[30]

Other predictors of growth and intervention have been found in the literature, albeit with less consistency. These include age <60, white race, Marfan Syndrome, elliptical or saccular formation of the true lumen, presence of only one entry tear, large entry tear (>10mm) located in the proximal portion of the dissection, false lumen located at the inner aortic curvature, and end stage renal disease, which has also been shown to be a risk factor for mortality.[26,31–34]

Conclusion

Uncomplicated acute type B aortic dissection is clearly not a benign disease. Although medical management has long been the gold standard for its treatment due to its superior survival over open repair, it leaves patients at risk for future aneurysmal degeneration and intervention. Comorbid profiles and anatomic factors of the dissection have been found to be predictive of mortality and future intervention but current large multicentre trials will shed new light on the validity of the premise that early intervention with TEVAR will reduce mortality and in which patient populations it should be applied.

Summary

- Medical management, while successful in the short term, subjects a substantial number of patients to future interventions, and there is an emerging consensus that late survival is better with early intervention when compared with continued medical management.

- Maximal aortic diameter >35mm and continued patency of the false lumen are independent risk factors for aortic growth.

- Maximal aortic diameter >44mm and end stage renal disease are independent risk factors for mortality.

- Maximal aortic diameter >44mm and false lumen diameter >22mm are associated with decreased intervention free survival.

- Current prospective investigation will determine if early thoracic endografting confers protection against mortality compared with medical management in uncomplicated dissection.

References

1. Olsson C, Thelin S, Ståhle E, et al. Thoracic aortic aneurysm and dissection: increasing prevalence and improved outcomes reported in a nationwide population-based study of more than 14,000 cases from 1987 to 2002. Circulation 2006; 114 (24): 2611–8.
2. Morris C, Henly W, DeBakey M. Correction of acute dissecting aneurysm of aorta with valvular insufficiency. JAMA 1963; 184 (1): 63–4.
3. Gurin D, Bulmer J, Derby R. Diagnosis and operative relief of arterial obstruction due to this cause. N State J Med 1935; 35: 1200.
4. Abbott OA. Clinical experiences with the application of polythene cellophane upon the aneurysms of the thoracic vessels. J Thorac Surg 1949; 18 (4): 435–61.
5. DeBakey ME, Cooley DA, Creech O. Surgical considerations of dissecting aneurysm of the aorta. Ann Surg 1955; 142 (4): 586–610; Discussion, 611–2.
6. Palmer RF, Wheat MW. Treatment of dissecting aneurysms of the aorta. Ann Thorac Surg 1967; 4 (1): 38–52.
7. DeBakey ME, McCollum CH, Crawford ES, et al. Dissection and dissecting aneurysms of the aorta: twenty-year follow-up of five hundred twenty-seven patients treated surgically. Surgery 1982; 92 (6): 1118–34.
8. Dialetto G, Covino FE, Scognamiglio G, et al. Treatment of type B aortic dissection: endoluminal repair or conventional medical therapy? Eur J Cardio-Thorac Surg 2005; 27 (5): 826–30.
9. Suzuki T, Mehta RH, Ince H, et al. Clinical profiles and outcomes of acute type B aortic dissection in the current era: lessons from the International Registry of Aortic Dissection (IRAD). Circulation 2003; 108 Suppl 1: II312–7.
10. Tsai TT, Fattori R, Trimarchi S, et al. Long-term survival in patients presenting with type B acute aortic dissection insights from the international registry of acute aortic dissection. Circulation 2006 Nov 21; 114 (21): 2226–31.
11. Nienaber CA, Zannetti S, Barbieri B, et al. Investigation of stent grafts in patients with type B aortic dissection: design of the INSTEAD trial—a prospective, multicenter, European randomized trial. Am Heart J 2005 Apr; 149 (4): 592–9.

12. Estrera AL, Miller CC, Safi HJ, *et al.* Outcomes of medical management of acute type B aortic dissection. *Circulation* 2006 Jul 4; **114** (1 Suppl): I384–9.

13. Umaña JP, Lai DT, Mitchell RS, *et al.* Is medical therapy still the optimal treatment strategy for patients with acute type B aortic dissections? *J Thorac Cardiovasc Surg* 2002 Nov; **124** (5): 896–910.

14. Winnerkvist A, Lockowandt U, Rasmussen E, Rådegran K. A prospective study of medically treated acute type B aortic dissection. *Eur J Vasc Endovasc Surg Off J Eur Soc Vasc Surg* 2006 Oct; **32** (4): 349–55.

15. Durham CA, Cambria RP, Wang LJ, *et al.* The natural history of medically managed acute type B aortic dissection. *J Vasc Surg* 2015 May; **61** (5): 1192–8.

16. Lauterbach SR, Cambria RP, Brewster DC, *et al.* Contemporary management of aortic branch compromise resulting from acute aortic dissection. *J Vasc Surg* 2001 Jun; **33** (6): 1185–92.

17. Juvonen T, Ergin MA, Galla JD, *et al.* Risk factors for rupture of chronic type B dissections. *J Thorac Cardiovasc Surg* 1999 Apr; **117** (4): 776–86.

18. Fattori R, Montgomery D, Lovato L, *et al.* Survival after endovascular therapy in patients with type B aortic dissection: a report from the International Registry of Acute Aortic Dissection (IRAD). *JACC Cardiovasc Interv* 2013 Aug; **6** (8): 876–82.

19. Durham CA, Aranson NJ, Ergul EA, *et al.* Aneurysmal degeneration of the thoracoabdominal aorta after medical management of type B aortic dissections. *J Vasc Surg* 2015 Oct; **62** (4): 900–6.

20. Limet R, Sakalihassan N, Albert A. Determination of the expansion rate and incidence of rupture of abdominal aortic aneurysms. *J Vasc Surg* 1991; **14** (4): 540–8.

21. Sueyoshi E, Sakamoto I, Hayashi K, *et al.* Growth rate of aortic diameter in patients with type B aortic dissection during the chronic phase. *Circulation* 2004 Sep 14; **110** (11 Suppl 1): II256–61.

22. Onitsuka S, Akashi H, Tayama K, *et al.* Long-term outcome and prognostic predictors of medically treated acute type B aortic dissections. *Ann Thorac Surg* 2004 Oct; **78** (4): 1268–73.

23. Kelly AM, Quint LE, Nan B, *et al.* Aortic growth rates in chronic aortic dissection. *Clin Radiol* 2007; **62** (9): 866–75.

24. Nienaber CA, Kische S, Rousseau H, *et al.* Endovascular repair of type B aortic dissection: long-term results of the randomized investigation of stent grafts in aortic dissection trial. *Circ Cardiovasc Interv* 2013 Aug; **6** (4): 407–16.

25. Ray HM, Durham CA, Ocazionez D, *et al.* Predictors of intervention and mortality in patients with uncomplicated acute type B aortic dissection. *J Vasc Surg*; In Press.

26. Tolenaar JL, van Keulen JW, Jonker FHW, *et al.* Morphologic predictors of aortic dilatation in type B aortic dissection. *J Vasc Surg* 2013 Nov; **58** (5): 1220–5.

27. Marui A, Mochizuki T, Koyama T, Mitsui N. Degree of fusiform dilatation of the proximal descending aorta in type B acute aortic dissection can predict late aortic events. *J Thorac Cardiovasc Surg* 2007 Nov; **134** (5): 1163–70.

28. Akutsu K, Nejima J, Kiuchi K, *et al.* Effects of the patent false lumen on the long-term outcome of type B acute aortic dissection. *Eur J Cardio-Thorac Surg* 2004; **26** (2): 359–66.

29. Conrad MF, Crawford RS, Kwolek CJ, *et al.* Aortic remodeling after endovascular repair of acute complicated type B aortic dissection. *J Vasc Surg* 2009; **50** (3): 510–7.

30. Lombardi JV, Cambria RP, Nienaber CA, *et al.* Prospective multicenter clinical trial (STABLE) on the endovascular treatment of complicated type B aortic dissection using a composite device design. *J Vasc Surg* 2012; **55** (3): 629–40.e2.

31. Jonker FHW, Trimarchi S, Rampoldi V, *et al.* Aortic expansion after acute type B aortic dissection. *Ann Thorac Surg* 2012; **94** (4): 1223–9.

32. Evangelista A, Salas A, Ribera A, *et al.* Long-term outcome of aortic dissection with patent false lumen: predictive role of entry tear size and location. *Circulation* 2012 Jun 26; **125** (25): 3133–41.

33. Sueyoshi E, Sakamoto I, Uetani M. Growth rate of affected aorta in patients with type B partially closed aortic dissection. *Ann Thorac Surg* 2009; **88** (4): 1251–7.

34. Tolenaar JL, van Keulen JW, Trimarchi S, *et al.* Number of entry tears is associated with aortic growth in type B dissections. *Ann Thorac Surg* 2013; **96** (1): 39–42.

Aortic remodelling after standard TEVAR in chronic type B dissection

AV Kamman, JA van Herwaarden, FL Moll
and S Trimarchi

Introduction

Thoracic endovascular aortic repair (TEVAR) is currently the standard of care for complicated acute and subacute type B aortic dissections.[1] For uncomplicated cases, optimal medical therapy is associated with satisfactory short-term results; in-hospital mortality is reported to be up to 13% within the first week of hospitalisation.[2] However, up to 20–50% of these uncomplicated patients require invasive treatment during follow-up after developing complications.[3–5] These complications sometimes include malperfusion, but more frequently include aneurysmal degeneration and rapid aortic enlargement.[4]

For chronic type B dissections, the optimal management strategy is unknown. This is mainly due to a lack of randomised trials that compare treatment modalities, such as open surgical repair, standard TEVAR or branched/fenestrated TEVAR.[1] Open surgical repair is associated with greater operative risks compared with other approaches but is rarely affected by anatomical restraints. Furthermore, it has the benefit of the diseased sections of the aorta being excised (Figure 1). While TEVAR is a less invasive intervention than open repair, it is not suitable for all patients.

Under a new temporal classification, "chronic" dissections are now described as those that present more than three months after the onset of symptoms. Previously, a dissection was labelled as chronic if it presented more than two weeks after the onset of symptoms.[6,7] This change in description is important for assessing remodelling after standard TEVAR for a dissection because a repair of a two-day or three-week-old dissection will have different results compared with a repair of a 12-month-old dissection in terms of false lumen thrombosis and aortic remodelling.

TEVAR for chronic type B dissections

The goal of TEVAR in aortic dissections is to cover the primary entry tear and stop perfusion of the false lumen, thereby relieving malperfusion and preventing rupture and propagation of the dissection to promote false lumen thrombosis and remodelling. If this goal is attained, progressive enlargement of the aorta is halted and, therefore, the risk of aortic rupture is reduced. In the acute phase, the true lumen is usually compressed (either dynamically or statically); but in the

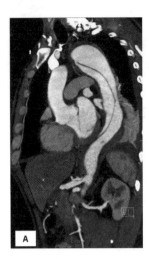 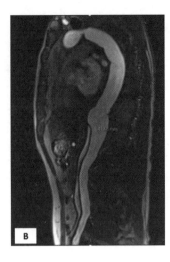

Figure 1: Chest computed tomography (CT); sagittal views. Chronic type B aortic dissection (A) before and (B) after surgical excision of dissected thoracic aorta from the left hemiarch to the mid descending thoracic aorta.

chronic phase, true lumen is usually small due to a chronic compression (Figure 2). Moreover, scarring and thickening of the intimal flap occurs and this makes true lumen expansion and aortic remodelling after TEVAR more challenging compared with after TEVAR in the acute phase.[1]

Because of these stiff and narrow lumens, endovascular repair is not always possible and factors such as short landing zones, involvement of the visceral vessels and important angulation of the aorta could further inhibit its use. Therefore, open surgical repair is still an important method of treating these chronic cases; in particular, younger patients and those affected by connective tissue disorders.

Experiences with TEVAR for chronic dissections have been frequently reported. The INSTEAD (Investigation of stent grafts in aortic dissection) trial showed no survival benefit of TEVAR compared with optimal medical therapy in uncomplicated subacute and chronic patients after up to two years of follow-up.[8] However, at the five-year follow-up point, TEVAR was associated with an improved aorta-related mortality compared with medical therapy alone.[9] It should be noted that this study was underpowered and sponsored, which needs to be considered when interpreting the results.

In a recent multicentre study from China, patients with chronic dissections undergoing TEVAR had lower aorta-related mortality compared with those treated with medical therapy alone. However, they did not have improved all-cause survival or a lower rate of aorta-related adverse events during follow-up.[10]

Aortic remodelling in chronic type B aortic dissections

The "old" definition of chronic dissection is frequently used in studies reporting aortic remodelling after TEVAR. This is important because some of these patients are consequently treated in the subacute phase, which seems the most appropriate timing for TEVAR in acute type B aortic dissections.[11] Therefore, in this patient cohort, remodelling rates may be higher compared with truly chronic patients.

One of the other issues that arise when assessing remodelling after TEVAR is the variety of terminology that is used. This can include "true and false lumen", "volume or diameter change", "false lumen status" (complete, partial or no thrombosis) or "aortic remodelling" in general. A recent systematic review stated

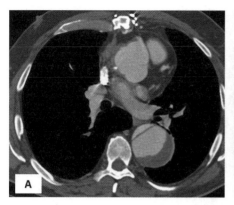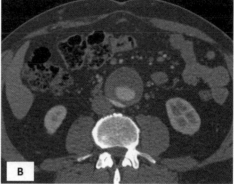

Figure 2: Chest CT; axial views. Chronic type B aortic dissection. (A) Partial false lumen thrombosis determining compression of true lumen of mid descending thoracic aorta and (B) more evident true lumen compression at the level of abdominal aorta, associated with subtotal false lumen thrombosis.

that great heterogeneity was present in reporting standards for aortic remodelling after TEVAR in chronic type B dissections.[12] For example, some authors mentioned false lumen status in the aortic sections adjacent to the stent graft, but others report the status of the entire false lumen. Another primary outcome to assess is the patency of the distal aortic segment because the segments below the diaphragm may still be patent and show growth over time.

Expansion of the true lumen and decrease of the false lumen after TEVAR for chronic dissections is often reported (Figure 3).[13–17] Andacheh *et al* showed an increase in true lumen volume of 38%, 46%, 71% and 114% at one-, three-, six- and 12-month follow-up, respectively. But, the false lumen volume decreased by -65%, -68%, -84% and -84%.[13] Song *et al* reported a general decrease of the thoracic aortic volume of 9% and 22% at one and twelve months.[17] Another study showed a decrease of the size of the false lumen in 26% of the patients.[15] A further recent case series demonstrated aneurysm shrinkage or stabilisation in 65% of cases.[16] A systematic review of several of these studies identified false lumen expansion in 15% and true lumen expansion in 66%, with a median follow-up of 30 months.[12]

Another outcome parameter after TEVAR is the aortic diameter. A study showed that true lumen increased by up to 10% during follow-up while false lumen diameter decreased by a maximum of 30%.[13] Interestingly, in this study, in patients with infrarenal dissection involvement, an increase of the infrarenal diameter was noted in up to 17%.[13] Kang *et al* showed a decrease of the maximal aortic diameter during follow-up, and this was the same for limited and extensive dissections. However, in extensive dissections, abdominal aortic diameters increased significantly. Furthermore, in 15% of patients, an increase of aortic diameter in the stented section has been also reported.[18] Reduction of the false lumen diameter was seen in 80% of patients in a recent systematic review.[12] Overall, the maximum diameter of the aorta expanded in 3%, reduction was seen in 18%, and no change in 13%.[12]

Complete false lumen thrombosis during follow-up of the entire lumen has been described as ranging from as low as 5% to as high as 89%.[14,16,18–21] Kang *et al* observed complete thrombosis of the entire false lumen in 39% of patients, and

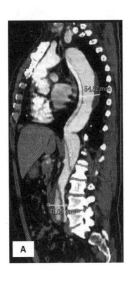 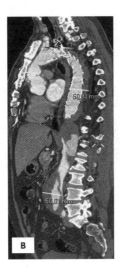

Figure 3: Chest CT; sagittal views. Aortic remodelling after TEVAR for chronic type B aortic dissection. Comparison of aortic diameters (A) before and (B) after TEVAR. The stented portion of dissected aorta shows reduction of total aortic diameter. In the not-stented abdominal aorta, there is an expansion of false lumen with increase of total aortic diameter.

this was mostly in limited dissections compared to extensive dissections (78% vs. 13%). Furthermore, this thrombosis was more frequently seen in proximal and mid-thoracic aorta.[18] Most of the patients without complete false lumen thrombosis had involvement of the visceral arteries.[16]

Complete false lumen thrombosis rates can be between 39% and 100%,[12] and has been reported to be 45% at one-year follow-up and 50% after two years.[22] The rates for partial false lumen thrombosis were 55% and 50%, respectively.[22] Additionally, complete thrombosis of the false lumen at the stented section has been seen in 64% within one month and 100% after 12 months of follow-up.[17] Whereas in two other studies described, thrombosis at the stented sections ranged between 25% and 86%.[20,23]

Aortic remodelling is associated with a similar wide range of results. During follow-up, observed rates of complete aortic remodelling were between 5% and 89%.[10,14,15,19,24,25] Czerny et al, with a remodelling rate of 35%, observed incomplete remodelling and continued perfusion of the false lumen at the abdominal level in 43% of patients.[14] Another experience reported that all of the abdominal false lumens were patent, even though complete resolution of the thoracic false lumen was achieved in 75% of cases.[15] Similarly, 95% of patients in another study showed partial remodelling or distal reperfusion.[19] Chen et al reported 93% of complete false lumen thrombosis and evidence of remodelling within six months, in both the true and false lumen.[26] Likewise, 87% of patients with imaging beyond six months showed remodelling in the region of the previous aneurysm in a different case series.[27]

The VIRTUE trial showed that in the chronic group, the true lumen increased over time and the false lumen decreased. The false lumen area change was less significant in the chronic patients compared with the acute, showing both reduction and increase in false lumen area at different time points and anatomical areas. In terms of remodelling, an overall increase of false lumen area was observed. It is of interest to note that there was no difference in false lumen thrombosis rates between the acute and chronic patients in the proximal section of the aorta up to the diaphragm, but in the segment between the diaphragm and coeliac axis, chronic patients showed significantly lower false lumen thrombosis rates.[11]

Long-term results of the INSTEAD (Investigation of stent grafts in aortic dissection) trial showed that morphological results were significantly improved by TEVAR. Expansion of the true lumen was seen, as well as reduction of the false lumen diameter up to five years of follow-up. Complete false lumen thrombosis was seen in 90% of patients at the thoracic level, with evidence of remodelling in 80% after five years. Medical therapy was associated with expansion of the maximum aortic diameter and false lumen thrombosis and remodelling was hardly noticed. During follow-up, about 16% of patients who were on optimal medical therapy required a crossover to TEVAR because of adverse events.[9]

Conclusion

TEVAR for chronic aortic dissections can promote remodelling of the diseased aorta. However, reporting standards for aortic remodelling are not homogeneous, making the comparison between studies difficult and contributing to the wide range of results. Furthermore, it is important to note continued perfusion of the distal aortic segments after TEVAR for chronic dissections is often described. Possibly, a longer section of the aorta needs to be stented, which poses a problem with the current standard stent grafts because they are not designed to cover also the visceral segments. Therefore, the long-term results of dedicated branched and fenestrated devices are highly anticipated. Until then, the choice between open or endovascular repair should be a patient-specific decision and should be based on anatomy of the dissection, extension of the dissection, as well as on the condition of the patient.

Summary

- The optimal treatment strategy for chronic type B aortic dissections, open surgical repair or standard TEVAR, is unknown.

- TEVAR in the chronic phase poses several technical difficulties due to scarring/thickening of the intimal flap and chronically compressed true lumens.

- False lumen thrombosis and aortic remodelling can be achieved after TEVAR for chronic type B aortic dissections.

- Reporting standards of aortic remodelling differ greatly within the literature, making it hard to present clear data and contribute to a wide range of results.

- Patency of the distal aortic segments is often seen after TEVAR for chronic type B dissections, even when remodelling in the false lumen of the stented segments is observed.

- Stenting a longer section of the aorta may be necessary in chronic type B aortic dissection patients. Branched and fenestrated devices could be the solution, and long-term results are highly anticipated.

References

1. Erbel R, Aboyans V, Boileau C, et al. 2014 ESC Guidelines on the diagnosis and treatment of aortic diseases: Document covering acute and chronic aortic diseases of the thoracic and abdominal aorta of the adult. The Task Force for the Diagnosis and Treatment of Aortic Diseases of the European Society of Cardiology (ESC). Eur Heart J 2014; **35** (41): 2873–926.

2. Tsai TT, Trimarchi S, Nienaber CA. Acute aortic dissection: perspectives from the International Registry of Acute Aortic Dissection (IRAD). *Eur J Vasc Endovasc Surg* 2009; **37**: 149–59.

3. Dialetto G, Covino FE, Scognamiglio G, *et al.* Treatment of type B aortic dissection: endoluminal repair or conventional medical therapy? *Eur J Cardiothorac Surg* 2005; **27**: 826–30.

4. Moulakakis KG, Mylonas SN, Dalainas I, *et al.* Management of complicated and uncomplicated acute type B dissection. A systematic review and meta-analysis. *Ann Cardiothorac Surg* 2014; **3** (3): 234–46.

5. Qin YL, Deng G, Li TX, *et al.* Treatment of acute type-B aortic dissection: thoracic endovascular aortic repair or medical management alone? *JACC Cardiovasc Interv* 2013; **6**: 185–91.

6. Booher AM, Isselbacher EM, Nienaber CA, *et al.* The IRAD classification system for characterizing survival after aortic dissection. *Am J Med* 2013; **126**: 730, e19–24.

7. Dake MD, Thompson M, van Sambeek M, *et al,* Investigators D. DISSECT: a new mnemonic-based approach to the categorization of aortic dissection. *Eur J Vasc Endovasc Surg* 2013; **46**: 175–90.

8. Nienaber CA, Rousseau H, Eggebrecht H, *et al.* Randomized comparison of strategies for type B aortic dissection: the INvestigation of STEnt Grafts in Aortic Dissection (INSTEAD) trial. *Circulation* 2009; **120**: 2519–28.

9. Nienaber CA, Kische S, Rousseau H, *et al.* Endovascular repair of type B aortic dissection: long-term results of the randomized investigation of stent grafts in aortic dissection trial. *Circ Cardiovasc Interv* 2013; **6**: 407–16.

10. Jia X, Guo W, Li TX, *et al.* The results of stent graft *versus* medication therapy for chronic type B dissection. *J Vasc Surg* 2013; **57**: 406–14.

11. Investigators VR. Mid-term outcomes and aortic remodelling after thoracic endovascular repair for acute, subacute, and chronic aortic dissection: the VIRTUE Registry. *Eur J Vasc Endovasc Surg* 2014; **48**: 363–71.

12. Thrumurthy SG, Karthikesalingam A, Patterson BO, *et al.* A systematic review of mid-term outcomes of thoracic endovascular repair (TEVAR) of chronic type B aortic dissection. *Eur J Vasc Endovasc Surg* 2011; **42**: 632–47.

13. Andacheh ID, Donayre C, Othman F, *et al.* Patient outcomes and thoracic aortic volume and morphologic changes following thoracic endovascular aortic repair in patients with complicated chronic type B aortic dissection. *J Vasc Surg* 2012; **56**: 644–50.

14. Czerny M, Roedler S, Fakhimi S, *et al.* Midterm results of thoracic endovascular aortic repair in patients with aneurysms involving the descending aorta originating from chronic type B dissections. *Ann Thorac Surg* 2010; **90**: 90–94.

15. Kim U, Hong SJ, Kim J, *et al.* Intermediate to long-term outcomes of endoluminal stent-graft repair in patients with chronic type B aortic dissection. *J Endovasc Ther* 2009; **16**: 42–47.

16. Scali ST, Feezor RJ, Chang CK, *et al.* Efficacy of thoracic endovascular stent repair for chronic type B aortic dissection with aneurysmal degeneration. *J Vasc Surg* 2013; **58**: 10–17 e1.

17. Song TK, Donayre CE, Walot I, *et al.* Endograft exclusion of acute and chronic descending thoracic aortic dissections. *J Vasc Surg* 2006; **43**: 247–58.

18. Kang WC, Greenberg RK, Mastracci TM, *et al.* Endovascular repair of complicated chronic distal aortic dissections: intermediate outcomes and complications. *J Thorac Cardiovasc Surg* 2011; **142**: 1074–83.

19. Oberhuber A, Winkle P, Schelzig H, *et al.* Technical and clinical success after endovascular therapy for chronic type B aortic dissections. *J Vasc Surg* 2011; **54**: 1303–09.

20. van Bogerijen GH, Patel HJ, Williams DM, *et al.* Propensity adjusted analysis of open and endovascular thoracic aortic repair for chronic type B dissection: a twenty-year evaluation. *Ann Thorac Surg* 2015; **99**: 1260–06.

21. Yang CP, Hsu CP, Chen WY, *et al.* Aortic remodeling after endovascular repair with stainless steel-based stent graft in acute and chronic type B aortic dissection. *J Vasc Surg* 2012; **55**: 1600–10.

22. Guangqi C, Xiaoxi L, Wei C, *et al.* Endovascular repair of Stanford type B aortic dissection: early and mid-term outcomes of 121 cases. *Eur J Vasc Endovasc Surg* 2009; **38**: 422–26.

23. Czerny M, Zimpfer D, Rodler S, *et al.* Endovascular stent-graft placement of aneurysms involving the descending aorta originating from chronic type B dissections. *Ann Thorac Surg* 2007; **83**: 1635–39.

24. Kitamura T, Torii S, Oka N, *et al.* Key success factors for thoracic endovascular aortic repair for non-acute Stanford type B aortic dissection. *Eur J Cardiothorac Surg* 2014; **46**: 432–37.

25. Shimono T, Kato N, Yasuda F, *et al.* Transluminal stent-graft placements for the treatments of acute onset and chronic aortic dissections. *Circulation* 2002; **106** (12 Suppl 1): I241–47.

26. Chen SL, Zhu JC, Li XB, *et al.* Comparison of long-term clinical outcome between patients with chronic *versus* acute type B aortic dissection treated by implantation of a stent graft: a single-center report. *Patient Preference and Adherence* 2013; **7**: 319–27.

27. Parsa CJ, Williams JB, Bhattacharya SD, *et al.* Midterm results with thoracic endovascular aortic repair for chronic type B aortic dissection with associated aneurysm. *J Thorac Cardiovasc Surg* 2011; **141**: 322–27.

Retrospective analysis of chronic type B dissection intervention— future prediction of intervention defined

D Böckler, M Ante and MS Bischoff

Introduction

Patients with aortic type B dissections present to physicians on a daily basis in different ways: complicated or uncomplicated acute type B or chronic type B dissection, either primary classic or residual after prior type A dissection. Although thoracic endovascular aortic repair (TEVAR) is a valuable treatment option for complicated aortic dissection both in the acute and chronic setting, controversy has existed for years regarding the management of acute and subacute uncomplicated type B aortic dissections.[1-4] Unstable false lumen and branch artery obstruction are important causes of early death. According to current guidelines,[5-7] best medical therapy remains the recommended standard treatment modality for uncomplicated type B dissections. Intervention is, therefore, reserved for patients who present with complications such as malperfusion or aortic rupture. Despite the initial success of best medical therapy in the acute management of type B dissections, long-term complications from aortic degeneration, disease progression and aortic-related mortality remain of concern. Some studies indicate that 20–50% of patients with uncomplicated type B aortic dissection will require future intervention.[8,9] Estimated rupture rates rise to 30% once the aortic diameter expands 6cm, and mortality is considered to be 20–40% at five years.[10-13]

The importance of clinical factors such as refractory pain and uncontrollable hypertension in the setting of acute type B aortic dissection is well known to be associated with increased in-hospital mortality.[11] Furthermore, the identification of imaging predictors of poor prognosis is potentially very helpful to select patients in whom a more aggressive management may be beneficial. Current tasks of preoperative imaging are to identify impending rupture and arterial compromise, and to detect vulnerable anatomy, anticipating complications.

This chapter focuses on factors predicting late aortic events in patients treated conservatively for acute type B dissections, based on initial preoperative imaging.

Furthermore, a comprehensive summary of published trials and current treatment algorithms are given.

Results with TEVAR *versus* best medical therapy

Currently, there are only two prospective randomised trials on uncomplicated dissection: ADSORB (Acute dissection treatment with stent graft or best medical therapy) for acute dissections and INSTEAD (Investigation of stent grafts in aortic dissection) for dissections between 14 days and one year (chronic).

ADSORB is the only randomised trial on acute type B dissection. This European study comparing the use of TEVAR with Gore's TAG thoracic endoprosthesis in addition to best medical therapy *versus* best medical therapy alone, enrolled 61 patients (31 in the best medical therapy alone group and 30 in the TEVAR plus best medical therapy group) and excluded patients with malperfusion or rupture.[12] During the first 30 days, no deaths occurred in either group but there were three crossovers from best medical therapy to TEVAR (all due to progression of disease within one week). Incomplete false lumen thrombosis was found in 13 (43%) TEVAR patients and in 30 (97%) best medical therapy cases (p<0.001). The false lumen reduced and true lumen increased in size in the TEVAR group (p<0.001). In conclusion, uncomplicated aortic dissection can be safely treated with the TAG device. Remodelling with thrombosis of the false lumen and reduction of its diameter is induced by the stent graft, but long-term results are needed.

The INSTEAD trial was published in 2009 and enrolled 136 patients with type B chronic dissection. It failed to show an improvement regarding two-year survival and a reduction in adverse event rates with TEVAR, but did show that stent graft repair was associated with expansion of true lumen (which was not seen in the conservative group). Furthermore, it found that stent graft repair was associated with lower all-cause and aortic-related mortality than best medical treatment alone at five years.[10]

The INSTEAD-XL trial showed improved five-year aortic-related survival and delayed disease progression. The risk of all-cause mortality (11.1% *versus* 19.3%; p=0.13), aorta-specific mortality (6.9% *versus* 19.3%; p=0.04), and progression (27.0% *versus* 46.1%; p=0.04) after five years was lower with TEVAR than with best medical therapy alone. Results showed a benefit of TEVAR with regard to

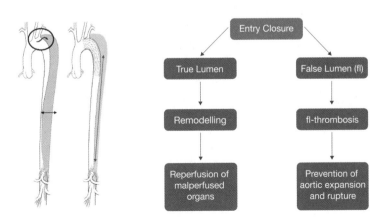

Figure 1: Treatment goals for TEVAR in aortic type B dissection.

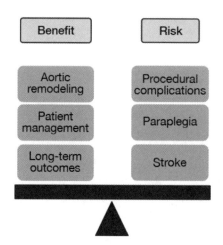

Figure 2: Benefit/risk evaluation of endovascular interventional treatment in aortic type B dissection

all-cause mortality (0% vs. 16.9%; p=0.0003), aorta-specific mortality (0% vs. 16.9%; p=0.0005), and disease progression (4.1% vs. 28.1%; p=0.004) between two and five years. Following TEVAR, 90.6% of patients had stent graft induced false lumen thrombosis (p<0.0001). The conclusion of the trialists was that TEVAR was recommended in stable cases of type B dissection with suitable anatomy in addition to best medical therapy.[13]

Current treatment paradigm of acute type B aortic dissections

The aim of treating acute type B aortic dissections is to maintain or restore perfusion of the vital organs and to prevent progression of the dissection and/or aortic rupture (Figure 1). Therefore, it is important to make a detailed risk assessment at an early stage to determine the merits of medical, endovascular or surgical intervention. In the acute setting, patients may present with clinical conditions characterised by absence of complications in almost 50% of cases.[14] Despite initial stable conditions, these patients may suffer from in-hospital mortality of up to 10%.[15] In the presence of complications such as visceral, renal and limb ischaemia and/or aortic rupture, mortality rises to 20% by day two and 25% by day 30. According to current guidelines, endovascular repair should be considered as a first interventional option for complicated acute type B aortic dissection (Class IIA; Level B).[7]

Although TEVAR results are promising, the procedure-related complications can be devastating and may require open correction/reintervention.[16] Stroke is reported to occur in 3–10% due to the manipulation of catheters in the arch and ascending aorta and is more common in patients with severe arch atheroma.[17] Although rare in acute type B aortic dissection patients, spinal cord ischaemia has shown to be related to the extent of aortic coverage, previous aortic surgery and hypotension at presentation. Arm ischaemia, paraparesis or paraplegia may occur from branch vessel occlusion. In the case of left subclavian artery over-stenting, left subclavian artery revascularisation can prevent stroke, paraplegia and death. Therefore, it is recommended in stable patients.[5]

Retrograde type A dissection has been reported to occur in less than 2% of patients but is associated with poor outcome. The risk is increased with balloon

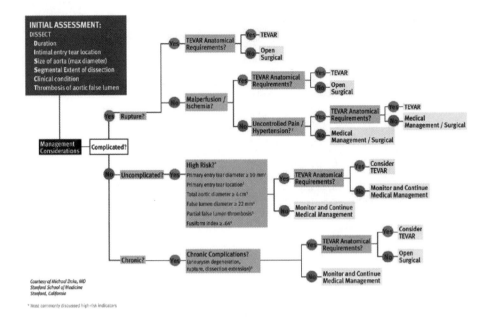

Figure 3: Treatment algorithm for patients with aortic dissection, proposed by Michael Dake and DEFINE Investigators.[19]

dilation, proximal bare stents and rigid non-compliant devices.[18] Given these complications and the fact that there is no robust evidence about the superiority of TEVAR over best medical therapy for acute uncomplicated and asymptomatic type B dissections, a careful balance of benefits and risks is necessary when making decisions in clinical practice (Figure 2). Specifically in asymptomatic patients with uncomplicated type B dissections, it is crucial to evaluate the potential advantage of an interventional treatment preventing early and late aortic-related complications. This so-far unpredictable benefit has to be balanced with the TEVAR-associated risks or even open surgery. Morphological classification of type B dissections (DeBakey and Stanford) were developed more than 40 years ago and represented the foundation for clinical decision over decades. These traditional classification schemes may potentially be outdated today, as endovascular techniques are more frequently used, even as the first-choice modality.

The "DISSECT" classification (Figure 3) is a new mnemonic-based categorisation of aortic dissections. Published by Dake M *et al,*[19] the algorithm may provide a more specific and reproducible approach to future management of aortic type B dissections.

Literature-based predictors for progression of acute type B dissection

The following "high-risk" predictors—primary entry tear diameter >10mm, primary entry tear location, total aortic diameter >40mm, false lumen diameter >22mm, partial false lumen thrombosis, and fusiform index >0.64 for late aortic events in patients with type B acute aortic dissection—are reported in the literature. All authors conclude that patients fulfilling one or more of these predictors predictors should undergo early intervention, or at least very close follow-up.

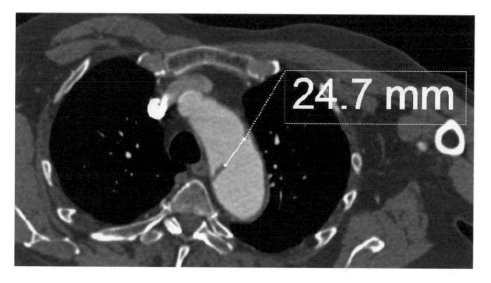

Figure 4: Axial view of a CT scan demonstrating a large proximal primary entry.

Evangelista *et al* demonstrated that patients, besides those presenting with persistent patent false lumen and Marfan syndrome, who have a large entry tear (Figure 4) located in the proximal part of the dissection are a high-risk subgroup that may benefit from earlier and more aggressive therapy. The proposed optimal cut-off value of entry size for prediction of aortic complications was >10mm (hazard ratio [HR] 5.8; p>0.001).[20]

Loewe *et al* identified a new high-risk subgroup of a total of 65 patients with the primary entry tear at the concavity of the distal aortic arch. There was a significant difference with regard to the incidence of primary complications of type B dissections (convexity 21% vs. concavity 61%; p=0.003) and time of appearance (convexity 9 days vs. concavity 0 days; p=0.02). Concavity was the only predictor of primary and secondary complications after acute type B aortic dissection (HR 1.8. 95% confidence interval [CI] 1.0–3.2).[21] Similar observations were reported by others.[22]

In 1995, Kato *et al* performed an univariate and multivariate factor analysis in order to determine the predominant predictors for chronic-phase enlargement (≥60mm) of the dissected aorta.[23] The predominant predictors for aortic enlargement in the chronic phase were the existence of a maximum aortic diameter of >40 mm during the acute phase (p<0.001) and a patent primary entry site in the thoracic aorta (p=0.001). The values of actuarial freedom from aortic enlargement for the patients with a large aortic diameter (≥40mm) during the acute phase and a patent primary entry site in the thoracic aorta at one, three, and five years were 70%, 29% and 22%, respectively. No aortic enlargement was observed in the other patients throughout the entire follow-up period. These data suggest that patients with acute type B dissection who have a large aortic diameter (≥40mm) and a patent primary entry site in the thorax should be treated early (at that time surgically) during the acute phase. The same predictors (maximum aortic diameter >40mm) were confirmed by other groups.[24–26] In addition, cox regression analysis showed that the presence of ulcer-like projections (p=0.016) was a predictor for late aortic events.

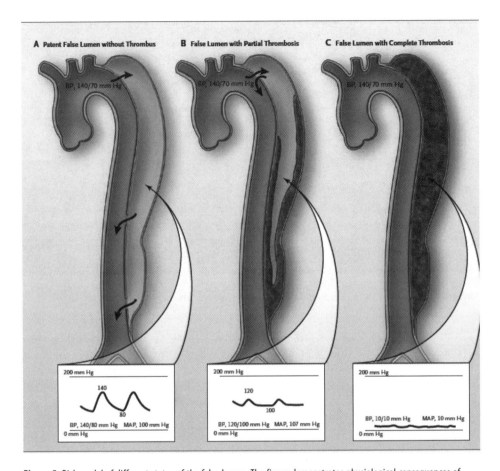

Figure 5: Risk model of different status of the false lumen. The figure demonstrates physiological consequences of false-lumen patency or thrombosis[29]

Song and colleagues concluded that a large false lumen diameter >22mm at the upper descending thoracic aorta on the initial computed tomography (CT) scan predicts late aneurysm dilatation and adverse outcome, warranting early intervention in this group of patients (p<0.001). Aneurysmal dilatation occurred in 28% with highest growth rates in the upper descending aorta of 3.43+3.66mm/ year. In addition, Marfan syndrome and maximum diameter in the mid descending thoracic aorta were independent predictors.[27]

The influence of false lumen status including partial false lumen thrombosis was investigated by two groups. Tanaka et al demonstrated that the need for intervention was higher in patients with patent false lumen but did not alter long-term mortality. Intervention (surgical or interventional) was required in 0% of patients with complete thrombosis, 16% with partial thrombosis and 26% with patent false lumen.[28]

In contrast, Tsai TT et al demonstrated that partial thrombosis of the false lumen, as compared with complete patency, is a significant independent predictor for post-discharge mortality (HR 2.69 95%, CI 1.45-4.98; p=0.002)—three-year mortality for patients with a patent false lumen was 13.7+7.1%; 31.6+12.4% for those with partial thrombosis; and 22.6+22.6% for those with complete thrombosis (median follow-up 2.8 years; p=0.003).[29]

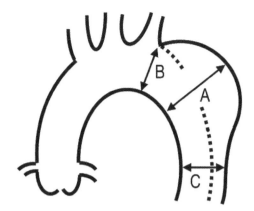

Figure 6: Definition and calculation of the fusiform index

Fusiform index (FI) = A / (B +C)

This is explained by obstructed re-entry tears causing a blind sac, leading to elevated mean and diastolic blood pressure levels (Figure 5). Bernhard Y *et al* had already shown in 2001 that patency of the aorta false lumen within the descending aorta is responsible for progressive aortic dilation.[30]

Marui *et al* developed the "fusiform index", which expresses the degree of fusiform dilatation of the proximal descending aorta during the acute phase of aortic type B dissection (Figure 6). The authors investigated whether late aortic events can be predicted on the basis of index. The fusiform index is calculated by: maximum diameter of the proximal descending aorta at the pulmonary level divided by the diameter of the distal arch plus the diameter of the descending aorta at the pulmonary level. A fusiform index value of >0.64 was considered to be the threshold for late aortic events.[31]

Further evidence identifying another high-risk patient subgroup was recently published. Lavingia *et al* concluded in a five-year retrospective single centre study on 164 uncomplicated type B patients that volumetric analysis of the initial index CT scan is able to predict growth. The natural history of uncomplicated type B dissection and need for future intervention.[32] A true lumen volume/false lumen volume ratio <0.8 was highly predictive for requiring an intervention (sensitivity 69%, specificity 84%, positive predictive value 71%, negative predictive value 81%, odds ratio 12.2, 95% CI 5-26; p<0.001).

Open questions

Despite increasing evidence, there remain debatable questions in patients classified as high-risk by imaging who might benefit from early intervention.

- Is the closure of the primary entry site alone sufficient to induce aortic remodeling or is there a need for extended aortic coverage using multiple devices?
- What is the ideal stent graft to conform to the challenging anatomy of aortic dissections? Preliminary analyses were published recently but need further investigation.[33]

- What is the optimal timing for intervention to achieve complete aortic remodelling in TEVAR? A newly published article revealed different outcomes in those patients receiving TEVAR between two weeks and three months, indicating that this time period could be defined as subacute instead of chronic.[34]
- What is the optimal follow-up schedule for both, conservatively and interventionally treated patients?
- Is CT scanning or magnetic resonance imaging (MRI) angiography (including MRI elastography or 4D-MRI the best modality?[35]

Conclusion

In current clinical practice, endovascular therapy is increasingly considered as an alternative to medical management in selected cases of acute uncomplicated type B dissection. Several groups identified predictive factors based on imaging and were consequently able to define high risk subgroups of patients who may benefit from earlier and more aggressive therapy. Further retrospective and prospective studies are needed in order to fully understand and confirm independent predictors of adverse outcome. The use of a new system for categorisation of aortic dissection (DISSECT) implements those predictors in order to support management decisions based on these specific features of aortic disease progression.

Summary

- ADSORB and INSTEAD trials are the only randomised trials addressing acute and subacute aortic type B dissection.

- Guidelines still recommend surveillance and best medical therapy in the management of acute uncomplicated type B aortic dissections.

- Despite current guidelines there is a trend towards early intervention in subgroups of patients considered to be at higher risk.

- Imaging-based predictors for acute and late adverse events are published in retrospective single centre series.

- These imaging-based predictors are implemented in a new categorisation scheme titled as DISSECT.

- Future studies in larger patient cohorts are needed to confirm reproducibility of these predictors.

- Correct timing, simultaneous or staged TEVAR and post-interventional follow-up schemes remain open for debate and investigation.

References

1. Dake MD, Miller DC, Mitchell RS, *et al.* The 'first generation' of endovascular stent-grafts for patients with aneurysms of the descending thoracic aorta. *J Thorac Cardiovasc Surg* 1998; **116**: 689–704
2. Nienaber CA1, Fattori R, Lund G, *et al.* Nonsurgical reconstruction of thoracic aortic dissection by stent-graft placement. *N Engl J Med* 1999 20; **340** (20):1539–45
3. Umana JP, Lai DT, Mitchell RS, *et al.* Is medical therapy still the optimal treatment strategy for patients with acute type B aortic dissections? *J Thorac Cardiovasc Surg* 2002; **124**: 896–10.

4. Böckler D, Hyhlik-Dürr A, Hakimi M, *et al.* Type B aortic dissections: treating the many to benefit the few? *J Endovasc Ther* 2009; **16** (Suppl 1): I80–89.

5. Hiratzka LF, Bakris GL, Beckman JA, *et al.* 2010 ACCF/AHA/AATS/ACR/ASA/SCA/SCAI/SIR/STS/SVM guidelines for the diagnosis and management of patients with thoracic aortic disease. *Circulation* 2010; **121**: 266–69.

6. Svensson LG, Kouchoukos NT, Miller DC, *et al.* Society of Thoracic *Surgeons* Endovascular Surgery Task Force. Expert consensus document on the treatment of descending thoracic aortic disease using endovascular stent-grafts. *Ann Thorac Surg* 2008; **85** (1 Suppl): S1–41.

7. Riambau R, Böckler D, Brunkwall J, *et al.* Management of Descending Thoracic Aorta Diseases. Clinical Practice Guidelines of the European Society for Vascular Surgery. In press.

8. Fattori R, Tsai TT, Myrmel T, *et al.* Complicated acute type B dissection: is surgery still the best option? A report from the International Registry of Acute Aortic Dissection. *JACC Cardiovasc Interv* 2008; **1**: 395–402.

9. Kusagawa H, Shimono T, Ishida M, *et al.* Changes in false lumen after transluminal stent-graft placement in aortic dissections: six years' experience. *Circulation* 2005; **111**: 2951–57.

10. Nienaber CA, Kische S, Rousseau H, *et al.* Endovascular repair of type B aortic dissection: long-term results of the randomized investigation of stent grafts in aortic dissection trial. *Circ Cardiovasc Interv* 2013; **6**: 407–16.

11. Sueyoshi E, Sakamoto I, Uetani M. Growth rate of affected aorta in patients with type B partially closed aortic dissection. *Ann Thorac Surg* 2009; **88**: 1251–57.

12. Kato M, Bai H, Sato K, *et al.* Determining surgical indications for acute type B dissection based on enlargement of aortic diameter during the chronic phase. *Circulation* 1995; **92** (Suppl): II107–12.

13. Onitsuka S, Akashi H, Tayama K, *et al.* Long-term outcome and prognostic predictors of medically treated acute type B aortic dissections. *Ann Thorac Surg* 2004; **78**: 1268–73.

14. Nienaber CA, Rousseau H, Eggebrecht H, *et al.* Randomized comparison of strategies for type B aortic dissection: the INvestigation of STEnt Grafts in Aortic Dissection (INSTEAD) trial. *Circulation* 2009; **120** (25): 2519–28.

15. Trimarchi S, Eagle KA, Nienaber CA, *et al.* Importance of refractory pain and hypertension in acute type B aortic dissection: insights from the International Registry of Acute Aortic Dissection (IRAD). *Circulation.* 2010; **122** (13): 1283–89.

16. Brunkwall J, Kasprzak P, Verhoeven E, *et al*, ADSORB Trialists. Endovascular repair of acute uncomplicated aortic type B dissection promotes aortic remodelling: 1 year results of the ADSORB trial. *Eur J Vasc Endovasc Surg* 2014; **48** (3): 285–91.

17. Nienaber CA, Kische S, Rousseau H, *et al*; INSTEAD-XL trial. Endovascular repair of type B aortic dissection: long-term results of the randomized investigation of stent grafts in aortic dissection trial. *Circulation: Cardiovascular Interventions* 2013; **6** (4): 407–16.

18. Tsai TT, Fattori R, Trimarchi S, *et al.* Long-term survival in patients presenting with type B acute aortic dissection: insights from the International Registry of Acute Aortic Dissection. *Circulation* 2006; **114**: 2226–31

19. Suzuki T, Mehta RH, Ince H, *et al.* Clinical profiles and outcomes of acute type B aortic dissection in the current era: lessons from the International Registry of Aortic Dissection (IRAD). *Circulation* 2003; **108** (Suppl 1): II312-17.

20. Böckler D, Schumacher H, Ganten M, *et al.* Complications after endovascular repair of acute symptomatic and chronic expanding Stanford type B aortic dissections. *J Thorac Cardiovasc Surg.* 2006; **132** (2): 361–68.

21. Maldonado TS, Dexter D, Rockman CB, *et al.* Left subclavian artery coverage during thoracic endovascular aortic aneurysm repair does not mandate revascularization. *J Vasc Surg* 2013; **57**: 116–24.

22. Eggebrecht H, Thompson M, Rousseau H, *et al.* European Registry on Endovascular Aortic Repair Complications. Retrograde ascending aortic dissection during or after thoracic aortic stent graft placement: insight from the European registry on endovascular aortic repair complications. *Circulation* 2009; **120** (11 Suppl): S276–81.

23. Dake MD, Thompson M, van Sambeek M, *et al.* DEFINE Investigators. DISSECT: a new mnemonic-based approach to the categorization of aortic dissection. *Eur J Vasc Endovasc Surg* 2013; **46** (2): 175–90.

24. Evangelista A, Salas A, Ribera A, *et al.* Long-term outcome of aortic dissection with patent false lumen: predictive role of entry tear size and location. *Circulation* 2012; **125** (25): 3133–41.

25. Loewe C, Czerny M, Sodeck GH, *et al.* A new mechanism by which an acute type B aortic dissection is primarily complicated, becomes complicated, or remains uncomplicated. *Annals of Thoracic Surgery* 2012; **93** (4): 1215–22.

26. Weiss G, Wolner I, Folkmann S, *et al.* The location of the primary entry tear in acute type B aortic dissection affects early outcome. *European Journal of Cardiothoracic Surgery* 2012; **42** (3): 571–76

27. Kato M, Bai H, Sato K, *et al*. Determining surgical indications for acute type B dissection based on enlargement of aortic diameter during the chronic phase. *Circulation* 1995; **92** (9) Supp II: 107–12.

28. Onitsuka S, Akashi H, Tayama K, *et al*. Long-term outcome and prognostic predictors of medically treated acute type B aortic dissections. *Annals Thoracic Surgery* 2004; **78** (4): 1268–73.

29. Takahashi J, Wakamatsu Y, Okude J, *et al*. Maximum aortic diameter as a simple predictor of acute type B aortic dissection. *Annals of Thoracic & Cardiovascular Surgery* 2008; **14** (5): 303–10.

30. Kudo T, Mikamo A, Kurazumi H, *et al*. Predictors of late aortic events after Stanford type B acute aortic dissection. *J Thorac Cardiovasc Surg* 2014; **148**: 98–104.

31. Song JM, Kim SD, Kim JH, *et al*. Long-term predictors of descending aorta aneurysmal change in patients with aortic dissection. Journal of the American College of Cardiology 2007; **50** (8): 799–804.

32. Tanaka A, Sakakibara M, Ishii H, *et al*. Influence of the false lumen status on clinical outcomes in patients with acute type B aortic dissection. *Journal of Vascular Surgery* 2014; **59** (2): 321–26.

33. Tsai TT, Evangelista A, Nienaber CA, *et al;* International Registry of Acute Aortic Dissection. Partial thrombosis of the false lumen in patients with acute type B aortic dissection. *New England Journal of Medicine* 2007; **357** (4): 3495–99.

34. Bernard Y, Zimmermann H, Chocron S, *et al*. False lumen patency as a predictor of late outcome in aortic dissection. *Am J Cardiol* 2001 15; **87** (12):1378–82.

35. Marui A, Mochizuki T, Koyama T, Mitsui N. Degree of fusiform dilatation of the proximal descending aorta in type B acute aortic dissection can predict late aortic events. *Journal of Thoracic & Cardiovascular Surgery* 2007; **134** (5): 1163–70.

36. Lavingia KS, Larion S, Ahanchi SS, *et al*. Volumetric analysis of the initial index computed tomography scan can predict the natural history of acute uncomplicated type B dissections. *J Vasc Surg* 2015; **62** (4): 893–99.

37. Bischoff MS, Müller-Eschner M, Meisenbacher K, et al.Device Conformability and Morphological Assessment After TEVAR for Aortic Type B Dissection: A Single-Centre Experience with a Conformable Thoracic Stent-Graft Design. *Med Sci Monit Basic Res* 2015; **21**: 262–70

38. Steuer J, Bjorck M, Mayer D, *et al*. Distinction between acute and chronic type B aortic dissection: is there a sub-acute phase? *Eur J Vasc Endovasc Surg* 2013; **45** (6): 627–31.

39. Clough RE, Zymvragoudakis VE, Biasi L, Taylor PR. Usefulness of new imaging methods for assessment of type B aortic dissection. *Ann Cardiothorac Surg* 2014; **3** (3): 314–18.

Great Debate: In chronic type B dissection, there is no place for false lumen embolisation—true lumen TEVAR is preferred—for the motion

PJ Mossop

Introduction

While placement of a proximal endograft to seal a primary entry tear reduces the risk of rupture and shorter-term expansion of the thoracic aorta, the presence of more distal re-entries is often not addressed, with further distal growth seen in about 40% of patients.[1] It is our contention that through the evolution of new approaches and technologies, the inadequacies of conventional thoracic endovascular aortic repair (TEVAR) will be overcome and that these strategies will be reconstructive techniques of the native aortic true lumen rather than false lumen based embolic therapies.

The STABLE concept

Staged total aortic and branch vessel endovascular repair (STABLE) was one of the first suggested concepts re-imagining the mechanism for dissection repair by encompassing a complete true luminal and branch reconstruction when dealing with complex dissection.[2] It addresses the intrinsic shortcomings of conventional TEVAR and, through the use of simple available stent and stent graft technology, allows repair to be extended to the abdominal segment. Therefore, it addresses the issues of residual distal re-entries, pressurisation and retrograde perfusion of the thoracic false lumen.

The technique, while using a composite approach of endograft and bare dissection stents, is unlike the subsequently described "PETTICOAT" (provisional extension to induce complete attachment) procedure,[3] which focuses on bare stent re-expansion of the collapsed true lumen rather than also using it as scaffold to allow further reconstruction of the aorta. While similar to STABLE, PETTICOAT's composite use of bare stents with proximal endograft alone is unlikely to prevent distal aortic false lumen perfusion and its consequences.

In STABLE, the stent scaffold converts the abdominal dissection lamella into a "do it yourself fenestrated endograft *in situ*". Deploying covered stents between the stented aortic true lumen and branch vessel then seals re-entries related to branch

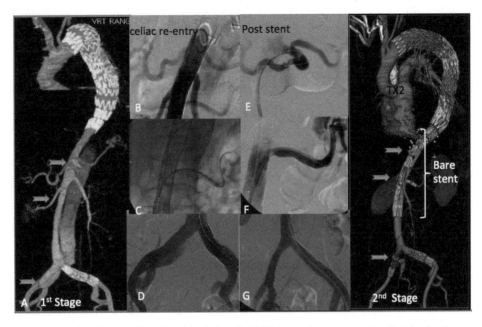

Figure 1: Staged total aortic and branch endoluminal repair; initial closure of primary entry tear (first stage) with residual coeliac, renal and iliac re-entries (A, B, C, D). After aortic dissection bare stenting to thoracoabdominal region, residual re-entries are closed (E, F, G, H) by covered (V12 and iliac branched) stents eliminating false lumen (2nd stage).

vessel ostia. Direct aortic or intra-branch re-entries are dealt with by spot endograft extension or branch graft (Figure 1).

The STABLE technique can also encompass the use of fenestrated or branched grafts, which can be deployed in conjunction with the bare stent remodelled true lumen and can be useful in eliminating direct entry tears that occur closely related to visceral branches that cannot be addressed by simple aortic extension pieces. Alternatively, as these focal entries can be closed by deployment of an Amplatzer closure device (St Jude Medical) across the intimal tear[4] or coil embolisation of the bare stent remodelled false lumen, which has a reduced volume and narrowed cross-sectional profile (Figure 2). Thus, aortic bare stenting makes embolisation technically easier and more effective.

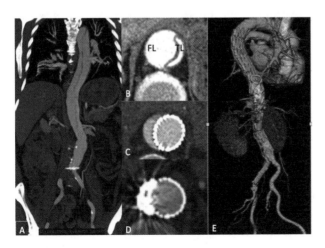

Figure 2: False lumen reduction to enhance embolisation. (A) CTA (coronal view) chronic TBAD. (B) Axial view of suprarenal aorta showing collapsed true lumen (TL). (C) Post proximal entry closure and distal dissection stent showing stent re-expansion of true lumen and reduced false lumen volume. (D) CTA (axial image) post catheter delivery of coils into false lumen at the level of peri-renal entry tear shows a compact coil mass occluding re-entry flow. 3D CTA reconstruction (E) at 3 years post embolisation showing complete false lumen reabsorption.

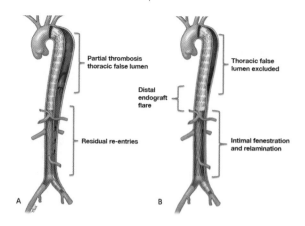

Figure 3: STABILISE. (A) Post initial repair with endograft and dissection stents. (B) Post dilation of the distal graft and bare stent segment disrupting the intimal lamella to create a uni-luminal space.

Labels in figure:
Partial thrombosis thoracic false lumen
Distal endograft flare
Residual re-entries
Thoracic false lumen excluded
Intimal fenestration and relamination
A
B

In particular, the more limited endograft coverage and staged approach using this technique was predicted to reduce overall morbidity and the risk of spinal ischaemia.[5] This coincides with our experience with no incidence of transient or permanent paresis following a STABLE procedure. A comparison of patients undergoing STABLE with a similar group undergoing TEVAR also showed STABLE to be associated with fewer late reinterventions (11% vs. 43%), no distal late aortic reintervention (0% vs. 19%), fewer late adverse events (3% vs. 10%) and lower late aortic mortality (3% vs. 9%). Aortic remodelling has also reflected aortic survival, with thoracic and abdominal aortic dimensions at long-term follow-up remaining stable.[6]

While STABLE is indicated for use in all forms of complicated dissection, our practice is now to apply it in degenerate chronic dissection involving the thoracic and abdominal aorta.

Fenestrated and branched endografts

A number of studies have recently documented encouraging outcomes of this technique for aneurysmal chronic dissection management.[7–9] Overall positive remodelling was reported with low mortality and complication rates. Although this is tempered by evidence of high reintervention rates, small patient numbers and lack of long-term follow-up, the use of fenestrated endovascular aneurysm repair is attractive. Potential drawbacks exist, including cost, availability of devices, required experience level, and procedural complexity.

As such, they may not be appropriate for some patients. In our experience, fenestrated or branched devices are used in 20–30% of chronic cases. In practice after commencing a staged reconstruction, fenestrated devices are used when issues arise. These instances include: absence or suboptimal position of an intimal fenestration in relation to its adjacent branch (making reconnection more difficult); persistent re-entry jets adjacent to major visceral origins (making their closure with simple endograft extension piece difficult); re-entries at bifurcation points (particularly the common iliac); and when aneurysm involvement of the arch or visceral segment makes branched grafting desirable.

STABILISE concept

The evolution of STABLE over the last decade has resulted in the stent and balloon-induced intimal disruption and relamination (STABILISE) concept (Figure 3,4).[10] The aim with STABILISE is to create more rapid and complete repair method for dissection, particularly where aneurysmal change of the abdominal aorta has not yet occurred. Balloon dilation of the distal endograft is performed initially to sequester the upstream thoracic false lumen. We refer this process to as "FLARE" (false lumen amputation by radial expansion) of the distal endograft. Subsequently, balloon and stent expansion causes fenestration or division along the length of the intimal flap distal to the zone of endograft coverage. Stent based re-apposition of intima to the aortic wall with creation of a uni-luminal aorta results in complete elimination of the false lumen space.

Using this approach, haemodynamic drivers of false lumen expansion (i.e. false lumen, shear flow and pressurisation) are eliminated. Furthermore, this approach appears more straightforward than other endovascular techniques and eliminates the need for embolotherapy as a means of occluding the false lumen. In our experience, this approach is applicable in at least 50% of dissections currently treated.

Early and intermediate results of this technique were initially reported in 11 patients having appropriate morphology and undergoing repair of complicated aortic dissection. There were no intraprocedural complications and no early incidence of stroke, spinal or visceral ischaemia. Median follow up was 18 months (range, four to 54 months). No late adverse events or aortic-related deaths occurred. Complete false lumen obliteration occurred in 90% of patients.[10]

The technique now has a maximum follow-up of 60 months (median 33 months) in 21 patients and is associated with an aortic specific survival of 95% (mortality due to ascending aortic anastomotic leak and unrelated to the endovascular repair). No branch vessel loss has been seen and no late aortic or branch reinterventions have occurred. Stability or positive remodelling of both the thoracic and abdominal total aortic diameters has occurred in 90% of patients.

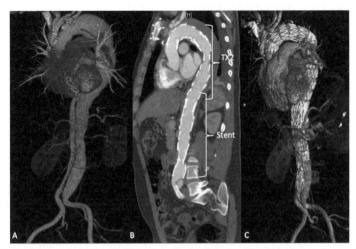

Figure 4: STABILISE. (A) CT angiography chronic type B aortic dissection (prior ascending aortic repair). (B) Post proximal TX2 endograft and distal dissection bare stenting with intimal disruption and relamination. The false lumen is thrombosed proximally and obliterated distally as shown on coronal CT angiography. (C) Follow up CT angiography at three years.

Embolisation

Embolisation for dissection can be directed at eliminating localised flow with the false lumen or more frequently directed at creating a baffle or occlusion to retrograde false lumen flow at the distal level of the previously treated thoracic aorta. Coils, glue and covered stents have been used. For the purposes of this discussion, only commercially available non-investigational devices will be considered.

Coil-based embolisation

Coil embolisation seems reasonable to further enhance false lumen thrombosis but is usually limited to a stage in treatment following elimination of all major re-entries and the development of partial thrombosis of the false lumen space. Our group published one of the first and largest of only a small number of reported series examining embolotherapy for dissection and found it efficacious for elimination of local re-entries and localised flow.[11] Overall morbidity was low and procedural success high, with stabilisation of growth in 90% of patients; however, a death occurred (due to a pressurising type II thoracic endoleak) following occlusion of the distal thoracic false lumen.

Occluder-mediated embolisation

The second approach, that of occlusion of the false lumen at the distal extent of the proximally placed endograft, potentially allows a more simple and attractive way of sealing the thoracic false lumen following initial TEVAR. Placement usually needs to be in the thoracoabdominal junction region, as other more distal abdominal re-entries usually exist.

A recent report using a variety of commercial iliac blockers demonstrated this to be relatively effective in blocking retrograde flow in chronic aneurysmal type B dissection.[12] Rate of complete thrombosis in the thoracic segment was 71% with reduction of maximal descending thoracic diameter in 62%. While encouraging, the 30-day mortality was 4.7%. It is of note that the mortality in this group occurred after closure of the thoracic false lumen space while an unrecognised residual re-entry pressurised the dissection with rupture. This parallels our own experience.

Conclusion

The inadequacy of conventional TEVAR for aortic dissection has driven consideration of other approaches including embolic solutions. However, the use of stent-based reconstructive techniques has allowed far more complete reconstruction of the dissected aorta than previously possible and, with increasing evidence, they are the primary way forward in the management of dissection. There is no doubt that embolotherapy has a place in dissection management. However, a number of potential problems exist.

With respect to coil and glue embolisation, false lumen flow and morphology may limit the stability of a coil mass and procedural success. The use of glue can be pro-inflammatory and a liquid embolic maybe potentially hazardous to the spinal circulation. Reported complications have included paresis, aortitis and aorto-oesophageal fistula.[13]

With respect to occlusive approaches, if residual re-entries exist distal to a blocked thoracic false lumen and the abdominal false lumen volume is large, alteration of flow dynamics may accelerate degeneration of the more distal abdominal segment. In this case, it is likely these re-entries would need to be eliminated longer term by more complete aortic reconstructive to prevent such degeneration. Furthermore, once distally occluded, access to the thoracic false lumen may be compromised in the event of a pressurising proximal endoleak.

Alternatively, if aneurysmal change is localised to the thoracic aorta, then complete elimination the false lumen by proximal endograft and distal (abdominal) intimal fenestration and relamination (STABILISE) is more effective.

The current evidence for any form of embolotherapy is at best limited with small heterogeneous studies, non-uniform indications, different methods and no long-term or high-level data. Additionally, some of the devices used have neither been specifically designed nor tested for use in dissection treatment. Therefore (apart from use of conventional embolic techniques for local entry flow in selected cases) clear indications for its more general use are unlikely for some time.

Summary

- Aortic dissection, in all its forms, requires a total and flexible approach using a variety of endovascular techniques to achieve the most complete repair.

- Staged stent and endograft technologies including fenestrated EVAR allow reconstruction of the entire dissection and are applicable particularly where thoracoabdominal aortic enlargement has occurred.

- In chronic dissection with thoracic aneurysm, STABILISE seals the thoracic segment while obliterating the distal false lumen creating a uni-luminal state and largely avoiding the need for further distal aortic interventions.

- A minority of treated patients may require embolotherapy as an adjunct if after true lumen reconstruction persistent re-entry flow is present. While this may be effective in eliminating false lumen perfusion, high-level data are lacking. Impact on long-term survival is unclear and occlusive devices are not specifically designed for use in dissection.

References

1. Eggebrecht H, Nienaber CA, Neuhauser M, *et al.* Endovascular stent-graft placement in aortic dissection: a meta-analysis. *Eur Heart J* 2006; **27**: 489–98.
2. Mossop PJ, McLachlan CS, Amukotuwa SA, Nixon IK. Staged endovascular treatment for complicated type B aortic dissection. *Nat Clin Pract Cardiovasc Med* 2005; **2** (6): 316–22.
3. Nienaber CA, Kische S, Zeller T, *et al.* Provisional extension to induce complete attachment after stent-graft placement in type B aortic dissection: the PETTICOAT concept. *J Endovasc Ther* 2006; **13** (6): 738–46.
4. Hu J, Yang J, Atrial septal defect occluder for the distal re-entry tear in type B aortic dissection. *Int J Cardiol* 2014; **176** (2): e70–72.
5. Hofferberth SC, Foley PT, Newcomb AE, *et al.* Combined proximal endografting with distal bare-metal stenting for management of aortic dissection. *Ann Thorac Surg* 2012; **93** (1): 95–102.
6. Hofferberth SC, Newcomb AE, Yii MY, *et al.* Combined proximal stent grafting plus distal bare metal stenting for management of aortic dissection: Superior to standard endovascular repair? *J Thorac Cardiovasc Surg* 2012; **144** (4): 956–62.
7. Oikonomou K, Kopp R, Katsargyris A, *et al.* Outcomes of fenestrated/branched endografting in post-dissection thoracoabdominal aortic aneurysms. *Eur J Vasc Endovasc Surg* 2014; **48** (6): 641–48.

8. Sobocinski J1, Spear R, Tyrrell MR, *et al.* Chronic dissection - indications for treatment with branched and fenestrated stent-grafts. *J Cardiovasc Surg* (Torino) 2014; **55** (4): 505–17

9. Kitagawa A, Greenberg RK, Eagleton MJ, *et al.* Fenestrated and branched endovascular aortic repair for chronic type B aortic dissection with thoracoabdominal aneurysms. *J Vasc Surg* 2013; **58** (3): 625–34.

10. Hofferberth SC, Nixon IK, Boston RC, *et al.* Stent-assisted balloon-induced intimal disruption and relamination in aortic dissection repair: the STABILISE concept. *J Thorac Cardiovasc Surg* 2014; **147** (4): 1240–45.

11. Hofferberth SC, Nixon IK, Mossop PJ. Aortic false lumen thrombosis induction by embolotherapy (AFTER) following endovascular repair of aortic dissection. *J Endovasc Ther* 2012; **19** (4): 538–45.

12. Idrees J, Roselli EE, Shafii S, *et al.* Outcomes after false lumen embolization with covered stent devices in chronic dissection. *J Vasc Surg* 2014; **60** (6): 1507–13.

13. Riesenman PJ, Farber MA, Mauro MA, *et al.* Aortoesophageal fistula after thoracic endovascular aortic repair and transthoracic embolization. *J Vasc Surg* 2007; **46**: 789–91.

Great Debate: In chronic type B dissection, there is no place for false lumen embolisation—true lumen TEVAR is preferred—for the motion

J Sobocinski, RE Clough, R Spear, A Hertault, T Martin-Gonzalez, R Azzaoui and S Haulon

Introduction

Thoracic endovascular aortic repair (TEVAR) is the first-line therapy for patients with acute type B aortic dissections complicated with malperfusion of aortic branches and/or aortic rupture. In such complications, the placement of at least one stent graft in the descending thoracic aorta is performed, provided that a suitable non-dissected proximal landing zone is available.[1] The placement of a stent graft in the proximal aorta redirects aortic flow towards the true lumen and thus promotes a drop of pressure in the false lumen that will partially or completely thrombose. This will improve true lumen and thus aortic branch perfusion.

Although the early outcomes of complicated type B aortic dissection are more favourable following endovascular treatment and medical management compared with medical management alone,[2,3] questions still remain regarding the mid- and long-term results of this treatment.[4] Initially successful treatment with TEVAR is not necessarily associated with favourable remodelling of the entire dissected aorta during follow-up.[5] The mechanisms involved in aortic remodelling after extensive acute aortic dissections are not yet completely understood. TEVAR may induce positive aortic remodelling, but this is usually limited to the aortic segment covered by the stent graft and frequently, the diameter of the aorta in the distal thoracic and abdominal segment will enlarge over time.[1,6,7] Extensive coverage of the thoracic aorta usually results in early thoracic aorta remodelling, at least at the level of the stent graft.[8] However, the additional risks of extensive coverage (such as spinal cord ischaemia) must be balanced against the risk of long-term aortic growth in each individual patient.[9]

In medically-treated patients with type B aortic dissection at five years from onset, up to 73% of patients face significant aortic growth that justifies secondary intervention regardless of the initial management strategy.[10] Significant dilatation of the distal aorta exposes the patient to the risk of aortic rupture and the long-term

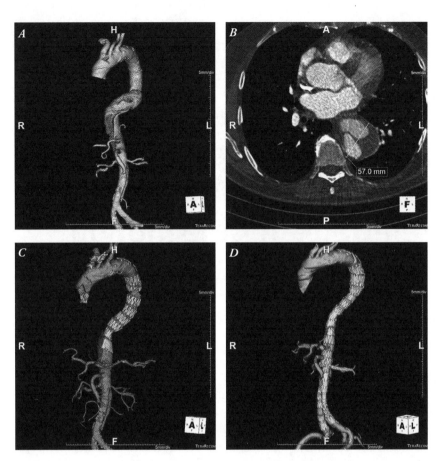

Figure 1: (A) CT-scan of a patient with chronic type b aortic dissection in 3D-VR; (B) 14 months after the onset the patient got a significant enlargement of the thoraco-abdominal aortic segment. (C) The first stage of the surgical treatment included the proximal deployment of a thoracic stent graft to exclude the proximal tear; and (D) the second stage of the treatment included the exclusion of the distal thoracic and the abdominal aorta by a fenestrated custom-made stent graft.

results from IRAD (International registry of acute aortic dissections) indicate that more than 60% of patients at five years develop aortic dilatation or aneurysm formation after TEVAR for acute type B aortic dissection.[1] When considering treated type A aortic dissection with residual dissection of the descending aorta, the rate is lower but still important with up to 49% of patients presenting with significant enlargement of the remaining native aorta during follow-up.[11] When the aortic lesion extends through the thoracoabdominal segment of the aorta, based on the experience with degenerative aneurysm, surgery is usually considered when the maximal diameter is larger than 6cm or 7cm.[12]

Technology to recreate a complete true lumen

Since the early 2000s, less invasive therapies than open surgery have been developed to treat extensive aortic aneurysmal disease, which include the use of "custom-made" fenestrated and/or branched stent grafts.[13] Recently they have been proposed as a less invasive alternative to standard open surgery when treating dissections that extend either to the aortic arch and/or through the thoracoabdominal aorta.[14]

The main challenges when treating dissection with an endovascular approach is the narrow true lumen, the fact that aortic branches may arise from the false lumen, and the absence of a proper distal sealing zone for the stent graft. The applicability of this technique requires suitable aortic morphology including an adequate proximal sealing zone. No compromise can be accepted in this sealing zone and meticulous preoperative analysis is required to evaluate it. It should be longer than 25mm in a non-angulated and non-diseased aortic segment. The preferred strategy in the absence of adequate proximal sealing zone at the level of the distal arch is to consider open arch repair. If the patient is deemed suitable for such a repair, then an elephant trunk is used to create an optimal proximal sealing zone for further stent grafting. The proximal stent graft is generally tapered distally to match the maximum diameter of the true lumen. The morphological appearance of the visceral aorta is better suited to endovascular treatment using fenestrated devices rather than branched stent grafts. The narrow workspace of the true lumen can preclude the correct deployment of the side branches of custom-made thoracoabdominal stent grafts. It is acknowledged that even fenestrated devices can be difficult to position and manoeuvre accurately in aortic dissections (Figure 1). The use of preloaded catheters through renal fenestrations to simplify access to these target vessels, and the addition of double-reducing ties at the posterior aspect of the device to limit expansion of the device during target vessel cannulation can be helpful adjuncts. The management of aortic branches that arise from the false lumen requires careful preoperative imaging analysis. In cases where the intimal tear(s) could not be identified on the preoperative computed tomography (CT)-scan at the level of the origin of a visceral perfused by the false lumen, a "neo-fenestration" can be created. Small fenestrations of the dissection flap can be enlarged with a 12mm balloon before deployment of the fenestrated device. In our experience, 25% of patients require interventions to prepare the target aortic branches prior to deployment of the fenestrated device (Figure 2).[14] A staged strategy is recommended in cases of extensive aortic repair to reduce the postoperative morbidity, especially the occurrence of spinal cord ischaemia.[15]

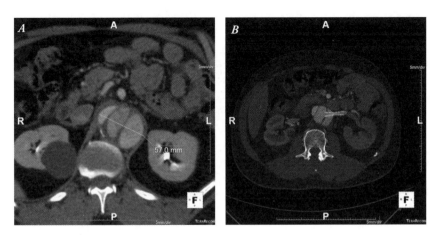

Figure 2: (A) CT-scan of a patient with chronic type B aortic dissection in MPR; the initial presentation of the initial flap was not adequate to be directly excluded by a fenestrated stent graft; (B) a neofenestration assisted by the deployement of a self-expansible stent was thus completed.

Fusion software can assist intraprocedural navigation, in particular by locating the origin of the aortic branches and distinguishing the true from the false lumen. These techniques have also been shown to significantly reduce procedure duration and the amount of radiation to both the patient and the operative team.[16] There are few but encouraging data available to describe the outcome of patients with chronic type B aortic dissections treated with fenestrated stent grafts. Kitagawa *et al* from the Cleveland Clinic Foundation, Verhoeven *et al*, and our centre have all reported their initial experience (15, six and 23 patients respectively)[15–18] and these reports confirm the feasibility of the technique with good short-term outcomes. Early mortality and spinal cord ischaemia rates ranged from 0% to 9.6 %, and 0% and 12.6%, respectively.

Conclusion

Early evidence supports the use of fenestrated aortic stent grafts to safely and successfully treat post-dissection aneurysms. These aortic lesions are more challenging compared with degenerative aortic aneurysm and, therefore, patient selection, device and procedural planning and procedural strategy have to be carefully considered for each patient. Longer-term data is required to further determine the role of fenestrated endovascular technology in the treatment of chronic aortic dissections.

Summary

- TEVAR at the onset of acute type B aortic dissection will generally offer long-term aortic remodelling limited to the aortic segment covered by the stent graft.

- Large number of patients will then be exposed to significant enlargement of the distal aorta during follow-up.

- Fenestrated (not branched) custom-made aortic stent grafts can be applied for the treatment of chronic aortic dissection.

- Patient selection, device planning and procedural strategies have to be adapted to the specific setting of the aortic dissection.

- Small cohorts of patients have proven favourable short-term outcomes and confirmed the feasibility of the technique.

- Longer term data is required to further evaluate the use of fenestrated technology for the management of chronic aortic dissections.

References

1. Fattori R, Montgomery D, Lovato L, *et al*. Survival after endovascular therapy in patients with type B aortic dissection: a report from the International Registry of Acute Aortic Dissection (IRAD). *JACC Cardiovasc Interv* 2013; **6**: 876–82.
2. Zeeshan A, Woo EY, Bavaria JE, *et al*. Thoracic endovascular aortic repair for acute complicated type B aortic dissection: superiority relative to conventional open surgical and medical therapy. *J Thorac Cardiovasc Surg* 2010; **140**: S109–15.

3. Rogers AM, Hermann LK, Booher AM, *et al.* Sensitivity of the aortic dissection detection risk score, a novel guideline-based tool for identification of acute aortic dissection at initial presentation: results from the international registry of acute aortic dissection. *Circulation* 2011; **123**: 2213–18.
4. Steuer J, Eriksson MO, Nyman R, *et al.* Early and long-term outcome after thoracic endovascular aortic repair (TEVAR) for acute complicated type B aortic dissection. *Eur J Vasc Endovasc Surg.* 2011; **41**: 318–23.
5. The Virtue Registry Investigators. Mid-term outcomes and aortic remodelling after thoracic endovascular repair for acute, subacute, and chronic aortic dissection: the VIRTUE Registry. *Eur J Vasc Endovasc Surg* 2014; **48**: 363–71.
6. Eggebrecht H, Nienaber CA, Neuhäuser M, *et al.* Endovascular stent-graft placement in aortic dissection: a meta-analysis. *Eur Heart J* 2006; **27**: 489–98.
7. Sobocinski J, Dias NV, Berger L, *et al.* Endograft repair of complicated acute type B aortic dissections. *Eur J Vasc Endovasc Surg* 2013; **45**: 468–74.
8. Sayer D, Bratby M, Brooks M, *et al.* Aortic morphology following endovascular repair of acute and chronic type B aortic dissection: implications for management. *Eur J Vasc Endovasc Surg* 2008; **36**: 522–29.
9. Griepp RB, Griepp EB. Spinal cord protection in surgical and endovascular repair of thoracoabdominal aortic disease. *J Thorac Cardiovasc Surg* 2015; **149**: S86–90.
10. Jonker FH, Trimarchi S, Rampoldi V, *et al.* Aortic expansion after acute type B aortic dissection. *Ann Thorac Surg* 2012; **94**: 1223–29.
11. Tsai TT, Fattori R, Trimarchi S, *et al.* Long-term survival in patients presenting with type B acute aortic dissection: insights from the International Registry of Acute Aortic Dissection. *Circulation* 2006; **114**: 2226–31.
12. Coady MA, Rizzo JA, Hammond GL, *et al.* What is the appropriate size criterion for resection of thoracic aortic aneurysms? *J Thorac Cardiovasc Surg* 1997; **113**: 476–91.
13. Faruqi RM, Chuter TA, Reilly LM, *et al.* Endovascular repair of abdominal aortic aneurysm using a pararenal fenestrated stent-graft. *J Endovasc Surg* 1999; **6**: 354–58.
14. Spear RS, Settembre N, Tyrrell MR, *et al.* Early Experience of Endovascular Repair of Post-dissection Aneurysms Involving the Thoraco-abdominal Aorta and the Arch. *Eur J Vasc Endovasc Surg* 2015:In Press
15. O'Callaghan A, Mastracci TM, Eagleton MJ. Staged endovascular repair of thoracoabdominal aortic aneurysms limits incidence and severity of spinal cord ischemia. *J Vasc Surg* 2015; **61**: 347–54.
16. Maurel B, Hertault A, Sobocinski J, *et al.* Techniques to reduce radiation and contrast volume during EVAR. *J Cardiovasc Surg* (Torino) 2014; **55**: 123–31.
17. Oikonomou K, Kopp R, Katsargyris A, *et al.* Outcomes of fenestrated/branched endografting in post-dissection thoracoabdominal aortic aneurysms. *Eur J Vasc Endovasc Surg* 2014; **48**: 641–48.
18. Kitagawa A, Greenberg RK, Eagleton MJ, *et al.* Fenestrated and branched endovascular aortic repair for chronic type B aortic dissection with thoracoabdominal aneurysms. *J Vasc Surg* 2013; **58**: 625–34.

Great Debate: In chronic type B dissection, there is no place for false lumen embolisation— true lumen TEVAR is preferred—against the motion

F Rohlffs, N Tsilimparis, S Debus and T Kölbel

Introduction

The hallmark of aortic dissection is that the disease is dynamic in time. Despite a myriad of new developments in therapy, definite treatment—especially in chronic aortic dissection—remains challenging. The concept of standard thoracic endovascular aortic repair (TEVAR) with occlusion of the proximal entry tear, as applied in acute dissection, is not sufficient for chronic disease. As reported in literature, single TEVAR in chronic dissection is associated with high long-term morbidity and mortality rates.[1]

Hence, treatment strategy in chronic dissection should consider the morphologic and haemodynamic changes that occur because of chronicity which include: rigid dissection membrane; reduced remodelling capacity;[2] and false lumen back-flow

Of the aforementioned changes, back-flow into the thoracic false lumen from distal entry tears should be considered as the main factor for progression of the disease with aneurysm formation. Presumably, the principle behind this persistent flow consists of continuous run-off through spinal or intercostal arteries with continued pressure transmission into the false lumen, especially at the thoracic level.

This affects patients with type B aortic dissection, residual dissection after surgical repair of a DeBakey type I aortic dissection, or those with dissection after ascending aortic repair for other pathologies. Therefore, it is evident that strategies to achieve false lumen occlusion are of increasing importance and that novel techniques have been introduced to solve the problem of persisting false lumen perfusion.

Indication for treatment

Chronic aortic dissection carries a high risk of late complications. Mainly, false lumen enlargement and subsequent rupture pose a significant risk for affected patients. A ruptured thoracic false lumen aneurysm is one of the most challenging conditions for open and endovascular repair. This emergency situation should be prevented according to current treatment recommendations. Malperfusion is a relatively rare finding in the later stage of aortic dissection, but may become symptomatic due to late morphological changes (i.e. with claudication).

Current indications for operative treatment as proposed by a recent international expert consensus are:[3] rupture or bleeding; false lumen aneurysm of >5.5–6cm; false lumen growth 5mm/year and more; and malperfusion.

If treatment is indicated, several techniques exist to achieve false lumen occlusion. Which approach should generally be chosen—open surgical or endovascular therapy—remains unclear yet.[4] As a basic principle, open surgical approaches should be preferred in patients with connective tissue disease as Marfan-Syndrome, whereas endovascular procedures are more favourable in the older and multimorbid patient because of less procedural harm.

Strategies to occlude the false lumen

Irrespective of complete open surgical aortic repair, there are five main principles of how to occlude the false lumen in chronic aortic dissection: extended aortic coverage combined with visceral debranching (hybrid-procedure); extended aortic coverage by branched or fenestrated stent-grafts; embolisation of intercostal or bronchial arteries; fenestration of the dissection membrane followed by TEVAR; and direct false lumen occlusion (embolisation; new endovascular techniques).

Extension of aortic coverage

Regarding false lumen occlusion, extending aortic coverage distally increases the possibility of entry-tear sealing at the abdominal, especially visceral, branch bearing aortic segment. Hybrid procedures as well as branched or fenestrated endovascular aneurysm repair (EVAR) procedures enable long aortic segment coverage, preserving unimpaired flow to the reno-visceral arteries. Compared with branched/fenestrated EVAR, hybrid repair is still associated with a high mortality and morbidity rate of up to 34% at 30-day follow up.[5]

Limitations of branched/fenestrated EVAR are described as difficulties of manoeuvring the fenestrated graft in a small true lumen—as commonly present in chronic dissection—and in catheterisation of the branched/fenestrations. Lumen expansion cannot be expected immediately in chronic dissection due to the adverse tissue changes. This is particularly in the case of overlapping graft components as it requires more material to fit into the small true lumen, there is a risk for graft-occlusion. Complex stent graft planning and individualised concepts are required (Figure 1). With this complex technique, long-segment coverage of the aorta is required and increases the risk for spinal cord ischaemia.[6]

High technical demands and elaborate logistics of both hybrid repair and branched/fenestrated EVAR indicate reasons that could make a broad use of this method unlikely.

Occlusion of intercostal or bronchial arteries

Proximal runoff arteries arising from the thoracic false lumen—most commonly, intercostal or bronchial vessels—have to be present to preserve a continuous retrograde flow through the false lumen arising from downstream entry tears. Following this concept, embolisation of these run-off arteries should be considered a feasible method to interrupt false lumen perfusion and pressurisation of the false lumen. Nevertheless, this strategy is not established in clinical practice but remains a potential future approach.

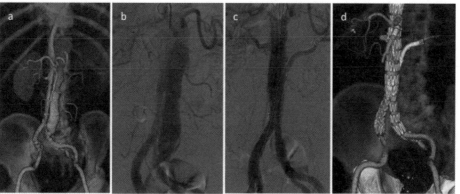

Figure 1: (A) CT-volume rendering of a complex chronic type B aortic dissection with perfusion of the left kidney from the false lumen. (B and C) Angiography and repair of the dissection with a custom-made stent graft with three fenestrations for the coeliac trunk, superior mesenteric artery and the right renal artery and an inverted branch crossing the dissection membrane to reconnect the left kidney to the true lumen. Final angiogramm shows good perfusion of all renovisceral branches (D) CT-volume rendering showing the postprocedural result with adequate expansion of the true lumen.

Fenestration of the dissection membrane followed by TEVAR

The presence of the dissection-membrane prevents distal sealing of tubular stent grafts that are placed in the true lumen as the endograft cannot expand to the outer aortic wall. False lumen backflow can be prevented by fenestration of the dissection-membrane, creating a single lumen at an aortic segment to allow the endograft to seal the false lumen aneurysm distally.

Open surgical fenestration of the dissection-membrane to create a distal sealing zone can be performed using sternotomy, thoracotomy or laparotomy. Roselli *et al* delivered the first description of open fenestration at the level of the descending aorta in 24 patients after an elephant trunk procedure with good results of 92% survival at two years.[7] Konings *et al* described a subxyphoid incision for supraceliac fenestration of the dissection membrane.[8]

However, open surgical fenestration techniques as described require open surgical access with aortic cross-clamping. Nevertheless, the same can be achieved by endovascular fenestration with subsequent TEVAR.[9]

Direct false lumen occlusion

Direct false lumen occlusion is used in addition to a standard TEVAR procedure. Embolisation materials such as coils, plugs and glue are positioned into the false lumen occluding it like a "cork in the bottle neck". This technique was primarily described by Loubert *et al*[10] Several similar approaches have been successfully performed since then. But, this technique is limited to patients with smaller false lumen diameters at the level of the diaphragm since materials for arterial embolisation are not commercially available for large diameters.

New endovascular developments

To overcome the above mentioned limitations, new endovascular strategies were introduced to allow false lumen occlusion in a less invasive, endovascular fashion and without a long procedural time.

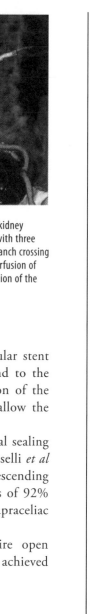

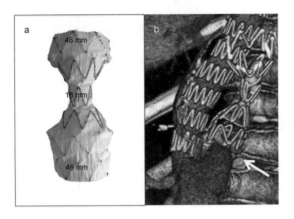

Figure 2: (A) Photograph of a Candy-Plug. The Candy-Plug (Cook Medical) is available as a CMD device. The large proximal and distal diameter makes it suitable for the occlusion of large false lumen diameter pathologies. The central narrowing can be occluded by a Vascular Plug after removing the loading system of the graft. (B) CT-volume rendering: distal alignment of the thoracic stent graft (true lumen) and the Candy-Plug (false lumen) at the level of the celiac trunk. The Candy-Plug prevents false lumen back-flow to the thoracic level (white arrow).

The Candy-Plug technique

The Candy-Plug was introduced to address the problem of large false lumen diameters, not suitable for materials such as described in the "cork in the bottle neck" technique.[11] It may have a proximal and distal diameter of up to 50mm and a central narrowing to 18mm, which gives the typical candywrapper-like appearance (Figure 2a). The Candy-Plug in the false lumen should be used additionally to a stent graft in the true lumen. Both stent grafts should land immediately above the celiac trunk, where the TEVAR opens and stabilises the true lumen and the Candy-Plug occludes the false lumen to interrupt thoracic back-flow (Figure 2b). This new technique has already been successfully applied to 11 patients with technical and clinical success rate of 100% at 30-day follow up and appears very promising.

Knickerbocker technique

The Knickerbocker technique is a completely endovascular fenestration technique without the need for open surgery. The concept is based on the dilation of the middle part of a large diameter stent graft that is placed in the true lumen of the descending aorta ending immediately above the coeliac trunk. A short segment of the stent graft is forcefully dilated using a compliant balloon, aiming to rupture the dissection membrane and extending the stent graft to the false lumen. Instead of an oversized standard tubular stent graft, a double-tapered graft construction with a bulbous section can be used.[12] After stent graft placement in the right orientation a compliant balloon is advanced to deploy the bulbous section for septum rupture and false lumen occlusion.

Conclusion

The principle in chronic aortic dissection should be to thrombose the false lumen to successfully exclude the false lumen aneurysm. There are many approaches to achieve this goal, but most concepts are limited by either high technical and logistic demands to the surgeon or high rates of mortality and morbidity. New endovascular concepts as the Candy-Plug and the Knickerbocker-Technique are developed to address these limitations with promising early results.

Summary

- Chronic aortic dissection is a challenging disease that requires individualised treatment concepts.

- Standard TEVAR procedures are barely sufficient.

- False-lumen perfusion and pressurisation counts as a main risk factor for aneurysm formation and hazardous complications in chronic aortic dissection.

- The main principle in treatment should be to occlude the false lumen.

- Novel promising endovascular strategies have evolved to solve the problem of false lumen back flow, giving new directions in regard to treatment indications and strategies in chronic type B aortic dissection.

References

1. Mani K, Clough RE, Lyons OT, *et al.* Predictors of outcome after endovascular repair for chronic type B dissection. *Eur J Vasc Endovasc Surg* 2012; **43** (4): 386–91.

2. Haulon S, Greenberg RK, Spear R, *et al.* Global experience with an inner branched arch endograft. *J Thorac Cardiovasc Surg* 2014; **148** (4):1709–16.

3. Fattori R, Cao P, De Rango P, *et al.* Interdisciplinary expert consensus document on management of type B aortic dissection. *J Am Coll Cardiol* 2013; **61** (16):1661–78.

4. Tian DH, De Silva RP, Wang T, *et al.* Open surgical repair for chronic type B aortic dissection: a systematic review. Ann Cardiothorac Surg 2014; **3** (4):340–50.

5. Idrees J, Roselli EE, Shafii S, *et al.* Outcomes after false lumen embolization with covered stent devices in chronic dissection. *J Vasc Surg* 2014; **60** (6):1507–13.

6. Oikonomou K, Kopp R, Katsargyris A, *et al.* Outcomes of fenestrated/branched endografting in post-dissection thoracoabdominal aortic aneurysms. *Eur J Vasc Endovasc Surg* 2014; **48** (6): 641–48.

7. Roselli EE, Sepulveda E, Pujara AC, *et al.* Distal landing zone open fenestration facilitates endovascular elephant trunk completion and false lumen thrombosis. *Ann Thorac Surg* 2011; **92** (6): 2078–84.

8. Konings R, de Bruin JL, Wisselink W. Open fenestration of the distal landing zone via a subxyphoid incision for subsequent endovascular repair of a dissecting thoracic aneurysm. *J Endovasc Ther* 2013; **20** (1): 28–31.

9. Kolbel T, Diener H, Larena-Avellaneda A, *et al.* Advanced endovascular techniques for thoracic and abdominal aortic dissections. *J Cardiovasc Surg* (Torino) 2013; **54** (1 Suppl 1): 81–90.

10. Loubert MC, van der Hulst VP, De Vries C, *et al.* How to exclude the dilated false lumen in patients after a type B aortic dissection? The cork in the bottleneck. *J Endovasc Ther* 2003; **10** (2): 244–48.

11. Kolbel T, Lohrenz C, Kieback A, *et al.* Distal false lumen occlusion in aortic dissection with a homemade extra-large vascular plug: the candy-plug technique. *J Endovasc Ther* 2013; **20** (4): 484–89.

12. Kolbel T, Carpenter SW, Lohrenz C, *et al.* Addressing persistent false lumen flow in chronic aortic dissection: the knickerbocker technique. *J Endovasc Ther* 2014; **21** (1): 117–22.

Great Debate: In chronic type B dissection, there is no place for false lumen embolisation— true lumen TEVAR is preferred—against the motion

F Fanelli and A Cannavale

Introduction

Thoracic endovascular aortic repair (TEVAR) is these days considered to be the treatment of choice for both acute and chronic dissections.[1–4] The aim of endovascular treatment is to exclude the primary entry tear with a consequent remodelling of the thoracic aorta. This phenomenon is secondary to the progressive reduction of the false lumen and contemporary enlargement of the true lumen during follow-up, without enlargement of the total aortic diameter. Several factors play a role in this process but not all of them are clear.[1–6]

Acute aortic dissections are associated with a higher degree of remodelling compared with chronic aortic dissections; however, procedural factors that may affect further clinical outcome, morphologic changes and the risk of endoleaks have not been fully explored.[3–6] Also, survival rate is reported to be higher in those patients who achieved aortic remodelling with a 5mm reduction in the maximum descending thoracic aorta diameter.[1,5] By contrast, TEVAR does not significantly modify the aortic morphology in chronic dissections.[7]

Evidence base

The INSTEAD (Investigation of stent grafts in aortic dissection)-XL trial has highlighted the efficacy of TEVAR in facilitating aortic remodelling. In this study, TEVAR in uncomplicated aortic dissections was associated with greater aorta remodelling and less aorta-related mortality compared with medical therapy.[2]

Stent graft oversizing is one factor that can intervene to modify the morphology of the aorta after stent graft deployment. In the case of thoracic aortic dissections, especially in the acute setting, stent graft oversizing should be minimal ($\leq$20%).[2,8,9] Minimal stent graft oversizing reduces the barotrauma on the fragile aortic wall, reducing the risk of antegrade dissection or aortic rupture. Larger oversizing may be associated with endograft collapse (infolding) and consequent incomplete sealing.[10,11] A recent report found that stent graft oversizing of $\geq$20% was a significant predictive factor for re-intervention.[12]

A retrospective analysis[13] was performed in 60 consecutive patients (mean age 69±3.5; 40 males, 20 females) who underwent endovascular treatment for acute and chronic Stanford type B aortic dissections. Twenty-nine patients (48.3%) had acute aortic dissection group and 31 (51.7%) had chronic dissections. Computed tomography (CT)-angiography, axial images, were evaluated on: short axis diameter, whole aorta, and true and false lumens at seven different levels (3cm and 1cm above the stent graft; superior edge of the stent graft; mid-level of the stent graft; inferior edge of the stent graft; 1cm and 3cm below the stent graft). The aortic changes, regarding morphology and diameter of the true and false lumen, were assessed and compared with the pre-treatment CT-angiography findings.

False lumen thrombosis was more evident in the acute group within the first 18 months after treatment. These outcomes are similar to the results of other recent studies that stress the higher capacity of remodelling of acute dissections after TEVAR.[5,9,12–14]

The results confirmed that with acute dissections, false lumen thrombosis and shrinkage is directly proportional to the absence of major adverse events and endoleaks. However, the false lumen thrombosis in chronic dissections is less prominent initially and, at the same time, had a weak correlation with major adverse events and endoleak occurrence. This finding is probably related to the fact that a higher incidence of type II endoleak was secondary to left subclavian artery intentional coverage.

Apart from false lumen and true lumen changes in size, which are well known, the whole lumen of the aorta above the stent graft had not been analysed in previous studies.[15,16] Our results showed that the whole aortic lumen increases significantly above the stent graft (+4.5mm in 36 months) in acute dissections but does not increase in chronic dissections. This may be related to the increased active remodelling of the aortic wall that is typical of acute dissections and may also be associated with increased shear stress forces above the stent graft, which may lead to aneurysm formation or retrograde type A dissection.

Regarding stent graft oversizing, we observed that it was not associated with endoleaks in either the acute dissections group or in the chronic dissections group, nor was stent graft oversizing associated with major adverse events.

Univariate and multivariate analysis confirmed that stent graft oversizing in both acute dissections and chronic dissections did not influence aortic remodelling, endoleak or major adverse events. In the acute setting: stent graft oversizing, univariate hazard ratio (HR) (95% confidence interval [CI]) 1.12 p=0.915; balloon dilatation after stent deployment, univariate HR (95% CI) 0.36 p=0.031—multivariate HR (95% CI) 0.81 p=0.754. In the chronic dissections, stent graft oversizing: univariate HR(95% CI) 1.08 p=0.971; balloon dilatation after stent deployment univariate HR (95% CI) 0.31 p=0.11.[13]

The endovascular treatment of acute dissections resulted in a significant increase of true lumen diameter over the time (from a mean value of 20.4mm—calculated from all indicated aorta levels—to 28mm after 36 months; p=0.02) and a significant decrease of the false lumen diameter (from a mean value of 9.1mm—calculated from all indicated aorta levels—to 5mm at 36 months; p=0.01).

However, the total maximum diameter of the aorta in acute dissections was not significantly altered at level of the stent graft and below (from level 4 to 7) from a mean value of 28.8mm to 29.3mm at 36 months (p>0.05), with a mean overall enlargement of +0.47mm. However, we noted a significant enlargement of the aorta diameter above the stent graft (from level 1 to 3) from a mean value of 31.5mm to 35.5mm at 36 months (p=0.05), with a mean overall evolution of +4.5mm.

In chronic dissections, TEVAR did not significantly modify the total aortic calibre (mean of all levels: from 31.8mm at discharge to 33.3mm at 36 months; mean enlargement of +1.1mm, p>0.05). This was also the case with true and false lumen—either at the level of the stent graft (true lumen mean enlargement of +3mm at 36 months, p>0.05; false lumen mean shrinkage of -0.73mm, p>0.05) or in the aorta below the endograft (true lumen mean enlargement of +2.5mm, p>0.05; false lumen mean shrinkage of -1.5mm, p>0.05).

We investigated the relationship between stent graft dilatation, clinical outcomes, complications rate and aorta remodelling in both acute dissections and chronic dissections. In case of acute dissections, at 36 months, significant false lumen thrombosis rates were observed in those patients where a dilatation has been performed. Also in this case, the difference was more evident within the first 18 months after the procedure. From these results, we might suggest that stent graft dilatation improves false lumen thrombosis especially in acute dissections (95% of acute patients vs. 70% chronic patients with complete false lumen thrombosis; p<0.01). However, there is not a statistical difference for endoleak development and major adverse events in patients who underwent post dilatation and in patients who did not (p=0.09). On the contrary, in the chronic dissection group, no significant difference of the false lumen thrombosis rate was observed between patients who underwent stent graft dilatation and those who did not (72% percutaneous transluminal angioplasty vs. 68% for no percutaneous transluminal angioplasty; p>0.05). An explanation can be correlated to the higher stiffness of the aorta in chronic dissections that does not allow stent-graft dilatation to influence the aortic remodelling.

Conclusion

Aorta remodelling after TEVAR can be related to the characteristics of the dissection and to the procedural technique. In particular, acute dissections seem to be more sensitive, in comparison to chronic dissections, for aortic remodelling and development of endoleaks.

Summary

- Acute aortic dissections show a higher degree of remodelling when compared with chronic aortic dissections.

- False lumen thrombosis was more evident in acute dissections within the first 18 months after treatment.

- In acute dissections, false lumen thrombosis and shrinkage is directly proportional to the absence of major adverse events and endoleaks. However, the false lumen thrombosis in chronic dissections is less prominent initially and at the same time has a weak correlation with major adverse events and endoleaks occurrence.

- Stent graft dilatation improves false lumen thrombosis especially in acute dissections; in the chronic group, no significant difference of the false lumen thrombosis rate was observed between patients who undergo stent graft dilatation and those who did not.

References

1. Patterson BO, Cobb RJ, Karthikesalingam A, *et al.* A systematic review of aortic remodeling after endovascular repair of type B aortic dissection: methods and outcomes. *Ann Thorac Surg* 2014; **97**: 588–95.

2. Nienaber CA, Kische S, Rousseau H, *et al;* INSTEAD-XL trial. Endovascular repair of type B aortic dissection: long-term results of the randomized investigation of stent grafts in aortic dissection trial. *Circ Cardiovasc Interv* 2013; **6**: 407–16.

3. Qin YL, Deng G, Li TX, *et al.* Treatment of acute type-B aortic dissection: thoracic endovascular aortic repair or medical management alone? *JACC Cardiovasc Interv* 2013; **6**: 185–91.

4. Grabenwöger M, Alfonso F, Bachet J, *et al.* Thoracic Endovascular Aortic Repair (TEVAR) for the treatment of aortic diseases: a position statement from the European Association for Cardio-Thoracic Surgery (EACTS) and the European Society of Cardiology (ESC), in collaboration with the European Association of Percutaneous Cardiovascular Interventions (EAPCI). *Eur J Cardiothorac Surg* 2012; **42**: 17–24.

5. Sigman MM, Palmer OP, Ham SW, *et al.* Aortic morphologic findings after thoracic endovascular aortic repair for type B aortic dissection. *JAMA Surg* 2014; **149**: 977–83.

6. Eriksson MO, Steuer J, Wanhainen A, *et al.* Morphologic outcome after endovascular treatment of complicated type B aortic dissection. *J Vasc Interv Radiol* 2013; **24**: 1826–33.

7. Watanabe Y, Shimamura K, Yoshida T, *et al.* Aortic remodeling as a prognostic factor for late aortic events after thoracic endovascular aortic repair in type B aortic dissection with patent false lumen. *J Endovasc Ther* 2014; **21**: 517–25.

8. Sze DY, van den Bosch MA, Dake MD, *et al.* Factors portending endoleak formation after thoracic aortic stent-graft repair of complicated aortic dissection. *Circ Cardiovasc Interv* 2009; **2**: 105–12.

9. Rohlffs F, Tsilimparis N, Diener H, *et al.* Chronic type B aortic dissection: indications and strategies for treatment. *J Cardiovasc Surg* (Torino). 2015; **56**: 231–38.

10. Fanelli F, Dake MD. Standard of Practice for the Endovascular Treatment of Thoracic Aortic Aneurysms and Type B Dissections. Cardiovasc Intervent Radiol 2009; **32**: 849–60.

11. Huang X, Huang L, Sun L, *et al.* Endovascular repair of Stanford B aortic dissection using two stent grafts with different sizes. *J Vasc Surg* 2015; **62**: 43–48.

12. Kasirajan K, Dake MD, Lumsden A, *et al.* Incidence and outcomes after infolding or collapse of thoracic stent grafts. *J Vasc Surg* 2012; **55**: 652–58.

13. Fanelli F, Cannavale A, O'Sullivan GJ, *et al.* Endovascular Repair of Acute and Chronic Aortic Type B Dissections: Main Factors Affecting Aortic Remodeling and Clinical Outcome. *JACC Cardiovasc Interv* 2016; **9**: 183–91

14. Jonker FH, Schlosser FJ, Geirsson A, *et al.* Endograft collapse after thoracic endovascular aortic repair. *J Endovasc Ther* 2010; **17**: 725–34.

15. Conrad MF, Carvalho S, Ergul E, *et al.* Late aortic remodeling persists in the stented segment after endovascular repair of acute complicated type B aortic dissection. *J Vasc Surg* 2015; **62** (3): 600–05.

16. Lombardi JV, Cambria RP, Nienaber CA, *et al;* on behalf of the STABLE investigators. Aortic remodeling after endovascular treatment of complicated type B aortic dissection with the use of a composite device design. *J Vasc Surg* 2014; **59**: 1544–54.

TEVAR follow-up

15 years' experience of TAAA—similar 30-day mortality endovascular and open and similar paraplegia rates

R Chiesa, G Melissano, Y Tshomba, M Leopardi, C Ferrer, P De Rango, F Verzini and P Cao

Introduction

The possibility of managing aortic aneurysms by endovascular means has been one of the major innovations of the past 15 years in vascular surgery. Currently endovascular repair has become the predominant treatment option for thoracic and abdominal aortic aneurysms that comply with morphological feasibility criteria.[1-4] Open surgery still remains the gold standard in case of complex aortic aneurysms involving visceral vessels; nevertheless, there are relatively few vascular surgeons undertaking open surgery for thoracoabdominal aortic aneurysm (TAAA) offering patients low mortality and morbidity risk exposure (Figure 1).[5-7] Similarly, there are only few centres involved in endovascular repair who report encouraging results with branched and fenestrated stent grafts in thoracoabdominal aneurysms (Figure 2).[8] Reliable unbiased data comparing open and endovascular technique for complex aneurysms involving the thoracoabdominal aorta are lacking. The aim of this study was to compare early and mid-term results of open and endovascular procedures for the treatment of such aneurysms in equivalent-risk populations.

Methods

A comparative analysis of outcome after endovascular repair and open surgery for patients with thoracoabdominal aneurysms, referred at three tertiary Italian vascular centres from 2007 to 2014, was performed. The study was based on retrospective institutional review analysis of a prospectively maintained database including preoperative demographics and risk factors, operative details and follow-up outcome data. The study was performed in accordance with the Institutional Ethical Committee rules and individual consent for this retrospective analysis was waived. All patients provided consent for intervention. The extent of aortic repair was classified according to Crawford's classification. Treatment selection for repair was based on clinical and morphological characteristics and left to the discretion of the local operator team. Computed tomography (CT) angiography was performed at one and six months and then yearly to monitor the early and late development of complications (endoleak, stent

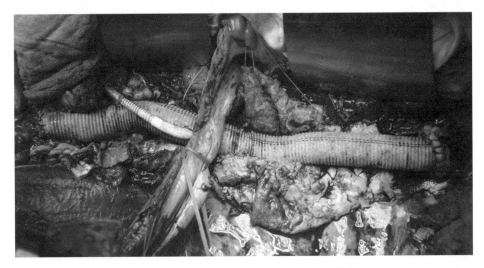

Figure 1: Intraoperative thoracoabdominal aortic open repair. Selective reimplant of left renal artery.

graft disconnection, loss of integrity or migration, aneurysm growth) of endovascular repair. The primary endpoints of this study were mortality and paraplegia. Secondary endpoints included any spinal cord ischaemia, renal and respiratory insufficiency and the composite of these complications or death as recorded at 30 days or in-hospital when occurring during hospitalisation protracted beyond 30 days. Renal insufficiencies were defined as the need of temporary or permanent dialysis after the procedure. Respiratory insufficiency was any prolonged intubation (longer than 72 hours) or need for re-intubation. Spinal cord ischaemia was defined as any neurological deficit related to spinal cord ischaemia, regardless of the severity and the duration.

Statistical analysis

Patients in the open surgery group were matched to patients in the endovascular repair group on the basis of propensity score (i.e. the conditional probability of receiving a particular treatment given the set of confounders).[9–11] Endovascular repair was commonly offered to older patients with higher comorbidity burden (cardiac, pulmonary, renal, diabetes) while open repair was more suitable for more extensive aneurysms or females (likely small vessels unfit for endovascular repair), leading to the following variables of selection: age, sex, hypertension, coronary disease, chronic pulmonary disease, diabetes, aneurysm extent, and renal function. Comparative data were expressed as odds ratio (OR) and corresponding 95% confidence interval (CI). A value of <0.05 was used for significance. Survival and reintervention rates were analysed with Kaplan Meier curves and a log rank test. Data were reported up to standard error <0.1.

Results

During the study period, 341 procedures involving thoracoabdominal aorta were identified. A total of 257 patients, referred to one of the three centres, underwent open surgery, while 84 referred to the other two centres, concurrently underwent endovascular repair. Before the propensity matching process, patients in the endovascular repair group were significantly older and more frequently affected by coronary artery disease. After

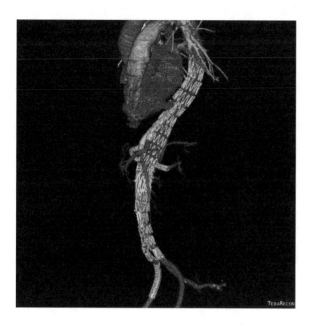

Figure 2: 3D Reconstruction of thoracoabdominal endovascular repair with a four branch stent graft.

propensity matching, there were 65 patients in the endovascular repair group and 65 in the open surgery group with correction of all differences in baseline characteristics. In the open surgery group, six patients (9.2%) had a chronic dissection, two of which (3.1%) related to connective tissue disorders; all the remaining patients were affected by degenerative aneurysms. In the endovascular repair group, one patient (1.5%), with Marfan's syndrome and previous multiple operations, was treated for a post-dissection aneurysm. In the endovascular repair group, one patient (1.5%) with symptomatic aneurysms was urgently treated with an off-the-shelf device, while three patients (4.6%) underwent urgent open surgery. There were not relevant differences with respect to the included endovascular repair and open surgery cohorts with the exception of age that was lower in the open surgery group. Thirty-day mortality[1] and paraplegia were 7.7% in the endovascular repair group and 6.2% in the open surgery group (p=1) and 9.2% and 10.8% (p=1), respectively. The rate of the composite endpoint, was significantly lower in the endovascular repair group (18.5% vs. 36.9%; p=0.03). The risk of any spinal cord ischaemia (12.3% in endovascular repair and 20% in open surgery; p=0.34) and renal insufficiency (9.2% in endovascular repair and 12.3% in open surgery; p=0.78), when individually analysed, did not significantly differ between the two groups; however, the 30-day rate of respiratory insufficiency was significantly reduced in the endovascular repair group (0% vs. 12.3%; p=0.006). Additionally, intensive care unit stay and total hospitalisation time were significantly shorter in the endovascular repair group (1.6 days vs. 2.8 days, p=0.01; and 6.3 days vs. 16.3 days, p<0.001; in the endovascular repair and open surgery groups, respectively). There were overall nine deaths: among the five deaths (7.7%) in endovascular repair group, two were due to haemorrhagic stroke, two to bowel ischaemia and one to multiorgan failure. Four deaths (6.2%) after open surgery were due to multiorgan failure. Twenty-one patients presented neurological deficit due to spinal cord ischaemia regardless of the severity and duration (12.3% in endovascular repair vs. 20% in open surgery; p=0.34). Permanent paraplegia was observed in six patients after endovascular repair (9.2%) and seven after open surgery (10.8%, p=1). Fourteen patients (six in the endovascular repair group and eight in the open surgery group) required dialysis immediately after the procedure, but only one patient per group (1.5%, p=1) required permanent dialysis.

Mid-term results were assessed at median follow-up of 21.6 months. According to Kaplan-Meier estimates, all-cause survival at 24 and 42 months was 82.8% in the endovascular repair group and 84.9% in the open surgery group (p=0.9) (Figure 3). No aorta-related late deaths occurred after endovascular repair, while one patient in the open surgery group died from sepsis secondary to an aorto-bronchial fistula. Other causes of late death included haemorrhagic stroke (n=2), cancer (n=2) and respiratory failure (n=1) in the endovascular repair group, and cardiac disease (n=2) and cancer (n=2) in the open surgery group.

During follow-up, 10 reinterventions were performed in the endovascular repair group and eight in the open surgery group. In the endovascular repair group, five patients underwent successful embolisation (n=1) or bridging stent realignment (n=4) for type III endoleak, one patient required an iliac extension cuff for type Ib endoleak, two patients underwent a surgical revision of the access site for bleeding, and two patients had cross-over femoro-femoral bypasses for iliac leg occlusion. In the open surgery group, two patients required an early surgical revision for bleeding. During follow-up, thoraco-laparotomy related redo surgery was required in four patients after open surgery. The other two patients in the open surgery group were retreated by endovascular means: bilateral renal stenting was required for a patient with inadequate renal perfusion, and aorto-uni iliac stent graft and cross-over femoro-femoral bypass for a patient with distal anastomotic pseudoaneurysm. Freedom from reintervention rates were 91% in endovascular repair *versus* 89.7% in open surgery, and 80% in endovascular repair *versus* 79.9% in open surgery (p=0.3) at 24 and 42 months, respectively.

Discussion

The treatment of patients with thoracoabdominal aneurysms is technically demanding and represents an area of ongoing development. The present study shows comparative results between open surgery and fenestrated-branched devices when applied to

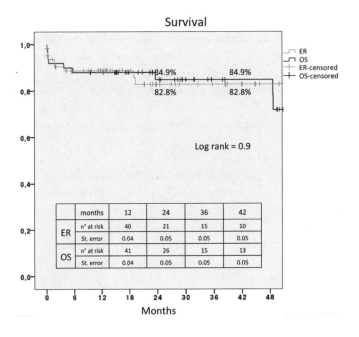

Figure 3: Kaplan-Meier curve of all-cause survival at 24 and 42 months. ER =endovascular repair; OS=open surgery.

matched comparable patients. Based on our results, both the endovascular repair and open surgery groups of patients had similar rates of perioperative mortality (7.7% vs. 6.2%) and renal complications (9.2% vs. 12.3%). The incidence of spinal cord ischaemia was 12.3% in the endovascular repair and 20% in the open surgery group, a difference that was not statistically significant and disappeared when only rates of permanent paraplegia were considered (9.2% vs. 10.8% in endovascular repair and open surgery, respectively). However, open surgery exposed the patients to a major overall morbidity burden as shown by the two-times higher rate of the composite endpoint compared to the endovascular group: 36.9% *versus* 18.5% after endovascular repair and open surgery, respectively. Furthermore, as expected, the 30-day rate of respiratory insufficiency was significantly lower in endovascular repair (0% vs. 12.3%; p=0.006). These findings may help selecting the open *versus* endovascular treatment for aneurysms tailored to the single patient specifically with respect to the effect of an open surgery on respiratory function. However, the findings of this study should be interpreted with caution: propensity analysis did not allow for a totally balanced comparison as by a randomised trial, and resulted in a well-matched albeit smaller subset of our overall aneurysms population for which 30-day and mid-term outcomes were evaluated. The numbers of comparable patients decreased the power in detecting difference in treatment efficacy.

A recent large multi-institutional nationwide analysis involving more than 390 sites based on American College of Surgeons National Surgical Quality Improvement Program (ACS-NSQIP) database investigating 1,091 open surgery and 1,264 fenestrated endograft for complex aortic aneurysms, performed between 2005 and 2010, found that only 26% of the fenestrated endograft procedures were applied to patients deemed ASA IV according to American Anesthesiologists Association (ASA classification) and thereby implying "excessive surgical risk" or "unsuitability" for surgery. Most of the repairs, either open or fenestrated endograft were on patients with average risk, scoring III or less according to ASA classification.[12] The reported 30-day mortality was significantly lower for fenestrated endograft (5.4% vs. 0.8%; p=0.001). Even though the reasons why fenestrated endograft was performed in this study in patients at average-risk was unclear, the results of the study confirmed the possibility to apply today a less invasive alternative to open surgery in patients fit for major surgery and should be considered in the decision making for management of complex aortic diseases and thoracoabdominal aneurysms. The selection of best suitable cases is paramount to achieve safety outcomes in these not high-risk settings. However, balanced and solid information with fenestrated/branched devices compared to open surgery specifically for the treatment of thoracoabdominal aneurysms is currently missing. Lack of adjustments influenced the published results leading to uneven comparisons of outcomes between these two treatment modalities and conflicting results. Data showing limited mortality and morbidity rates are available from studies performed in high-volume centres with extensive experience with fenestrated/branched devices,[12–15] but there are also recent reports still showing excess mortality rates compared to open surgery.[16] Differences in the propensity-selected populations may probably explain the different findings of our study with respect to others. In a combined French and American institutions' experience, the comparison of 147 open and 42 fenestrated repairs for juxtarenal aneurysms with propensity score matching, showed unsatisfying results for the endovascular approach. Mortality (9.2% vs. 2%; p=0.05) and procedural complications (24% vs. 7%; p<0.01) were significantly higher in the endovascular than in the open repairs. Despite the fact that the comparison was focused on patients with juxtarenal aneurysms, and thoracoabdominal aneurysms were excluded, reflecting less challenging diseases to be treated, endovascular approach was independently associated with fivefold increased 30-day mortality risk (odds ratio 5.1; 95% 1.1–24; p=0.04).[16]

The technique with endovascular devices was progressively refined: there was a preference for staging the procedure (the branched component or the bridging stents deployed after seven or more days of the first stage); furthermore, a full relining with bare metal stent was preferred in case of branched stent graft needing long self-expandable bridging stents or when longer landing in the target vessels was needed. There is evidence that changes with the fenestrated technique based on accumulated experience have prompted decreased risk of spinal cord ischaemia after fenestrated/branched thoracoabdominal aneurysms repairs.[15] The French experience of 204 endovascular thoracoabdominal aneurysms repairs using custom-made devices manufactured with branches and fenestrations from 2004 to 2013 reported outcomes after the implementation of an innovative protocol since 2010 that included optimisation of the device implantation technique (early restoration of arterial flow to the pelvis and lower limbs, staged approach) and the systematic application of the proactive spinal cord protective protocol. Authors found that the introduction of the new protocol allowed a significant decrease of spinal cord ischaemia risk from 14% *versus* 1.2% (p<0.01) and a benefit in halving the 30-day mortality, from 11.6% to 5.6%, even though not statistically relevant (p=0.09). The benefit was particularly evident in the reducing rates of spinal cord ischaemia following type I-III thoracoabdominal aneurysmsendovascular repair (excluding type IV): 25% (6/24 patients) before the protocol and 2.1% (2/95 patients) after the protocol (p<0.01).[15] Our data for reinterventions are partially in disagreement with previous studies showing uncertainty regarding the durability of endovascular repair and reporting a need for reintervention as high as 26% at a mean follow-up of two years after the endovascular procedure for complex aortic disease even though most reinterventions were required for type III endoleak, similar to other reports.[14,17,18]

The two centres performing endovascular procedures shared the same team leader and thereby similar training and techniques and the three hospitals all applied the standard postoperative care used by high-volume centres performing thoracoabdominal aneurysms repairs, there may be some subtle differences in populations and hospital facilities that could not have been captured as with a random assignment.

Conclusion

The present study suggests that in matched patient populations with thoracoabdominal aneurysms, endovascular and open repair may be associated with a similar 30-day and two-year mortality. Permanent spinal cord ischaemia may be also comparable with the two treatments and around 10% at 30 days, highlighting the uncertainty regarding the best management to prevent this complication after repair.

Nevertheless, the 30-day overall morbidity may be two times lower using endovascular repair. The impact of respiratory stress and age remain of paramount relevance in planning open repair for thoracoabdominal aneurysms even in average-risk patients. These findings may help identifying the best suited approach for individual patients.

Summary

- Comparison of open and endovascular procedures for the treatment of thoracoabdominal aneurysms.

- Multicentric comparative analysis with propensity score matching.

- Endovascular and open repair may be associated with a similar 30-day and two-year mortality.

- 30-day overall morbidity may be two times lower using endovascular repair.

References

1. Demers P, Miller DC, Mitchell RS, *et al.* Midterm results of endovascular repair of descending thoracic aortic aneurysms with first-generation stent grafts. *J Thorac Cardiovasc Surg* 2004; **127**: 664–73.
2. Cheng D, Martin J, Shennib H, *et al.* Endovascular aortic repair *versus* open surgical repair for descending thoracic aortic disease a systematic review and meta-analysis of comparative studies. *J Am Coll Cardiol* 2010; **55**: 986–1001.
3. Giles KA, Pomposelli F, Hamdan A, *et al.* Decrease in total aneurysm-related deaths in the era of endovascular aneurysm repair. *J Vasc Surg* 2009; **49**: 543–51.
4. Schwarze ML, Shen Y, Hemmerich J, Dale W. Age-related trends 1 in utilization and outcome of open and endovascular repair for abdominal aortic aneurysm in the United States, 2001-2006. *J Vasc Surg* 2009; **50**: 722–29.
5. Jacobs MJ, Mommertz G, Koeppel TA, *et al.* Surgical repair of thoracoabdominal aortic aneurysms. *J Cardiovasc Surg* (Torino). 2007; **48**: 49–58.
6. Coselli JS, Bozinovski J, LeMaire SA. Open surgical repair of 2286 thoracoabdominal aortic aneurysms. *Ann Thorac Surg.* 2007; **83**: S862–64;.
7. Kazen UP, Blohmé L, Olsson C, Hultgren R. Open Repair of Aneurysms of the Thoracoabdominal Aorta. *Thorac Cardiovasc Surg* 2015 DOI: 10.1055/s-0035-1564450
8. Greenberg R, Eagleton M, Mastracci T. Branched endografts for thoracoabdominal aneurysms. *J Thorac Cardiovasc Surg.* 2010; **140** (6 Suppl): S171–78.
9. Parsons L. Using SAS software to perform a case-controlled method for bias reduction in an observational study. In: Proceedings of the Twenty-Fifth Annual SAS Users Group International Conference. Cary, NC: SAS Institute, Inc; 2000. p. 1166–71.
10. Rosenbaum PR, Rubin DB. Reducing bias in observational studies using subclassification on the propensity score. *J Am Stat Assoc* 1984; **79**: 516–24.
11. Blackstone EH. Comparing apples and oranges. *J Thorac Cardiovasc Surg* 2002; **123**: 8–15.
12. Tsilimparis N, Perez S, Dayama A, Ricotta JJ 2nd. Endovascular repair with fenestrated branched stent grafts improves 30-day outcomes for complex aortic aneurysms compared with open repair. *Ann Vasc Surg* 2013; **27**: 267–73.
13. Greenberg RK, Lytle B. Endovascular repair of thoracoabdominal aneurysms. *Circulation* 2008; **117**: 2288–96.
14. Austermann M, Donas KP, Panuccio G, Troisi 1 N, Torsello G. Pararenal and thoracoabdominal aortic aneurysm repair with fenestrated and branched endografts: lessons learned and future directions. *J Endovasc Ther* 2011; **18**: 157–60.
15. Maurel B, Delclaux N, Sobocinski J, *et al.* The impact of early pelvic and lower limb reperfusion and attentive peri-operative management on the incidence of spinal cord ischemia during thoracoabdominal aortic aneurysm endovascular repair. *Eur J Vasc Endovasc Surg* 2015; **49**: 248–54.
16. Raux M, Patel VI, Cochennec F, *et al.* A propensity-matched comparison of outcomes for fenestrated endovascular aneurysm repair and open surgical repair of complex abdominal aortic aneurysms. *J Vasc Surg* 2014; **60**: 858–63
17. Haulon S, Greenberg RK. Part two: treatment of type IV thoracoabdominal aneurysms—fenestrated stent-graft repair is now the best option. *Eur J Vasc Endovasc Sur* 2011; **42**: 4–8
18. Troisi N, Donas KP, Austermann M, *et al.* Secondary procedures after aortic aneurysm repair with fenestrated and branched endografts. *J Endovasc Ther* 2011; **18**: 146–53.

Long-term survival after TEVAR depends on indications

K Mani, T Hellgren and A Wanhainen

Introduction

Stent graft implantation for treatment of thoracic aortic disease was first performed for a chronic aortic transection aneurysm by Volodos in Ukraine.[1] Since then, thoracic endovascular aortic repair (TEVAR) has been tested and proven effective in treatment of various elective and acute disorders of the descending thoracic aorta.[2-4] TEVAR has revolutionised surgical treatment of diseases in this aortic segment, and endovascular repair is currently the treatment of choice in patients with complicated acute type B dissection, acute and elective thoracic aortic aneurysm, and aortic transection.[5] Stent graft insertion is also increasingly used in treatment of chronic dissection aneurysms.[6] In England, the incidence of descending aortic aneurysm and dissection repair more than doubled after 2006, due to the broad introduction of TEVAR, with the sharpest increase occurring in the elderly population.[7]

The scientific evidence for TEVAR in treatment of descending aortic pathology is mainly based on single- or multicentre reports, and registry based comparisons of endovascular repair to open surgery.[8,9] In the short term, TEVAR is associated with lower mortality and morbidity rates than open descending aortic surgery. The minimally invasive treatment also enables surgical intervention in patients who would otherwise not be considered fit for open aortic repair (Figure 1). In this chapter, the short- and long-term results of TEVAR for different indications are discussed.

Patient demographics and short-term outcome

The perioperative mortality and morbidity rates of TEVAR are naturally related to indication and the acuteness of the intervention. Emergency repair for acute type B dissection, ruptured aneurysm or traumatic transection is associated with mortality due to the systemic effects of the acute aortic syndrome, or present comorbidities. Patient characteristics often differ with indication for TEVAR. In a joint registry-based analysis of all patients treated with TEVAR with Medtronic devices in five prospective registries and a single institution series, mean age was approximately 10 years older for patients treated for aneurysmal disease compared with those treated for dissection disease in the aorta.[10] The same trend was present in an analysis of all TEVARs performed at Uppsala University Hospital 1999–2013. A total of 250 patients were included in this analysis. Patients treated for acute or chronic dissection were in their mid-60s, while patients treated for intact or

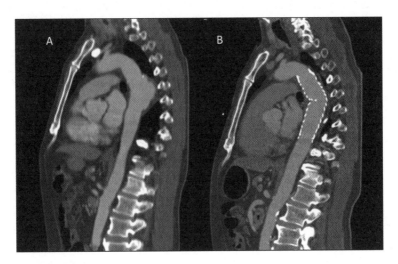

Figure 1: Descending thoracic aortic aneurysm (A) in an elderly patient with cardiac and pulmonary comorbidity prohibiting open surgical repair. After TEVAR (B), the aneurysm is sealed and the aorta has remodelled.

ruptured aneurysm were on average 72 and 75 years old respectively. Traumatic transection patients are a different category, with an over-representation of young male patients. In a multicentre analysis, mean patient age was 41 years, with 84% male patients.[11]

The perioperative mortality after elective TEVAR for thoracic aortic aneurysm or chronic dissection is reported at 3–5%.[10,12] Neurological events such as spinal cord ischaemia and stroke occurs in approximately 5% of the patients, and the rate is higher in patients treated for aneurysmal disease, compared to those treated for dissection.[10] For patients treated with an acute indication, mortality is highest among those treated for ruptured aortic aneurysm. Non-elective aneurysm mortality was 18% in the 38 patients in the Medtronic registries, and reached in excess of 25% in the Uppsala experience of ruptured thoracic aneurysms. The results are better for traumatic ruptures, where 30-day mortality was 9% in the multicentre report,[11] with most deaths related to concomitant trauma injuries. For patients with acute complicated type B dissection, 30-day mortality is reported at 10% in large registries,[8] with higher mortality in patients treated for mesenteric malperfusion or ruptured dissection. The neurological event rate is significantly higher in patients treated for ruptured aneurysm, with spinal cord injury occurring in up to one tenth of the patients.[10] This is related to the combination of hypotension and extensive aortic coverage with TEVAR. Other predictors of early mortality after TEVAR include high age, presence of comorbidities (especially renal failure), and presence of spinal cord injury post repair.

Long-term outcome

Relevant parameters for successful long-term outcome after TEVAR include age and comorbidity, and freedom from aortic complications and from reinterventions. Based on the experience from abdominal aortic aneurysm repair, the main concern with an expanding TEVAR practice is that the patients may remain at a higher risk of late aortic complications or reinterventions after endovascular repair compared with what would be the case after open surgery. In addition, the increasing rate of intervention among patients who are not regarded as suitable for open surgery may result in TEVAR treatment of patients who would not benefit from the repair due to high risk of death as a result of high age and/or comorbidities.

Type B dissection

For patients with type B dissection, the five-year survival after TEVAR is approximately 80–90%.[8,13] Although this is an excellent result, it should be underlined that the survival of aortic dissection patients still remains lower than that of an age matched population. Survival after acute complicated type B dissection repair is higher with an endovascular technique than with open surgery, which is the rationale for preference for TEVAR in this setting.[8] The five-year survival rate is comparable in patients with acute complicated type B dissection and those treated for chronic dissection aneurysms.[10] Successful long-term outcome of TEVAR for dissection includes aortic remodelling, with thrombosis of the false lumen and reduction of the false lumen volume as a surrogate marker for success. Aortic remodelling occurs more often in those treated with TEVAR in the acute or subacute phase of the disease, and in patients in whom the dissection is confined to the thoracic aorta above the diaphragm.[14]

Aortic related reinterventions are common after TEVAR for type B dissection. Approximately one-third of patients require aortic reinterventions, most of which can be performed with an endovascular technique.[13,15] Reinterventions are more common in patients treated for acute type B dissection than in those treated for chronic disease, and in those with an extensive dissection including the thoracoabdominal aorta.[10,15,16] This mandates vigorous follow-up with regular imaging to identify possible complications or need for reinterventions timely. Late aortic death remains a rare event after TEVAR for type B dissection, indicating that the treatment is successful.[10] There are, however, indications that lack of aortic remodelling after TEVAR may be associated with worse outcome with risk of late aortic-related death.[15]

Thoracic aortic aneurysm

Patients with thoracic aortic aneurysm have a lower five-year survival rate compared to those treated for dissection disease. The five-year survival rate for thoracic aortic aneurysm patients was <60% in the Medtronic registries,[10] which mainly included elective repairs. In the Uppsala cohort, the five-year survival for intact thoracic aortic aneurysms was 65%. This is comparable to the long-term survival of patients treated for intact abdominal aortic aneurysm, which was 69% at five years in a Swedish cohort.[17]

Thoracic aneurysm patients are older than dissection patients, and have a higher atherosclerotic disease burden, explaining this higher mortality rate. In the Medtronic registries, aneurysm patients had a significantly higher rate of renal impairment, chronic obstructive pulmonary disease, and cardiac disease than those treated for dissection disease. The cause of death analysis in this cohort indicated that aortic-related death constituted only 9% of the late deaths, while most late deaths being attributable to cardiac disease.

Data regarding long-term survival of patients treated with TEVAR for ruptured thoracic aortic aneurysm is scarce. In a national analysis from England based on

Hospital Episode Statistics data, 97 patients treated with TEVAR and 44 patients treated with open repair for ruptured thoracic aortic aneurysm were identified.[18] Thirty-day mortality was equal for those treated with open repair and TEVAR, and long-term survival was not reported specifically for the ruptured group. Patients treated with TEVAR had a higher rate of re-interventions than those treated with open surgery. This study also assessed the turn down rate of ruptured thoracic aneurysms in England over a 12-year period, and concluded that the proportion of patients being offered repair after thoracic aortic rupture had increased from 7% in 1999 to 51% in 2010, mainly due to a high proportion of patients being treated with TEVAR.

In a single-centre analysis, the long-term survival of TEVAR for aortic rupture in Uppsala was assessed (Figure 2). Despite acceptable perioperative results, only less than one third of the patients treated for aortic rupture were alive at three years after repair, and none of the patients survived five years after the repair. As a comparison, the crude five-year survival rate after ruptured abdominal aortic aneurysm repair was 42% in Sweden.[17] Expansion of TEVAR to treat patients unfit for surgery in this field has, therefore, resulted in an improved short-term outcome after rupture, but long-term survival remains low in these patients with multiple comorbidities.

Aortic transection

Patients treated for aortic transection are much younger compared with the other indications for TEVAR. When assessing the results up to 10 years after TEVAR, survival rate was approximately 80%, and most reinterventions were stent graft related and occurred within the first year after implantation.[11] However, the long-term results in these patients will be related to possible device-related complications, such as device failure and stent graft induced aortic wall degeneration, 20 to 50 years after implantation. Furthermore, aortic diameter increases with age, and one of the concerns is how the small stent grafts put into young patients with aortic transection will behave with increasing age.

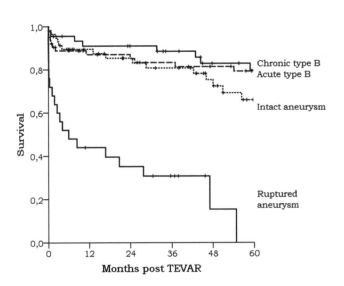

Figure 2: Long-term survival after TEVAR based on indication in a single-centre analysis at Uppsala University Hospital.

Conclusion

Repair of thoracic aortic disease has been transformed with TEVAR, which is currently the first-line treatment for various indications. Short- and mid-term outcomes of TEVAR are excellent for patients with dissection of the descending aorta, and intact thoracic aortic aneurysms, and aortic transection. For patients with thoracic aneurysm rupture, TEVAR offers an opportunity to treat patients with acceptable short-term outcome, and expands treatment options to many patients who were not regarded as surgical candidates previously. However, the long-term survival of these patients is dismal, due to excessive cardiopulmonary comorbidity. When assessing long-term outcome of TEVAR, it is important to report results separately based on indication, rather than based on surgical technique.

Summary

- In the short-term, TEVAR offers lower mortality and morbidity rates than that of open surgery for thoracic aortic disease.

- Perioperative mortality after elective TEVAR is 3–5%, with higher rate of neurological events in patients treated for aneurysmal disease than those treated for dissection.

- For acute TEVAR, short-term mortality is in the range of 10% after acute complicated dissection and aortic transection, and 20–25% for ruptured thoracic aneurysm.

- Long-term survival after TEVAR is highly dependent on indication, with five year survival at 80% for dissections and transections, and 60–65% for elective aneurysms.

- In patients treated for ruptured thoracic aneurysm, data on long-term survival is scarce. A single centre analysis indicates that less than one third of the patients remain alive at three years after TEVAR.

- The expansion of TEVAR to offer intervention in non-surgical candidates may therefore result in acceptable short-term outcomes, but high mortality in the long term.

References

1. Volodos NL. Historical perspective: The first steps in endovascular aortic repair: how it all began. *J Endovasc Ther* 2013; **20** Suppl 1: I3–23.
2. Dake MD, Miller DC, Semba CP, *et al*. Transluminal placement of endovascular stent-grafts for the treatment of descending thoracic aortic aneurysms. *N Engl J Med* 1994; **331** (26): 1729–34.
3. Dake MD, Kato N, Mitchell RS, *et al*. Endovascular stent-graft placement for the treatment of acute aortic dissection. *N Engl J Med* 1999; **340** (20): 1546–52.
4. Semba CP, Kato N, Kee ST, *et al*. Acute rupture of the descending thoracic aorta: repair with use of endovascular stent-grafts. *J Vasc Interv Radiol* 1997; **8** (3): 337–42.
5. Clough RE, Mani K, Lyons OT, *et al*. Endovascular treatment of acute aortic syndrome. *J Vasc Surg* 2011; **54** (6): 1580–87.
6. Thrumurthy SG, Karthikesalingam A, Patterson BO, *et al*. A systematic review of mid-term outcomes of thoracic endovascular repair (TEVAR) of chronic type B aortic dissection. *Eur J Vasc Endovasc Surg* 2011; **42** (5): 632–47.

7. von Allmen RS, Anjum A, Powell JT. Incidence of descending aortic pathology and evaluation of the impact of thoracic endovascular aortic repair: a population-based study in England and Wales from 1999 to 2010. *Eur J Vasc Endovasc Surg* 2013; **45** (2): 154–59.

8. Fattori R, Tsai TT, Myrmel T, *et al.* Complicated acute type B dissection: is surgery still the best option?: a report from the International Registry of Acute Aortic Dissection. *JACC Cardiovascular interventions* 2008; **1** (4): 395–402.

9. Desai ND, Burtch K, Moser W, *et al.* Long-term comparison of thoracic endovascular aortic repair (TEVAR) to open surgery for the treatment of thoracic aortic aneurysms. *J Thorac Cardiovasc Surg* 2012; **144** (3): 604–609; Discussion 609–11.

10. Patterson B, Holt P, Nienaber C, *et al.* Aortic pathology determines midterm outcome after endovascular repair of the thoracic aorta: report from the Medtronic Thoracic Endovascular Registry (MOTHER) database. *Circulation* 2013; **127** (1): 24–32.

11. Steuer J, Bjorck M, Sonesson B, *et al.* Editor's Choice - Durability of endovascular repair in blunt traumatic thoracic aortic injury: Long-term outcome from four tertiary referral centers. *Eur J Vasc Endovasc Surg* 2015; **50** (4): 460–65.

12. Patel HJ, Williams DM, Drews JD, *et al.* A 20-year experience with thoracic endovascular aortic repair. *Ann Surg* 2014; **260** (4): 691–97.

13. Steuer J, Eriksson MO, Nyman R, *et al.* Early and long-term outcome after thoracic endovascular aortic repair (TEVAR) for acute complicated type B aortic dissection. *Eur J Vasc Endovasc Surg* 2011; **41** (3): 318–23.

14. Patterson BO, Cobb RJ, Karthikesalingam A, *et al.* A systematic review of aortic remodeling after endovascular repair of type B aortic dissection: methods and outcomes. *Ann Thorac Surg* 2014; **97** (2): 588–95.

15. Mani K, Clough RE, Lyons OT, *et al.* Predictors of outcome after endovascular repair for chronic type B dissection. *Eur J Vasc Endovasc Surg* 2012; **43**: 386–91.

16. Eriksson MO, Steuer J, Wanhainen A, *et al.* Morphologic outcome after endovascular treatment of complicated type B aortic dissection. *J Vasc Interv Radiol* 2013; **24** (12): 1826-33.

17. Mani K, Bjorck M, Lundkvist J, Wanhainen A. Improved long-term survival after abdominal aortic aneurysm repair. *Circulation* 2009; **120** (3): 201–11.

18. von Allmen RS, Anjum A, Powell JT. Outcomes after endovascular or open repair for degenerative descending thoracic aortic aneurysm using linked hospital data. *Br J Surg* 2014; **101** (10): 1244–51.

Radiation damage to the pioneer operators

Endovascular total aorta replacement challenges

T Resch

Introduction

Endovascular aneurysm repair (EVAR) has been an established procedure for over 20 years. What began as an almost inconceivably simple approach to aortic repair, championed by Volodos and Parodi in the late 1980s and 1990s, has evolved into the primary choice for the standard repair of infrarenal aortic aneurysms. Its efficacy, durability and clinical success has been established in several randomised trials that clearly show the technique to be favourable to conventional open repair, when patients are anatomically suitable for standard infrarenal EVAR.[1] In the setting of aneurysm rupture, robust trial data have, understandably, been more difficult to produce. In the recently published IMPROVE trial, and the following subanalyses, the authors find that although EVAR provides no significant short-term mortality advantage over open repair, patients ultimately treated with EVAR have a significantly lower perioperative mortality.[2] In addition, patients undergoing EVAR have significantly better quality of life, and a higher chance of hospital discharge. In addition, EVAR has a significant cost-effectiveness benefit over open repair. Therefore, the authors ultimately advise that all patients suitable for EVAR should have the procedure.

In parallel to the evolution of infrarenal abdominal aortic aneurysm treatment, endovascular strategies were developed in the early 1990s to tackle pathologies involving the thoracic aorta, including aortic dissections, aneurysms, ulcers and traumatic aortic transections. It has since been widely established that thoracic endovascular aneurysm repair (TEVAR) is the preferred treatment modality for the vast majority of these pathologies as well.[3,4] A less traumatic event than open thoracic repair—often requiring thoracotomy as well as bypass adjuncts—TEVAR has led to decreased rates of mortality and of morbidity, including respiratory complications, spinal cord ischaemia issues, and cardiac complications.

Dissection treatment is still a controversial topic, but when invasive treatment is indicated, an endovascular approach is generally highly favoured.[5] In most cases of classical Stanford type B dissections, proximal TEVAR covering the primary entry tear in the proximal descending thoracic aorta is the recommended treatment. However, the absolute indications for TEVAR in the acute setting, apart from rupture and clinical malperfusion, remain controversial. Some reported data indicate that interventions might be warranted, even in uncomplicated dissections, to prevent long-term aortic failure. Solid data, however, are largely lacking. Similarly, the timing of intervention for type B dissections is less than clear-cut. Some authors suggest that treatment should be performed in the subacute phase

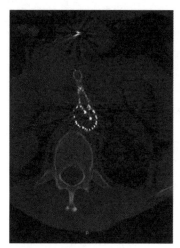
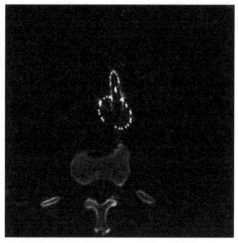

Figure 1a: Completion cone-beam CT showing compression of stent in the superior mesenteric artery after fenestrated endografting.

Figure 1b: Repeat cone-beam CT after percutaneous transluminal angioplasty of superior mesenteric artery stent showing good stent configuration.

(two weeks to three months after symptom onset) to minimise risk and optimise positive aortic remodelling.

Aortic segments involving branching vessels represent a particular challenge for all aortic repair; endovascular as well as open. John Anderson and colleagues first described fenestrated aortic repair in 1999. By designing a stent graft (Zenith, Cook Medical) with fenestrations in the position of aortic branching target vessels, the aortic repair could be extended into the juxta and pararenal position, while preserving branch vessel flow. This technique has subsequently been applied to more extensive thoracoabdominal aneurysms, as well as pathologies involving the aortic arch. Many studies have established the role for fenestrated aortic repair as a valid option in many patients.[6,7] Other platforms have also been developed such as the Anaconda (Vascutek) and the e-Vita (Jotec) devices.

Another option for preserving branch vessel flow is the use of directional branches instead of fenestrations. The use of branches for thoracoabdominal aortic aneurysm repair was first described by Tim Chuter, University of California, San Francisco, USA.[8] This technology was later also applied in the aortic arch as well as in the iliac bifurcation.[9] For the iliac bifurcation, branch devices have become the technique of choice.[10]

Fenestrations and branches can be used in combination to achieve a repair that is optimally designed to fit the specific aortic anatomy. There is no clear evidence favouring the use of fenestrations *versus* branches in the thoracoabdominal aorta but, rather, surgeon preference and device availability dictates choice.[11]

It is becoming evident that the technological development of aortic stent grafts has now enabled treatment of the vast majority of aortic pathologies, from the aortic valve, down to the common femoral artery. Some areas, such as infrarenal EVAR and descending TEVAR, are more mature than others with regards to evaluation and long-term outcomes. But, data are accumulating even for more complex treatments, and we are beginning to have more specific treatment algorithms defined.

With the increasing width, depth and complexity of aortic repair, as well as an increased understanding of the natural history of aortic disease, we are also learning more about the potential risks of the adjuncts that are necessary for the successful practice of endovascular repair.

All phases of endovascular repair—preoperative planning, repair and follow-up—rely to some degree on imaging. Imaging is vital to accurately analyse the aortic morphology, to tailor graft planning preoperatively, to precisely and safely implant the endovascular device, and to evaluate the repair during follow-up.[12] With the use of imaging, the concepts of radiation and contrast use are central. One must always consider the possible negative side-effects they might have for both patients and operators. With more challenging aortic repairs, the use of radiation and contrast tend to increase.

The aim of this chapter is to outline the possible advantages and disadvantages of radiation and contrast use during all phases of EVAR, and to outline some developments and strategies to maximise the utility of imaging while minimising the risks.

Contrast use during EVAR and potential side-effects

Contrast-enhanced computed tomography (CT) angiography is the gold standard for pre- and postoperative imaging during EVAR. Modern protocols for pre- and postoperative EVAR imaging use multidetector scanners with 64–128 rows. Images are acquired at 0.6–1.25mm slice thickness at a pitch of 1.0–1.5, and a reconstruction interval of 0.5-0.625. For follow up imaging, a delayed scan of the same format is acquired after one minute in order to detect any type II endoleaks. As ionised contrast has a potentially nephrotoxic effect, particularly when used repeatedly, it must be used with caution. One must also realise that acceptance of an inferior preoperative CT angiography, in the attempt to reduce contrast load and nephrotoxicity, might potentially lead to improper planning and a more challenging operation requiring excessive amounts of intraoperative contrast to guide and adjust the implantation. In the preoperative evaluation in patients with renal insufficiency, protocols utilising lower contrast doses are available. To achieve adequate imaging quality and resolution, scanner settings can be adapted to run at lower voltage (80kV), which allows for a higher enhancement of the iodine contrast maintaining the diagnostic potential. Another option is to use intra-arterial contrast administration via a catheter. Although this requires invasive catheter placement, the amount of contrast is reduced, and the scan following a CT scan can be limited to the segment of interest where the highest resolution is needed.

Intraoperatively, excessive amounts of contrast should be avoided. Reducing the concentration of contrast, and using a power injector, can often achieve more precise imaging at a lower contrast load. Higher concentrations of contrast can be reserved for areas of particular interest. Using alternative contrast agents, such as carbon dioxide, can also dramatically decrease the total amount of contrast during a procedure. This can be effectively used for gross orientation of devices as opposed to using repeat runs of ionised contrast. Proper use of preoperative imaging can drastically reduce the use of contrast intraoperatively as well. With proper evaluation of the anatomy, proper angulation of the C-arm intraoperatively can be used to achieve optimal visualisation of vital structures and targets without the need for repeat contrast injections.

During follow-up, the best way of avoiding contrast use is to avoid performing contrast-enhanced CT studies if not specifically indicated. After standard EVAR, duplex ultrasound follow-up has proven very effective for the vast majority of routine imaging, including surveillance of target vessel flow after fenestrated and branched EVAR for pathologies involving the visceral aortic segment. Contrast-enhanced ultrasound has a high specificity for endoleak detection and delineation, and thus CT angiography can be reserved for situations when focused ultrasound is inconclusive.

The situation is different in the thoracic aorta, including the aortic arch. Ultrasound is not suitable for evaluation, and CT angiography and magnetic resonance remain the main options in this area.

Radiation effects and how to minimise them to operators and patients during EVAR

The effects of radiation can be divided into deterministic and stochastic effects. Deterministic effects are those that arise as a direct consequence of excessive radiation in the short- and midterm. Damage occurs at threshold values. In patients, inflammatory changes in the skin are most relevant and can be avoided by minimising repeat high exposure to the skin. Most modern equipment will come with warning systems to indicate when a critical skin dose has been reached. For the operator, the most relevant deterministic outcome is subcapsular induced cataracts. Recent studies indicate that there is no threshold value for cataract development. Appropriate use of shields, protective eye wear, and positioning in the operating room, is critical to minimise the risks.

Stochastic effects have no threshold values, often occur many years after exposure and include malignant development. The radiation effect is cumulative and, as such, the significance for the operators and staff is generally greater than to the EVAR patient. The highest risk to the patients is prolonged and repeated CT follow-up, which has been clearly associated with the development of malignancies. This is

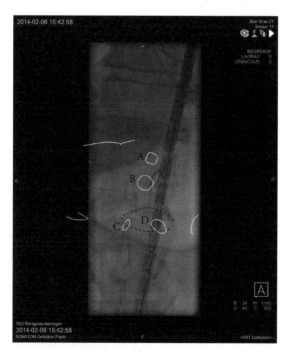

Figure 2: (A) Coeliac artery; (B) superior mesenteric artery; (C) Right renal artery; and (D) left renal artery. Interrupted ring marker denotes aortic outline just below renal arteries (to avoid parallax during stentgraft delivery).

particularly important to consider in the younger patient population undergoing EVAR/TEVAR, where alternate follow-up modalities should be used whenever possible. For most aneurysm patients, repeat CT exposures are of less risk simply because the time until malignant development is quite long, and because this patient population is generally elderly.

Intraoperative techniques to minimise radiation use
The first, and perhaps most important, means by which to reduce intraoperative radiation exposure is the proper use of imaging equipment and X-ray protection. Use of low-dose settings on C-arms can significantly reduce radiation exposure, and should be used as default. Appropriate image collimation, avoiding C-arm angulations and working with minimal magnification, as well as use of lead shield to protect from scatter radiation from the patient, is critical.[13]

The radiation exposure decreases by the inverse squared distance from the patient. Using a power injector and leaving the room during digital subtraction angiography runs can prove very effective. Limiting the use of digital subtraction angiography runs and replacing them with injections using only fluoroscopy can be sufficient and will reduce the overall exposure as well.

Advanced Intraoperative imaging
Fusion imaging works by importing the preoperative imaging data (mostly from CT angiography) into the angiographic equipment. A 3D volume or a 2D dataset is then recorded at the start of the procedure, and used to fuse the preoperative image dataset by using bony landmarks or calcium outlines in the vessel. This fusion volume then automatically follows the table and detector movement. During the procedure, the fusion overlay can be corrected to adapt to configurational changes imposed by the introduction of the stent graft. Using fusion allows for placement and vessel catheterisation without using further angiographic runs for orientation, thus reducing the overall radiation exposure (Figure 2).[14]

Cone-beam CT provides a scan by employing a 5–8 second C-arm rotation around the patient. The volume image set is processed in a workstation, allowing the operator to view the images as they would a standard CT in axial, sagittal or coronal views (Figure 1). Advanced post-processing of the images in 3D rendering is also available to help the operator to detect kinks or stent graft compression that can be difficult to interpret when conducting the final angiogram.[15] During complex EVAR, the cone-beam CT in completion state also gives the operator the chance to detect compressions and kinks in the mating stents of the stent graft, which is often difficult to detect by digital subtraction angiography alone.[16] This improved diagnostic tool allows for treatment of potential failures immediately, thereby potentially reducing the need for early reinterventions after EVAR, given that most early reintervention is due to technical or stent graft-associated problems.

The current drawbacks of cone-beam CT are the higher amounts of radiation exposure, and the sometimes sub-optimal image quality. Recent studies indicate that one cone-beam CT might provide radiation equivalent to a standard three phase, postoperative CT angiography.[17] Clearly, clinical judgment is needed in every situation to maximise patient benefit whilst minimising exposure according to the "as low as reasonably achievable" (ALARA) principle. Studies indicate that the reduced need for reinterventions when using cone-beam CT, and perhaps also the reduced need for early postoperative CT angiography, might compensate for the increase in perioperative radiation exposure.

A recent study evaluating the combined use of the techniques described in this paper indicates that it can lead to significant reductions in radiation and exposure to both patients and operators during EVAR.[18] Reduction of the frame rate setting alone (from 7.5f/second to 3.75f/second) reduced the dose area product by 22%. Contrast volume and iodine dose were reduced by 75% and 50%, respectively, despite unchanged operating and fluoroscopic times.

Summary

- EVAR and TEVAR are well established for infrarenal aortic aneurysms and descending thoracic aortic pathologies.

- Endovascular repair of areas including aortic branch vessels, such as iliac bifurcation, visceral aorta and the aortic arch, is evolving rapidly.

- Proper use and evaluation of preoperative imaging for planning is vital to minimise contrast and radiation exposure during complex EVAR.

- Operators and staff are at high risk for radiation exposure during complex cases.

- Proper use of X-ray equipment, X-ray protection and understanding of fundamental principles of minimising radiation exposure is critical to minimise risk.

- Advanced imaging using fusion technology and intraoperative cone beam CT has the possibility of reducing exposure and improving outcome.

References

1. United Kingdom ETI, Greenhalgh RM, *et al.* Endovascular *versus* open repair of abdominal aortic aneurysm. *The New England Journal of Medicine* 2010; **362**: 1863–71.
2. Investigators IT, Powell JT, *et al.* Endovascular or open repair strategy for ruptured abdominal aortic aneurysm: 30 day outcomes from IMPROVE randomised trial. *BMJ* 2014; **348**: f7661.
3. Steuer J, *et al.* Editor's choice - Durability of endovascular repair in blunt traumatic thoracic aortic injury: Long-term outcome from four tertiary referral centers. *European Journal of Vascular and Endovascular Surgery* 2015; **50**: 460–65.
4. Bicknell C, Powell JT. Aortic disease: thoracic endovascular aortic repair. Heart 2015; **01**: 586–91.
5. Scott AJ, Bicknell CD. Contemporary management of acute type B dissection. *European Journal of Vascular and Endovascular Surgery* 2015; doi: 10.1016/j.ejvs.2015.10.026.
6. Kristmundsson T, *et al.* Outcomes of fenestrated endovascular repair of juxtarenal aortic aneurysm. *Journal of Vascular Surgery* 2014; **59**: 115–20.
7. Rao Vallabhaneni S, *et al.* Global collaborators on advanced stent-graft techniques for aneurysm repair (GLOBALSTAR) project. *Journal of Endovascular Therapy* 2007; **14**: 352–6.
8. Chuter TA, *et al.* An endovascular system for thoracoabdominal aortic aneurysm repair. *Journal of Endovascular Therapy* 2001; **8**: 25–33.
9. Haulon S, *et al.* Global experience with an inner branched arch endograft. *The Journal of Thoracic and Cardiovascular Surgery* 2014; **148**: 1709–16.
10. Oderich GS, Greenberg RK. Endovascular iliac branch devices for iliac aneurysms. *Perspectives in Vascular Surgery and Endovascular Therapy* 2011; **23**: 166–72.
11. Conway BD, *et al.* Renal artery implantation angles in thoracoabdominal aneurysms and their implications in the era of branched endografts. *Journal of Endovascular Therapy* 2010; **17**: 38–7.

12. Tornqvist P, Dias NV, Resch T. Optimizing imaging for aortic repair. *The Journal of Cardiovascular Surgery* 2015; **56**: 189–95.

13. Maurel B, *et al*. Techniques to reduce radiation and contrast volume during EVAR. *The Journal of Cardiovascular Surgery* 2014; **55**: 123–31.

14. Hertault A, *et al*. Impact of hybrid rooms with image fusion on radiation exposure during endovascular aortic repair. *European Journal of Vascular and Endovascular Surgery* 2014; **48**: 382–90.

15. Tornqvist P, *et al*. Utility of intraoperative cone beam computed tomography in endovascular treatment of aortoiliac occlusive disease. *European Journal of Vascular and Endovascular Surgery* 2015; **61**: 13S.

16. Tornqvist P, *et al*. Intra-operative cone beam computed tomography can help avoid reinterventions and reduce CT follow up after infrarenal EVAR. *European Journal of Vascular and Endovascular Surgery* 2015; **49**: 390–5.

17. Tornqvist P, unpublished data.

18. Dias N, *et al*. The effects of combining fusion imaging, low-frequency pulsed fluoroscopy, and low-concentration contrast agent during EVAR. *Journal of Vascular Surgery* 2015; **61**: 17S–18S.

Endovascular radiation protection training: Reduction of radiation exposure to patients and staff

M Strøm, L Konge, TV Schroeder, HN Waltenburg and LB Lönn

Introduction

Interventional procedures are performed using ionising radiation for visualising structures. The patient, operator and staff are all exposed to radiation directly from the X-ray tube, and to scattered radiation from the patient and the surroundings. The use of X-ray follows the "as low as reasonably achievable" (ALARA) principle as part of radiation protection.[1] Several steps can, and must, be taken to reduce stochastic and deterministic effects of radiation exposure to the patient as well as to the staff. The optimal use of X-ray intensity, contrast and collimation primarily aims to reduce the amount of radiation delivered to ensure "good enough" X-ray images for clinical work. The use of absorbers aims to reduce the amount of scattered radiation produced secondarily to the intervention. Personal protective equipment, such as lead augmented aprons, glasses, thyroid collars and gloves, add further shield to operators and staff where it is not practicable to avoid the presence of operators and staff close to the patient. However, not even the optimal suit of armour provides protection for incautious behaviour, and distance from radiation is a significant factor in radiation intensity. Thus, there is a need to educate all members of staff to ensure optimal radiation protection behaviour, and thereby reduce the cumulated exposure endured throughout a career. Legislation in Europe, and the recommendations from the International Commission On Radiological Protection advise that all staff exposed to radiation should be educated in radiation protection and credentialed through national legislation.[2] In Denmark, accreditation is obtained though specialist training. The National Society for Interventional Radiology advocates post-certification training, as proposed in the Cardiovascular and Interventional Radiological Society of Europe (CIRSE) syllabus.[3,4]

Education in the field of radiation protection can be achieved at several levels in concordance with Miller's pyramid for learning clinical competence from "knows" to "does".[5] Understanding the equipment used, radiation physics and tissue absorption is fundamental for acting within the borders of caution. Knowledge of this can be achieved from textbook materials. Adequate behaviour during radiation can be trained live by a proctor, in a mock up setting, or in an off-site simulated environment where the trainee can learn how to position himself according to table position and C arm angulation. These modes of training will be discussed in this chapter.

Background

Occupational radiation doses of staff working in interventional radiology are in general higher than for staff working in other areas of radiology. This is due to the fact that interventional radiology staff must work inside the room and close to the patient during radiation exposure, while the staff working in diagnostic radiology will, in the vast majority of cases, stay outside of the room during exposure. Use of lead augmented aprons is standard and mandatory for staff working in an X-ray room and this lowers the absorbed doses to the main parts of the body considerably. However, the hands and the eyes remain outside the protection of lead augmented aprons, which is of special concern because of the proximity from hands to the radiation field, and the particular sensitivity of the eyes to radiation. Over-representation of cataract has been observed, for example, in US radiological technologists exposed to high eye lens doses.[6] This, and similar observations, have led to a lowering of the dose limit to the lens of the eye from 150mSv/year to 20mSv/year.[7]

Radiation exposure affects human cells, which may lead to acute (deterministic) effects, which will be manifest within hours to weeks, and to late (stochastic) effects, which show a latency period of several years. For deterministic effects—such as skin burns and hair loss—dose thresholds exist, and the effects should not occur in cases of dosage below the threshold. The occupational dose limits are set below these thresholds and, by good practice, deterministic effects should be avoidable for staff.

Low-dose exposures are associated with a long-term risk of cancer, which is considered to be proportional to the dose, without a threshold (Linear-no-threshold

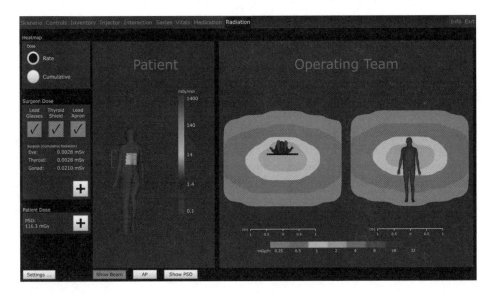

Figure 1: Dose heatmap from simulator showing radiation to patient and operator. Copyright: AB Mentice, Gothenburg, Sweden.

(LNT) theory). Therefore, doses to staff should be kept as low as possible to minimise such risk. For patients, the benefits of medical procedures using radiation must outweigh the risks of radiation exposure for the procedure to be justified. Procedures carried out as part of the treatment of severe or life-threatening conditions are of course justified; the cancer risk will by far be outweighed by the risks of not performing the procedure. For very long interventional procedures, there will also be a risk of causing skin burns to the patient. In most cases, these effects will be avoidable, e.g. by limiting the dose to individual parts of the skin by changing the entrance field of the X-ray field.

Methods

Radiation protection is a minor component of the basic medical curricula at Danish universities. In the specialist education for radiology, a 10-hour course in radiation protection is included (seven hours of theory and three hours of practical training). Otherwise, the antiquated master-apprentice scheme—"see one, do one, teach one"—is predominant. There is a current shift in medical education towards a "mastery" style of learning, in contrast to this method, in which the learner trains and then is tested and retested until a proficiency standard is reached.[8] A contemporary issue in clinical practice is how to train clinical procedures.

Simulation-based training cannot replace clinical *in vivo* learning for skills-based specialties. Metric-based simulation training can, however, supplement the early part of the learning curve. Thus, training or acquiring knowledge of an endovascular procedure can be acquired by the use of a high fidelity virtual reality simulator.[9] By using a simulator, the trainee can learn the procedural steps, and how to handle the endovascular instruments. Most importantly, the trainee can also learn how to use fluoroscopy, the collimators, and other tools, to manage the (virtual) radiation dose. The simulated setup allows the trainee to make errors first-hand, without endangering the patient, and without exposing themselves to radiation.[10-14] The setup can be very basic—with just the endovascular training interface for instrument insertion and monitors for fluoroscopy images—or more elaborate, with an entire faux endosuite including an interactive C-arm, replicating full-scale procedures allowing full or partial team training.[15]

A wide range of endovascular interventions can be trained, including all endovascular specialists and their team members. The simulator conveys fluoroscopy images, and shows the interaction of the instruments with the virtual anatomy. Real endovascular instruments—with their active tips removed—are used, and the simulator emulates the tip and its interaction. Simulation cases can either be developed by the simulator manufacturer, or can be real cases based on computed tomography (CT) angiography; segmented and added to the simulator. It is thereby possible to rehearse on actual patient data before the real procedure.[9]

The simulator can also be used as a proxy to convey desirable handling of instruments and operator positioning while performing endovascular procedures. The simulator alone can relay the handling of tools in rotary and longitudinal motions, and deliver metrics in form of fluoroscopy time, contrast use, C-arm angulation, and amount of radiation delivered. By using an experienced proctor, the trainee can also be judged on instrument interaction by observation of their hand positioning, as well as their positioning in relation to the C-arm.[13] This extends training from just simple task training to full procedure training, where issues such as protective distance from the C-arm, and the effect of angulation of the C-arm to exposure, can be discussed and learned without exposing the patient, trainee, or proctor to radiation.

It is possible to extend the traditional endovascular virtual training to also include radiation protection. The big advantage is that this training is completely safe, since no actual radiation is present in this virtual environment. The simulator system has during the entire procedure full knowledge of the position of the C-arm, how and when it is activated to generate images, the position of the table, the anatomy of the patient, and all settings of the fluoroscope and more. A model of how the radiation affects the patient and the operating team and detailed information about radiation exposure can be obtained and presented to the user. Both real time "dose rate" information and "accumulated dose" can be calculated both for the patient, and the staff (depending on where in the operating room a team member has been positioned). The amount of information the simulator system has knowledge about exceeds the information available to a real cathlab system (since for example the patient anatomy is known in detail to the simulator), so the simulator estimation of radiation exposure can be very detailed.

Preliminary results of an ongoing study by the Danish Health Authority, Radiation Protection, indicated that eye doses depend very much on the kind of fluoroscopy-guided procedures carried out by staff. In the study, these doses were assessed by two different extra dosimeters; one ordinary personal dosimeter placed at shoulder level, and a dedicated eye lens dosimeter worn on the forehead with a headband. For many types of procedures, doses were observed well below the dosage limits. For staff carrying out endovascular procedures, however, the doses were around—and even above—established radiation dose limits set by the authorities.

There are commercial systems available for endovascular simulation supporting radiation safety training, such as the Mentice AB (from Sweden) and 3D Systems (Simbionix from the USA). Typically, the radiation safety module is an add-on functionality that can be applied to any simulated endovascular procedure, to supply the trainee with many details regarding radiation exposure, including estimates of applicable dose values. At least one simulator system replicates many of the C-arm/table control available on real cathlab equipment, like collimators, dosage settings, table height, cineloops, etc., and takes all these settings into account when modelling the patient and scattered radiation exposure.

Discussion

The development of medical knowledge and technical complex procedures is challenging traditional ways of educating medical trainees. Heavy demands on competence and clinical skills are placed on physicians in order to master specialised and advanced procedures. Furthermore, patients have a legitimate claim for competent physicians and are less willing to be in the care of a trainee.

The physician and team always aim to execute the procedure with excellence in order to deliver optimal care. Additionally, endovascular operators must perform procedures under consideration of exposing the patient, themselves, and their surroundings to radiation. To weigh the benefits of "intense" radiation to image quality against the adverse effects of direct and scattered radiation is a delicate task.

Furthermore, the opportunities to learn and practice in clinical settings are limited. Residents have less time to do clinical work than in the past and, currently, senior doctors have less time to supervise due to high demands of service.[16]

In the cath lab, the trainee can learn to handle the C-arm and, under direct observation, perform various positioning tasks without engaging radiation. Based on textbook knowledge, the implication of various angulations can be discussed. However, integrating the use of C-arm, radiation exposure, collimation and table position with the use of endovascular instruments requires a phantom, a glass model vasculature, or a real patient in order to have working angiographic images. This form of training allows the trainee to learn how to operate the entire range of cath lab equipment, at the expense of radiation exposure. Learning to use radiation by using radiation essentially opposes the ALARA principle. However, training is necessary in order to reach proficiency. On top of this, communication with the patient and within the team is necessary.

In this context, simulation–based training meets the current challenges and furthers the movement towards mastery learning.

The simulated system allows for additional levels of training compared to the traditional methods. Radiation safety can be practised using practical exercises with a simulated C-arm, a virtual patient, and an estimate of the scattered radiation. Explicit training on radiation safety can show the trainee the effects of interacting with the C-arm on scattered radiation. Implicit training on radiation safety can involve performing a simulated endovascular procedure, where radiation exposure is continuously tracked during the procedure. After the complete procedure, the radiation exposure performance of the physician can be studied, making note of not only accumulated doses but when, and why, the peak doses were obtained.

A simulated setting allows for the delivery of a direct radiation response to the patient, and a calculated estimate of the scattered radiation delivered to operators.

Cath lab and simulator training offer different approaches to training and have different benefits and drawbacks.

The cath lab offers full procedural freedom and, thus, the trainee must navigate the whole picture while reducing the amount of radiation and not risk adverse effects for the patient. This is where the proficient learner can fine-tune his or her operational skills. For a novice learner, this may all be overwhelming and causing cognitive load.[17] The simulated setting will, whilst lacking the full physical setup, allow the trainee to handle the equipment, angulate the C-arm and table, and learn the relationship of radiation, angulation and contrast to image quality.

While dosimeters can be used to show the radiation dose delivered to operator and staff, the simulator can calculate the dose delivered to the patient and the scattered dose delivered to the operator. This can be illustrated with a dynamic heat map showing the direct implications of altering angulation, collimation, and intensity, etc.

Furthermore, in the simulated setup tasks can be trained in-part. The adverse effect of "poor decisions" and bad planning can be illustrated without endangering patient or staff.

For a team approach, the simulated setup can be used as a frame for the procedure. However, the estimated scatter is not dynamically related to the surrounding staffs' movements and, thus, feedback will be restricted to an interpretation of the heat map and feedback from the instructor. In the cath lab, team training with live

Conclusion

Radiation protection training is an important part of the education of endovascular operators.

Both classical training and simulations training offer advantages and drawbacks. The simulated setting is radiation-free, and allows the trainee to try different approaches and learn from mistakes while receiving dynamic feedback on delivered radiation. Simulated radiation protection training, based on a proficiency standard, could potentially be used as part of the accreditation of new interventional operators in the future.

Acknowledgments: Henrik Storm (chief technology officer at Mentice AB) for his technological input.

Summary

- Currently, a shift in medical education is taking place from the classical apprenticeship model towards mastery learning with accrediting to a proficiency standard.

- CIRSE recommends that all staff exposed to radiation should be educated in radiation protection.

- Interventional procedures are generally performed using ionising radiation, which is absorbed in the patient and scattered amongst the operator and the surrounding staff.

- In order to reduce deterministic and stochastic effects, the amount of delivered radiation should be as low as reasonable achievable to create acceptable working images, whilst behaviour and use of personal protective gear should be optimised for safety.

- Radiation protection concept can be trained in an endosuite without radiation. Additionally, C-arm handling with a phantom, with or without radiation exposure, can be used to comprehensively train students how to interact with the angio equipment.

- Simulations can be used for partial-task training and full-scale team training in a total radiation-free environment. The simulator can continually estimate the radiation dose delivered to patient, operator and staff.

References

1. Moores BM. Cost-risk-benefit analysis in diagnostic radiology: A theoretical and economic basis for radiation protection of the patient. *Radiat Prot Dosimetry* 2015; doi: 10.1093/rpd/ncv506.
2. Wrixon AD. New ICRP recommendations. *J Radiol Prot* 2008; **28** : 161–68.
3. Nielsen AP, Graumann. Et europæisk Interventionsradiologisk Uddannelsesprogram 2012.
4. Belli A, Bezzi M, Nicholson A. European curriculum and syllabus for interventional radiology. Cardiovascular and Interventional Radiological Society of Europe 2013.
5. Miller GE. The assessment of clinical skills/competence/performance. *Acad Med* 1990; **65**: S63–7.

Endovascular radiation protection training: Reduction of radiation exposure to patients and staff • M Strøm, L Konge, TV Schroeder, HN Waltenburg and LB Lönn

186

6. Chodick G, *et al.* Risk of cataract after exposure to low doses of ionizing radiation: A 20-year prospective cohort study among US radiologic technologists. *Am J Epidemiol* 2008; **168**: 620–31.

7. The Council of The European Union. Council Directive 2013/59/EURATOM.

8. Mcgaghie WC. Mastery learning : It is time for medical education to join the 21st century. *Acad Med* 2015; **90**: 1–4.

9. Desender L, *et al.* Patient-specific rehearsal prior to EVAR: a pilot study. *Eur J Vasc Endovasc Surg* 2013; **45**: 639–47.

10. Våpenstad C, Buzink SN. Procedural virtual reality simulation in minimally invasive surgery. *Surg Endosc* 2013; **27**: 364–77.

11. Berry M, *et al.* The use of virtual reality for training in carotid artery stenting: a construct validation study. *Acta radiol* 2008; **49**: 801–5.

12. Coates PJB, Zealley IA, Chakraverty S. Endovascular simulator is of benefit in the acquisition of basic skills by novice operators. *J Vasc Interv Radiol* 2010; **21**: 130–4.

13. Bech B, *et al.* Construct validity and reliability of structured assessment of endovascular expertise in a simulated setting. *Eur J Vasc Endovasc Surg* 2011; **42**: 539–48.

14. Chaer RA, *et al.* Simulation improves resident performance in catheter-based intervention: results of a randomized, controlled study. *Ann Surg* 2006; **244**: 343–52.

15. Rudarakanchana N, *et al.* Virtual reality simulation for the optimization of endovascular procedures: current perspectives. *Vasc Health Risk Manag* 2015; **11**: 195–202.

16. Antiel RM, *et al.* Effects of duty hour restrictions on core competencies, education, quality of life, and burnout among general surgery interns. *JAMA Surg* 2013; **148**: 448–55.

17. Naismith LM, *et al.* Practising what we preach: using cognitive load theory for workshop design and evaluation. *Perspect Med Educ* 2015; doi: 10.1007/s40037-015-0221-9.

Aortic transection challenges and a conundrum

The Kommerell conundrum: Diverticulum or aneurysm, and when and how to treat

FJ Criado

Introduction

In 1936, German radiologist Burckhard Friedrich Kommerell (1901–1990) reported the case of an aortic diverticulum giving rise to an aberrant right subclavian artery.[1,2] His was the first clinical, rather than post-mortem, diagnosis of an aberrant right subclavian artery—a vascular anomaly first noted in 1735 but not fully related to the clinical syndrome of dysphagia caused by extrinsic compression of the oesophagus until 1761, when Bayford provided a full narrative.[3] The Latin term *lusus naturae* (freak of nature) was used as a descriptor, reflecting the anomalous anatomy and the absence of an intrinsic oesophageal lesion. The syndrome was called *dysphagia lusoria* by Autenrieth and, in 1926 Arkin suggested the term *arteria lusoria* as an appropriate label for the aberrant right subclavian artery.[4]

Kommerell's diverticulum, or diverticulum of Kommerell, is the term widely used today to denote the presence of a funnel-shaped widening at the origin and most proximal segment of the subclavian artery, whether right or left. It represents an embryological defect resulting from failure of regression with persistence of a remnant of the fourth primitive right or left dorsal arch in cases of, respectively, left-sided "normal" arch or right-sided anomalous arch.[5] The "double aortic arch" is another rare but related anomaly that continues to confuse as it can also cause *dysphagia lusoria*.[6]

Classification and Incidence

The classification of aortic diverticula proposed by Salomonowitz *et al*[7] is most useful and deserving of universal embrace:

- Type 1: Diverticulum occurring in left (so-called "normal") aortic arch in association with an aberrant right subclavian artery (Figure 1)
- Type 2: Diverticulum in right (anomalous) aortic arch associated with aberrant left subclavian artery (Figure 2)
- Type 3: Diverticulum emerging from the isthmus (ductal zone) of the thoracic aorta, not associated with the subclavian artery: non-Kommerell (or ductal) diverticulum (Figure 3).

Type 1 diverticula tend to be conical in shape while those associated with a right arch (type 2) often adopt a more rounded and larger configuration.

The reported prevalence of normal left side aortic arch with aberrant right subclavian artery is 0.7–2% of the population, and 0.04–0.4% for right-sided arch with aberrant left subclavian artery. The presence of a Kommerell's diverticulum has been reported in 20–60% of individuals with an aberrant subclavian artery.[4] Many experts believe the true prevalence of these anomalies to be higher than historical estimates in light of current experience where such lesions can be easily uncovered with computed tomography (CT) and magnetic resonance (MR) imaging. In terms of gender differences, female predominance has been noted with left aortic arch-aberrant right subclavian artery, and male predominance with right arch-aberrant left side artery.[8] Anatomically, aberrant subclavian arteries course behind the oesophagus in 80% of instances, and between the trachea and the oesophagus in 15%. A pre-tracheal course has been noted in 5% of cases.[9] From a clinical perspective, respiratory symptoms are common in the paediatric population because of the softness of their trachea, whereas dysphagia and blood pressure mismatch in the upper limbs tend to predominate in the adult population. Kommerell aneurysms can attain large size and cause severe compressive symptoms (Figure 4). However, only 5% of adults with aberrant subclavian arteries are clinically symptomatic, being a purely imaging-based incidental diagnosis for the vast majority. There is reason to believe patients with right side arch are more prone to present with rupture (or dissection) than those with a normal-configuration left arch.[10]

Natural history and sizing

The natural history of Kommerell's diverticulum remains undefined, mainly because of the rarity of the condition. The literature fails to provide clear-cut information on a critical size threshold for rupture, but 4cm or larger is the figure described in a preponderance of reported cases,[4] leading to the recommendation for elective treatment of diverticula measuring >3cm.[11] Difficult to justify as it may be, some authors espouse a policy of elective treatment for all aortic diverticula based on the unpredictable behaviour and perceived high rupture risk, but many more (this author included) favour a selective approach. Added to these challenges are the notorious difficulties regarding best sizing and measurement techniques as they remain non-standardised and vary widely in published reports. The situation is

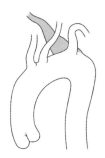

Figure 1: Type 1 Kommerell associated with a normal-configuration left arch and aRSA.

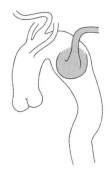

Figure 2: Type 2 Kommerell: note right and left carotid arteries arising as separate individual vessels, normal right subclavian, and aberrant left subclavian artery.

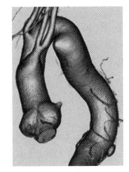

Figure 3: Non-Kommerell ductal diverticulum on a patient with right-sided arch.

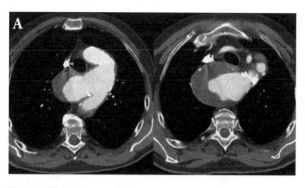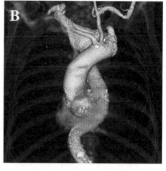

Figure 4: (A) 7cm Kommerell's aneurysm causing severe compression of the esophagus, associated with aRSA and (B) left side arch.

definitely improving at present thanks to the superb anatomical definition and display capabilities afforded by advanced CT and MR imaging. Among the various approaches reported in the recent past, the author finds the measurement techniques proposed by Idrees *et al*[12] to be most reasonable and practically useful (Fig. 5), as are their suggested size thresholds for elective treatment in the adult population: 5cm or larger for total diameter and >3cm at the base with total diameter likely being the more important of the two. These guidelines would be applicable in all Kommerell cases, including (presumably) non-Kommerell type 3 ductal diverticula.

For the paediatric patient population, Backer *et al* proposed to designate as significant (and deserving of treatment) any diverticulum that is more than 1.5 times the diameter of the subclavian artery distal to it.[13]

Surgical treatment

Various surgical approaches have been described including median sternotomy alone, right thoracotomy alone, left thoracotomy alone, bilateral thoracotomy, and median sternotomy plus thoracotomy.[14] Numerous operative strategies have been

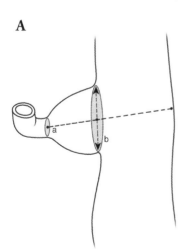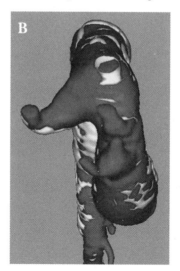

Figure 5: (A) Total diameter from apex to opposite normal aortic wall (a), diameter at the base where diverticulum originates off the aorta (b). (B) Recommended measurement technique as used on a patient with left arch and aRSA

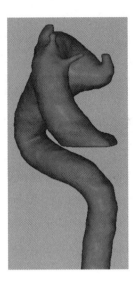

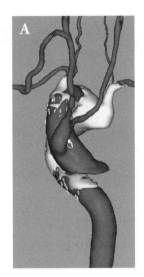

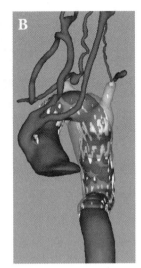

Figure 6: 58-year-old man presenting with right side arch (and right descending thoracic aorta) and a large type 2 Kommerell's associated with aLSA.

Figure 7: Staged repair consisted of: first, arch debranching via median sternotomy and side-graft bypass from the root of the ascending aorta to the right and left common carotid arteries. The second stage (several weeks later) involved a right carotid-axillary artery bypass, trans-femoral endograft deployment across the arch, and left trans-brachial vascular-plug closure of the left subclavian artery just beyond the diverticulum (A, B).

applied for resection of the diverticulum and arch repair, with continuing concern regarding technical complexity and risks of complications and even mortality.

Hybrid strategies

Less invasive hybrid approaches combining surgical and endovascular techniques have emerged in the more recent past. Treatment of "patient G" (Figures 6 and 7) serves to illustrate one such strategy. He was referred for management of a large type II Kommerell's associated with right side aortic arch and aberrant left subclavian artery. This author has managed three additional type II patients with the same general approach, but including an aorto-right axillary artery bypass at the time of arch debranching.

Two other hybrid strategies for diverticula associated with aberrant left subclavian artery in right arch cases are worthy of description. They both emphasise antegrade delivery of the thoracic endograft to facilitate precise deployment across the sharply angulated anatomy that often creates severe challenges when using the standard trans-femoral access technique:

- Single-stage frozen elephant trunk with antegrade delivery of the endograft through an open aortotomy approach[12] (Figure 8) or
- Single-stage median-sternotomy with arch debranching and simultaneous antegrade delivery and deployment of the thoracic stent graft across the arch to cover the aberrant left subclavian artery (Figure 9).

Closure of the subclavian artery (with coils or a vascular plug) just beyond the diverticulum is an important component in both.

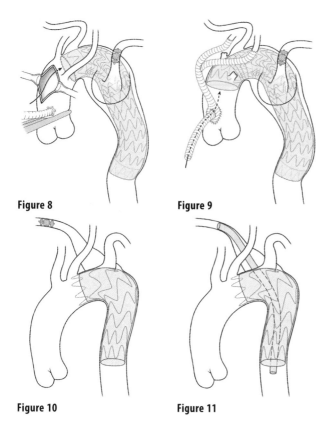

Figure 8

Figure 9

Figure 10

Figure 11

Figure 8: Single-stage frozen elephant-trunk technique via open aortotomy in type II anatomy: median sternotomy and cardio-pulmonary bypass required. Note antegrade delivery of endograft (arrow) under direct visualization, and vascular-plug closure of left subclavian artery just beyond the Kommerell aneurysm.

Figure 9: Arch debranching and simultaneous antegrade delivery and deployment of thoracic stent-graft for type II lesions.

Figure 10: Endografting of arch and proximal descending thoracic aorta with coverage of the normal left subclavian artery and aRSA, and vascular-plug closure just beyond the aneurysm. Not illustrated is the required revascularisation of one or both subclavian.

Figure 11: Transfemoral placement of a periscope parallel graft into the aRSA, together with aortic endografting to exclude Kommerell aneurysm and preserve normal antegrade flow.

Treatment of type I diverticula associated with aberrant right subclavian artery in left side arch tends to be more straightforward, as the normal arch configuration allows for standard transfemoral deployment of the thoracic stent graft device. The frequent anatomic proximity of the aberrant right subclavian artery to the origin of the normal left subclavian artery is such that coverage of both vessels is necessary in the majority of these cases, implying the need for preliminary debranching and revascularisation of one or both. Closure of the aberrant right subclavian artery beyond the diverticulum is necessary to secure complete exclusion (Figure 10). This treatment plan has been used successfully in three type I patients managed by the author.

Lastly, it is worth mentioning the recently described and innovative subclavian periscope technique[15] that can be used in the treatment of type 1 lesions, especially in situations where debranching and cervical bypass operations are deemed impractical or unfeasible (Figure 11).

Conclusion

Aberrant subclavian arteries and Kommerell diverticula are relatively rare vascular anomalies, but their prevalence may well be considerably higher than early estimates. The potential for rupture (and dissection) is quite real and somewhat unpredictable, and these risks grow exponentially with increasing size. In this regard, adopting the term Kommerell's aneurysm instead of the more obscure "diverticulum" would be helpful (in the author's view) and probably lead to a better understanding of the clinical implications and need for treatment. The measurement techniques described in this chapter are felt to represent the best approach to sizing and decision-making in a given case.

It is important and practically useful to classify Kommerell aneurysms into two main groups: type I—normal-configuration left arch with aberrant right subclavian artery; and type II—anomalous right arch with aberrant left subclavian artery. More rare still and belonging with the latter from a repair strategy viewpoint is the ductal non-Kommerell diverticulum (type 3).

Various surgical approaches have been proposed for adult Kommerell patients, with much success in many reported cases. However, these are truly formidable operations that can only be performed with the required expertise and safety at a handful of centres of excellence around the world. The still-evolving hybrid strategies represent an important effort at lessening invasiveness and lowering risks. Various options exist, including those illustrated in this chapter. Reported results are encouraging at this time and the endovascular techniques are undoubtedly appealing, but careful analysis of a larger collective experience with longer patient follow-up must be awaited before we can proclaim with confidence that a new standard of care has arrived.

Summary

- Kommerell's diverticula are infrequent but probably not as rare as predicted by previous estimates.

- They remain a conundrum of sorts because of lingering uncertainties as to their nature, the potential for catastrophic complications, and the indications for treatment.

- Abandoning the term diverticulum and using, instead, the proposed Kommerell aneurysm as a descriptor would be helpful.

- The ability to measure these lesions precisely and reproducibly is felt to be crucially important, and a historical barrier to appropriate management. The techniques described in the chapter emerge as best and should become standard.

- Classification of Kommerell lesions into types I and II is very helpful and with important implications as to anatomy and repair options.

- Surgical treatment is the historical gold standard, but the involved operative approaches are frequently complex and risky.

- Emerging hybrid surgical-endovascular strategies are appealing and may prove safer for some patients presenting with aortic diverticula of all types.

References

1. Kommerell B. Verlagerung des Osophagus durch eine abnorm verlaufende Arteria subclavia dextra (Arteria lusoria). *Fortschr Geb Roentgenstrahlen* 1936; **54**: 590–95.
2. van Son JAM, Konstantinov IE. Burckhard F Kommerell and Kommmerell's Diverticulum. *Tex H Inst J* 2002; **29**: 9–12.
3. Miller JM, Miller KS. A note on the historical aspects of dysphagia lusoria. *Am Surg* 1992; **58**: 502–03.
4. Tanaka A, Milner R, Ota T. Kommerell's diverticulum in the current era: a comprehensive review. *Gen Thorac Cardiovasc Surg* 2015; **63**: 245–59.
5. Edwards JE. Anomalies of the derivatives of the aortic arch system. Med Clin North Am 1948; **32**: 925–49.

6. Han MT, Hall DG, Manche A, *et al.* Double aortic arch causing tracheoesophageal compression. *Am J Surg* 1993; **165**: 628–31.
7. Salomonowitz E, Edwards JE, Hunter DW, *et al.* The three types of aortic diverticula. *Am J Roentgenol* 1984; **142**: 673–79.
8. Molz G, Burri B. Aberrant subclavian artery (arteria lusoria): sex differences in the prevalence of various forms of the malformation. Evaluation of 1378 observations. *Virchows Arch A Pathol Anat Histol* 1978; **380**: 303–15.
9. Gomes MM, Bernatz PE, Forth RJ. Arteriosclerotic aneurysm of an aberrante right subclavian artery. *Dis Chest* 1968; **54**: 549-52 .
10. Austin EH, Wolfe GW. Aneurysm of aberrant subclavian artery with a review of the literature. *J Vasc Surg* 1985; **2**: 571–77.
11. Cina CS, Althani H, Pasenau J, *et al.* Kommerell's diverticulum and right-sided aortic arch: a cohort study and review of the literature. *J Vasc Surg* 2004; **39**: 131–39.
12. Idrees J, Keshavamurthy S, Subramanian S, *et al.* Hybrid repair of Komerell diverticulum. *J Thorac Cardiovasc Surg* 2014; **147**: 973–76.
13. Backer CL, Russell HM, Wurlitzer KC, *et al.* Primary resection of Kommerell diverticulum and left subclavian artery transfer. *Ann Thorac Surg* 2012; **94**: 1612–17.
14. Tsukui H, Aomi S, Yamazaki K. Surgical strategy for Kommerell's diverticulum: total arch replacement. *J Thorac Cardiovasc* 2014; **148**: 1423–27.
15. Lachat M, Mayer D, Pfammatter T, *et al.* Periscope endograft technique to revascularize the left subclavian artery during thoracic endovascular aortic repair. *J Endovasc Ther* 2013; **20**: 728–34.

Juxtarenal challenges

Challenging and short infrarenal neck

The value of hybrid debranching

R Chiesa, A Kahlberg, R Castellano, D Mascia, Y Tshomba and G Melissano

Introduction

Although great strides in morbidity and mortality reduction have been made in the surgical treatment of thoracoabdominal aortic aneurysm,[1] visceral and renal ischaemic complications are still present, even in the most specialised centres.[2]

Multiple aetiopathological factors are supposed to be involved in perioperative visceral and renal dysfunction, but the most important are definitely the time of organ ischaemia during artery reattachment, and the associated atherosclerotic vessel disease, such as ostial stenosis or dissection. These factors account for a significant increase in technical difficulty, prolonged time of anastomosis, and increased global risk of intraoperative organ injury.

Covered self-expanding stents are being used to perform "sutureless anastomoses" on visceral aortic branches during debranching procedures, obviating the need for technically demanding vessel exposure and anastomoses, thereby reducing the duration of flow interruption and simplifying the performance of complex aortic repair.[3] Lachat and colleagues named this method "VORTEC" (Viabahn open revascularisation technique), as they used a "standard" covered stent graft (Viabahn, Gore).

The Gore Hybrid Vascular Graft is a novel expanded polytetrafluoroethylene (ePTFE) vascular prosthesis that includes a nitinol reinforced self-expanding section at one of its extremities, allowing a "sutureless" endovascular anastomosis. In this chapter we report a recent update on the experience with this graft for visceral revascularisation during thoracoabdominal aortic aneurysm open repair.

Device description, indications, and surgical technique

We previously reported our standard surgical techniques and outcomes for open repair and visceral vessels management.[4]

The Gore Hybrid Vascular Graft received the US Food and Drug Administration (FDA) approval on March 2010, and obtained the CE mark in July 2012. This device is currently commercially available in the USA, Europe, Russia, and few Middle Eastern countries. It is an ePTFE vascular prosthesis that has a distal section reinforced with nitinol. The nitinol-reinforced section is partially constrained to allow for easy insertion and deployment into a vessel. Its lumen is continuous with the Carmeda bio-active surface consisting of a stable covalently bonded, reduced molecular weight heparin of porcine origin. An embedded low permeability film provides a barrier to ultrafiltration. The graft is available with the nitinol reinforced section length of 5cm and 10cm, and diameter of 6mm, 7mm, 8mm and 9mm.

Our indications to use the Gore Hybrid Vascular Graft for revascularisation of renal and splanchnic vessels are:

- Inclusion in an aortic patch (e.g. Carrel patch) not deemed adequate, because of artery ostium anatomical location or poor quality of the surrounding aortic wall
- Anatomical location of the artery ostium considered demanding for performing a conventional anastomosis
- Severe atherosclerotic disease of the proximal tract of the artery (including the presence of highly calcified or disrupted plaque, critical stenosis, or local dissection).

The choice to use the Gore Hybrid Vascular Graft was guided by the intention to decrease technical complexity and duration of the distal anastomosis, reduce accidental damage to the arterial wall, concurrently treat stenotic or dissected arteries, and prevent early kinking of bypassed vessels during visceral derotation.

Sizing of the nitinol-reinforced section was performed using a 10% to 20% oversizing compared with the diameter of the target vessel, as measured at preoperative computed tomography (CT) angiography and confirmed by intraoperative finding. The distance between the origin and the first bifurcation of the target artery was always measured at preoperative CT angiography, in order to avoid unintentional coverage of renal/splanchnic artery branches during Gore Hybrid Vascular Graft deployment.

Contraindications to the use of the Gore Hybrid Vascular Graft include: target artery diameter <5mm or >9mm, the presence of anomalous major collaterals of the target artery originating in its proximal tract, and the presence of a severe stenosis of the distal tract of the target artery.

With the patient on cerebrospinal fluid drainage, positioned in a right lateral decubitus, thoraco-phreno-laparotomy is performed and the thoracoabdominal aorta is exposed following our standard surgical technique.[4] After institution of

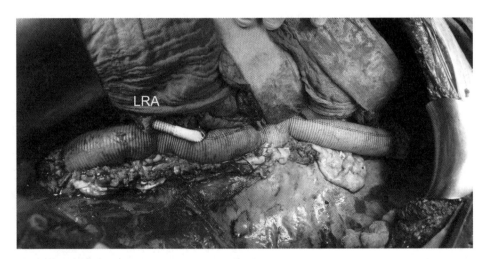

Figure 1: Intraoperative result after type II thoracoabdominal aortic aneurysm open repair, with revascularisation of the coeliac trunk, superior mesenteric artery and right renal artery by means of Carrel patch inclusion, and separate bypass to the left renal artery using a 7mm Gore Hybrid Vascular Graft.

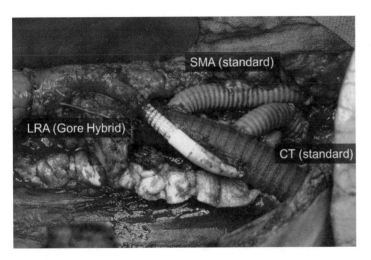

Figure 2: Customised reconstruction of the visceral vessels during open repair for type V thoracoabdominal aortic aneurysm, using conventional bypass to revascularise the coeliac trunk and the superior mesenteric artery, and the Gore Hybrid Vascular Graft with distal "sutureless" anastomosis to the left renal artery.

labile high blood pressure, the proximal anastomosis is performed and critical intercostal arteries are reattached using a sequential clamping technique. Then, the distal clamp is moved below the renal arteries and the visceral aorta is opened. Visceral normothermic haematic perfusion is then delivered by the pump with 9Fr irrigation-occlusion catheters (LeMaitre Vascular) into the coeliac trunk and the superior mesenteric artery (400mL/min). Selective perfusion of the renal arteries is performed with cold (4 degrees Celsius) crystalloid solution enriched with Histidine-Tryptophan-Ketoglutarate (Custodiol).[5] Visceral arteries that are not deemed to require a separate reattachment are usually firstly reimplanted by means of a Carrel patch. Then, the distal aortic anastomosis is performed, and the aortic clamps are removed.

After identification of the Gore Hybrid Vascular Graft-target vessel, the perfusion-catheter is temporarily removed. A flexible steerable J-tip guidewire (usually 0.035") is inserted into the target artery. The constrained stented segment of the Gore Hybrid Vascular Graft is gently placed into the artery for 2cm to 3cm, with respect to the distances measured at preoperative CT angiography, with the deployment line facing upwards. The stent is released pulling the deployment line parallel to the vascular graft section. Care must be taken to hold it firm in place during this manoeuvre. Stent post-dilatation is performed in all cases after Gore Hybrid Vascular Graft distal segment deployment, using a non-compliant balloon advanced on the guidewire through the conduit. Perfusion-catheter is then immediately reinserted into the graft to reduce organ ischaemia. The Gore Hybrid Vascular Graft is then sewn in place with at least three single circumferential monofilament polypropylene stitches. Finally the proximal anastomosis to the main aortic graft is completed in the usual fashion after cutting the proximal unstented section of the graft at the proper length.

After blood flow restoration, protamine is administered to completely reverse heparin. Red blood cells, platelets, and plasma transfusions are aggressively used to correct severe thrombocytopenia and coagulation derangements. Anastomoses are carefully checked for bleeding and reinforced when needed. Mild initial bleeding from ePTFE needle-holes usually resolved spontaneously after few minutes. In case of major suture-hole bleeding, haemostasis is obtained by manual compression with surgical gauze and oxidised cellulose pads.

Antiplatelet therapy (usually aspirin) is routinely initiated by the third postoperative day, if not contraindicated. Dual antiplatelet therapy (adding ticlopidine or clopidogrel) is then started by the tenth postoperative day, and continued after discharge for at least one month.

In vivo experience

A series of 108 consecutive patients who underwent elective thoracoabdominal aortic aneurysm open repair, including revascularisation with the Gore Hybrid Vascular Graft of at least one of the coeliac trunk, the superior mesenteric artery, the right renal or left renal artery between September 2012 and December 2015, was included in the present analysis. During this period, 187 other patients were submitted to thoracoabdominal aortic aneurysm open repair using standard renal revascularisation techniques, because the Gore Hybrid Vascular Graft was deemed contraindicated or not necessary by the operating surgeon.

At preoperative CT angiography, all Gore Hybrid Vascular Graft patients had patent coeliac trunk and superior mesenteric artery, 105 patients had two functioning kidneys with both patent renal arteries, while three patients had only one functioning kidney, for a total of 429 patent visceral vessels in this group. Visceral artery stenosis was defined as a >50% lesion as documented by CT angiography. Acute renal failure was defined as both a doubling of serum creatinine level and an absolute value greater than 3mg/dL.[6]

All CT angiography performed after the operation were carefully reviewed, in order to ascertain patency of the visceral vessels and of the implanted grafts, identify graft migration, stenosis, kinking or twisting, stent fractures, and instances of bleeding or renal/bowel infarctions.

In the analysed period, at least one Gore Hybrid Vascular Graft was used for revascularisation in 37% of patients submitted to thoracoabdominal aortic

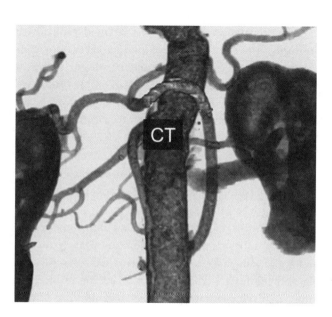

Figure 3: Three-dimensional reconstruction of follow-up CT scan following thoracoabdominal aortic aneurysm open repair associated with aorto-coeliac bypass using the Gore Hybrid Vascular Graft.

aneurysm open repair. In this group of patients, among the 213 patent renal arteries, 100 were revascularised with the Gore Hybrid Vascular Graft (76 left, and 24 right), and 113 using standard surgical techniques (105 by means of Carrel patch reimplantation, and eight by means of conventional aorto-renal bypass). Among 108 patent coeliac trunks and 108 patent superior mesenteric arteries, five coeliac trunks and seven superior mesenteric arteries were revascularised with the Gore Hybrid Vascular Graft, respectively, the other being all included in a Carrel patch. Indications to the use of the Gore Hybrid Vascular Graft included intraoperative detection of a remote location of the ostium of the visceral artery (75% of cases), severe atherosclerotic wall degeneration or dissection (62% of cases), and visceral artery stenosis (27% of cases).

All intended target vessels were treated without technical concerns with the Gore Hybrid Vascular Graft. No significant bleeding from ePTFE needle-holes or from the graft anastomoses was observed. Total surgical and total renal ischaemic times were 262±79 minutes, and 51±23 minutes, respectively. Cold renal perfusional time was 27±13 minutes. No adjunctive unplanned endovascular or surgical procedures were required on the Gore Hybrid Vascular Graft-treated vessels. Prior to revascularisation, a balloon-expandable stent was directly implanted at the ostium of 17 visceral arteries (6.4% of non-Gore Hybrid Vascular Graft revascularised visceral arteries).

Thirty-day mortality was 5.5%, including one patient who died on postoperative day six for myocardial infarction, one patient who died due to coagulopathy and bleeding, and five other patients who suffered from multiorgan failure.

Perioperative complications included acute renal failure, occurring in 10 patients (9.3%), and requiring dialysis in four (temporary dialysis in three cases, and permanent dialysis in one). Occlusion of the Gore Hybrid Vascular Graft at subsequent CT angiography was found to be the main causative factor of renal failure in three of these patients. In one case, early thrombosis of a right renal Gore Hybrid Vascular Graft was found on postoperative day eight, successfully treated by means of urgent endovascular recanalisation and stenting of the distal endpoint. No cases of Gore Hybrid Vascular Graft-related bowel ischaemia were observed.

Follow-up CT angiography was available in 92 patients at a mean follow-up of 16±9 months, including 94 Gore Hybrid Vascular Graft revascularised arteries. Gore Hybrid Vascular Graft patency rate was 91% (86/94). The observed eight occluded Gore Hybrid Vascular Grafts were all left aorto-renal bypass grafts. A kinking/twisting of the non-stented segment was observed in three cases, and a compressed/narrowed lumen of the stented-segment was observed in two cases. No other Gore Hybrid Vascular Graft-related complications, reintervention or cases of new-onset renal failure requiring dialysis were reported at follow-up in available patients.

Conclusion

Our currently updated experience on 108 patients confirmed that this technique was technically feasible in all planned cases, irrespective of visceral artery anatomical location and quality. The specific indications to the use of Gore Hybrid Vascular Graft included the "most feared" situations of the renal and splanchnic arteries (remote access to the ostium, poor quality of the vessel wall, ostial stenosis or dissection), leading to the use of this device in about one third of thoracoabdominal aortic aneurysm operated patients. Nevertheless, the supposed advantages of this approach were confirmed, such as the ability to perform the aorto-visceral bypass in a timely fashion (thanks to the distal "sutureless" anastomosis), the ability of reaching remote arterial ostia without the need of extensive exposure of the artery (typically of the right renal artery), the aptitude to avoid kinking or twisting of the revascularised vessel (especially the left renal artery) after viscera derotation, resulting in perioperative good clinical outcomes and acceptable patency rates at mean follow-up of about 15 months.

Summary

- Renovisceral ischaemic damage is still one of the most feared complications of thoracoabdominal aortic aneurysm open repair, and is a strong predictor for early and late mortality.

- The techniques used to perform renovisceral vessels reattachment play an important role in reducing organ ischaemic times and avoiding permanent damage or vessel subsequent occlusion.

- The Gore Hybrid Vascular Graft with distal sutureless anastomosis is an effective tool for separate reattachment of one or more renovisceral vessels during thoracoabdominal aortic aneurysm open repair, based on recent data collected on more than 100 patients.

References

1. Piazza M, Ricotta JJ 2nd. Open surgical repair of thoracoabdominal aortic aneurysms. *Ann Vasc Surg.* 2012; **26** (4): 600–05.
2. Lemaire SA, Jones MM, Conklin LD, *et al.* J Randomized comparison of cold blood and cold crystalloid renal perfusion for renal protection during thoracoabdominal aortic aneurysm repair. *Vasc Surg* 2009; **49** (1): 11–19.
3. Lachat M, Mayer D, *et al.* New technique to facilitate renal revascularization with use of telescoping self-expanding stent grafts: VORTEC. Vascular 2008; **16** (2): 69–72.
4. Chiesa R, Melissano G, Civilini E, *et al.* Video-atlas of open thoracoabdominal aortic aneurysm repair. *Ann Cardiothorac Surg* 2012; **1** (3): 398–403.
5. Tshomba Y, Kahlberg A, Melissano G, *et al.* Comparison of renal perfusion solutions during thoracoabdominal aortic aneurysm repair. *J Vasc Surg* 2014; **59**: 623–33.
6. Kashyap VS, Cambria RP, Davison JK, L'Italien GJ. Renal failure after thoracoabdominal aortic surgery. *J Vasc Surg*1997; **26** (6): 949–55.

EVAR repair with parallel graft use

RR Kolvenbach, R Karmeli and A Rabin

Introduction

In most cases of infrarenal abdominal aortic aneurysms, endovascular aneurysm repair (EVAR) is now the treatment of choice. When EVAR was first introduced, the patient had to have a sufficiently long infrarenal landing zone for the procedure. However, gradually, patients with challenging anatomy—e.g. short infrarenal necks of less than 1cm and severe angulation—have begun to be treated with commercially available endografts.

While open repair is often still considered to be the gold standard for patients with hostile neck and/or juxtarenal aneurysms, surgery in older patients is suboptimal in many cases because of the presence of multiple comorbidities. But despite the introduction of new grafts with more active fixation, a hostile neck can still be a major obstacle to long-term success with EVAR; adjuncts, such as balloon-expandable stents, only solve a minority of problems. Fenestrated grafts, though mostly only outside the USA, are now available and be ordered from several manufacturers. Only one of these is labelled as an "off-the-shelf" device and all others are still custom made with a manufacturing time of at least two months even if only one scallop is ordered. Therefore, the optimal approach to the suprarenal or juxtarenal aortic aneurysm, often with severely compromised proximal necks, remains controversial.

Parallel grafts

Endovascular repair in the setting of adverse anatomy has been the focus of much research over the past decade and is an evolving field. An off-the-shelf aortic stent graft for exclusion of juxtarenal aneurysms was taken off the market (again) after problems associated with the renal arteries. A branched endograft that can be used in patients with thoracoabdominal aortic aneurysms is available in Europe, but the instructions for use do not permit deployment for a large number of patients.

Although parallel graft techniques are feasible and are associated with low morbidity and mortality, robust data supporting their use are lacking. But endovascular challenges, particularly in the aortic arch and in thoracoabdominal aortic aneurysms, make parallel grafts an attractive alternative to other endovascular techniques or open surgical procedures.

A custom-made parallel graft device can take up to three months to be manufactured, which is not an option for symptomatic patients or those with ruptured aneurysms. For these patients, off-the-shelf endografts are readily available.

However, there is some confusion regarding terminology and configuration of these devices. Greenberg *et al* first described a chimney graft as a bare metal stent introduced from a transbrachial approach to secure inflow into the renal artery in patients with juxtarenal aneurysms (Figure 1).[1,2] Alternatively, a covered stent can be used unilaterally or for both renal arteries for this top fenestrating technique. Also, a downward facing chimney or periscope graft can be deployed from a transfemoral access into the visceral and renal arteries or into the aortic arch.[3]

A third technique that has been recently gaining more popularity is the sandwich technique in which the parallel graft is running in a gutter between two stent grafts (Figure 2).

Chimney technique

The chimney technique involves placement of bare metal stents or covered grafts in parallel to the main aortic stent graft. In many cases, the space between the parallel stent, the aortic graft and the origin of the renal artery is only a few millimetres in length, which resembles a top fenestration technique.[4-7] Particularly in cases in which bare metal stents are used, selective engagement of the renal artery can be technically challenging because of wire entrapment inside the struts of the stents involved. In cases in which only a top fenestration is required, a bare metal stent can be the easiest solution to maintain organ perfusion. In more complex cases, the authors prefer covered self-expandable stents over bare metal stents. Re-interventions should be easier when a covered stent is in place compared with bare metal stents. The main disadvantage is the need for large sheath placement into the brachial or subclavian artery.

With a chimney graft deployment, antegrade visceral access is obtained from open exposure of the subclavian, axillary, or proximal brachial arteries—either separately or in combination, depending on their diameter and the number of planned chimney grafts.[8,9] When two or more chimney grafts are required, we either perform a cutdown of the contralateral axillary artery or use a downward facing periscope graft that is deployed inside at least one renal artery. Other groups,

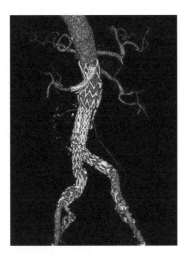

Figure 1: Dorsal view of chimney graft in the left renal artery in combination with a Cordis aortic stent graft.

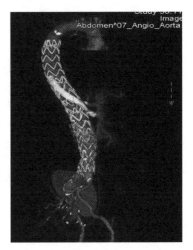

Figure 2: Sandwich technique in a renal transplant patient. ViaBahn self-expanding parallel graft in the superior mesenteric artery. Long overlap of self-expanding visceral artery graft.

such as Mario Lachat (Cardiothoracic Surgery, University of Zurich, Zürich, Switzerland) and colleagues, have discussed performing these procedures using a purely percutaneous access.

Through the antegrade sheaths, the targeted renal and visceral branches are cannulated using 260cm length hydrophilic guidewires and a 125cm JB1 catheter (Cook Medical). Once cannulated, the sheaths are advanced coaxially into the target artery orifice. If possible, we prefer to use Viabahn self-expanding covered stents (Gore Medical). These are advanced through the sheaths into the target branch vessel. If self-expanding covered stents are used, additional bare metal balloon-expandable stents are placed within the graft to reinforce the snorkel stent.[10]

Particularly in the USA, some surgeons prefer to use homemade fenestrations because of the lack of available custom-made branched devices. In our experience, this can be accomplished with most aortic endografts as long as care is taken to meticulously reload the graft.[11] These techniques can be combined in those cases in which a graft with a scallop for the superior mesenteric artery and the coeliac trunk are used with two chimney grafts for the renal arteries.

Intraoperative quality control of the various chimney grafts is essential and wires in the parallel self-expanding grafts should stay in place until the end of the procedure. This permits selective angiography of all branches and, if necessary, pressure measurements. In those cases where there is a kink of the graft, reinforcement with a self-expanding stent can be performed to improve long-term patency. Additionally, platelet inhibition with aspirin and clopidogrel (Plavix, Bristol-Myers Squibb/Sanofi Aventis) should be prescribed for at least six months.

Current studies

There are only a few reports describing mid-term results of parallel grafting and there are none with long-term results. In one of the first publications, Bruen *et al* published results for 21 patients with juxtarenal aortic aneurysms. Outcomes, including 30-day mortality, were identical to a matched group of patients who underwent open repair. There was one asymptomatic superior mesenteric artery stent occlusion and partial compression of a second superior mesenteric artery stent, requiring balloon angioplasty. Primary patency was 84% at 12 months with no type I endoleaks.[10] In another series, with a larger patient cohort, Donas *et al* used a balloon-expandable chimney graft. They compared their results (37 patients) with those of a group in Zurich that used self-expanding Viabahn grafts in all of their cases (35). There were no significant differences in outcomes with regard to the stent used. The success rate for target vessel preservation was 97% for the balloon-expandable and was 100% for the self-expanding stent.[12]

In our own experience, we have found that anything more than two chimney grafts can cause leakage and will potentially weaken the proximal seal.[13–15] There are also anecdotal reports of good results after filling the gutters between the chimneys with liquid embolisation material such as Onyx (Covidien).

Correct sizing of the aortic stent graft and the chimneys is another important consideration; we oversize routinely by 30% plus half the diameter of each parallel graft in millimetres.

Long-term durability

The long-term durability of chimney grafts is unclear; we can assume that they will perform similar to most branched or fenestrated devices. This is confirmed by the most recent publication of the PERICLES (Performance of the chimney technique for the treatment of complex aortic pathologies) registry, which is a multicentre registry that involves more than 500 patients across the US and Europe. The authors of this registry concluded that, with regard to the different endpoints such as aneurysm exclusion and graft patency, the results are as good as those published from branched and fenestrated graft registries. This study is an important milestone in the evaluation of parallel grafts in a real-life setting.[16]

Theoretically the chimney graft compromises sealing of the aortic endograft creating a gutter between the aortic graft and the vessel wall. In the long term, this could be an advantage of sandwich grafts where the chimney is in direct contact with an endograft and eliminating the gutter between the aortic wall and the abdominal or thoracic stent graft. We believe we will see more techniques used in combination with parallel grafts that actively seal these gutters, such as liquid embolising agents, coils, or endovascular staplers. Reducing the number of chimney grafts whenever possible is another option to securely avoid type I and III endoleaks.

Conclusion

The whole concept of chimney grafts to exclude juxtarenal aneurysms depends on thrombosis of the gutters between the parallel grafts and the aortic stent graft. The importance of long gutters and chimneys must be emphasised as this is probably one of the most essential factors that promote sealing.[17] When this can be accomplished in combination with excellent long-term branch patency rates, this technique will be a widely accepted alternative to branched or fenestrated devices.

Summary

- Endovascular repair of juxtarenal aneurysms will gradually replace open surgery in a majority of cases. Off-the-shelf parallel grafts will play a key role in this setting.

- Long-term durability and target vessel patency are still to be determined. According to recent registries mid-term branch patency can be compared to custom made branched or fenestrated devices.

- Gutters are still the most controversial issue of any parallel graft technique. Active sealing of gutters will play an increasing role in the future.

- Challenges particularly in the aortic arch and in thoracoabdominal aortic aneurysms currently make parallel grafts an attractive alternative to other endovascular techniques or open surgical procedures.

References

1. Greenberg RK, Clair D, Srivastava S, *et al.* Should patients with challenging anatomy be offered endovascular aneurysm repair? *J Vasc Surg* 2003; **38**: 990–96.

2. Greenberg RK, Sternbergh WC III, Makaroun M, *et al.* Intermediate results of a United States multicenter trial of fenestrated endograft repair for juxtarenal abdominal aortic aneurysms. *J Vasc Surg* 2009; **50**: 730–37.

3. Greenberg R, Eagleton M, Mastracci T. Branched endografts for thoracoabdominal aneurysms. *J Thorac Cardiovasc Surg* 2010; **140** (6 Suppl): S171–78.

4. Ohrlander T, Sonesson B, Ivancev K, *et al.* The chimney graft: a technique for preserving or rescuing aortic branch vessels in stent-graft sealing zones. *J Endovasc Ther* 2008; **15**: 427–32.

5. Criado FJ. A percutaneous technique for preservation of arch branch patency during thoracic endovascular aortic repair (TEVAR): retrograde catheterization and stenting. *J Endovasc Ther* 2007; **14**: 54–58.

6. Ricci C, Ceccherini C, Leonini S, *et al.* Double renal chimney graft using only femoral approach. *J Cardiovasc Surg* (Torino) 2011; **52**: 93–97.

7. Larzon T, Eliasson K, Gruber G. Top-fenestrating technique in stent grafting of aortic diseases with mid-term follow-up. *J Cardiovasc Surg* (Torino) 2008; **49**: 317–22.

8. Allaqaband S, Jan MF, Bajwa T. The chimney graft—A simple technique for endovascular repair of complex juxtarenal abdominal aortic aneurysms in no-option patients. *Cath Cardiovasc Interv* 2010; **75**: 1111–15.

9. Hiramoto JS, Chang CK, Reilly LM, *et al.* Outcome of renal stenting for renal artery coverage during endovascular aneurysm repair. *J Vasc Surg* 2009; **49**: 1100–06.

10. Bruen KJ, Feezor JR, Daniels JM, *et al.* Endovascular chimney technique *versus* open repair of juxtarenal and suprarenal aneurysms. *J Vasc Surg* 2011; **53**: 895–905.

11. Oderich GS, Ricotta JJ. Modified fenestrated stent grafts: device design, modifications, implantation, and current applications. *Perspect Vasc Surg Endovasc Ther* 2009; **21**: 157–67.

12. Donas KP, Pecoraro F, Torsello G, *et al.* Use of covered chimney stents for pararenal aortic pathologies is safe and feasible with excellent patency and low incidence of endoleaks. *J Vasc Surg* 2012; **55**: 659–65

13. Kolvenbach RR, Yoshida R, Pinter L, *et al.* Urgent endovascular treatment of thoraco-abdominal aneurysms using a sandwich technique and chimney grafts—a technical description. *Eur J Vasc Endovasc Surg* 2011; **41** (1): 54–60.

14. Schwierz E, Kolvenbach RR, Yoshida R, *et al.* Experience with the sandwich technique in endovascular thoracoabdominal aortic aneurysm repair. *J Vasc Surg* 2014; **59** (6): 1562–69.

15. Coscas R, Kobeiter H, Desgranges P, Becquemin JP. Technical aspects, current indications, and results of chimney graft for juxtarenal aortic aneurysms. *J Vasc Surg* 2011; **53**; 1520–27.

16. Donas KP, Lee JT, Lachat M, *et al;* PERICLES investigators. Collected world experience about the performance of the snorkel/chimney endovascular technique in the treatment of complex aortic pathologies: the PERICLES registry. *Ann Surg* 2015 Sep; **262** (3): 546–53.

17. Kolvenbach R. The role of periscopes and chimneys in complex aneurysm cases. *J Endovasc Ther* 2011; **18** (5): 661–65.

Use of polymer seal with complex aortic aneurysm necks and use of parallel grafts

KM Stenson and MM Thompson

Introduction

The widespread use of endovascular aneurysm repair (EVAR) to treat infrarenal abdominal aortic aneurysm has reduced perioperative risk compared with open surgical repair.[1,2,3] Despite this, concerns remain regarding the durability of EVAR in the long term; in particular with respect to the development of endoleak, which may lead to sac enlargement and subsequent rupture.[4,5,6] Although reintervention rates vary, about one in eight patients will require a further procedure following EVAR;[7] this is commonly due to recurrent or persistent aneurysm sac flow, either because of failed proximal sealing (type 1a endoleak) or aortic branch flow (type 2 endoleak). Endovascular aneurysm sealing (EVAS) was developed as a novel way of treating aneurysms, the rationale being to seal the entire aneurysm sac. Therefore, the aim is to reduce the incidence of type 2 endoleak and, subsequently, the need for reintervention. The technique involves the use of two stent grafts surrounded by polymer-filled endobags, which creates a sealing zone in the aortic neck and both common iliac arteries and provides anatomical fixation within the aneurysm sac itself.[8]

Parallel stents or "chimneys" were initially developed as a rescue manoeuvre to maintain patency in branch vessels that were unintentionally covered during the EVAR procedure to gain adequate proximal seal.[9] Chimneys comprise stents that are placed parallel to the aortic stent graft to maintain perfusion through vital aortic branches. When used in combination with conventional EVAR, the use of chimney stents is associated with a significant risk of type 1 endoleak because of "guttering".[10] This risk might potentially be decreased when the chimney stent is used in conjunction with EVAS as the polymer within the endobags may conform to the shape of the chimney stents while maintaining a proximal seal at the aneurysm neck. EVAS with parallel stents may potentially be used as an alternative to fenestrated EVAR for the treatment of juxtarenal aneurysms.

Polymer seal

The Nellix EVAS system (Endologix) consists of two identical catheter-based devices with a 10mm flow lumen, consisting of two balloon-expandable polytetrafluoroethylene-covered cobalt-chromium stents surrounded by polyurethane endobags. Once deployed in the appropriate position, the endobags are filled with a polyethylene glycol-based hydrogel that conforms to the aneurysm flow lumen and cures within minutes to produce a seal at the proximal and distal extents of the aneurysm with anatomical fixation within the sac (Figure 1).[11] Filling of the endobags is carried out under pressure monitoring, thus allowing the polymer to be instilled to a pressure of 180mm to 220mmHg.

The Nellix EVAS system was commercialised and gained its CE mark in 2013. Multicentre data published in 2015 were encouraging: for 171 patients with a median follow-up of five months, technical success was achieved in 99%.[12] Low levels of endoleak were observed: type 1a endoleak was seen in 4% of patients; type 1b seen in 2%; and type 2 in 2%. Limb occlusions were seen in 5% of patients. Overall, the aneurysm-related reintervention rate was 9%. In this study, there were no reported ruptures or open surgical conversions.

Hostile aneurysm morphology is still a significant obstacle to the universal use of endovascular techniques to treat aneurysms. Reintervention following EVAR is more probable in cases where there is adverse aortic morphology, in particular adverse morphology of the aneurysm neck.[13,14] Aneurysms demonstrating short, wide, angulated or conical necks are associated with higher rates of proximal type 1 endoleaks and are thus more likely to require reintervention.

A morphological analysis published in 2013 compared the aneurysm morphologies of patients with aneurysms who underwent EVAR with those of patients who underwent open repair, fenestrated EVAR or no procedure.[15] Overall, 70% of patients were considered to be morphologically suitable for a Nellix device. Of those patients treated with infrarenal EVAR (94.1%), 73% of morphologies fell within the instructions for use for the Nellix device, compared with rates of 29% to 68% for three other EVAR systems in frequent use. Not only does the EVAS system appear to be applicable to a wide range of aneurysm morphologies, it also seems to be a viable option for when the anatomy of a given aneurysm falls outside of the instructions for use of conventional EVAR devices.

Early results with EVAS have so far been encouraging, with high rates of aneurysm exclusion and low rates of complications. Our own institution is due to report one-year follow-up data for over 100 patients treated with the Nellix device in the near future, and the results of the ongoing EVAS FORWARD Global Registry are also awaited.

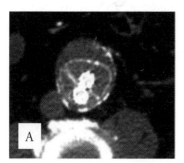 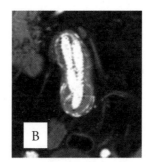 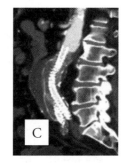

Figure 1: (A) The two stent grafts deployed within an infrarenal aneurysm. (B) Polymer is instilled into the endobags to create an anatomical seal. (C) Sagittal view of polymer-filled endobags surrounding stent grafts.

Parallel grafts

Successful EVAR necessitates an adequate proximal sealing zone. In patients with a juxtarenal aneurysm, conventional treatment is either open repair or fenestrated EVAR. However, a technique using parallel grafts may be an option for patients who are unfit for open repair, have aneurysm morphology unfavourable for fenestrated EVAR, or whose aneurysm requires urgent treatment.

The delay associated with creating a bespoke graft for a fenestrated EVAR procedure is unacceptable for an emergent case (such as a rapidly-expanding or symptomatic aneurysm). The components for EVAR with chimney grafts are available "off the shelf". In the setting of aneurysms, chimneys grafts can be inserted into one or both renal arteries, the superior mesenteric artery and the coeliac axis.

The results from the multicentre PERICLES (Performance of the chimney technique for the treatment of complex aortic pathologies) were reported in 2015.[16] In this study, 517 patients underwent chimney EVAR with a total of 898 chimney stents, with a mean follow-up time of 17 months. Overall, survival in this high-risk group of patients was 79%, with a 94% primary chimney patency rate and a 95% secondary patency rate. These data would seem to indicate that chimney EVAR is a valid off-the-shelf and immediately available technique for the treatment of complex aneurysms.

Type 1a endoleak is a significant concern after chimney EVAR procedures,[17] and this outcome is likely to be the result of "guttering" (i.e. the formation of a channel around the chimney graft but outside the main aortic stent graft). The development of a proximal type 1 endoleak may be affected by a number of technical factors:[18] oversizing the main stent graft should decrease the risk of endoleak, but excessive oversizing may lead to unacceptable infolding of the stent graft; the use of large chimney stents with a relatively small diameter endograft could lead to compression of the main endograft; and the use of balloon-expandable chimney stents will cause

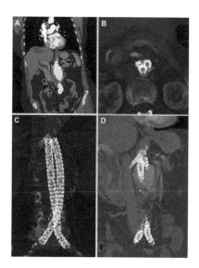

Figure 2: (A) Coronal computed tomography (CT) image showing juxtarenal aneurysm morphology. (B) Axial CT image showing the two Nellix stents and right renal artery chimney. (C) 3D reconstruction of CT image showing the sealed aneurysm sac and patent chimney. (D) Three-month follow-up CT image showing stable appearance of the sealed sac and patent stents.

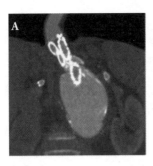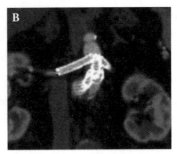

Figure 3: (A) Coronal CT image showing the two Nellix stents with three chimney grafts in both renal arteries and the superior mesenteric artery (six-month follow-up scan). (B) Coronal CT image showing the two Nellix stents with two chimney grafts, one in each renal artery (six-month follow-up scan).

less compression but larger gutters. This problem may potentially be obviated by using chimney stents in combination with the EVAS system.

Because of the way that EVAS achieves its fixation, chimney EVAS may result in polymer conformation around the chimney stent(s) while maintaining a proximal seal. The polymer creates a wrap around the chimney stent, thus fixing it in position and forming a motionless environment around the endograft and stents following curing. To prevent compression of the chimneys, the chimney balloons remaining inflated during the polymer-curing process (Figure 2). The forthcoming multicentre ASCEND (Aneurysm study for complex AAA: evaluation of Nellix durability) registry will yield definitive data regarding the use of chimney EVAS.

Conclusion

Unfavourable aortic anatomy has been a thorn in the side of EVAR since its inception in the early 1990s. EVAR devices have evolved to allow the treatment of a somewhat wider range of aneurysms since then. However, EVAS—with its novel approach to fixation within the aneurysm sac—would appear to offer a new paradigm in the treatment of infrarenal aneurysms. It could not only potentially reduce the need for reintervention, but it also could widen the spectrum of aneurysm morphologies that may be treated with an endovascular approach.

The use of chimney grafts in combination with endovascular devices offers a treatment option to patients with juxtarenal aneurysms who are either unfit to undergo open repair, have morphology unsuitable for fenestrated EVAR, or need urgent intervention. Chimney EVAR is an effective procedure but may be associated with a significant risk of proximal type I endoleak. This risk may potentially be

Summary

- Reintervention is relatively common following EVAR due to endoleak.

- EVAS is a novel treatment to treat aneurysms that may reduce the incidence of type II endoleak, in particular, and, therefore, reduce the reintervention rate.

- EVAS may treat a wider range of aneurysm morphologies than conventional EVAR.

- Chimney EVAR offers an endovascular treatment option for high-risk patients with juxtarenal aneurysms requiring urgent treatment.

- Chimney EVAS may reduce the risk of type I endoleak associated with chimney EVAR.

References

1. Greenhalgh RM, Brown LC, Kwong GPS, *et al.* Comparison of endovascular aneurysm repair with open repair in patients with abdominal aortic aneurysm (EVAR trial 1), 30-day operative mortality results: randomised controlled trial. *Lancet* 2004; **364**: 843–48.

2. Prinssen M, Verhoeven ELG, Buth J, *et al.* A randomized trial comparing conventional and endovascular repair of abdominal aortic aneurysms. *N Engl J Med* 2004; **351**(16): 1607–18.

3. Lederle F, Freischlag J, Kyriakides TC, *et al.* Outcomes following endovascular vs open repair of abdominal aortic aneurysm: a randomized trial. *JAMA* 2009; **302**: 1535–42.

4. Greenhalgh RM, Brown LC, Powell JT, *et al.* Endovascular *versus* open repair of abdominal aortic aneurysm. *N Engl J Med* 2010; **362**: 1863–71.

5. De Bruin JL, Baas AF, Buth J, *et al.* Long-term outcome of open or endovascular repair of abdominal aortic aneurysm. *N Engl J Med* 2010; **362**: 1881–89.

6. Lederle F, Freischlag J, Kyriakides TC, *et al.* Long-term comparison of endovascular and open repair of abdominal aortic aneurysm. *N Engl J Med* 2012; **367**: 1988–97.

7. Karthikesalingam A, Holt PJE, Hinchliffe RJ, *et al.* Risk of reintervention after endovascular aortic aneurysm repair. *Br J Surg* 2010; **97**: 657–63.

8. Donayre CE, Zarins CK, Krievins DK, *et al.* Initial clinical experience with a sac-anchoring endoprosthesis for aortic aneurysm repair. *J Vasc Surg* 2011; **53**: 574–82.

9. Ohrlander T, Sonesson B, Ivancev K, Resch T, Dias N, Malina M. The chimney graft: a technique for preserving or rescuing aortic branch vessels in stent-graft sealing zones. *J Endovasc Ther* 2008; **15**: 427–32.

10. Malkawi AH, de Bruin JL, Loftus IM, Thompson MM. Treatment of a Juxtarenal Aneurysm With the Nellix Endovascular Aneurysm Sealing System and Chimney Stent. *J Endovasc Ther* 2014; **21**: 538–40.

11. Brownrigg JRW, de Bruin JL, Rossi L, *et al.* Endovascular Aneurysm Sealing for Infrarenal Abdominal Aortic Aneurysms: 30-Day Outcomes of 105 Patients in a Single Centre. *Eur J Vasc Endovasc Surg* 2015; **50**: 157–64.

12. Böckler D, Holden A, Thompson M, *et al.* Multicenter Nellix EndoVascular Aneurysm Sealing system experience in aneurysm sac sealing. *J Vasc Surg* 2015; **62**: 1–9.

13. Karthikesalingam A, Holt PJ, Vidal-Diez A, *et al.* Predicting aortic complications after endovascular aneurysm repair. *Br J Surg* 2013; **100**: 1302–11

14. Patterson BO, Hinchliffe RJ, Holt PJ, *et al.* Importance of aortic morphology in planning aortic interventions. *J Endovasc Ther* 2010; **17**: 73–77.

15. Karthikesalingam A, Cobb RJ, Khoury A, *et al.* The Morphological Applicability of a Novel Endovascular Aneurysm Sealing (EVAS) System (Nellix) in Patients with Abdominal Aortic Aneurysms. *Eur J Vasc Endovasc Surg* 2013; **46**: 440–45.

16. Donas KP, Lee JT, Lachat M, *et al.* Collected world experience about the performance of the snorkel/chimney endovascular technique in the treatment of complex aortic pathologies: the PERICLES registry. *Ann Surg* 2015; **262**: 546–53; discussion 552–53.

17. Coscas R, Kobeiter H, Desgranges P, Becquemin J-PP. Technical aspects, current indications, and results of chimney grafts for juxtarenal aortic aneurysms. *J Vasc Surg* 2011; **53**: 1520–27.

18. Rouer M, El Batti S, Julia P, *et al.* Chimney Stent Graft for Endovascular Sealing of A Pararenal Aortic Aneurysm. *Ann Vasc Surg* 2014; **28**: 1936: e15–e1936.e18.

Configuration affects parallel graft results

M Shames, A Tanious and M Wooster

Introduction

The use of parallel stent grafts in conjunction with endovascular aneurysm repair (EVAR) was initially described as a method of increasing aortic neck length by raising the ostium of the renal artery in a salvage procedure, after renal artery coverage with an EVAR device.[1] Whilst these early reports yielded mixed results, contemporary reports of parallel stent grafts in conjunction with EVAR demonstrate favourable mid-term results in challenging aneurysm morphology.[2–9]

The technique has been expanded to include the aortic arch, thoracoabdominal aorta and even the iliac bifurcation, in both urgent and elective aneurysm repairs.[10–12] Successful parallel graft procedures have been reported using a variety of formulas to determine optimal device oversizing, length of overlap, graft type and parallel graft orientation. However, there is no consensus as to the optimal configuration and operative technique. [7,11,13–16]

Proponents of the chimney graft procedure describe its utility as easily available technology and potentially cost-effective, *versus* fenestrated, branched and custom endografts.[17–19] There are, however, many arguments against the use of chimney grafts, which particularly focus on the rate of endoleaks and branch thrombosis with a bias toward fenestrated and branched endografts for the management of complex aortic pathology.[19]

We present a concise review of the chimney, periscope, and snorkel techniques, with their optimal configurations based on currently available literature and personal experience.

Preoperative planning

A computed tomography (CT) angiogram of the chest, abdomen, iliac, and femoral arteries is necessary to understand the anatomy of the vessels being treated. A thorough evaluation of the size of the vessels, tortuosity, length prior to branching, degree of calcification/stenosis, and angulation are all vital to achieving technical success. Assessment of the upper extremity arterial anatomy is also crucial, as a brachial or axillary access is necessary for deployment of the chimney grafts.

Bilateral femoral access is used for all cases (except for prior known iliac occlusion with planned aorto-uni-iliac reconstruction). Our preference is to use a left brachial access (open or percutaneous) in cases with only one chimney graft. For two or more chimney grafts we employ an axillary conduit, which has been previously described.[20] Alternative access techniques describe using bilateral brachial

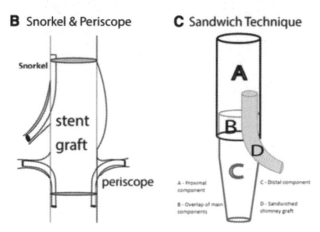

Figure 1: Chimney graft orientation.[11]

access, or multiple direct punctures into the axillary artery, with clinical success.[21,22] Manipulation in the arch should be minimised as observations of stroke during these procedures has been reported as high as in 3.1% of cases. Our technique has resulted in minimal arterial or nerve injuries, and minimises the risk of stroke associated with crossing the innominate and left carotid artery.

Graft orientation and sizing

Since the chimney graft technique requires the interaction of multiple stent grafts with the aortic wall, the configuration of the devices and the resulting "gutters" impact the success of the technique. Chimney graft orientation can by defined by the direction of flow into the target vessel. Simplified cartoons describing these graft orientations can be seen in Figure 1.[11] Appropriate orientation, oversizing of the stent grafts, and sufficient graft overlap must be obtained to avoid "gutter leaks" and optimise the graft/vessel wall interaction. The type of EVAR device and chimney graft used probably plays a part on the outcome of the procedure. However, to date, no single configuration has been demonstrated to be superior to another.

Graft oversizing

Optimal graft oversizing is critical to avoid creating large "gutters" in the space between the endograft and the chimney graft. Mestres *et al* performed *in vitro* experiments with the Endurant (Medtronic) and Excluder (Gore) endografts using Atrium balloon expandable stents (Atrium) and Viabahn (Gore) self-expandable stents.[27] Each endograft was tested with one chimney graft (either Viabahn or Atrium) in three oversizing conditions; normal oversizing (15%), excessive oversizing (30%), and over-excessive oversizing (>30%). The results found that there is better endograft-chimney graft stent apposition, and a smaller gutter area, when excessive oversizing is used. Mario Lachat proposed an equation for a two-vessel snorkel case to optimise sealing between the parallel stent grafts, stating "Stent graft diameter for a two-chimney procedure should be equal to the circumference of an ellipse with major diameter (A) equal to the sum of the aortic diameter

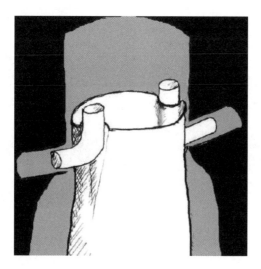

Figure 2: Optimal configuration for chimney grafts.

plus the chimney graft's diameters and minor diameter (B) equal to the aortic diameter". For three chimney grafts, 1.5 times the mean of the grafts' diameters is added to the aortic diameter to calculate the optimal stent graft diameter.[15] With respect to the chimney graft itself, a 1–2mm oversizing is generally recommended, based on target vessel diameter.[11]

Antegrade grafts (chimneys/snorkels)

Chimney grafts provide antegrade flow into upgoing vessels, typically in the aortic arch. A systematic review of chimney grafts for aortic arch pathologies demonstrates acceptable outcomes with this technique.[28]

Snorkel grafts provide antegrade perfusion to the visceral and renal vessels in a downward orientation. The procedure typically allows for up to four chimney grafts placed alongside a standard EVAR device, to preserve the visceral and renal arteries in juxtarenal and pararenal aneurysms.

Access to the visceral arteries is approached from an axillary or brachial approach, while the EVAR is deployed in the standard fashion. An alternative approach describes an initial retrograde chimney graft (periscope) deployment from the femoral access site, followed by a "lift" to reverse the chimney graft orientation to an antegrade snorkel graft.[29]

Data from the PERICLES (Performance of the chimney technique for the treatment of complex aortic pathologies) registry on 517 patients undergoing chimney grafts reported a primary patency of 9% and type Ia endoleak rate of 5.7% at 17 months follow up.[16] These data showed improved outcomes as compared to previously reported single centre experiences.[4,11,18] The PROTAGORAS (Study to evaluate the performance of the Endurant stent graft for patients with pararenal pathologic processes treated by the chimney/snorkel endovascular technique) trial using a prospective defined protocol and a single device combination (Endurant, Medtronic, and iCAST, Atrium) demonstrates the best published results to date with respect to endoleak (1.6%) and branch patency(95.7%).[24] In order to minimise the risk of gutter leaks and maximise graft/aortic wall seal, a minimum of 20mm is recommended for chimney grafts,[11] more than the 10–15mm required for seal

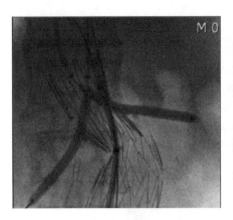 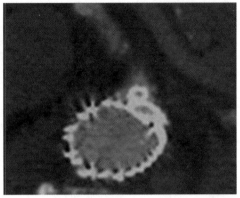

Figure 3: Clustering of chimney grafts with increase "gutters".

in standard EVAR. In ideal circumstances, the chimney graft will lay parallel with the endograft (Figure 2), but it is not uncommon for the graft to take a spiralled course to the target vessel (Figure 3). This configuration may increase the risk of "gutters" and may require a longer length chimney graft. Caution must be taken not to obstruct the origin of adjacent vessels with the top of the graft.

Retrograde configuration (periscopes)

Originally described by Rancic *et al* in 2010, the retrograde configuration of parallel stent grafts describes the positioning of a parallel stent graft running caudally into the distal neck of an endovascular thoracoabdominal aneurysm repair, allowing for retrograde blood flow into the target vessel. The authors advocate for covered stents, specifically Viabahn stents, over bare-metal stents to prevent against type Ib endoleaks.[15,30] They do admit to difficulty with sealing off the distal neck intraoperatively, with low-flow type Ib endoleak sealing postoperatively without required intervention. Retrograde grafts have also been described to revascularise the left subclavian artery in thoracic endovascular aneurysm repair (TEVAR) procedures.[31]

Combined antegrade and retrograde configuration

Lachat *et al* reviewed two-year data, using both antegrade and retrograde chimney grafts for the treatment of juxtarenal and type VI thoracoabdominal aortic aneurysms with a two-year follow up and a 99% technical success rate. Ninety-five per cent of aneurysms showed stability or decreasing size.[15] On postoperative CT angiographies, 20 patients (25%) had a type II or III endoleak.[15] At 16 months only three patients (4%) had endoleaks, with 13 of the 20 (65%) patients requiring endovascular salvage techniques. At 36 months, patency rates approached 98%.

Sandwich/terrace configuration

The technique originally described by Lobato *et al* in 2010 provides an "off-the-shelf" endovascular solution to treat type I–VI thoracoabdominal aneurysms.[32] Employing the use of two main-body stent grafts, visceral snorkel/chimney grafts are deployed between the thoracic and abdominal aortic main body stents, with total endovascular exclusion of the thoracoabdominal pathology. Lobato *et al*

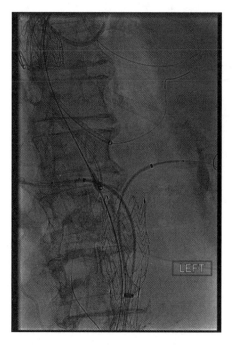

Figure 4a: Combination of antegrade and retrograde chimney grafts to treat thoracoabdominal aneurysm.

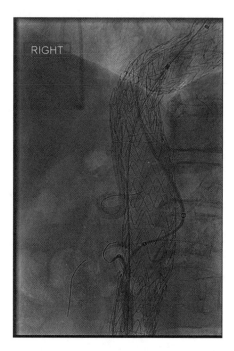

Figure 4b: Final terrace graft with antegrade coeliac and SMA and retrograde renal chimney grafts using Viabhan and Gore CTAG and C3 endografts.

initially described a 93% technical success rate and a 20% mortality rate in a 15-patient cohort. This series reported a 47% endoleak rate (seven endoleaks out of 15 patients with 48 total visceral stent placements), two of which required return to the operating room for treatment.[24]

Schweirz *et al* published their experience with this technique with a cohort twice the size, with twice as many visceral chimney grafts.[21] They described an 87% technical success rate with a 7% 30-day mortality and a 17% 18-month mortality rate. The majority of patients required three chimney/snorkel stents (57%) or four visceral stents (35%). They report a 35% endoleak rate, with type I endoleaks being more common in patients with three or four chimney grafts; however, this was not statistically significant. Chimney graft patency was much improved with three or less chimney stents.

Both groups advocate for Viabahn stents to be used for the chimney grafts. The chimney stents were oversized by 1mm, and extra-long stents were used to allow for 7–9cm of overlap between the chimney stent and the main body stent.[21] The two groups differed in the approach to renal *versus* visceral stents. Lobato described a completely antegrade chimney/snorkel stent approach for all reno-visceral vessels, while Schweirz initially advocated for a periscope technique when approaching the renal arteries and a snorkel technique when approaching the visceral vessels. We have used the combination antegrade/retrograde technique using a conformable Gore TAG thoracic endoprosthesis, and the Gore C3/Viabahn chimney graft combination with variable success (Figure 4a and 4b). Limited distal overlap has resulted in an excessive type Ib endoleak rate and the retrograde renal configuration has had a significant thrombosis rate. Schweirz has abandoned the retrograde renal configuration, and the group now use the "lift" technique described by Lachat *et al* to allow simultaneous axillary and femoral access. Both groups agreed on a 30% oversizing of the distal main body stent graft, to be deployed just inferior to the covered snorkel and/or periscope reno-visceral covered stents.[29]

In our experience, it is difficult to obtain adequate overlap using the retrograde renal approach described by Schwierz, due to limitations of the length of the aortic endograft main body. Using the 36mm C3 device, a maximum of 5–6cm of overlap can be obtained in the main body. Longer chimney grafts risk extending into the iliac limb, which in our experience is associated with early chimney graft thrombosis. An additional limitation is the fixed length of Viabahn grafts. The 10cm graft can occasionally be too short in large aneurysms while the 15cm graft extends too far into the iliac limb. For this reason, we have limited the use of retrograde renal grafts, and prefer all four vessels to be oriented antegrade.[20]

Discussion

Parallel stent graft techniques expand the indication for EVAR and TEVAR procedures. The results of these procedures vary widely based on the techniques used, graft configurations and indications for treatment. In order for chimney graft procedures to stand up to scrutiny and compare favourably to other techniques for complex abdominal aortic aneurysm repair, a well described set of rules is required to describe the optimal graft/chimney graft configuration. To date no such consensus exists.

Continued investigation and analysis of these procedures is required to determine the optimal device configurations. The configurations are most likely to differ based on the anatomy of the aneurysm and number of vessels being treated.

Summary

- Preoperative imaging is critical to procedure planning.

- Optimal oversizing is 30% for endograft and 1–2mm for chimney grafts. More excessive oversizing may be required when more chimney grafts are used.

- No significant difference exists between balloon expandable and self-expanding stents for chimney grafts.

- Antegrade and retrograde configuration both have acceptable patency rates and freedom from endoleak.

- There is no advantage to any type of endograft.

- The terrace/sandwich technique may have application in patients with thoracoabdominal aneurysms that cannot be treated with open or branched/fenestrated endografts.

- Chimney grafts continue to have a significant role in the endovascular management of complex aneurysm pathology.

References

1. Greenberg RK, Clair D, Srivastava S *et al*. Should patients with challenging anatomy be offered endovascular aneurysm repair? YMVA 2003; **38**: 990–96.

2. Lee JT, Greenberg JI, Dalman RL. Early experience with the snorkel technique for juxtarenal aneurysms. *Journal of Vascular Surgery* 2012; **55**: 935–46.

3. Usai MV, Torsello G, Donas KP. Current evidence regarding chimney graft occlusions in the endovascular treatment of pararenal aortic pathologies: a systematic review with pooled data analysis. *J Endovasc Ther* 2015; **22**: 396–400.

4. Scali ST, Feezor RJ, Chang CK, *et al.* Critical analysis of results after chimney endovascular aortic aneurysm repair raises cause for concern. *J Vasc Surg* 2014; **60**: 865–75.

5. Bruen KJ, Feezor RJ, Daniels MJ, *et al.* Endovascular chimney technique *versus* open repair of juxtarenal and suprarenal aneurysms. *J Vasc Surg* 2011; **53**: 895–905.

6. Siani A, Accrocca F, Gabrielli R, Marcucci G. Is the chimney graft technique a safe and feasible approach to treat urgent aneurysm and pseudoaneurysm of the abdominal aorta? An analysis of our experience and technical considerations. *Interact Cardiovasc Thorac Surg* 2013; **16**: 692–94.

7. Donas KP, Pecoraro F, Torsello G, *et al.* Use of covered chimney stents for pararenal aortic pathologies is safe and feasible with excellent patency and low incidence of endoleaks. *J Vasc Surg* 2012; **55**: 659–65.

8. Moulakakis KG, Mylonas SN, Avgerinos E, *et al.* The chimney graft technique for preserving visceral vessels during endovascular treatment of aortic pathologies. *J Vasc Surg* 2012; **55**: 1497–503.

9. Lindblad B, Bin Jabr A, Holst J, Malina M. Chimney grafts in aortic stent grafting: Hazardous or useful technique? Systematic review of current data. *Eur J Vasc Endovasc Surg* 2015; **50**: 722–31.

10. Lobato AC, Camacho-Lobato L *et al.* Endovascular treatment of complex aortic aneurysms using the sandwich technique. *J Endovasc Ther* 2012; **19**: 691–706.

11. Patel RP, Katsargyris A, Verhoeven EL, *et al.* Endovascular aortic aneurysm repair with chimney and snorkel grafts: Indications, techniques and results. Cardiovasc Intervent Radiol 2013; **36**: 1443–51.

12. Lobato AC. Sandwich technique for aortoiliac aneurysms extending to the internal iliac artery or isolated common/internal iliac artery aneurysms: A new endovascular approach to preserve pelvic circulation. *J Endovascular Ther* 2011; **18**: 106–11.

13. Dorsey C, Chandra V, Lee JT. The "Terrace Technique"-"Totally endovascular repair of a type IV thoracoabdominal aortic aneurysm. *Annals of Vascular Surgery* 2014; **28**: e11-6.

14. Lee JT, *et al.* EVAR deployment in anatomically challenging necks outside the IFU. European Journal of Vascular & Endovascular Surgery 2013; **46**: 65–73.

15. Lachat M, *et al.* Chimney and periscope grafts observed over 2 Years After Their Use to Revascularize 169 Renovisceral Branches in 77 Patients With Complex Aortic Aneurysms. *J Endovascular Ther* 2013; **20**: 1–9.

16. Donas KP, Lee JT, Lachat M, *et al.* Collected world experience about the performance of the snorkel/chimney endovascular technique in the treatment of complex aortic pathologies: the PERICLES registry. *Ann Surg* 2015; **262**: 546–53.

17. Ohrlander T, Sonesson B, Ivancev K, *et al.* The chimney graft: A technique for preserving or rescuing aortic branch vessels in stent-graft sealing zones. *J Endovasc Ther* 2008; **15**: 427–32.

18. Banno H, Cochennec F, Marzelle J, Becquemin JP, *et al.* Comparison of fenestrated endovascular aneurysm repair and chimney graft techniques for pararenal aortic aneurysm. *Journal of Vascular Surgery* 2014; **60**: 31–39.

19. Hertault A, Haulon S, Lee JT. Debate: Whether branched/fenestrated endovascular aneurysm repair procedures are better than snorkels, chimneys, or periscopes in the treatment of most thoracoabdominal and juxtarenal aneurysms. *Journal of Vascular Surgery* 2015; **62**: 1357–65.

20. Wooster M, Powell A, Back M, *et al.* Axillary artery access as an adjunct for complex endovascular aortic repair. *Annals of Vascular Surgery* 2015; **29**: 1543–47.

21. Schwierz E, Kolvenbach RR, Yoshida R, *et al.* Experience with the sandwich technique in endovascular thoracoabdominal aortic aneurysm repair. *Journal of Vascular Surgery* 2014; **59**: 1562–69.

22. Lee JT, Greenberg JI, Dalman RL. Early experience with the snorkel technique for juxtarenal aneurysms. *Journal of Vascular Surgery* 2012; **55**: 935–46.

23. Coscas R, Kobeiter H, Desgranges P, Becquemin JP. Technical aspects, current indications, and results of chimney grafts for juxtarenal aortic aneurysms. *Journal of Vascular Surgery* 2011; **53**: 1520–27.

24. Donas KP, Torsello GB, Piccoli G, *et al.* The PROTAGORAS study to evaluate the performance of the Endurant stent graft for patients with pararenal pathologic processes treated by the chimney/snorkel endovascular technique. *Journal of Vascular Surgery* 2015; **63**: 1–7.

25. Hiramoto JS, Chang CK, Reilly LM, *et al.* Outcome of renal stenting for renal artery coverage during endovascular aortic aneurysm repair. *Journal of Vascular Surgery* 2009; **49**: 1100–06.

26. Donas KP, Pecoraro F, Torsello G, *et al.* Use of covered chimney stents for pararenal aortic pathologies is safe and feasible with excellent patency and low incidence of endoleaks. *Journal of Vascular Surgery* 2012; **55**: 659–65.

27. Mestres G, Uribe JP, García-Madrid C, *et al.* The best conditions for parallel stenting during EVAR: an in vitro study. *Eur J Vasc Endovasc Surg* 2012; **44**: 468–73.

28. Yang J, Xiong J, Liu X, *et al*. Endovascular chimney technique of aortic arch pathologies: a systematic review. *Annals of Vascular Surgery* 2012; **26**: 1014–21.

29. Lachat M, Bisdas T, Rancic Z, *et al*. Chimney endografting for pararenal aortic pathologies using transfemoral access and the lift technique. *J Endovasc Ther* 2013; **20**: 492–97.

30. Montelione N, Pecoraro F, Puippe G, *et al*. A 12-year experience with chimney and periscope grafts for treatment of type I endoleaks. *Journal of Endovascular Therapy* 2015; **22**: 568–74.

31. Lachat M, Mayer D, Pfammatter T, *et al*. Periscope endograft technique to revascularize the left subclavian artery during thoracic endovascular aortic repair. *J Endovascular Ther* 2013; **20**: 728-34.

32. Lobato AC, Camacho-Lobato L. A new technique to enhance endovascular thoracoabdominal aortic aneurysm therapy—the sandwich procedure. *Semin Vasc Surg* 2012; **25**: 153–60.

Debate: More than two parallel grafts relates to poorer outcome—for the motion

K Stavroulakis, G Torsello and KP Donas

Introduction

The chimney or snorkel technique is an increasingly popular means for the endovascular aneurysm repair (EVAR) of complex aortic pathological processes. The main principle of this alternative approach is the creation of an adequate proximal or distal sealing zone in cases of insufficient neck using off-the-self devices by placement of mainly covered stents parallel to and outside of the main abdominal endograft. Consequently, we create an adequate sealing zone and the endograft can be placed proximately at the origin of the non-stented aortic side branches.

Although initially proposed as a bailout technique for an inadvertent coverage of aortic side branches or for urgent situations,[1,2] nowadays chimney EVAR is up to 80% employed in elective cases.[3] Recently, the PERICLES (Performance of the chimney technique for the treatment of complex aortic pathologies) registry collected the global experience of 13 high- and low-volume international US and European centres in more than 500 patients and confirmed reproducible results[4] providing impetus for further use of the chimney technique.

On the other hand, despite the broad applicability and the growing interest in chimney EVAR, there is a paucity of data concerning various aspects of this technique. For instance, it remains unclear if the application of more than two parallel grafts is associated with poorer clinical and radiological outcomes.

Performance of one/two versus multiple chimney grafts

Literature review

Up to now, only two studies evaluated the performance of multiple *versus* single/two chimney grafts. PROTAGORAS (Study to evaluate the performance of the Endurant stent graft for patients with pararenal pathologic processes treated by the chimney/snorkel endovascular technique) registry evaluated the performance of Endurant stent graft (Medtronic) as a standard abdominal device for pararenal aortic disease in two European centres prospectively.[5] Subgroup analysis of graft patency and chimney graft-related reinterventions did not reveal any significant differences between single and multiple chimneys procedures. However, it is important to mention that the percentage of patients treated by three or more chimney grafts was only 7.9% of this cohort and, therefore, even if we have a trend of similar outcomes, a robust conclusion cannot be drawn.

Another study reporting on the "sandwich technique", as a modified chimney procedure for the treatment of thoracoabdominal aortic disease, showed a higher incidence of adverse events between patients treated by multiple chimney grafts.[6] In particular, the incidence of chimney or periscope graft occlusion tended to be higher in patients with three/four chimney grafts than those treated by two. However, the number of patients was too small for the log-rank test to reveal significant differences. Although again not statistically significant, the incidence of initial type I endoleak was higher in patients treated by three or four chimney grafts. Additionally, a more apparent postoperative renal function decline was noticed in the multiple-chimney group.

Institutional experience

According to our internal and published algorithm[7] chimney EVAR is the preferable treatment option in case of juxtarenal and pararenal disease with involvement of one or two visceral branches. If more than two side branches are involved, we usually perform fenestrated EVAR. Main reasons are the better fixation of the endograft and the lower risk for neurological complications due to the option to treat the patient transfemorally. However, in case of symptomatic/ruptured aortic aneurysm with no time for delay or hostile iliac vessels, use of parallel grafts for all four renovisceral vessels remains our preferable option. Consequently, a chimney EVAR with more than two chimney conduits was indicated in almost 30% of our last 150 chimney cases (unpublished data).

Based on this experience, the following technical aspects should be taken into consideration in case of multiple chimney aneurysm repair:

1. Undetected compression of previous deployed chimney grafts with consecutive early occlusion
2. Insufficient oversizing of the abdominal endograft
3. Placement of chimney grafts from the dorsal face of the abdominal endograft creating a more horizontal and not parallel fashion.

Figures Ia and b shows these important parameters leading to type Ia endoleak.

Discussion

Despite the fact that a comparison of one/two *versus* more than two chimney grafts chimney EVAR is not suitable due to the different underlying diseases such as juxtarenal for the single/double chimney cases *versus* suprarenal or infradiaphragmatic aneurysms for the multiple cases, various aspects should be considered.

The inevitable formation of gutters because of chimney graft deployment parallel to and outside of the main abdominal endograft can theoretically lead to a type Ia endoleak. On the other hand, the formation of a persistent or new-onset type Ia endoleak is rare based on the literature.[4] The creation of a sufficient sealing zone of 20mm and the use of compatible chimney covered stents and main abdominal endografts seems to be crucial in order to minimise the risk of persistent needed reintervention type Ia endoleaks.[5]

However, placement of more than two chimney grafts raises specific technical challenges in order to create this sufficient neck. The most market available abdominal main bodies/cuffs have a maximum proximal diameter of 36mm. Thus an aortic diameter >29mm in the renovisceral segment burdens the applicability of chimney EVAR due to the recommended oversizing between 20% and 30%. Of note, insufficient oversizing was associated with late ruptures following chimney EVAR.[8]

Furthermore, the available stent grafts, as they are not specially designed for chimney EVAR, were not created to mould around each other to achieve a seal. Use of devices with a nitinol endoskeleton seems to perform better compared to stainless steel endoskeleton. However, the clinical impact of this difference seems to be limited, as the PERICLES registry showed. There is no doubt that placement of multiple chimneys can be the reason for insufficient moulding around the deployed devices leading to a type Ia endoleak (Figure 1a–b; Figure 2a-c).

Moreover, concerns are raised about the relatively high incidence of ischaemic stroke following chimney EVAR. In a meta-analysis from Katsargyris *et al* including pararenal and thoracic chimneys, the ischaemic stroke rate reported was 3.2%.[9] By contrast, the observed rate in the recently published PERICLES registry, including only pararenal pathologies, was 1.7%.[4] There is no doubt that an upper extremity access increases the risk for iatrogenic stroke. Particularly in cases of multiple chimneys where a bilateral upper extremity access and the extensive navigation of multiple arterial sheaths in the aortic arch are needed, the risk for ischaemic stroke is present.

On the other hand, the risk of an ischaemic cerebral event is not associated with chimney EVAR, but related to the upper extremity access. Comparable stroke rates were observed in studies evaluating the performance of fenestrated endografting such as the French multicentre experience of fenestrated aortic endografts and the Windows trial.[10,11]

In our institution, a duplex ultrasound scan of the supra-aortic vessels was routinely performed in order to exclude a relevant stenosis of the carotid artery. In elective cases, a carotid revascularisation should be performed prior to chimney EVAR. Moreover, we prefer a single upper extremity access through the left axillary artery and double puncture of the vessel in case of double chimneys, avoiding access from the right upper extremity. Further, the "lift" technique with placement of a flexible self-expanding covered stent (Viabahn, Gore) via transfemoral access may also reduce the risk of stroke in inappropriately calcified and stenotic supra-aortic vessels.[12]

Although Usai *et al* did not find any correlation between the number of chimneys deployed and the incidence of chimney graft occlusions, it should be noted that the only lethal occlusions reported were related to superior mesenteric artery grafts.[3,13]

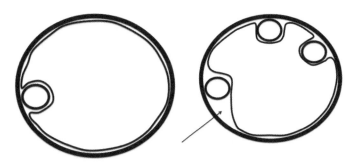

Figure 1a and b: Increased gutters in cases of multiple chimney (arrow) as a result of an inadequate abdominal graft and aortic wall contact in case of insufficient oversizing (<20%) or short new neck length (<20mm).

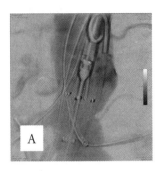 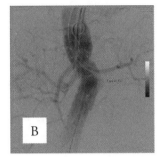 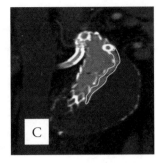

Figure 2: Type Ia endoleak following triple chimney aortic reconstruction for pararenal abdominal aortic aneurysm in a male patient: (A) and (B) Placement of the sheath for the left renal artery behind the aortic endograft and final intraoperative angiography; (C) Postoperative CT angiography with suboptimal contact of the aortic endograft and the aortic wall due to limited oversizing and placement of the chimney graft for the left renal artery between them.

Moreover, despite the theoretical description of a parallel course of the chimney graft to the main abdominal endograft, chimney stents usually have a tortuous course. Thus, multiple chimney deployment could lead to a mechanical interaction between the grafts, increasing the mechanical stress applied and consequently the risk of a graft occlusion.

Interestingly, in our recently published work about chimney EVAR to save failed EVAR and type Ia endoleaks, a superior mesenteric artery chimney occlusion was observed due to mechanical compression from the right renal chimney graft.[14] The patient suffered postoperatively from diarrhoea and was treated by retrograde recanalisation of the occluded superior mesenteric artery through the coeliac trunk and the gastroduodenal artery. After successful AngioJet (Possis Medical) embolectomy, an additional bare metal stent (ev3 Protégé, Covidien) was deployed into the recanalised Advanta/iCAST V12 covered stent (Maquet). As there is no way to predict or exclude a mechanical interaction/compression between the chimney grafts, we routinely perform a kissing-balloon dilation between the aortic and chimney stent grafts in cases of more than two chimney conduits.

Finally, a possible decline of the renal function could complicate multiple chimney procedures. Overall, the incidence of acute kidney injury in the PERICLES registry amounted to 17.5% but no subgroup analysis was performed concerning the number of grafts deployed. Given the increased complexity of the multiple chimney procedures and the necessity of repeated angiographic controls intraoperatively, there is an increased risk of periprocedural acute kidney injury. Indeed, as mentioned above, a significantly higher postoperative acute kidney injury was observed in patients treated by multiple chimneys compared with patients with two chimneys only for thoracoabdominal aneurysms.[6] Notably, recent studies suggest that chronic kidney disease and acute kidney injury are closely interconnected, as acute kidney injury is a risk factor for the development of chronic kidney disease, and both acute kidney injury and chronic kidney disease are risk factors for cardiovascular disease.[15] However, a meticulous evaluation of renal function following chimney EVAR in the long run is missing.

Conclusion

Chimney EVAR represents a durable technique for the endovascular treatment of complex aortic pathological processes. However, many aspects of this treatment modality, such as the performance of more than two parallel conduits, remain unclear. It seems that the application of more than two chimney grafts can potentially increase the risk of postoperative type Ia endoleak, cerebral ischaemic events and acute kidney injury, whereas its effect on graft occlusion seems to be equal with the group of single chimneys. Anyhow, in the absence of profound evidence, no robust conclusions can be drawn.

Summary

- Increasing evidence in the current literature (PERICLES registry) shows reproducible results providing safety of the chimney technique for the treatment of complex aortic pathologic processes.

- Use of more than two chimney grafts can be associated with higher rates of postoperative type Ia endoleak, cerebral ischaemic events and acute kidney injury due to the need of bilateral access from the upper extremity and the limitation of inadequate oversizing. Further studies are warranted to evaluate the performance of multiple vs. single chimneys.

- At the moment, multiple chimney EVAR is recommended in cases of symptomatic/ruptured aortic aneurysms or in patients, who are unfit for open repair or anatomically unsuitable for branched/fenestrated EVAR.

References

1. Greenberg RK, Clair D, Srivastava S, *et al.* Should patients with challenging anatomy be offered endovascular aneurysm repair? *J Vasc Surg* 2003; **38**: 990e6.

2. Criado FJ. Chimney grafts and bare stents: aortic branch preservation revisited. *J Endovasc Ther 2007*; **14** (6): 823–4.

3. Lindblad B, Jabr A. Bin, Holst J, Malina M. Chimney grafts in aortic stent grafting: Hazardous or useful technique? Systematic review of current data. *Eur J Vasc Endovasc Surg* 2015; **50**: 722e731.

4. Donas K, Lee J, Lachat M, *et al* on behalf of the PERICLES investigators. Collected world experience about the performance of the snorkel/chimney endovascular technique in the treatment of complex aortic pathologies. The PERICLES Registry. *Ann Surg* 2015; **262** (3): 546–53.

5. Donas K, Torsello G, Piccoli G, *et al.* The PROTAGORAS study to evaluate the performance of the Endurant stent graft for patients with pararenal pathologic processes treated by the chimney/snorkel endovascular technique. *J Vasc Surg* 2016; **63** (1): 1–7.

6. Schwierz E, Kolvenbach R, Yoshida R, *et al.* Experience with the sandwich technique in endovascular thoracoabdominal aortic aneurysm repair. *J Vasc Surg* 2014; **59** (6): 1562–9.

7. Donas KP, Eisenack M, Panuccio G, *et al.* The role of open and endovascular treatment with fenestrated and chimney endografts for patients with juxtarenal aortic aneurysms. *J Vasc Surg* 2012; **56** (2): 285–90.

8. Schiro A, Antoniou GA, Ormesher D, *et al.* The chimney technique in endovascular aortic aneurysm repair: late ruptures after successful single renal chimney stent grafts. *Ann Vasc Surg* 2013; **27** (7): 835–43.

9. Katsargyris A, Oikonomou K, Klonaris C, *et al.* Comparison of outcomes with open, fenestrated, and chimney graft repair of juxtarenal aneurysms: are we ready for a paradigm shift? *J Endovasc Ther* 2013; **20** (2): 159–69.

10. Haulon S Amiot S, Magnan PE, *et al;* Association Universitaire de Recherche en *Chirurg*ie Vasculaire (AURC). An analysis of the French multicentre experience of fenestrated aortic endografts: medium-term outcomes. *Ann Surg* 2010; **251** (2): 357–62.

11. Marzelle J, Presles E, Becquemin JP; WINDOWS trial participants. Results and factors affecting early outcome of fenestrated and/or branched stent grafts for aortic aneurysms: a multicenter prospective study. *Ann Surg* 2015; **261** (1): 197–206.

12. Lachat M, Bisdas T, Mayer D, *et al.* Chimney endografting for pararenal aortic pathologies using transfemoral access and the lift technique. *J Endovasc Ther* 2013; **20**: 492–95.

13. Usai MV, Torsello G, Donas KP. Current evidence regarding chimney graft occlusions in the endovascular treatment of pararenal aortic pathologies: a systematic review with pooled data analysis. *J Endovasc Ther* 2015; **22** (3): 396–400.

14. Donas KP, Telve D, Torsello G, *et al.* Use of parallel grafts to save failed prior endovascular aortic aneurysm repair and type Ia endoleaks. *J Vasc Surg* 2015; **62**: 578–84.

15. Chawla L, Eggers P, Star R, *et al.* Acute kidney injury and chronic kidney disease as interconnected syndromes. *N Engl J Med* 2014; **371**: 58–66.

Debate: More than two parallel grafts relates to poorer outcome—against the motion

HWL de Beaufort, JA van Herwaarden and FL Moll

Introduction

The endovascular deployment of a graft in an aortic side branch, parallel to the aortic main device, was first reported as a method to preserve renal artery perfusion for endovascular aneurysm repair (EVAR) patients with short aortic necks.[1] The technique can also be used during thoracic endovascular aortic repair (TEVAR), where it was first performed as a salvage method for unintentional coverage of a left carotid artery.[2] It allows deployment of the aortic main body proximal to the ostium of any aortic side branch to ensure a proximal sealing zone of sufficient length. Only readily available, "off-the-shelf" endovascular devices with relatively low profile delivery systems are required for parallel grafting, which makes it an appealing treatment option for high surgical risk patients with complex aortic disease.

Concerns about using multiple parallel grafts

Despite good initial short-term results with parallel grafting, concerns about the durability of the technique have existed from its outset. Neither the aortic main device nor the parallel grafts have been designed for or tested in the parallel graft configuration. In particular, occlusion of one of the parallel grafts is a cause for concern, especially if there is a high degree of angulation between the side branch and the aorta, or if the parallel graft is long and small in diameter. Moreover, multiple parallel grafts hamper visualisation, and can make it impossible to determine the exact location of each of the grafts with standard fluoroscopy. The most important concerns, however, are caused by the so-called gutter areas. These are the areas between the aortic wall, parallel graft and aortic main device that are invariably created when deploying a parallel graft. These gutters can vary in size and volume, and when they are small, there is little or no flow through them. If on top of that, the gutter areas "run blind" into an area where the aortic main body is fully deployed against the aortic wall, they are most likely to thrombose spontaneously, ensuring adequate sealing. On the other hand, if there is high flow through the gutters, or if any graft migration occurs, they are a potential source of type I endoleak. When more than two parallel grafts are used, the gutter area and volume are obviously increased. Additionally, the procedure becomes technically more difficult, and there is an increased risk of a crossing configuration of the grafts, instead of deployment precisely parallel to the aortic main body. This crossing configuration increases gutter size—hence the risk of endoleak.

Experience with multiple parallel grafts

Parallel grafting can be performed to revascularise any number of side branches during endovascular repair of the aorta. Most physicians refrain from using more than two parallel grafts, and experience with multiple parallel grafts is limited. In the aortic arch, parallel grafting is most commonly performed for a single supra-aortic vessel, usually the left subclavian artery or left common carotid artery. Multiple parallel grafts in the aortic arch are rare.[3] This is firstly because aortic motion over the cardiac cycle is most obvious in the ascending aorta and arch, and long-term effects on graft integrity might be most pronounced here. Secondly, much experience has been gained with the use of extra-anatomical bypasses of the supra-aortic vessels, which offer a reliable alternative for branch vessel perfusion. The use of more than two parallel grafts is therefore exceptionally rare in the arch, and available evidence is confined to case reports.[4,5]

More experience exists with multiple parallel grafts for visceral vessel preservation in endovascular aortic repair of the thoracoabdominal aorta. A review of 93 patients found an increased risk of type I endoleak with bilateral renal parallel grafts compared to a single renal parallel graft,[6] but in a more recent series of 128 patients treated with parallel grafting, the use of two, three or four parallel grafts did not seem to be associated with a higher risk of graft-related reinterventions or decreased graft patency at midterm follow-up.[7] The use of two renal parallel grafts is now generally accepted as safe and effective—in the short-term at least—and anatomical and clinical factors can guide the choice of treatment towards parallel graft repair of more visceral side branches, i.e. of the superior mesenteric artery and/or the coeliac trunk as well as one or both of the renal arteries. This has been reported at specialised centres and for small numbers of patients, with varying results.[8–17] The deployment of three or more parallel grafts is exceptional though, so comparison of three or more *versus* two or less parallel grafts has not been done. Nonetheless, a number of observations have been made for procedures with multiple parallel grafts. The requirement for right as well as left arm access was noted as an important drawback to applying the parallel graft technique to multiple

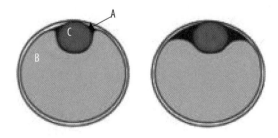

Figure 1: (A) Gutter area between (B) aortic main device, (C) parallel graft and aortic wall can vary in size and volume and are a potential source of type I endoleak, especially when they are large. (Source: Criado FJ, Duson, S. Parallel grafts in perspective: Definitions and a new classification. *Vasc Dis Manag* 2013; **10** (1): 16–19.)

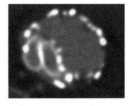

Figure 2: Crossing configuration of parallel grafts increases gutter area. (Source: Tolenaar JL, Zandvoort HJ, Moll FL, van Herwaarden JA. Technical considerations and results of chimney grafts for the treatment of juxtarenal aneurysms. *J Vasc Surg* 2013; **58**: 607–15.)

branch vessels, because it increases the risk of cerebral complications through wire manipulation in the arch.[12,18] A crossing configuration of the parallel grafts, due to the technical complexity of the procedure, was seen as another potential risk, as it increases gutter area.[14] Therefore, when more than two parallel grafts are used, modifications to the "standard" parallel graft procedure are usually employed. Some opt for a configuration with one or two proximal parallel grafts in the "chimney" or "snorkel" position, i.e. with the inflow proximal to the aortic main body, and one or two distal grafts in the "periscope" position, i.e. with the inflow at the distal end of the main device and pressure-driven, retrograde perfusion of the parallel graft.[10,19,20] Periscope grafts are mainly useful for juxtarenal aneurysms that do not extend too far distally. An advantage of periscope grafts is that femoral access can be used instead of upper extremity or carotid access. A disadvantage is that because the periscope relies on retrograde perfusion, any drop in flow or pressure in the distal aorta, which is already narrowed by the presence of the periscopes, could lead to end-organ ischaemia.

Alternatively, the sandwich technique involves deployment of the parallel grafts between two or three aortic main devices to increase stability of all different components, and is suited for any thoracoabdominal aneurysm repair.[21,22] In the double-two chimney configuration, both renal parallel grafts are deployed between two aortic main devices, but the two more proximal parallel grafts are deployed "normally", between the aortic main body and the aortic wall.[23] This technique is applicable to aneurysms that do not extend too far proximally to the coeliac trunk. Alternatively, the use of endoanchors to reduce the risk of migration and endoleak was proposed after good *in vitro* results, and has been reported for at least one patient.[24,25]

Proposed treatment strategy

Since its inception, various ways to perform the parallel graft technique have been adopted. Taking into account the theoretical background and the paucity of clinical evidence, we believe the following method reduces the risk of parallel graft related complications: the amount of main device oversizing should be about 30% when more than one parallel graft is needed. An *in vitro* study found this to be the optimal degree of oversizing for a single parallel graft.[26] Excessive oversizing might reduce gutter size, but will increase parallel graft compression, and can also increase the risk of main device collapse. Therefore, applying even more oversizing should probably be avoided, for single or for multiple parallel grafts.

A number of choices exist for the type of parallel graft, which can be covered or uncovered, self-expandable or balloon-expandable. Covered stents deserve preference because they reduce the pressure in the gutters and thus the risk of type I endoleak, especially if there is no aortic neck. The most commonly used covered stents are self-expandable, which generate slightly less radial force than balloon-expandable stents. Using multiple parallel grafts often means they need to be extended to reach a sufficient length. If this is necessary, deployment of an uncovered balloon-expandable stent at the level of the aortic lumen can be judicial. This will ensure sufficient radial strength and avoid kinking of the parallel graft. Additionally, regardless of the amount of parallel grafts, a proximal sealing length of at least 15mm should be adhered to, to ensure that the gutters running parallel

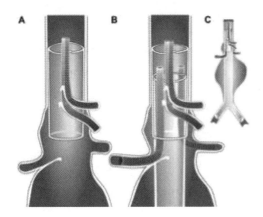

Figure 3: Double two-chimney technique for complete renovisceral revascularisation for endovascular repair of a suprarenal aneurysm. (Source: Buck DB, van Herwaarden JA, Schermerhorn ML, Moll FL. Endovascular treatment of abdominal aortic aneurysms. *Nat Rev Cardiol* 2014; **11**: 112–23.)

to the proximal sealing zone are long enough to induce gutter thrombosis. Finally, when deploying more than two parallel grafts, alternative configurations are likely to offer most durable results. Patient anatomy decides whether a double-two chimney, a sandwich configuration, or a part chimney/part periscope configuration should be adopted.

Conclusion

There is limited experience with parallel grafting using more than two parallel grafts, but it seems feasible for highly selected cases. Adjunctive procedures, such as the sandwich or double-two chimney techniques, are likely to increase the effectiveness of parallel grafting in these cases.

Summary

- Parallel grafting can be used to expand applicability of endovascular aortic repair for high-surgical risk patients with complex aortic disease with readily available devices.

- There are a number of concerns about the durability of parallel grafting. It involves off-label use of endovascular devices, and thus it could increase the risk of type I endoleak, graft migration, or graft occlusion.

- Parallel grafting using more than two parallel grafts potentially increases the risks of complications, especially type I endoleak, if a greater gutter area is created.

- Deployment of more than two parallel grafts seems feasible for selected patients. Adjunctive procedures like the sandwich or double-two chimney technique are likely to increase effectiveness of parallel grafting in these cases.

References

1. Greenberg RK, Clair D, Srivastava S, *et al.* Should patients with challenging anatomy be offered endovascular aneurysm repair? *J Vasc Surg* 2003; **38** (5): 990–6.
2. Criado FJ. A percutaneous technique for preservation of arch branch patency during thoracic endovascular aortic repair (TEVAR): retrograde catheterization and stenting. *J Endovasc Ther 2007*; **14** (1): 54–8.

3. Moulakakis KG, Mylonas SN, Dalainas I, et al. The chimney-graft technique for preserving supra-aortic branches: a review. Ann Cardiothorac Surg 2013; **2** (3): 339–46.

4. Yoshida RA, Kolvenbach R, Yoshida WB, et al. Total endovascular debranching of the aortic arch. Eur J Vasc Endovasc Surg 2011; **42** (5): 627–30.

5. Krankenberg H, Bader R, Sixt S, et al. Endovascular repair of ascending aortic aneurysm by transapical approach and periscope technique. J Endovasc Ther 2013; **20** (1): 13–7.

6. Moulakakis KG, Mylonas SN, Avgerinos E, et al. The chimney graft technique for preserving visceral vessels during endovascular treatment of aortic pathologies. J Vasc Surg 2012; **55** (5): 1497–503.

7. Donas KP, Torsello GB, Piccoli G, et al. The PROTAGORAS study to evaluate the performance of the Endurant stent graft for patients with pararenal pathologic processes treated by the chimney/snorkel endovascular technique. J Vasc Surg 2016; **63** (1): 1–7.

8. Scali ST, Feezor RJ, Chang CK, et al. Critical analysis of results after chimney endovascular aortic aneurysm repair raises cause for concern. J Vasc Surg 2014; **60** (4): 865–73; Discussion 73–5.

9. Ronchey S, Serrao E, Kasemi H, et al. Endovascular treatment options for complex abdominal aortic aneurysms. J Vasc Interv Radiol 2015; **26** (6): 842–54.

10. Pecoraro F, Pfammatter T, Mayer D, et al. Multiple periscope and chimney grafts to treat ruptured thoracoabdominal and pararenal aortic aneurysms. J Endovasc Ther 2011; **18** (5): 642–9.

11. Marino M, Kasemi H, Di Angelo CL, Fadda GF. Ruptured thoracoabdominal aneurysm treatment with modified chimney stent graft. Ann Thorac Surg 2014; **98** (2): e37–40.

12. Lee JT, Greenberg JI, Dalman RL. Early experience with the snorkel technique for juxtarenal aneurysms. J Vasc Surg 2012; **55** (4): 935–46; Discussion 45–6.

13. Filippi F, Ficarelli R, Tirotti C, Stella N, Taurino M. Emergent fully endovascular treatment of a free ruptured thoracoabdominal aneurysm. Ann Vasc Surg 2015; **29** (4): 842.e9–.e13.

14. Tolenaar JL, Zandvoort HJ, Moll FL, van Herwaarden JA. Technical considerations and results of chimney grafts for the treatment of juxtarenal aneursyms. J Vasc Surg 2013; **58** (3): 607–15.

15. Donas KP, Pecoraro F, Bisdas T, et al. CT angiography at 24 months demonstrates durability of EVAR with the use of chimney grafts for pararenal aortic pathologies. J Endovasc Ther 2013; **20** (1): 1–6.

16. Bin Jabr A, Lindblad B, Dias N, et al. Efficacy and durability of the chimney graft technique in urgent and complex thoracic endovascular aortic repair. J Vasc Surg 2015; **61** (4): 886–94.e1.

17. Banno H, Cochennec F, Marzelle J, Becquemin JP. Comparison of fenestrated endovascular aneurysm repair and chimney graft techniques for pararenal aortic aneurysm. J Vasc Surg 2014 ; **60** (1): 31–9.

18. Coscas R, Kobeiter H, Desgranges P, Becquemin JP. Technical aspects, current indications, and results of chimney grafts for juxtarenal aortic aneurysms. J Vasc Surg 2011; **53** (6): 1520–7.

19. Brechtel K, Ketelsen D, Endisch A, et al. Endovascular repair of acute symptomatic pararenal aortic aneurysm with three chimney and one periscope graft for complete visceral artery revascularization. Cardiovasc Interv Radiol 2012; **35** (2): 413–7.

20. Cariati M, Mingazzini P, Dallatana R, et al. Endovascular treatment of a symptomatic thoracoabdominal aortic aneurysm by chimney and periscope techniques for total visceral and renal artery revascularization. Cardiovasc Interv Radiol 2014; **37** (1): 251–6.

21. Lobato AC, Camacho-Lobato L. A new technique to enhance endovascular thoracoabdominal aortic aneurysm therapy-the sandwich procedure. Semin Vasc Surg 2012; **25** (3): 153–60.

22. Kolvenbach RR, Yoshida R, Pinter L, et al. Urgent endovascular treatment of thoraco-abdominal aneurysms using a sandwich technique and chimney grafts - A technical description. Eur J Vasc Endovasc Surg 2011; **41** (1): 54–60.

23. Tolenaar JL, Zandvoort HJ, Hazenberg CE, et al. The double two-chimney technique for complete renovisceral revascularization in a suprarenal aneurysm. J Vasc Surg 2013; **58** (2): 478–81.

24. Niepoth WW, De Bruin JL, Yeung KK, et al. A proof-of-concept in vitro study to determine if EndoAnchors can reduce gutter size in chimney graft configurations. J Endovasc Ther 2013; **20** (4): 498–505.

25. Galiñanes EL, Hernandez-Vila EA, Krajcer Z. Innovative chimney-graft technique for endovascular repair of a pararenal abdominal aortic aneurysm. Tex Heart Inst J 2015; **42** (1): 35–9.

26. Mestres G, Uribe JP, Garcia-Madrid C, et al. The best conditions for parallel stenting during EVAR: an in vitro study. Eur J Vasc Endovasc Surg 2012; **44** (5): 468–73.

Abdominal aortic aneurysm challenges

Lifestyle and aneurysm growth

Lifestyle risk factors and risk to develop abdominal aortic aneurysm

O Stackelberg and M Björck

Introduction

The prevalence of abdominal aortic aneurysms is 1.7% to 4.5% among men aged 65 years or older,[1-3] and 0.5% to 1.3% among women in the same age group.[4,5] Since the first presentation of the disease may be rupture, ultrasound screening among elderly men has been widely implemented to allow for elective repair. However, most aneurysms detected through screening are small,[1] and screening is warranted to find means of decreasing their growth rate to prevent rupture and need for repair. Advanced age, male sex, and heredity are major risk factors for the disease,[6] but modifiable risk factors have yet to be fully mapped. Dietary consumption, physical activity, obesity, and comorbidities are factors that may either interfere with, or facilitate, the inflammation, proteolysis, and degradation of elastin and collagen of the aortic wall that have been identified as key processes in aneurysm pathophysiology.[7,8] In this chapter, we aim to summarise the observed associations between modifiable lifestyle-related factors and the risk of aneurysm.

Smoking

Hammond and Horn first described an association between smoking and aneurysms in 1958.[9] A decade later, they reported that smoking was associated with aneurysm to an even larger extent than were other vascular diseases (e.g. coronary heart disease and cerebrovascular diseases)[10]—a finding that has been confirmed by a more recent study.[11] Current smoking seems to have the greatest effect and is associated with increased prevalence of the disease,[1,6] aneurysm growth rate,[12] and risk of rupture.[13] Furthermore, the excess prevalence associated with smoking has been reported to account for >70% of detected aneurysms.[1,6] Also, smoking cessation is one of the few medical strategies known to decrease the risk for expansion and rupture.[14-16] In Western Europe and North America, the frequency of active smoking among men has decreased, preceding a decline in aneurysm prevalence.[1]

Aneurysms are much less common[4,5] among women, who present with the condition at an older age than do men. Additionally, smoking affects women to a greater extent than it does men. For example, with an odds ratio of 2:1 for ever smoking, 18 out of 19 aneurysms detected in a population-based screening cohort of 70-year-old women were either current or former smokers.[5] One population-based cohort found that smoking women had twice the incidence of aneurysms compared with non-smoking men.[17] In that study, women experienced greater benefits of smoking cessation: the excess risk of continued smoking decreased to half after 11 years in women compared with 23 years in men.

Apart from affecting collagen synthesis, oxidative stress, and altered expression of metalloproteinases, smoking is thought to reduce oestrogenic effects,[18] ovarian function,[19] and age at menopause.[20] Furthermore, animal studies have reported that orchidectomy reduces the incidence of aneurysms in male mice,[21] and that the androgen- and oestrogen-related alpha-receptors in the aortic wall are down-regulated during early aneurysmal formation[22]—changes that might explain the increased vulnerability of aneurysms among smoking women compared with smoking men.

Obesity

Obesity induces a release of pro-inflammatory adipokines and cytokines from perivascular adipose tissue, which may influence aneurysm development.[23–25] However, a pathophysiological relation between obesity and aneurysms is complicated by the fact that diabetes has been reported to be inversely related to aneurysm prevalence in most studies.[26]

In a systematic review by Cronin *et al* (2012),[27] three out of five studies investigating body mass index (BMI) reported a positive association with aneurysms,[28–30] and two out of three studies investigating waist circumference, or waist to hip ratio, reported significant positive associations with aneurysm prevalence.[6,31] However, of the five studies, only Lederle *et al* accounted for both BMI and waist measures in their multivariate models. In their study, a positive association between waist circumference and larger aneurysms (≥40mm) was reported, suggesting that waist circumference may be of more interest than BMI. Furthermore, waist circumference—but not BMI—was associated with an increased risk of aneurysm diagnosis in a prospective population-based cohort study of 63,655 men and women.[32] Visceral abdominal fat, rather than general obesity, affects inflammation and formation of experimental aneurysms in animals[33] but whether adiposity affects aneurysm growth rate is not well studied. In a meta-analysis of five studies, involving 3,439 patients with aneurysms, a non-significant inverse association between BMI and growth rate of small aneurysms was observed.[13] BMI was not associated with mean aneurysm expansion rate in 567 patients in the Veterans Affair study.[34]

Diet

Diet may affect pathophysiology through several potential pathways, one of which is a reduction of oxidative stress.[35] Oxidative stress is increased in the aortic wall of patients with aneurysms and might contribute to formation through smooth muscle cell apoptosis, matrix proteolysis, increased mechanical forces attributable to hypertension, and recruitment of cytokines and other pro-inflammatory cells.[36] A reduction in the risk of aneurysm development might, therefore, be plausible through intake of antioxidants that have the potential to balance oxidative stress and, thereby, limit aortic wall inflammation. In the Life-Line Screening registry, data were reported for 3.1 million individuals screened at more than 20,000 sites across the USA.[29] In that study, Kent *et al* observed—respectively—a 9% and 10%

decrease in the odds ratio of an aneurysm being identified among individuals who were consuming fruits and vegetables and nuts more than three times a week. In a univariate analyses, meat and fast food were associated with a higher prevalence of aneurysms. In a Swedish cohort study of 80,426 participants, fruit consumption (but not vegetable consumption) was associated with a decreased risk of aneurysm development.[37] In that study, a more pronounced association of fruit consumption was observed with ruptured aneurysms compared with intact aneurysms. Given the complex pathophysiology of aneurysm formation, it is feasible that different dietary components may interfere in different steps of the progression of the disease. Other potential effects of diet are alternation of cholesterol metabolism—more specifically, high- and low-density lipoprotein (HDL/LDL) levels. In a screening study from the north of Sweden, both historically elevated LDL and reduced HDL levels were associated with the development of aneurysms.[38] No studies to date have investigated whether dietary consumption is directly associated with aneurysm growth rate.

Alcohol

A moderate consumption of alcohol is inversely associated with several cardiovascular comorbidities, such as myocardial infarction and stroke, but the three epidemiological studies investigating whether alcohol consumption is associated with aneurysms are inconsistent.

In a cardiovascular disease free population,[39] a significant trend toward a higher risk of aneurysm development with increasing consumption of alcohol was observed. That study also reported a non-significant increased risk of aneurysms among participants in the highest category of alcohol consumption. The second study,[40] including only male smokers, reported an indication of a J-shaped association between alcohol consumption and aneurysms. Moreover, a prospective cohort study from central Sweden[41] reported that a moderate consumption of alcohol was associated with a decreased risk of aneurysm development. That study is the only one to report associations for different types of alcohol and observed that wine and beer, but not spirits, were associated with a lower risk of aneurysm development.

Generally, light-to-moderate alcohol consumption is associated with a decrease in systemic inflammation and oxidative stress—two components of pathophysiology thought to be of major importance in the development of aneurysms. In addition to ethanol that promotes beneficial effects on lipid regulation,[42] polyphenolic content—mostly found in red, but also in white wine and beer—has been associated with further favourable effects on cellular redox state,[43] endothelial function,[44] and systemic inflammation.[45]

Physical activity

Physical activity is associated with a lower risk of coronary heart disease,[46] while sedentary behaviours have been associated with an increased risk, independent of leisure-time physical activity.[47] These associations are most probably explained by direct action on the heart, alterations of HDL and LDL levels, and effects on blood pressure, blood coagulability, and insulin sensitivity,[48] which potentially also affects the risk of developing aneurysms. Furthermore, a pure mechanistic effect due to adverse/pro-inflammatory haemodynamics in the abdominal aorta, which might be altered through physical exercise, may also be expected to have an impact on the progression of the disease. In a study of 10 patients with aneruysms,[49] the authors concluded that mild exercise might be sufficient to reduce oscillatory and stagnant haemodynamic conditions in the abdominal aorta, and thereby, slow the growth of an aneurysm. Epidemiological studies investigating associations between physical activity/inactivity and aneurysm risk are, however, very scarce. Kent *et al* reported from the Life-Line Screening registry that those who exercised more than once a week had 14% decreased risk of having an aneurysm.[29] In the Malmö preventive study,[50] in which factors for development of large aneurysms among middle-aged men were investigated, it was observed that those who were physically inactive (e.g. not walking or cycling to work) had an increased risk of developing an aneurysm.

Summary

- Smoking is a major risk factor for abdominal aortic aneurysms to a larger extent than for other vascular diseases. Women are more vulnerable to current smoking and experience greater benefits after smoking cessation.

- The association between obesity and aneurysm disease is complex. A predominant disposition of abdominal fat, rather than general obesity, seems to increase risk.

- Dietary consumption is likely to affect prevalence. A lower risk following a high consumption of fruits, fish, and nuts, have been reported. Associations with alcohol consumption remain inconsistent.

- Physical activity, and sedentary behaviours, may affect aneurysm prevalence.

- More studies are needed to investigate whether modifiable lifestyle-related factors also affect aneurysm growth rate, and whether changes in lifestyle may decrease intervention rate.

References

1. Dake MD, Miller DC, Semba CP, et al. Transluminal Placement of Endovascular Stent-Grafts for the Treatment of Descending Thoracic Aortic Aneurysms. *N Eng J Med* 1994; **331** (26): 1729–34.
2. Makaroun MS, Dillavou ED, Kee ST, et al. Endovascular treatment of thoracic aortic aneurysms: Results of the phase II multicenter trial of the GORE TAG thoracic endoprosthesis. *J Vasc Surg* 2005; **41** (1): 1–9.
3. Cambria RP, Crawford RS, Cho JS, et al. A multicenter clinical trial of endovascular stent graft repair of acute catastrophes of the descending thoracic aorta. *J Vasc Surg* 2009; **50** (6): 1255–64.
4. Najibi S, Terramani TT, Weiss VJ, et al. Endoluminal *versus* open treatment of descending thoracic aortic aneurysms. *J Vasc Surg* 2002; **36** (4): 732–37.
5. Schaffer JM, Lingala B, Miller DC, et al. Midterm survival after thoracic endovascular aortic repair in more than 10,000 Medicare patients. *J Thorac Cardiovasc Surg* 2015; **149** (3): 808–23.
6. Mitchell ME, Rushton Jr FW, Boland AB, et al. Emergency procedures on the descending thoracic aorta in the endovascular era. *J Vasc Surg* 2011; **54** (5): 1298–302.
7. Jonker FHW, Trimarchi S, Verhagen HJM, et al. Meta-analysis of open *versus* endovascular repair for ruptured descending thoracic aortic aneurysm. *J Vasc Surg* 2010; **51** (4): 1026–32.
8. Jordan Jr WD, Rovin J, Moainie S, et al. Results of a prospective multicenter trial of CTAG thoracic endograft. *J Vasc Surg* 2015; **61** (3): 589–95.
9. Cambria RP, Conrad MF, Matsumoto AH, et al. Multicenter clinical trial of the conformable stent graft for the treatment of acute, complicated type B dissection. *J Vasc Surg* 2015; **62** (2): 271–8.

10. Lee CJ, Rodriguez HE, Kibbe MR, *et al.* Secondary interventions after elective thoracic endovascular aortic repair for degenerative aneurysms. *J Vasc Surg* 2013; **57** (5): 1269–74.

11. LJ L, Harris PL, Buth J, Collaborators of the European collaborators registry (EUROSTAR). Secondary interventions after elective endovascular repair of degenerative thoracic aortic aneurysms: results of the European collaborators registry (EUROSTAR). *J Vasc Interv Radiol* 2007; **18** (4): 491–5.

12. Rolph R, Duffy JM, Waltham M. Stent graft types for endovascular repair of thoracic aortic aneurysms. Cochrane Database of Systematic Reviews 2015 (9): CD008448.

13. Bavaria JE, Brinkman WT, Hughes GC, *et al.* . Outcomes of Thoracic Endovascular Aortic Repair in Acute Type B Aortic Dissection: Results From the Valiant United States Investigational Device Exemption Study. *Ann Thorac Surg* 2015; **100** (3): 802–09.

14. Kim JB, Kim K, Lindsay ME, *et al.* Risk of Rupture or Dissection in Descending Thoracic Aortic Aneurysm. *Circulation* 2015; **132** (17): 1620–29.

15. Durham CA, Cambria RP, Wang LJ, *et al.* The natural history of medically managed acute type B aortic dissection. *J Vasc Surg* 2015; **61** (5): 1192–9.

16. Canaud L, Ozdemir BA, Patterson BO, *et al.* Retrograde Aortic Dissection After Thoracic Endovascular Aortic Repair. *Ann Surg* 2014; **260** (2): 389–95.

17. Hagan PG, Nienaber CA, Isselbacher EM, *et al.* The international registry of acute aortic dissection (irad): New insights into an old disease. *JAMA* 2000; **283** (7): 897–903.

18. White RA, Miller DC, Criado FJ, *et al.* Report on the results of thoracic endovascular aortic repair for acute, complicated, type B aortic dissection at 30 days and 1 year from a multidisciplinary subcommittee of the Society for Vascular Surgery Outcomes Committee. *J Vasc Surg* 2011; **53** (4): 1082–90.

19. Nienaber CA, Rousseau H, Eggebrecht H, *et al.* Randomized Comparison of Strategies for Type B Aortic Dissection: The INvestigation of STEnt Grafts in Aortic Dissection (INSTEAD) Trial. *Circulation* 2009; **120** (25): 2519–28.

20. Cooper DG, Walsh SR, Sadat U, *et al.* . Neurological complications after left subclavian artery coverage during thoracic endovascular aortic repair: A systematic review and meta-analysis. *J Vasc Surg* 2009; **49** (6): 1594–601.

21. Buth J, Harris PL, Hobo R, Collaborators of the European collaborators registry (EUROSTAR). . Neurologic complications associated with endovascular repair of thoracic aortic pathology: Incidence and risk factors. A study from the European Collaborators on Stent/Graft Techniques for Aortic Aneurysm Repair (EUROSTAR) Registry. *J Vasc Surg* 2007; **46** (6): 1103–11.e2.

22. Van Vickle-Chavez SJ, Tung WS, Absi TS, *et al.* Temporal changes in mouse aortic wall gene expression during the development of elastase-induced abdominal aortic aneurysms. *J Vasc Surg* 2006; **43**: 1010–20.

23. Barandier C, Montani JP, Yang Z. Mature adipocytes and perivascular adipose tissue stimulate vascular smooth muscle cell proliferation: effects of aging and obesity. *Am J Physiol Heart Circ Physiol* 2005; **289**: H1807–13.

24. Eringa EC, Bakker W, Smulders YM, *et al.* Regulation of vascular function and insulin sensitivity by adipose tissue: focus on perivascular adipose tissue. *Microcirculation* 2007; **14**: 389–402.

25. Chatterjee TK, Stoll LL, Denning GM, *et al.* Proinflammatory phenotype of perivascular adipocytes: influence of high-fat feeding. *Circ Res* 2009; **104**: 541–49.

26. Lederle FA. The strange relationship between diabetes and abdominal aortic aneurysm. *Eur J Vasc Endovasc Surg* 2012; **43**: 254–56.

27. Cronin O, Walker PJ, Golledge J. The association of obesity with abdominal aortic aneurysm presence and growth. *Atherosclerosis* 2013; **226**: 321–27.

28. Allison MA, Kwan K, DiTomasso D, *et al.* The epidemiology of abdominal aortic diameter. *J Vasc Surg* 2008; **48**: 121–27.

29. Kent KC, Zwolak RM, Egorova NN, *et al.* Analysis of risk factors for abdominal aortic aneurysm in a cohort of more than 3 million individuals. *J Vasc Surg* 2010; **52**: 539–48.

30. Long A, Bui HT, Barbe C, *et al.* Prevalence of abdominal aortic aneurysm and large infrarenal aorta in patients with acute coronary syndrome and proven coronary stenosis: a prospective monocenter study. *Ann Vasc Surg* 2010; **24**: 602–08.

31. Golledge J, Clancy P, Jamrozik K, Norman PE. Obesity, adipokines, and abdominal aortic aneurysm: Health in Men study. *Circulation* 2007; **116**: 2275–79.

32. Stackelberg O, Bjorck M, Sadr-Azodi O, *et al.* Obesity and abdominal aortic aneurysm. *Br J Surg* 2013; 100: 360–66.

33. Police SB, Thatcher SE, Charnigo R, *et al.* Obesity promotes inflammation in periaortic adipose tissue and angiotensin II-induced abdominal aortic aneurysm formation. Arterioscler Thromb Vasc Biol 2009; **29**: 1458–64.

34. Bhak RH, Wininger M, Johnson GR, *et al.* Factors associated with small abdominal aortic aneurysm expansion rate. *JAMA Surg* 2015; **150**: 44–50.

35. Miller FJ Jr, Sharp WJ, Fang X, *et al.* Oxidative stress in human abdominal aortic aneurysms: a potential mediator of aneurysmal remodeling. *Arterioscler Thromb Vasc* Biol 2002; **22**: 560–65.

36. McCormick ML, Gavrila D, Weintraub NL. Role of oxidative stress in the pathogenesis of abdominal aortic aneurysms. *Arterioscler Thromb Vasc Biol* 2007; **27**: 461–69.

37. Stackelberg O, Bjorck M, Larsson SC, *et al.* Fruit and vegetable consumption with risk of abdominal aortic aneurysm. *Circulation* 2013; **128**: 795–802.

38. Wanhainen A, Bjorck M, Boman K, *et al.* Influence of diagnostic criteria on the prevalence of abdominal aortic aneurysm. *J Vasc Surg* 2001; **34**: 229–35.

39. Wong DR, Willett WC, Rimm EB. Smoking, hypertension, alcohol consumption, and risk of abdominal aortic aneurysm in men. *Am J Epidemiol* 2007; **165**: 838–45.

40. Tornwall ME, Virtamo J, Haukka JK, *et al.* Life-style factors and risk for abdominal aortic aneurysm in a cohort of Finnish male smokers. *Epidemiology* 2001; **12**: 94–100.

41. Stackelberg O, Bjorck M, Larsson SC, *et al.* Alcohol consumption, specific alcoholic beverages, and abdominal aortic aneurysm. *Circulation* 2014; **130**: 646–52.

42. Mukamal KJ, Jensen MK, Gronbaek M, *et al.* Drinking frequency, mediating biomarkers, and risk of myocardial infarction in women and men. *Circulation* 2005; **112**: 1406–13.

43. Estruch R, Sacanella E, Mota F, *et al.* Moderate consumption of red wine, but not gin, decreases erythrocyte superoxide dismutase activity: a randomised cross-over trial. *Nutr Metab Cardiovasc Dis* 2011; **21**: 46–53.

44. Tousoulis D, Ntarladimas I, Antoniades C, *et al.* Acute effects of different alcoholic beverages on vascular endothelium, inflammatory markers and thrombosis fibrinolysis system. *Clin Nutr* 2008; 27: 594–600.

45. Estruch R, Sacanella E, Badia E, *et al.* Different effects of red wine and gin consumption on inflammatory biomarkers of atherosclerosis: a prospective randomized crossover trial. Effects of wine on inflammatory markers. *Atherosclerosis* 2004; **175**: 117–23.

46. Sattelmair J, Pertman J, Ding EL, *et al.* Dose response between physical activity and risk of coronary heart disease: a meta-analysis. *Circulation* 2011; **124**: 789–95.

47. Chomistek AK, Manson JE, Stefanick ML, *et al.* Relationship of sedentary behavior and physical activity to incident cardiovascular disease: results from the Women's Health Initiative. *J Am Coll Cardiol* 2013; **61**: 2346–54.

48. Manson JE. Prevention of myocardial infarction. New York: Oxford University Press; 1996.

49. Suh GY, Les AS, Tenforde AS, *et al.* Hemodynamic changes quantified in abdominal aortic aneurysms with increasing exercise intensity using mr exercise imaging and image-based computational fluid dynamics. *Ann Biomed Eng* 2011; **39**: 2186–202.

50. Lindblad B, Borner G, Gottsater A. Factors associated with development of large abdominal aortic aneurysm in middle-aged men. *Eur J Vasc Endovasc Surg* 2005; **30**: 346–52.

Population screening challenges

National population-based abdominal aortic aneurysm screening programmes remain a challenge for public health systems

L Capoccia and V Riambau

Introduction

Ruptured abdominal aortic aneurysms are still associated with significant mortality (up to 80% in some series).[1–3]

In recent years, screening programmes—with the aim of reducing the mortality and disability associated with aneurysms—have been carried out with good results; reductions in death and improved quality of life have been reported almost ubiquitously with such programmes.[4–7] Nevertheless, national population-based screening programmes, as part of public healthcare services, have some challenges that must be addressed if the best possible results are to be achieved with most effective use of limited resources.

Recent data have shown that to be cost-effective, screening programmes must focus on patients who are at highest risk of developing an aneurysm (and at the highest risk of dying of an aneurysm). Therefore, they should be based on data derived from previous programmes so that the subcategories of patients who are at highest risk are targeted.[8] At present, the key question with current and future screening programmes is how to continue to be cost-effective.

Benefits and harms of screening programmes

Data from four large randomised controlled trials[4–7] have demonstrated the benefit of screening programmes, showing a 40% reduction in mortality after approximately three to five years of follow-up.[9] For example, MASS (Multicentre aneurysm screening study), involving 67,770 men aged 65–74 with 1,334 aneurysms detected in those screened, showed a significant reduction of aneurysm-related mortality at 13 years (hazard ratio [HR] 0.58; 95% confidence interval [CI] 0.49–0.68).[4] Also, the Western Australia trial (which included 41,000 men between 65 and 83 years of age) found that the greatest benefit of screening was among those aged 65–74 years of age and those who smoked.[5] Smaller trials, such as the Viborg County Danish trial[6] and the Chichester trial,[7] have confirmed a benefit of screening for men older than 65 years in terms of preventing aneurysm-related deaths (HR 0.34

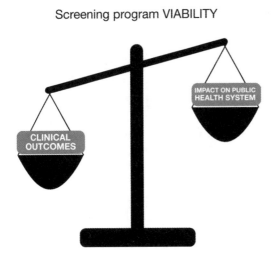

Screening program VIABILITY

Figure 1: Schema representing the conditions for a screening programme in a national public healthcare system. Clinical outcomes include the balance between benefits and harms. Impact on public healthcare system includes cost impact (cost-effectiveness involving costs of extra organisation and extra diagnoses and interventions) and the ethical impact (equity of access, impact on other care plans, increasing waiting lists).

95% CI 0.20-0.57, and HR 0.89 95% CI 0.6-1.32, respectively). Interestingly, the Chichester trial also randomised 9,342 women (between 1988 and 1991) but found that the rate of aneurysm-related mortality was very low among both the screening group and the control group (0.2% in both groups).[7]

In 1968, the World Health Organization (WHO) defined "screening" as "the presumptive identification of unrecognised disease or defect by the application of tests, examinations, or other procedures which can be applied rapidly".[10] However, these days, a national screening programme should also integrate detection-diagnosis, treatment and surveillance.[10,11] Additionally, a viable screening programme needs to offer more benefit than harm at a reasonable cost to public healthcare systems (Figure 1). Today's national healthcare systems are facing different challenges related to the ageing population, growing technology and financial issues for a sustainable service. As a consequence, the cost-effectiveness of a screening programme (if it is to be adopted and implemented at a national level) has become more and more important. But, the acceptable threshold of cost-effectiveness varies from country to country because it is related to the gross national income (GNI). This factor makes translating some specific healthcare approaches at a global level more difficult. Furthermore, before starting a national screening programme, the probable impact on the national healthcare system should be assessed. Therefore, resources for the structural organisation, the potential increased expenses for extra-treatments, the increase of waiting lists and the equity of access should be taken into account. Finally, all the resources invested in such programmes may lead to reductions in other public healthcare activities. Thus, understanding the real benefit of such programmes in terms of healthcare and resource savings is crucial for a clear appreciation of their cost-effectiveness.

Appropriate target population selection is key for such proposals. In order to assess the real impact and viability of a national screening programme, a pilot study in the same national territory is a good strategy to be considered.

The importance of age

Although male sex is a recognised risk factor for development of an aneurysm, any planned targeted programmes must also consider that some women may benefit from undergoing aneurysm screening. A 2015 report of a prospective population-based study of the incidence of acute aneurysms (identified between 2002 and 2014) in Oxfordshire (UK) found that hypertension in women aged more than 75 years was strongly associated with the occurrence of acute aneurysms events. Indeed, hypertension was the predominant risk factor for aneurysm acute event occurrence in women at all ages, but was found to be less important a risk factor for men. The report concluded that screening a woman aged 75 years with a known history of hypertension would prevent 27.4% of events, 30% of deaths, and 16.8% of life-years lost.[12]

The incidence of aneurysm-related mortality increases with age and given the progressive ageing of the world's population, the prevalence of aneurysms is expected to increase over time. However while it was predicted to show an aneurysm prevalence rate of 4.5% (based on data extrapolated from the UK, Danish, and Australian trials),[13] NAAASP (the UK National abdominal aortic aneurysm screening programme)[14] only showed a prevalence of 1.5%.

The drop in prevalence encountered in the most recent trials of screening can be regarded as a double-edged sword. If there is a rising public awareness of the risk factors for cardiovascular disease, leading to people living healthier lifestyles and paying stricter adherence to preventive antihypertensive and lipid-lowering medication regimens, it is also worth noting that published data for aneurysm screening programmes have not demonstrated to be effective at reducing all-cause mortality rates.[1–4,12] Therefore, cardiovascular risk factors among the ageing population (at risk for aneurysm development and for aneurysm-related mortality) are still far from being under control; so, aneurysm detection should be regarded as a starting point to modify other risk factors for cardiovascular morbidity and mortality. A possible explanation for the low rate of aneurysms identified among those screened in the aforementioned trials might relate to the difficulty of identifying all of the events of interest when dealing with aneurysm mortality (i.e. healthcare system coding problems) or to the low attendance rates of those invited to undergo screening; data show that around three-fourths of those invited to screening do not attend (non-attendance rate is around 21–22% in UK and Sweden).[15,16]

It has to be acknowledged that low attendance rate results in low benefit from screening and decreased cost-effectiveness, so improving the uptake rate of screening should be encouraged by redefining screening programmes. Howard et al[12] estimated that the impact of screening strategies in UK by determining the incidence and outcome of aneurysm acute events, current incidence trends, and population projections in 2020 and 2030. They identified a high number of events by matching coding data from in-hospital death records and out-of-hospital records. The authors started by collecting data for all cases described as acute aneurysm events (and this was possible by prospective and retrospective daily searches for acute events) in hospital, in general practice records, in coroner officer's records, in death certificates, and in International Classification of Diseases, 10th revision (ICD-10) death codes from the local department of public health. After this exhaustive search, they were able to assess an annual incidence of acute (no occlusive) aortic events: of 55 per 100,000 in men aged 65–74 years; of 112 per 100,000 in men aged 75–85; of 298 per 100,000 in men older than 85 years; and 82 per 100,000 in women older than 85 years. Howard et al found that rate of incident events was only 22.3% in men aged 65–74 and the rate of aneurysm-related deaths in this group was 13.1%.

Even if they were able to report an incidence of acute aneurysm and related death 30% to 40% higher than previous UK estimates, based on routine coding data, they confirmed a lower incidence in men aged 65 to 74 years of age compared with that seen in the MASS (Multicentre aneurysm screening study) data,[4] with two-thirds of acute aneurysms occurring in men aged >75 years.[12] Projecting a static total annual number of events, deaths, and life-years lost given a progressive decrease of age-specific incidence, Howard *et al* predicted that the proportion of all aneurysm-related deaths that occur by age >75 years would increase from 77.7% in 2010 to 91% by 2030. They also predicted that 56.3% of aneurysm events and 61.6% of aneurysm deaths will occur by age >85 years, with important differences with respect to projected data based on MASS trial findings.[4,12] The age-related incidence of aneurysms and of death from aneurysms has been well known and discussed in literature. This is why the ageing population and the resulting ageing population at risk of aneurysm-related acute events must be taken into consideration when planning a new screening programme. Extending current screening programmes to older populations might result in increases in the proportion of deaths prevented and life-years lost,[12] even taking into account a shorter life expectancy and a lower attendance rate in older people. Indeed, around 25% of elective aneurysm repairs in the UK are already performed in patients older than 80 years, with good functional outcomes in most cases.[17,18]

The importance of modifiable risk factors

Other features have to be considered when tailoring a screening strategy. Different screening programmes have demonstrated that current smoking is strongly associated with occurrence of acute aneurysms at younger ages.[4-7] Furthermore, current smoking increases rate of expansion of aneurysm by 15% to 20%, and it doubles the risk of rupture.[19] In the study by Howard *et al*, men aged 65–74 who smoked had an approximate 3% 10-year risk of developing an acute aneurysm, thus putting them in a very-high-risk group that should be among the first recipients of an aneurysm screening programme.[12] The authors also showed that screening current smokers, men aged 65 years and all men aged 75 years would result in an almost four-fold decrease in the number of deaths and a three-fold increase in the number of life-years saved compared with the current UK screening strategy.[8] Such an approach would also reduce the number of scans required by 20%,[12] thus dramatically increasing the cost-effectiveness of the programme.

The issue of surveillance of detecting small aneurysm or aortic ecstasy also needs to be addressed to increase cost-effectiveness. Current guidelines from the American Heart Association recommend follow-up imaging at five-year intervals for otherwise healthy patients with aortic diameters between 2.6cm and 2.9cm, at three years for those with diameters between 3cm and 3.4cm, annually for those with diameters between 3.5cm and 4.4cm, and every six months for those with aortic diameters greater than 4.5cm.[20] Such guidelines are extremely helpful in containing costs of surveillance, but they must be balanced against the psychological burden of those patients with a detected small aneurysm, who have a significant risk of overtreatment, and the subsequent risk of decreased cost-effectiveness.

Ethnic aneurysm-prevalence differences must also be taken into account when considering new screening strategies. Data from the southwest London area, within the NAAASP, collected between 2009 and 2013 showed an aneurysm prevalence of 1.18%, which dropped to lower rates in some ethnic categories.[15] It is worth noting that while this rate was 1.35% in Caucasians, it was reduced to 0.65% in black people, to 0.23% in South Asians, and to 0% in Chinese men.[15] When considering aneurysm prevalence among different ethnicities, a tailored screening strategy seems mandatory to keep being cost-effective.

Conclusion

Aneurysm rupture still carries a significant mortality, up to 80% in some series.[1–3] Recent randomised controlled trials on aneurysm screening have demonstrated their benefit in terms of aneurysm-related morbidity and mortality prevention, and screening programmes will continue to be cost-effective, in some countries, even with aneurysm prevalence rates as low as 0.5%.[21] Nevertheless, national screening programmes should offer more clinical benefits than harm at a reasonable cost for national public healthcare services. Since recent trials have demonstrated that aneurysm incidence is moving to older ages, it is of the outmost importance to plan new screening strategies to maximise benefit and optimise costs of screening and surveillance protocols. High-risk categories should be identified and a tailored screening strategy should be developed according to new data derived from population-based studies on aneurysm prevalence to improve cost-effectiveness of screening programmes.

Summary

National population-based aneurysm screening programmes remain a challenge for public health systems. To remain cost-effective in the general population:

- Abdominal scan attendance rate should be improved to sustain benefit and cost-effectiveness of screening.

- Small aneurysm surveillance should adhere to guidelines according to rupture risk rates.

- A tailored screening programme should be developed, thus offering the best prevention to the highest risk categories, by matching data on sex, age, familiar history, smoking current or previous status, race, blood pressure control, etc. To screen older (>75 years) men, limiting screening of younger population to those categories with significant adjunct risk factors for aneurysm development and aneurysm-related acute events (smokers, those with familial history or poor blood pressure control) would probably be the main point in order to increase cost-effectiveness of future screening programmes.

- A pilot study in the same territory is a strategy to be considered before to start a true national screening programme.

- Aneurysm screening should be the starting point to correct other cardiovascular risk factors that still play the most important role in all-cause mortality among patients recruited for screening programmes, so that healthcare education should be improved.

References

1. Heikkinen M, Salenius JP, Auvinen O. Ruptured abdominal aortic aneurysm in a well-defined geographic area. *J Vasc Surg* 2002; **36** (2): 291–96.

2. Ashton HA, Buxton MJ, Day NE, *et al.* The Multicentre Aneurysm Screening Study (MASS) into the effect of abdominal aortic aneurysm screening on mortality in men: a randomised controlled trial. *Lancet* 2002; **360** (9345): 1531–39.

3. Dueck AD, Kucey DS, Johnston KW, *et al.* Survival after ruptured abdominal aortic aneurysm: effect of patient, surgeon, and hospital factors. *J Vasc Surg* 2004; **39** (6): 1253–60.

4. Thompson SG, Ashton HA, Gao L, *et al;* Multicentre Aneurysm Screening Study (MASS) Group. Final follow-up of the Multicentre Aneurysm Screening Study (MASS) randomized trial of abdominal aortic aneurysm screening. *Br J Surg* 2012; **99** (12): 1649–56.

5. Jamrozik K, Norman PE, Spencer CA, *et al.* Screening for abdominal aortic aneurysm: lessons from a population-based study. Med J Aust 2000; **173** (7): 345–50.

6. Lindholt JS, Juul S, Henneberg EW, Fasting H. Is screening for abdominal aortic aneurysm acceptable to the population? Selection and recruitment to hospital-based mass screening for abdominal aortic aneurysm. J Public Health Med 1998; **20** (2): 211–17.

7. Scott RA, Bridgewater SG, Ashton HA. Randomized clinical trial of screening for abdominal aortic aneurysm in women. *Br J Surg* 2002; **89** (3): 283–85.

8. NHS Abdominal Aortic Aneurysm Screening Programme. Abdominal aortic aneurysm screening: 2014 to 2015 data tables. www.gov.uk/topic/population-screening-programmes/abdominal-aortic-aneurysm (date accessed 13 January 2016).

9. Cosford PA, Leng GC. Screening for abdominal aortic aneurysm. Cochrane Database Syst Rev. 2007; (2): CD002945.

10. Wilson JMG, Jungner G. Principles and practice of screening for disease. Geneva: WHO; n°34, 1968. http://apps.who.int/iris/bitstream/10665/37650/1/WHO_PHP_34.pdf (date accessed 13 January 2016).

11. Strong K, Wald NJ, Miller A, Alwan A. Current concepts in screening for noncommunicable disease: World Health Organization Consultation Group Report on methodology of noncomunicable disease screening. J Med Screen 2005; **12**: 12–19.

12. Howard DP, Banerjee A, Fairhead JF, *et al;* Oxford Vascular Study. Population-Based Study of Incidence of Acute Abdominal Aortic Aneurysms With Projected Impact of Screening Strategy. *J Am Heart Assoc* 2015; **4** (8): e001926.

13. Chichester Aneurysm Screening Group; Viborg Aneurysm Screening Study; Western Australian Abdominal Aortic Aneurysm Program; Multicentre Aneurysm Screening Study. A comparative study of the prevalence of abdominal aortic aneurysms in the United Kingdom, Denmark, and Australia. *J Med Screen* 2001; **8** (1): 46–50.

14. NHS Abdominal Aortic Aneurysm Screening Programme. Annual report 2011-12; summary. London: Public Health England, 2013. www.gov.uk (date accessed 13 January 2016).

15. Benson RA, Poole R, Murray S, *et al.* Screening results from a large United Kingdom abdominal aortic aneurysm screening center in the context of optimizing United Kingdom National Abdominal Aortic Aneurysm Screening Programme protocols. *J Vasc Surg* 2015. pii: S0741-5214(15)01841-8. Epub.

16. Linne A, Leander K, Lindström D, *et al.* Reasons for non-participation in population-based abdominal aortic aneurysm screening. *Br J Surg* 2014; **101** (5): 481–87.

17. Vascular services quality improvement programme. Outcomes after Elective Repair of Infra-renal Abdominal Aortic Aneurysm. www.vsqip.org.uk (date accessed 13 January 2016).

18. Pol RA, Zeebregts CJ, van Sterkenburg SM, Reijnen MM; ENGAGE Investigators. Thirty-day outcome and quality of life after endovascular abdominal aortic aneurysm repair in octogenarians based on the Endurant Stent Graft Natural Selection Global Postmarket Registry (ENGAGE). *J Vasc Surg* 2012; **56** (1): 27–35.

19. Sweeting MJ, Thompson SG, Brown LC, Powell JT; RESCAN collaborators. Meta-analysis of individual patient data to examine factors affecting growth and rupture of small abdominal aortic aneurysms. *Br J Surg* 2012; **99** (5): 655–65.

20. Anderson JL, Halperin JL, Albert NM, *et al.* Management of patients with peripheral artery disease (compilation of 2005 and 2011 ACCF/AHA guideline recommendations): a report of the American College of Cardiology Foundation/American Heart Association Task Force on Practice Guidelines. *Circulation* 2013; **127** (13): 1425–43.

21. Svensjö S, Mani K, Björck M, *et al.* Screening for abdominal aortic aneurysm in 65-year-old men remains cost-effective with contemporary epidemiology and management. *Eur J Vasc Endovasc Surg* 2014; **47** (4): 357–65.

The threshold for elective intervention for abdominal aortic and iliac aneurysm

Challenges in international harmonisation of abdominal aortic aneurysm treatment

K Mani, AW Beck and M Venermo

Introduction

Abdominal aortic aneurysm is a prevalent disease among the elderly Western population and is associated with a high mortality when ruptured. There has been much research into the optimum management of aortic aneurysms with the aim of identifying the most cost-effective approach for reducing the risk of rupture.

Several randomised trials, for example, have assessed the diameter threshold at which the benefit of repair (i.e. reducing the risk of rupture) exceeds the perioperative risk of mortality.[1–4] Also, multiple retrospective studies (as well as randomised trials) have reviewed the safety and efficacy of endovascular aneurysm repair (EVAR) compared with open repair for both elective and ruptured aneurysms.[5–8] Furthermore, population-based screening for aortic aneurysms to detect silent disease and allow for elective repair has been studied in both randomised and retrospective manners,[9–11] as have health economic aspects of management.[12,13] With avoidance of rupture (and subsequent mortality) as the aim of treatment, studies focused on aortic aneurysms have a firm outcome that is easy to monitor without the risk of confounders. In fact, abdominal aortic aneurysm is probably the most extensively studied vascular disease and one that clinicians have an abundance of evidence on which to base their decisions when managing individual patients.

Both the European Society for Vascular Surgery (ESVS) and the Society for Vascular Surgery (SVS) have produced guidelines, based on the available evidence, on the management of small aneurysms, diameter threshold for intervention, screening, and repair modalities. However, despite these guidelines and the extensive evidence base, international benchmarking studies of aneurysm repair indicate that there are considerable variations in the management of this well-studied disease.

Threshold for aneurysm repair

Elective intervention for aortic aneurysms should be performed in patients when the risk of rupture exceeds the risk of the repair itself and when the patient is felt to have a otherwise reasonable life expectancy. Two major randomised trials were performed in the late 1990s to determine whether open repair resulted in any survival benefit compared with surveillance for aneurysms <5.5cm in size.[2,14]

Both of these trials confirmed that repair at <5.5cm did not result in any benefit for the patient. The first of these studies—the UK Small Aneurysm Trial[1]—has been criticised for the high rate of perioperative mortality found in the repair arm (5.5%), but this result was confirmed in the second trial (with 2.7% perioperative mortality for elective repair).[2] Together, these trials showed that the risk of rupture for aneurysms <5.5cm in size is very low and, thus, repair is not warranted.

In the endovascular era, the European CAESAR (Comparison of surveillance *versus* aortic endografting for small aneurysm repair) trial and the American PIVOTAL (Positive impact of endovascular options for treating aneurysms early) trial compared EVAR with surveillance for small aneurysms.[3,4] Again, they did not find a survival benefit with early repair. Based on these studies, both the ESVS and SVS guidelines endorse a threshold of ≥5.5cm for elective repair in men.[15,16]

However, the indication for repair is less certain in women than it is in men because the number of women in the randomised controlled trials was low. The study of aneurysms among females is difficult because the prevalence of aneurysms in women is six times lower than that in men.[17] Therefore, because the risk of rupture is higher in women with small aneurysms than it is in men with small aneurysms, the European guidelines currently suggest a 5.2cm threshold for referring women for potential intervention. The SVS also provides endorsement of proceeding with repair in otherwise healthy patients, especially women, with aneurysms between 5cm and 5.4cm.[16]

Despite these guidelines, recent assessment of national and regional vascular surgical registries indicates that the proportion of patients with aneurysms of <5.5cm in size undergoing elective repair varies significantly among countries.[18] The proportion of patients with a maximum aortic diameter <5.5cm at time of repair varied from 6% in the UK to 27% in Australia among men, and from 9% in the UK to 48% in Hungary among women. Although uncertainties remain regarding the management of patients with rapid growth of aneurysms or symptomatic aneurysms as indications for repair, the variation in the number of patients with small aneurysms undergoing repair in different countries indicates that there are differences in the interpretation of the current evidence and guidelines. In this assessement, the perioperative mortality of intact repair in patients with small aneurysms was 0.7% for EVAR and 2.7% for open repair. Considering that the risk of rupture of small aneurysms is low (<1%), the benefit of repair in a general population is certainly debatable.

Endovascular and open repair

EVAR has surpassed open surgery as the primary technique for elective aneurysm repair in many countries.[19] It is associated with lower short-term mortality and morbidity than open surgery, but is associated with similar long-term survival.[5] The early benefit of EVAR compared with open repair is most prominent in female patients and in octogenarians. However, patients undergoing EVAR have a higher rate of late complications and are exposed to a higher risk of post-implantation aortic rupture than those undergoing open repair.[5] The risk of late complications after EVAR is associated with aneurysm anatomy.[20] Based on the instructions for use for currently available devices, approximately 50–60% of all elective aneurysm repairs are reported to be anatomically suitable for standard infrarenal EVAR.[21] But, this is a moving target with the development of new technology.

Although the use of EVAR for elective repair has increased dramatically in most countries over the past decade, significant differences in EVAR use remain (Figure 1). For example, while only one third of all intact repairs in Denmark were performed with EVAR in 2013, more than 70% of repairs in Australia and Germany were performed with EVAR. These variations are probably multifactorial and related not only to clinical differences, but also to differences in healthcare organisation and reimbursement. EVAR is associated with a significant device cost and the health economic benefit of this treatment has been debated, which may affect its use at some centres and in some countries.[12] In Denmark, provision of EVAR services has been centralised, which affects the use of endovascular repair. On the other hand, the use of EVAR in more than 70% of patients in Germany and Australia suggests that the physicians are prone to using EVAR in patients with difficult anatomy, which may be outside of the instructions for use for the devices. Therefore, these countries perhaps have less economic constraints than do other countries.

Screening for aneurysms

Most of the evidence for screening is based on MASS (UK Multicentre aneurysm screening study), which randomised more than 67,000 men aged 65–74 years old to screening or non-screening.[22]

This study demonstrated that screening reduced mortality from rupture by approximately half (48% relative risk reduction) in the group screened by ultrasound, and that the survival benefit was maintained up to 10 years after screening. Based on the results of this trial, aneurysm screening has been introduced on a national level in England, Wales, Scotland, Northern Ireland, and Sweden.[23] In these countries, a single screening scan with ultrasound is offered to men at age 65 as part of a national screening programme. Although the prevalence of aneurysms has

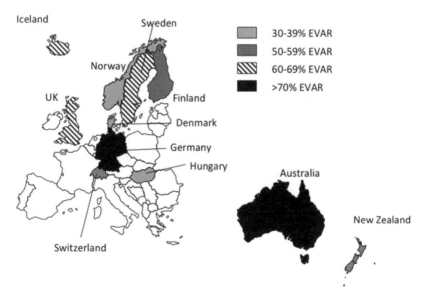

Figure 1: Rate of intact aortic aneurysm repair performed with EVAR in 2013, based on national and regional registry data. Source: Vascunet database.

been significantly lower in these populations than in the previous screening studies, screening is still to be considered cost-effective.[13]

In the USA, a one-time screening abdominal ultrasound is offered as part of the Medicare welcome package for men 65–75 years of age with a history of smoking more than 100 cigarettes in their life and also offered to both men and women with a family history of aneurysms. However, this health benefit is seldom used with only <1% of those eligible undergoing screening according to claim data.[24] National screening has not been documented in other countries, but further national and regional trials for screening are underway.[23]

The variation in screening practice is also reflected in management guidelines.[25] Some professional organisations recommend screening for all men at or above 65 years of age, while others focus screening on those who have smoked or have a family history. Recommendations regarding screening in women are even more diverse. Issues that affect introduction of screening include variations in healthcare delivery system, prevalence of disease, and health economic assessment of screening benefit.

Conclusion

Management of abdominal aortic aneurysms is based on well-performed clinical trials, but there remain significant international variations for all aspects of this disease, including screening, threshold for therapy and modality of treatment. International benchmarking of aneurysm treatment to monitor these variations in clinical practice will help identify remaining areas of uncertainty and direct future studies. Indeed, harmonisation of international treatment guidelines may lead to better management of patients worldwide.

Summary

- Despite the presence of several randomised trials and guidelines for management of patients with abdominal aortic aneurysms, significant variations remain in treatment across countries.

- The rate of elective repair below established treatment guidelines varies from 6% to 48% based on gender and country of treatment, indicating differences in interpretation of current evidence and guidelines.

- Although EVAR is used in >50% of elective repairs internationally, the proportion varies from 30% to >70% across countries.

- Screening has been established to save lives cost-effectively, but national screening is only established in a minority of the Western countries.

References

1. Powell JT, Brown LC, Forbes JF, et al. Final 12-year follow-up of surgery versus surveillance in the UK Small Aneurysm Trial. Br J Surg 2007; **94** (6):702–08.
2. Lederle FA, Wilson SE, Johnson GR, et al. Immediate repair compared with surveillance of small abdominal aortic aneurysms. N Engl J Med 2002; **346** (19): 1437–44.
3. Ouriel K, Clair DG, Kent KC, Zarins CK. Endovascular repair compared with surveillance for patients with small abdominal aortic aneurysms. J Vasc Surg 2010; **51** (5): 1081–87.

4. Cao P, De Rango P, Verzini F, *et al.* Comparison of Surveillance Versus Aortic Endografting for Small Aneurysm Repair (CAESAR): Results from a Randomised Trial. *Eur J Vasc Endovasc Surg* 2011; **41** (1): 13–25.

5. Greenhalgh RM, Brown LC, Powell JT, *et al.* Endovascular *versus* open repair of abdominal aortic aneurysm. *N Engl J Med* 2010; **362** (20): 1863–71.

6. Lederle FA, Freischlag JA, Kyriakides TC, *et al.* Long-term comparison of endovascular and open repair of abdominal aortic aneurysm. *N Engl J Med* 2012; **367** (21): 1988–97.

7. De Bruin JL, Baas AF, Buth J, *et al.* Long-term outcome of open or endovascular repair of abdominal aortic aneurysm. *N Engl J Med* 2010; **362** (20):1881–89.

8. Investigators IT. Endovascular strategy or open repair for ruptured abdominal aortic aneurysm: one-year outcomes from the IMPROVE randomized trial. *Eur Heart J* 2015; **36** (31): 2061–69.

9. Thompson SG, Ashton HA, Gao L, *et al.* Final follow-up of the Multicentre Aneurysm Screening Study (MASS) randomized trial of abdominal aortic aneurysm screening. *British Journal of Surgery* 2012; **99** (12): 1649–56.

10. Svensjo S, Bjorck M, Wanhainen A. Editor's choice: five-year outcomes in men screened for abdominal aortic aneurysm at 65 years of age: a population-based cohort study. *Eur J Vasc Endovasc Surg* 2014; **47** (1): 37–44.

11. Svensjo S, Bjorck M, Gurtelschmid M, *et al.* Low prevalence of abdominal aortic aneurysm among 65-year-old Swedish men indicates a change in the epidemiology of the disease. *Circulation* 2011; **124** (10): 1118–23.

12. Epstein D, Sculpher MJ, Powell JT, *et al.* Long-term cost-effectiveness analysis of endovascular *versus* open repair for abdominal aortic aneurysm based on four randomized clinical trials. *Br J Surg* 2014; **101** (6): 623–31.

13. Svensjo S, Mani K, Bjorck M, *et al.* Screening for Abdominal Aortic Aneurysm in 65-Year-old Men Remains Cost-effective with Contemporary Epidemiology and Management. *Eur J Vasc Endovasc Surg* 2014; **47** (4): 357–65.

14. The UK Small Aneurysm Trial Participants. Long-term outcomes of immediate repair compared with surveillance of small abdominal aortic aneurysms. *N Engl J Med* 2002; **346** (19): 1445–52.

15. Moll FL, Powell JT, Fraedrich G, *et al.* Management of abdominal aortic aneurysms clinical practice guidelines of the European society for vascular surgery. *Eur J Vasc Endovasc Surg* 2011; **41** Suppl 1: S1–S58.

16. Chaikof EL, Brewster DC, Dalman RL, *et al.* The care of patients with an abdominal aortic aneurysm: the Society for Vascular Surgery practice guidelines. *J Vasc Surg* 2009; **50** (4 Suppl): S2–49.

17. Scott RA, Bridgewater SG, Ashton HA. Randomized clinical trial of screening for abdominal aortic aneurysm in women. *Br J Surg* 2002; **89** (3): 283–85.

18. Mani K, Venermo M, Beiles B, *et al.* Regional Differences in Case Mix and Peri-operative Outcome After Elective Abdominal Aortic Aneurysm Repair in the Vascunet Database. *European Journal of Vascular and Endovascular Surgery* 2015; **49**: 646–52.

19. Mani K, Lees T, Beiles B, *et al.* Treatment of abdominal aortic aneurysm in nine countries 2005-2009: a vascunet report. *Eur J Vasc Endovasc Surg* 2011; **42** (5): 598–607.

20. Schanzer A, Greenberg RK, Hevelone N, *et al.* Predictors of abdominal aortic aneurysm sac enlargement after endovascular repair. *Circulation* 2011; **123** (24): 2848–55.

21. Sweet MP, Fillinger MF, Morrison TM, Abel D. The influence of gender and aortic aneurysm size on eligibility for endovascular abdominal aortic aneurysm repair. *J Vasc Surg* 2011; **54** (4): 931–37.

22. Thompson SG, Ashton HA, Gao L, Scott RA. Screening men for abdominal aortic aneurysm: 10 year mortality and cost effectiveness results from the randomised Multicentre Aneurysm Screening Study. *BMJ* 2009; **338**: b2307.

23. Stather PW, Dattani N, Bown MJ, *et al.* International variations in AAA screening. *Eur J Vasc Endovasc Surg* 2013; **45** (3): 231–34.

24. Olchanski N, Winn A, Cohen JT, Neumann PJ. Abdominal aortic aneurysm screening: how many life years lost from underuse of the medicare screening benefit? *Journal of General Internal Medicine* 2014; **29** (8): 1155–61.

25. Mussa FF. Screening for abdominal aortic aneurysm. *J Vasc Surg* 2015; **62** (3): 774–78.

The changing epidemiology of abdominal aortic aneurysms in Europe

D Sidloff, A Saratzis, M Bown and R Sayers

Introduction

Throughout the 20th century, there were well-documented escalations in the incidence and associated mortality of abdominal aortic aneurysms.[1] Contemporary data from the UK and many other developed countries[2] have, however, shown a steep decline in mortality associated with aneurysms. The Aneurysm Global Epidemiology Study[2] analysed abdominal aortic aneurysm mortality in 19 countries, and it found that the USA, UK, and Australia had the fastest declining male age-standardised mortality (at 6.7% 6.2%, and 6.2% per year, respectively) and that aneurysm mortality was declining overall. The largest reductions in female mortality were seen in the UK and USA: at 4% and 3.9% per year, respectively; therefore compared with men, women have had a diminished reduction in mortality.

However, not all countries have seen a decline in aneurysm mortality. For example, Hungary and Romania have both seen increases in male and female age-standardised mortality: 2.7% and 3.5% and 1.7% and 1%, respectively. The differences in aneurysm mortality between countries (i.e. why some saw a decrease and others saw an increase) were significantly associated with variations in traditional cardiovascular risk factors, including hypertension (p=0.028), hypercholesterolemia (p=0.0082), and smoking prevalence (p=0.017). This finding suggested that countries with focused public health measures to reduce cardiovascular risk factors had a related reduction in aneurysm mortality.

It is probable that the falling prevalence of aneurysms is associated with cardiovascular risk factor modification, and that the reduction in aneurysm mortality reflects this association. This view is supported by comparing findings from the randomised controlled trials of population-based aneurysm screening with more contemporary data.[3-6] The randomised controlled trials recruited patients between 1988 and 1999, demonstrating an aneurysm prevalence of between 7.6% and 4%.[3,5] However, more recent data from Sweden (2011; 1.7%, 95% confidence interval [CI]: 1.5 to 1.9), Denmark (2015; 3.3%, 95% CI: 3 to 3.6), and the UK (1.19%) show reduced prevalence compared with the randomised controlled trials.[7-9] In this chapter, we describe our up-to-date analysis of abdominal aortic aneurysm mortality in Europe and associations with smoking habits.

Methods

Data for age, gender, and cause-specific mortality relating to the International Classification of Diseases codes (10th Revision)—I71.3, I71.4, I71.5, I71.6, I71.8, and I71.9, respectively—that represent all abdominal aortic aneurysms and aortic aneurysms of unspecified site were obtained from the World Health Organization (WHO) mortality database (updated 25/11/2015) from 2000 to 2014, inclusive of all data published per country.[10] Data for thoracic aneurysms (without mention of an abdominal component) were excluded, and all data relating to countries within the common definition of Europe and available data were included.

International Classification of Diseases codes are generated through civil registration systems to ensure validity; only those countries with sufficient data coverage were included (above 95%). Data coverage[10] is calculated by WHO by dividing the total deaths reported by a country-year from the civil registration system by the total deaths (estimated by WHO) for that year for the national population.

Observed mortality was converted into deaths per 100,000 population and per age group, and age-standardised rates of mortality were calculated using the 2013 European Standard Population. This hypothetical population assumes that the age structure is the same in both genders, allowing comparisons to be made between geographical areas. Age-standardised mortality was plotted for each country and slopes of the regression lines used to calculate trends in age-standardised mortality. Data were further analysed by longitude, defined as the angular distance of any point on Earth measured east or west of the Greenwich meridian.

Tobacco use data were extracted from the International Mortality and Smoking Statistics (Version 4.10) and are presented as number of cigarettes per adult per day. Trends in cigarette consumption were calculated (1970–2013) and compared to trends in aneurysm mortality with linear regression performed.

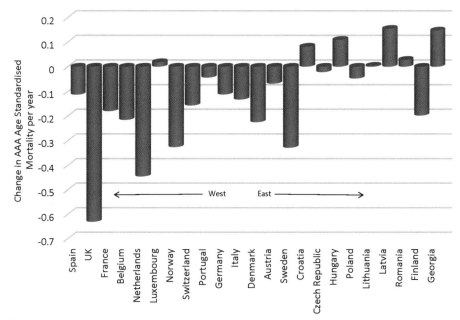

Figure 1: Trends in European aortic aneurysm age-standardised mortality by latitude.

Twenty three countries provided sufficient data to be included within the updated analysis, including Austria, Belgium, Croatia, Czech Republic, Denmark, Finland, France, Georgia, Germany, Hungary, Italy, Latvia, Lithuania, Luxembourg, Netherlands, Norway, Poland, Portugal, Romania, Spain, Sweden, Switzerland and the UK. The UK was subdivided into Scotland, Northern Ireland and England/ Wales for further analysis.

Results: Trends in aneurysm mortality across Europe

There are significant differences in age-standardised abdominal aortic aneurysm mortality trends across Europe (Figure 1). Similarly to what we found in our previous study, the UK had the fastest declining aneurysm mortality. It did, however, have the highest standardised mortality (14.8%) at the earliest time point of the study, declining to 7.8% in 2013. Furthermore, the UK's aneurysm mortality still remains high compared with much of Europe.

Comparatively, aneurysm mortality has fallen from 4.3% (2000) to 2.8% (2013) in Germany; while in the Netherlands, it has fallen from 11.7% (2000) to 5.1% (2013). As previously noted, some countries appear to have increasing aneurysm mortality—for example, age-standardised aneurysm mortality increased from 3% (2000) to 5% (2013) in Croatia, and has steadily increased from 2.8% (2000) to 4.5% (2013) in Hungary. Plotting trends in aneurysm mortality by latitude across Europe appears to suggest that, much like the trends in cigarette smoking, aneurysm mortality increases as you travel east.

Analysing the UK by "region" (Figure 2), England and Wales appear to demonstrate the highest aneurysm mortality (from 15.2% in 2001 to 7.9% in 2013) compared with Scotland (from 11.9% in 2001 to 6.7% in 2013) and Northern Ireland (from

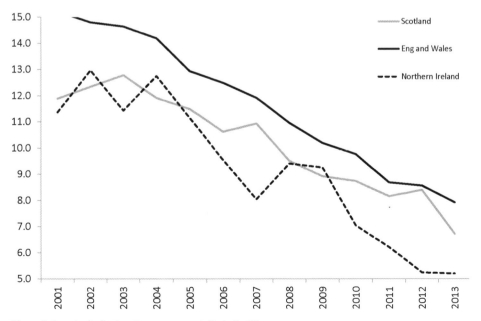

Figure 2: Age-standardised aortic aneurysm mortality in the UK.

11.4% in 2001 to 5.2% in 2013). All parts of the UK do, however, demonstrate a gradual decline in aneurysm mortality.

Abdominal aortic aneurysm mortality and smoking

Several studies have demonstrated a dose-dependent relationship between the risk of abdominal aortic aneurysm and smoking. Iribarren and colleagues[11] describe the relative risks of developing an aneurysm as, respectively, 3%, 5%, and 7% for current smokers who smoke less than one pack per day, those who smoke between one and two packs per day, and those who smoke three or more packs per day.

Another population-based study[12] demonstrated that approximately 50% of aortic aneurysm cases would not have occurred had tobacco smoke exposure been absent. Tobacco smoking is likely to be the most important predictor of future hospitalisation or death from aortic aneurysm and has well-established links with aneurysm expansion and rupture; therefore, it is not surprising that aneurysm mortality appears to mirror reductions in population cigarette smoking as can be seen in Figure 3 from the UK.

Interestingly, these data appear to demonstrate a lag period of approximately 30 years between changes in cigarette smoking habits and subsequent changes in aneurysm mortality. With more historical data for abdominal aneurysm mortality throughout Europe, it may be possible to further investigate this lag period. Similarly to that found in our previous study, trends in cigarette smoking remain closely related to trends in abdominal aortic aneurysm mortality (Figure 4). An analysis of the updated European data demonstrates a strong positive linear relationship (R2=0.6) whereby those countries with the largest reductions in cigarette exposure are also seeing the largest reductions in aneurysm mortality. This suggests that in Europe, further public health measures to reduce rates of smoking could further reduce the risks associated with abdominal aortic aneurysm probably through a reduction in prevalence.

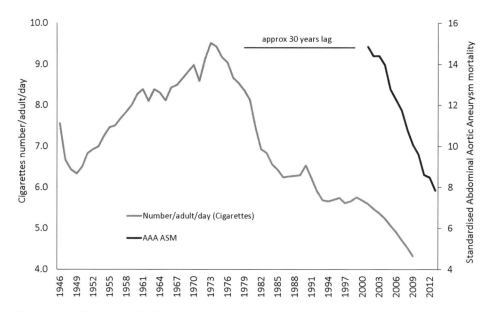

Figure 3: Cigarette smoking in the UK and standardised mortality from abdominal aortic aneurysm.

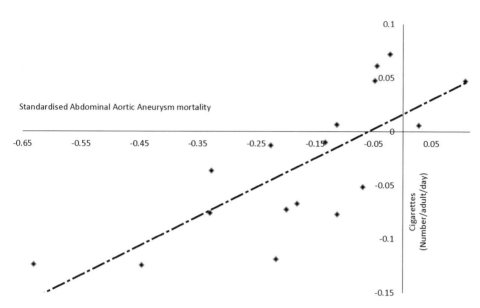

Figure 4: Linear regression suggesting a positive association between trends in the number of cigarettes adult/day (population average) and trends in standardised abdominal aortic aneurysm mortality, R2=0.6. Each dot represents a country.

Globally, this could be achieved by full implementation of the six components of "MPOWER": monitor tobacco use and prevention policies; protect people from tobacco smoke; offer help to quit tobacco use; warn about the dangers of tobacco; enforce bans on tobacco advertising, promotion and sponsorship; and raise taxes on tobacco. These components remain fundamental to the WHO Framework Convention on Tobacco Control and highlight the practically achievable steps in a vascular clinic, namely offering patients help to quit tobacco and warning patients about the dangers of tobacco use.

Limitations
One limitation of using mortality data is that aneurysm-related deaths could be missed unless post-mortem is performed. Throughout the European region, rates of post-mortem as a percentage of all deaths have remained steady over the last decade (2000=20.4%; 2012 =20.15%).[13] However, many countries do not routinely report these data and variation exists in those that do. For example, the Czech Republic reported post-mortem rates of 23.5% in 2013 compared with Finland (23.9%), Austria (14.1%), Luxembourg (1.9%), and Hungary (37.2%), which is one of the few countries with an increasing post mortem rate (up from 29% in 2000). All countries included had data coverage (2000–10) of between 97% and 100%. However, this system does not assess for accuracy of local civil registration system reporting.

Conclusion
Mortality from abdominal aortic aneurysm in Europe is generally declining. This is likely to reflect a reduction in the prevalence of aortic aneurysms secondary to large

population changes in the number of cigarettes smoked among other cardiovascular risk factor modifications.

Summary

- Aneurysm mortality is generally declining in Europe; this is likely to reflect a reduction in prevalence.

- Aneurysm mortality is increasing in some parts of Eastern Europe.

- Despite large reductions, abdominal aortic aneurysm mortality remains high in the UK.

- Reductions in population cigarette smoking may further reduce abdominal aneurysm mortality.

References

1. Filipovic M, Goldacre MJ, Roberts SE, *et al.* Trends in mortality and hospital admission rates for abdominal aortic aneurysm in England and Wales, 1979-1999. *Br J Surg* 2005; **92** (8): 968–75.

2. Sidloff D, Stather P, Dattani N, *et al.* Aneurysm global epidemiology study: public health measures can further reduce abdominal aortic aneurysm mortality. *Circulation* 2014; **129** (7): 747–53.

3. Scott RA, Wilson NM, Ashton HA, Kay DN. Influence of screening on the incidence of ruptured abdominal aortic aneurysm: 5-year results of a randomized controlled study. *Br J Surg* 1995; **82** (8): 1066–70.

4. Ashton HA, Buxton MJ, Day NE, *et al.* The Multicentre Aneurysm Screening Study (MASS) into the effect of abdominal aortic aneurysm screening on mortality in men: a randomised controlled trial. *Lancet* 2002; **360** (9345): 1531–39.

5. Lindholt JS, Juul S, Fasting H, Henneberg EW. Hospital costs and benefits of screening for abdominal aortic aneurysms. Results from a randomised population screening trial. *Eur J Vasc Endovasc Surg* 2002; **23** (1): 55-60.

6. Norman PE, Jamrozik K, Lawrence-Brown MM, *et al.* Population based randomised controlled trial on impact of screening on mortality from abdominal aortic aneurysm. *BMJ* 2004; **329** (7477): 1259.

7. Svensjo S, Bjorck M, Gurtelschmid M, *et al.* Low prevalence of abdominal aortic aneurysm among 65-year-old Swedish men indicates a change in the epidemiology of the disease. *Circulation* 2011; **124** (10): 1118–23.

8. Grondal N, Sogaard R, Lindholt JS. Baseline prevalence of abdominal aortic aneurysm, peripheral arterial disease and hypertension in men aged 65-74 years from a population screening study (VIVA trial). *Br J Surg* 2015; **102** (8): 902–06.

9. National Abdominal Aortic Aneurysm Screening Programme. http://bit.ly/1Qp8o7v (accessed 22 January 2016).

10. World Health Organization, Department of Health Statistics and Information Systems. http://www.who.int/healthinfo/statistics/mort/en/ (accessed 22 January 2016).

11. Iribarren C, Darbinian JA, Go AS, *et al.* Traditional and novel risk factors for clinically diagnosed abdominal aortic aneurysm: the Kaiser multiphasic health checkup cohort study. *Ann Epidemiol* 2007; **17** (9): 669–78.

12. Sode BF, Nordestgaard BG, Gronbaek M, Dahl M. Tobacco smoking and aortic aneurysm: two population-based studies. *Int J Cardiol* 2013; **167** (5): 2271–77.

13. World Health Organisation. http://bit.ly/1SBaHpq (date accessed 22 January 2016).

Internal iliac artery aneurysm does not rupture when the diameter is 3cm, but when it is 7cm

M Venermo, M Laine and K Mani

Introduction

The most common aortoiliac aneurysms are abdominal aortic aneurysms; aneurysms of the iliac arteries are less common and usually appear in the presence of a concomitant infrarenal aortic aneurysm. Approximately 10–20% of the patients with abdominal aortic aneurysms also have a concomitant aneurysm in the iliac arteries, and 10–12% of the iliac aneurysms present without a concomitant abdominal aortic aneurysm.[1,2] The most common location of an iliac aneurysm is the common iliac artery, followed by the internal iliac artery. Although they are often found in association with common iliac artery aneurysms, internal iliac artery aneurysms also occur as an isolated disease. Indeed, if an iliac artery aneurysm is found without involvement of the aorta, the most common location is the internal iliac artery.[3] Aneurysms of the external iliac artery are extremely rare, the suggested reason being the embryology of this artery as it originates later in development from a different cell population than other aortoiliac arteries.

Internal iliac artery aneurysms

Definition and epidemiology

An aneurysm is defined as a focal dilatation of the artery that is at least 50% larger than the expected normal diameter.[4] For abdominal aortic aneurysms, the transverse diameter of 3cm or greater has been used for practical reasons. Similarly, the definition of common iliac artery aneurysm has been a transverse diameter greater than 1.8cm, based on average values for normal individuals. No definition for internal iliac artery aneurysm can be found in the literature, but a transverse diameter of 1.8cm is useful in the iliac artery, although 1.5cm may be closer to the definition. The true prevalence and incidence of internal iliac artery aneurysms is unknown as these are most often asymptomatic and not felt in abdominal palpation. In autopsy studies the estimated prevalence of internal iliac artery aneurysms has been 0.003–0.4%.[1,3–5] The characteristics of the internal iliac artery aneurysm patients are similar to those of abdominal aortic aneurysm patients, and typical cases are those of males aged 70 years and older. The proportion of females has been reported at 5–15%.[3,6,7]

Aetiology, natural history and symptoms

Most of the aneurysms are degenerative atherosclerotic but as in other aortoiliac locations they may be of mycotic origin (caused most often by *Staphylococcus aureus*, E coli, Salmonella, *Pseudomonas* or tuberculosis; syphilic aneurysms are rare nowadays) or in patients with connective tissue disorder (such as Marfan syndrome, Ehler-Danlos syndrome, Behçet's disease, Takayasu's arteritis).[8,9]

The natural history of internal iliac artery aneurysms has not been described. The aneurysm is often asymptomatic and found at the time of rupture. When an internal iliac artery aneurysm is identified in an asymptomatic patient, by accident in an examination done because of other reasons, the diameter of the aneurysm is usually over the limit of elective treatment (3cm), and repaired, thus no surveillance data are available. Most probably the natural history reflects that of other aortoiliac aneurysms: the aneurysm grows slowly until it ruptures. The growth rate, however, is unknown.

Sometimes internal iliac artery aneurysms cause symptoms as the aneurysm compresses the adjacent anatomical structures such as the ureter, bladder, veins or lumbar nerves. The most common symptoms are urological due to the compression of the ureter and bladder.[9] These are difficulties in micturition and urinary retention leading to hydronephrosis, pyelonephritis and sometimes eventually to secondary renal failure.[9,10] Compression of the colon by the aneurysm may cause constipation and rectal pain. Lower limb symptoms can occur, such as ipsilateral hip or leg pain due to compression of the pelvic and lumbosacral nerves. Also deep venous thrombosis and pulmonary embolism have been described.[8,9]

Rupture

Because of their deep location in the pelvis, internal iliac artery aneurysms often remain asymptomatic until they rupture. Rupture is followed by hypotension and abdominal pain radiating to the groin and thigh. Rupture into the bladder and major bleeding secondary to ilio-rectal fistula have also been described.[11,12] Intraperitoneal rupture leading to rapid death is probably rarer than in the case of ruptured abdominal aortic aneurysms.

In 1988, Richardson and Greenfields published a report of 72 patients with one or more aneurysms in the iliac vessels; 22 of the patients had internal iliac artery aneurysms. Two-thirds of the patients had multiple aneurysms and isolated aneurysms were primarily found in the internal iliac artery. In the authors' series, 33% of the patients had a rupture.[5] The mean diameter of all aneurysms was 5.5cm (range 2.5–18cm); internal iliac aneurysms, however, were noted to be larger with a mean diameter of 7.7cm. They did not report separately the sizes of the ruptured cases. In a review article (2005), Dix and colleagues reported all 70 cases of isolated internal iliac aneurysms published in the literature.[3] Forty per cent of the cases presented with rupture. The median size of the aneurysms was 7.7cm (2–13cm). The median size of ruptured aneurysms was 7cm (5–13cm). In another study including 17 patients with isolated internal iliac artery aneurysm rupture, 29 patients with symptomatic internal iliac artery aneurysm including contained ruptures and nine asymptomatic patients, the mean aneurysm size was 8.3cm in ruptured aneurysms, 7.6cm in symptomatic and 5.1cm in asymptomatic patients.[13]

Treatment

A widely used threshold for elective repair is 3cm, as originally suggested by McCready *et al.*[6] Previously, aneurysms were always treated with open surgery and this included ligation of the aneurysm with or without endoaneurysmorrhaphy. Ligation should be performed both proximally and distally, as after proximal ligation alone the aneurysm usually continues to grow due to backflow from distal arteries. Nowadays, in many centres, endovascular treatment with embolisation and stenting has replaced open surgery. If other aneurysms are treated simultaneously, the treatment method is usually interposition bypass or endovascular stent grafting. However, also in these cases internal iliac artery is ligated or embolised.

Jeopardised flow to internal iliac arteries after surgery or endovascular treatment can cause significant morbidity including buttock claudication, buttock necrosis, impotence, as well as ischaemia of the colon or the spinal cord.[6] According to a recent review of the published cases, the incidence of ischaemic complications after occlusion of internal iliac arteries in vascular surgery patients was 37.4% and they were more common after endovascular treatment than open surgery.[6]

Multicentre data on ruptured internal iliac arteries

We collected retrospective data on 66 ruptured internal iliac artery cases from 28 vascular surgical centres in seven countries (Hungary, Sweden, Australia, New Zealand, Norway, Finland and Germany).[16] Patients' demographics and diameter of the internal iliac artery measured from the computed tomography (CT) images taken at the time of rupture were gathered (Figure 1). The earliest operation was from 1995 and the latest from 2015. The proportion of women was 15% and internal iliac artery aneurysm was bilateral in every fourth patient (24%). The majority of patients (62%) had an aneurysm also in the common iliac artery, and half of the patients in the infrarenal aorta. Twenty eight per cent (n=17) of the patients had an isolated internal iliac artery aneurysm, which were all except one that was unilateral (Figure 2).

The mean diameter at the time of rupture was 68mm (25–116mm) and women had slightly smaller internal iliac artery aneurysms (62mm, range 42–91mm) than men (68 mm, range 25–116mm). The mean age of patients was 77 years (range 48–93 years). There was a difference in diameter when comparing isolated internal iliac artery aneurysms and internal iliac artery aneurysm with concomitant aneurysms, the isolated aneurysms being smaller (57mm, range 38–110mm) than

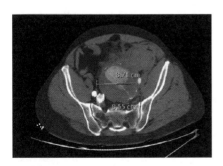

Figure 1: 65-year-old male with ruptured internal iliac artery aneurysm on the left side.

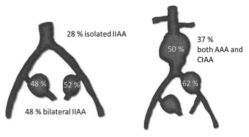

Figure 2: The prevalence of aortoiliac aneurysms in 66 patients with ruptured internal iliac artery aneurysm.

the internal iliac artery aneurysms with concomitant aneurysms (73mm, range 25–116mm; p=0.007). There was one rupture under 3cm (2% of the ruptures) and four under 4cm (6%).

All patients in this study were treated surgically—49 (74%) with open repair and 17 (26%) with endovascular repair. Open repair was usually carried out with ligation of the internal iliac artery, opening the aneurysm sac and oversuturing the back-bleeding ostia, while the most common endovascular technique was coiling the internal iliac artery aneurysm and placing a covered stent over the ostium of the internal iliac artery. Fifteen per cent of the patients died within 30 days after the operation (18% after open repair and 6% after endovascular treatment).

Discussion

The studies on internal iliac artery aneurysms are scarce due to the rarity of the condition. The existing literature consists primarily of case reports and small patient series. No prospective studies have been published. The widely used threshold for elective treatment is diameter of the aneurysm greater than 3cm. As endovascular treatment has developed it has replaced open surgery in many centres.

The view in the publications is that iliac aneurysms have a high rupture rate and mortality. However, on the basis of current literature the mean size of the aneurysm at the time of rupture is 7–8cm. As all aneurysms are in most cases over 3cm when they are diagnosed, no data on natural history of internal iliac artery aneurysm exists. In our data there was only one patient with a ruptured internal iliac artery aneurysm under 3cm and four patients under 4cm, which is 6% of all ruptures. Compared to ruptured abdominal aortic aneurysms, the proportion of small aneurysms is slightly smaller as 8% of abdominal aortic aneurysm ruptures are observed in patients with an aneurysm under the treatment threshold of 5.5cm. Although we are not able to calculate the rupture risk for internal iliac artery aneurysms according to size, the data available indicate that the rupture risk of internal iliac artery aneurysm under 4cm would not be higher than abdominal aortic aneurysms under 5.5cm.

When considering the relatively high incidence of ischaemic complications, after elective treatment as well as lower mortality at the time of rupture compared to abdominal aortic aneurysms, is seems reasonable to consider increasing the threshold for elective repair. Of course this is always dependent on the patient's condition, age and comorbidities as well as the aetiology of the aneurysm. In case of connective tissue disorders and mycotic aneurysms, the indications are different and the treatment threshold lower.

Conclusion

Internal iliac artery aneurysms are rare, and so is internal iliac artery aneurysm rupture. Although the presence of symptoms is more common than in the case of abdominal aortic aneurysms, internal iliac artery aneurysms are often asymptomatic. The most common symptoms are urologic and caused by compression of the bladder by the aneurysm. The current threshold for elective treatment is aneurysm diameter greater than 3cm. Because the size is usually greater than that at the time of diagnosis and aneurysms are then treated electively, no data on natural history are available. About 200 cases have been published in the literature so far, half of them being ruptured aneurysms. The mean size of the aneurysms at the time of rupture in the published cases has been 68–83mm. There are few ruptured cases reported where the diameter was under 4cm, and the aetiologies of these particular aneurysms are unknown.

Summary

- Internal iliac artery aneurysms are usually associated with other aneurysms, most often common iliac artery aneurysms and abdominal aortic aneurysm.

- The characteristics of patients with ruptured internal iliac artery aneurysm are the same as those in ruptured abdominal aortic aneurysm patients.

- The natural history and growth rate of an internal iliac artery aneurysm are unknown mostly because small aneurysms are often asymptomatic and the threshold for elective treatment is low, at 3cm.

- The mean size of the aneurysm at the time of rupture is 7cm and seldom below 4cm.

- Mortality after emergency treatment of ruptured internal iliac artery aneurysm is lower than after ruptured abdominal aortic aneurysms.

Acknowledgements
The authors of this chapter acknowledge the collaborators of the RIIAA study, Martin Björck, Uppsala University, Sweden; Barry Beiles, Western Hospital, Melbourne, Australia; Zoltán Szeberin, Semmelweis University, Hungary; Ian Thomson, University of Otago, Dunedin, New Zealand; Martin Altreuter, St Olavs Hospital, Trondheim, Norway; Sebastian Debus, University Heart Center, Hamburg, Germany; Gabor Menyhei, University Pécs Medical Centre, Hungary. Furthermore, we acknowledge the generosity of all the vascular surgeons who operated on the studied patients and so generously shared their experience by entering the data into the different vascular registries that were used to identify the operations.

References

1. Brunkwall J, Hauksson H, Bengtsson H, Bergqvist D, *et al.* Solitary aneurysms of the iliac arterial system: an estimate of their frequency of occurrence. *J Vasc Surg* 1989; **10**: 381–4.
2. Lawrence PF, *et al.* The epidemiology of surgically repaired aneurysms in the United States. *J Vasc Surg.* 1999; **30**: 632–640.
3. Dix FP1, Titi M, Al-Khaffaf H. The isolated internal iliac artery aneurysm–a review. *Eur J Vasc Endovasc Surg.* 2005; **30** (2): 119–29. .
4. Johnston KW, Rutherford RB, Tilson MD, Shah DM, *et al.* Suggested standards for reporting on arterial aneurysms. Subcommittee on Reporting Standards for Arterial Aneurysms, Ad Hoc Committee on Reporting Standards, Society for Vascular Surgery and North American Chapter, International Society for Cardiovascular Surgery. *J Vasc Surg* 1991; **13** (3): 452–8.
5. Richardson JW, Greenfield LJ. Natural history and management of iliac aneurysms. *J Vasc Surg* 1988; **8**: 165–71.
6. McCready RA, Pairolero PC, Gilmore JC, Kazmier FJ, *et al.* Isolated iliac artery aneurysms. *Surgery* 1983; **93**: 688–93.
7. Perdue GD, Mittenthal MJ, Smith RB, Salam AA. Aneurysms of the internal iliac artery. *Surgery* 1983; **93**: 243–246.

Interna iliac artery aneurysm does not rupture when the diameter is 3cm, but when it is 7cm • **M Venermo, M Laine and K Mani**

8. Krupski WC, Selzman CH, Floridia R, Strecker PK, *et al*. Contemporary management of isolated iliac aneurysms. *J Vasc Surg* 1998; **28**: 1–11

9. Ijaz S,Geroulakos G. Ruptured internal iliac artery aneurysm mimicking a hip fracture. *Int Angiol* 2000; **20** (2): 187–189

10. Kasulke RJ, Clifford A, Nichols WK, Silver D. Isolated atherosclerotic aneurysms of the internal iliac arteries: report of two cases and review of the literature. *Arch Surg* 1982; **117**: 73–77

11. Goff CD, Davidson JT, Teague N, Callis JT. Hematuria from arteriovesical fistula: unusual presentation of ruptured iliac artery aneurysm. *Am Surg* 1999; **65**: 421–22.

12. Karkos C, Oshodi T, Vimalachandran D, *et al*. Internal iliac aneurysm rupture into the rectum following endovascular exclusion. *J Endovasc Ther* 2002; **9**: 907–11.

13. Wilhelm BJ, Sakharpe A, Ibrahim G, Baccaro LM, *et al*. The 100-year evolution of the isolated internal iliac artery aneurysm. *Ann Vasc Surg* 2014; **28**: 1070–77.

14. Chitragari G, Schlosser FJ, Ochoa Chaar CI, Sumpio BE. Consequences of hypogastric artery ligation, embolization, or coverage. *J Vasc Surg* 2015; **62** (5): 1340–47.

15. Laine MT, Vänttinen T, Kantonen I, *et al*. Rupture of Abdominal Aortic Aneurysms in Patients under Screening Age and Elective Repair Threshold. *Eur J Vasc* 2015. In Press.

16. Laine M, Björck M, Beiles B, Szeberin Z, *et al*. Internal Iliac Aneurysms have a low Risk of Rupture under 4cm: A Multicentre Study. Annual meeting of the European Society for Vascular surgery 2015. Abstract book. Oral presentation.

Publication of surgeon level results and risk aversion

E Sim, A Karthikesalingam and I Loftus

Introduction

Mandatory public reporting of surgeon-specific mortality data has recently been introduced across nine surgical specialties in the UK, including vascular surgery.[1] Although outcome feedback to clinicians is widely accepted as important for iterative improvements to quality of care, the wider publication of surgeon-specific mortality data has received criticism from the surgical community, particularly in regards to the potential for risk-averse behaviour.[2] The first calls for surgeon-specific data came over two decades ago in the UK and provide important political and societal context for the present debate regarding whether surgeon-specific mortality is an appropriate or meaningful measure for abdominal aortic aneurysm repair in particular.

Description of topic

The 1994 Bristol Royal Infirmary Inquiry into mortality rates following paediatric cardiothoracic surgery provided an important catalyst for the reporting of surgeon-specific mortality in the UK.[1] The inquiry prompted the Government to mandate surgeon-specific mortality data for all cardiothoracic units in the UK. *The Guardian* newspaper subsequently gained access to mortality rates for coronary artery bypass grafting under the Freedom of Information Act, significantly accelerating the wider publication of such data.[2] Further attention, including the Francis Inquiry into failings at Mid Staffordshire Hospital, resulted in the National Health Service (NHS) publication entitled "Everybody Counts" in 2012.[1] This highlighted the need for greater transparency for NHS patients, and called for the publication of activity, quality and survival rates for every practising consultant across nine surgical specialties in the UK.[3] The concept was promoted as a "ground-breaking step towards ensuring the rights and pledges set out in the NHS Constitution, including patients' right to choose the most appropriate setting for care, are delivered".[3]

Over a similar timeframe, vascular surgery in the UK had attracted considerable attention, particularly in regards to elective abdominal aortic aneurysm repair.[4] The 2008 VASCUNET report suggested that the UK had a considerably higher mortality rate following elective abdominal aortic aneurysm repair (7.9%) than nine other European and Australasian countries (1.9–4.5%).[5] This prompted a significant reconfiguration of vascular services, which included centralisation of major arterial services, annual examination of institutional mortality rates for index procedures, quality improvement initiatives and greater uptake of endovascular technology.[4] These changes resulted in a fall in elective abdominal aortic aneurysm mortality to 1.8% by the end of 2012.[6] There is little evidence to suggest that the attribution of deaths to individual surgeons will further add to this success, and there is a need to examine the balance between the potential benefits of surgeon-specific mortality reporting (transparency and quality improvement) *versus* the potential risks (gaming and risk-averse behaviour).

Evidence for views

The public disclosure of surgeon-specific mortality for cardiac surgery generated considerable controversy in the UK and abroad. Although promoted as a means to enhance quality improvement and maintain patient autonomy, it has also been suggested that publication of surgeon-specific mortality has been associated with a number of unintended negative outcomes.[7] One potential consequence of public reporting for individual surgeons is "gaming", wherein surgeons (consciously or unconsciously) alter their practice (through case selection, ascertainment of risk, or reporting bias in data submission) in order to mitigate the potential of poor outcomes on their reputations.[7] Such alterations are made to reported data or case selection for surgery but do not improve patient care and include tactics such as up-coding of comorbidities or symptom status, the addition of trivial procedures to high-risk coronary artery bypass cases, or prolongation of life in postoperative patients requiring palliation.[7]

Perhaps the most important example of potential gaming is risk aversion. The hypothesis is that surgeons who are required to publicly disclose their mortality data will avoid treating high-risk patients in order to protect their professional standing and lower the expected operative risk of their personal practice.[1] This presents a significant public health issue, as in large abdominal aortic aneurysms, it is frequently the case that high-risk operative candidates may also have the greater potential gain from interventions. Viewed from this perspective, it is possible that risk-averse behaviour by individual surgeons can lead to paradoxically greater population mortality, which in turn could increase healthcare costs due to the implementation of less effective therapies.[7] Turndown rates for abdominal aortic aneurysm repair are already known to be inversely associated with the volume (caseload or experience) of procedures within an institution; and there is compelling epidemiological evidence that turndown rates for ruptured abdominal aortic aneurysm patients have a considerable impact on population mortality for the condition.[8]

Risk aversion has also been linked to racial or socioeconomic profiling in cases where surgeons may regard patients from minority groups as inherently high-risk.[9,10] It was reported that 62% of cardiothoracic surgeons at the height of surgeon-specific report cards in New York had refused to operate on at least one coronary artery bypass grafting (CABG) patient in the previous year due to public reporting.[11] Similar results were found in Philadelphia where 59% of physicians had increased difficultly referring high-risk risk patients and 63% of cardiac surgeons admitted that they were more likely to refuse such patients.[12] Proponents of surgeon-specific mortality data refute suggestions of widespread risk aversion by citing concerns regarding incomplete risk adjustment, ascertainment bias and a lack of information regarding patients who are refused surgery as confounders.[13] Contrarian evidence also exists in the literature to contest the presence of risk aversion, including reports that a higher percentage of high-risk patients were treated in US states with public reporting compared with those that did not have such programmes from 1994 to 1999.[14]

Risk aversion is particularly important for a condition such as abdominal aortic aneurysm, in which the proportion of patients denied surgery is an important determinant of outcomes.[4] Few studies have focused on the proportion of patients turned down for abdominal aortic aneurysm repair,[15–24] even though these data are required to place perioperative mortality in context and may be subject to considerably greater variation than operative mortality rates. The rate of aortic rupture is significant in patients with large unoperated abdominal aortic aneurysms and the decision to turndown aneurysm repair for physiological reasons is therefore not always justifiable; especially if the aneurysm is morphologically amenable to endovascular aneurysm repair (EVAR) and the patient expresses a strong preference for aneurysm repair. Patients with aneurysms larger than 8cm who are managed conservatively have a rupture rate of 26% within six months, and the rate of aneurysm rupture is 32.5% within a year for aneurysms exceeding 7cm diameter.[25] Common reasons for non-operative management of abdominal aortic aneurysms include medical comorbidity and hostile aneurysm morphology, as well as patient refusal. However, the clinician's refusal to operate on aneurysm patients is subjective and, therefore, may be incorrect or contested by their colleagues. Surgeon-specific mortality fails to capture turndown rates, aneurysm diameter, morphologic suitability for EVAR, non-aneurysm-related life expectancy and principle reasons for turndown. Because of this, the extent of selection bias for aneurysm repair remains unknown and subsequently, the presence of risk-averse behaviour cannot be excluded.

Accurate risk adjustment is another necessity for credible surgeon-specific mortality data. Operative mortality is determined by a number of factors for abdominal aortic aneurysm repair, including the type of operation, the institutions' structures and processes of care, and patient-specific risk factors. Inaccurate risk adjustment when analysing outcome data may result in either false assurances of satisfactory performance or alternatively, false identifications of poor-performing outliers with damaging consequences arising from widespread publicity. Risk-adjustment tools for cardiac surgery have been the subjects of considerable re-evaluation and the challenge is even greater for abdominal aortic aneurysm repair.[26,27] Determinants of outcome differ between EVAR and open repair of abdominal aortic aneurysms with the former being largely morphological and the latter being more commonly physiological.[28–30] Despite this, existing risk adjustment tools for aneurysm repair in the UK are based on surgeon-submitted data for both operations, rather than each operation in isolation. The current risk-adjustment tools used in the NHS for abdominal aortic aneurysm repair outcomes are not accurate due to their lack of adjustment of aneurysm morphology, rigorous external validation, quantified long-term durability and protection from aneurysm-related mortality for EVAR.[31,32] They also fail to account for the life expectancy of those patients refused aneurysm repair as a result of the application of these tools preoperatively. There remains an unmet need for an accurate and objective algorithm to predict which patients will benefit from aneurysm repair and this is the subject of considerable ongoing research funded by the National Institute for Health Research (NIHR HTA 09/91/39). In the absence of an accepted national algorithm to contextualise case selection, a policy of national public reporting for surgeon-specific mortality will continue to be contested.

Surgeon-specific mortality for aneurysm repair in particular can be difficult to interpret as it is widely acknowledged that institutions, rather than individual surgeons, have significantly more influence on patient outcomes. High-volume centres have been repeatedly shown to have lower mortality rates following aneurysm repair and this has been the underlying principle behind centralisation of aortic services.[33] Institution level outcome data may, therefore, be more appropriate and accurate. The fact that aneurysm repair is an increasingly complex and technological activity—often performed by a team with more than one consultant present—provides further support for institution-level outcome reporting.

Following the release of surgeon-specific mortality data by default in the USA, the President of the Institute for Healthcare Improvement, Donald Berwick, equated these data with "measurement for judgment" rather than "measurement for improvement".[34] He argued that poor outcomes were the result of system and process failure, not individuals. The Society of Thoracic Surgeons in the USA later took heed of this message and established a Quality Management Task Force that advised institution level reporting rather than SSMD. Berwick reiterated this opinion when commissioned to examine the NHS patient safety by the British Prime Minister following the Francis Inquiry into the Mid-Staffordshire Foundation Trust failings.[33]

Finally, mortality after abdominal aortic aneurysm repair often results from the failure to detect and expediently manage postoperative complications, rather than from the case selection or operative care itself.[35] Known as "failure to rescue", this concept is of great importance for surgeon-specific mortality reporting as it implies that many deaths after abdominal aortic aneurysm repair will remain unrelated to the designated primary operating surgeon, and are a wider reflection of institutional structures, processes and quality of care. Failure to rescue rates correlate with institution characteristics such as staffing and intensive care resource; and hospital-wide mortality data for a number of surgical conditions have been repeatedly shown to correlate with institutional characteristics that individual surgeons cannot be held responsible for, including the staffing, funding or bed ratios.[36]

Conclusion

The publication of outcome data is essential for accountability and transparency within a healthcare system. The validity of surgeon-specific reporting for abdominal aortic aneurysms, however, remains controversial due to concerns regarding whether it is an appropriate or meaningful measurement for quality of care in this particular case. Misinterpretation of surgeon-specific data has resulted in sensationalist journalism using the "ranking" of consultant surgeons by mortality rates to declare that some surgeons were "30 times worse than their colleagues".[37] This type of irresponsible journalism has potentially negative consequences for the care of patients and can affect surgeon behaviour, team dynamics and case selection, as well as impacting tertiary referral between centres. A comprehensive approach is still needed for abdominal aortic aneurysm repair and should look to include publicly accountable data regarding institutional structure/process factors, safety data (including failure to rescue, institutional reporting of adverse events), resource availability, and the uptake of endovascular technology, timeliness of care, equity of access to aneurysm repair, efficiency of care (length of stay and morbidity data), patient-reported outcomes, and, most importantly, turndown rates. Appropriate risk adjustment tools must be developed and include aneurysm morphology data. Until the potentially adverse impact of surgeon-specific mortality reporting can be monitored and understood, caution is advocated in the public attribution of deaths after aneurysm repair to individual surgeons.

Summary

- The validity of surgeon-specific reporting for abdominal aortic aneurysm remains controversial due to concerns regarding whether it is an appropriate or meaningful measurement for quality of care.

- Misinterpretation of surgeon-specific data has potentially negative consequences for the care of patients and can affect surgeon behaviour, team dynamics and case selection, as well as impacting tertiary referral between centres.

- A comprehensive approach is still needed for aneurysm repair and should look to include publicly accountable data regarding institutional structure/ process factors, safety data, resource availability, and the uptake of endovascular technology, timeliness of care, equity of access to aneurysm repair, efficiency of care, patient-reported outcomes, and, most importantly, turndown rates.

- Appropriate risk adjustment tools must be developed and include aneurysm morphology data.

- Until the potentially adverse impact of surgeon-specific mortality reporting can be monitored and understood, caution is advocated in the public attribution of deaths after aneurysm repair to individual surgeons.

References

1. Radford PD, Derbyshire LF, Shalhoub J, *et al.* Publication of surgeon specific outcome data: a review of implementation, controversies and the potential impact on surgical training. *Int J Surg* 2015; **13**: 211-6
2. Westaby S, De Silva R, Petrou M, *et al.* Surgeon-specific mortality data disguise wider failings in delivery of safe surgical services. *Eur J Cardiothorac Surg* 2015; **47** (2): 341e5.
3. NHS England. Everyone Counts: Planning For Patients 2013/2014. https://www.england.nhs.uk/wp-content/uploads/2012/12/everyonecounts-planning.pdf (date accessed: 4 February 2016).
4. Karthikesalingam A, Holt PJE, Loftus IM, *et al.* Risk aversion in vascular intervention: The consequences of publishing surgeon-specific mortality for abdominal aortic aneurysm repair. European *Journal of Vascular Surgery* 2015, http://dx.doi.org/10.1016/j.ejvs.2015.06.003.
5. European Society for Vascular Surgery. Second Vascunet report 2008.
6. Waton S, Johal A, Groene O, *et al.* Outcomes after elective repair of infra-renal abdominal aortic aneurysm. London: *The Royal College of Surgeons* of England, November 2013.
7. Shahian DM, Edwards FH, Jacobs JP, *et al.* Public reporting of cardiac surgery performance: Part 1 – history, rationale, consequences. *Ann Thorac Surg* 2011; **92** (Suppl. 3): S2e11.
8. Karthikesalingam A, Holt PJ, Vidal-Diez A, *et al.* Mortality from ruptured abdominal aortic aneurysms: clinical lessons from a comparison of outcomes in England and the USA. *The Lancet* 2014; **383** (9935): 2123–24.
9. Werner RM, Asch DA. The unintended consequences of publicly reporting quality information. *JAMA* 2005; **293** (10): 1239e 44.
10. Werner RM, Asch DA, Polsky D. Racial profiling: the unintended consequences of coronary artery bypass graft report cards. *Circulation* 2005; **111** (10): 1257e63.

11. Burack JH, Impellizzeri P, Homel P, *et al*. Public reporting of surgical mortality: a survey of New York State cardiothoracic surgeons. *Ann Thorac Surg* 1999; **68**: 1195–200.

12. Schneider EC, Epstein AM. Influence of cardiac-surgery performance reports on referral practices and access to care—a survey of cardiovascular specialists. *N Engl J Med* 1996; **335**: 251–56.

13. Bridgewater B, Grayson AD, Brooks N, *et al*. Has the publication of cardiac surgery outcome data been associated with changes in practice in northwest England: an analysis of 25,730 patients undergoing CABG surgery under 30 surgeons over eight years. *Heart* 2007; **93** (6): 744e8.

14. Hannan EL, Sarrazin MS, Doran DR, *et al*. Provider profiling and quality improvement efforts in coronary artery bypass graft surgery: the effect on short-term mortality among Medicare beneficiaries. *Med Care* 2003; **41**: 1164 –72.

15. Szilagyi DE, Smith RF, DeRusso FJ, *et al*. Contribution of abdominal aortic aneurysmectomy to prolongation of life. *Ann Surg* 1966; **164** (4): 678e99.

16. Bardram L, Buchardt Hansen HJ, Dahl Hansen AB. Abdominal aortic aneurysms. Early and late results after surgical and non-surgical treatment. *Acta Chir Scand Suppl* 1980; **502**: 85e93.

17. Perko MJ, Schroeder TV, Olsen PS, *et al*. Natural history of abdominal aortic aneurysm: a survey of 63 patients treated nonoperatively. *Ann Vasc Surg* 1993; **7** (2): 113e.

18. Ruberti U, Scorza R, Biasi GM, *et al*. Nineteen year experience on the treatment of aneurysms of the abdominal aorta: a survey of 832 consecutive cases. *J Cardiovasc Surg* (Torino) 1985; **26** (6): 547e53.

19. Campbell WB, Collin J, Morris PJ. The mortality of abdominal aortic aneurysm. *Ann R Coll Surg Engl* 1986; **68** (5): 275e8. 27

20. Woodburn KR, Chant H, Davies JN, *et al*. Suitability for endovascular aneurysm repair in an unselected population. *Br J Surg* 2001; **88** (1): 77e81

21. Heikkinen M, Salenius J, Zeitlin R, *et al*. The fate of AAA patients referred electively to vascular surgical unit. *Scand J Surg* 2002; **91** (4): 345e52.

22. Tambyraja AL, Stuart WP, Sala Tenna A, *et al*. Non-operative management of high-risk patients with abdominal aortic aneurysm. *Eur J Vasc Endovasc Surg* 2003;**26**(4):401e4.

23. Tanquilut EM, Veith FJ, Ohki T, *et al*. Nonoperative management with selective delayed sur- gery for large abdominal aortic aneurysms in patients at high risk. *J Vasc Surg* 2002; **36** (1): 41e6.

24. Hickey GL, Grant SW, Caiado C, *et al*. Dynamic prediction modeling approaches for cardiac surgery. Circ Cardiovasc Qual Outcomes 2013; **6** (6): 649e58.

25. Lederle FA, Johnson GR, Wilson SE, *et al*. Rupture rate of large abdominal aortic aneu- rysms in patients refusing or unfit for elective repair. *JAMA* 2002; **287** (22): 2968e72.

26. Hickey GL, Grant SW, Murphy GJ, *et al*. Dynamic trends in cardiac surgery: why the logistic EuroSCORE is no longer suitable for contemporary cardiac surgery and implications for future risk models. *Eur J Cardiothorac Surg* 2013; **43** (6): 1146e52.

27. Patterson BO, Hinchliffe RJ, Holt PJ, *et al*. Importance of aortic morphology in planning aortic interventions. *J Endovasc Ther* 2010; **17** (1): 73e7.

28. Patterson BO, Holt PJ, Hinchliffe R, *et al*. Predicting risk in elective abdominal aortic aneurysm repair: a systematic review of current evidence. *Eur J Vasc Endovasc Surg* 2008; **36** (6): 637e45.

29. Patterson BO, Karthikesalingam A, Hinchliffe RJ, *et al*. The Glasgow aneurysm score does not predict mortality after open abdominal aortic aneurysm in the era of endovascular aneurysm repair. *J Vasc Surg* 2011; **54** (2): 353e7.

30. Ambler GK, Gohel MS, Mitchell DC, *et al*. The abdominal aortic aneurysm statistically corrected operative risk evaluation (AAA SCORE) for predicting mortality after open and endovascular interventions. *J Vasc Surg* 2015; **61** (1): 35e43.

31. Grant SW, Grayson AD, Mitchell DC, *et al*. Evaluation of five risk prediction models for elective abdominal aortic aneurysm repair using the UK National Vascular Database. *Br J Surg* 2012; **99** (5): 673e9.

32. Karthikesalingam A, Hinchliffe RJ, Loftus IM, *et al*. Volume-outcome relationships in vascular surgery: the current status. *J Endovasc Ther* 2010; **17** (3): 356e65.

33. Department of Health. A promise to learn – a commitment to act. 2013. https://goo.gl/BWDO6e (date accessed 4 February 2016).

34. Berwick, DM. Quality comes home. *Ann Intern Med* 1996; **125** (10): 839–43.

35. Sinha S, Ata Ozdemir B, Khalid U, *et al*. Failure-to-rescue and interprovider comparisons after elective abdominal aortic aneurysm repair. *Br J Surg* 2014; **101** (12): 1541e50.

36. Ozdemir BA, Sinha S, Karthikesalingam A, *et al*. Mortality of emergency general surgical patients and associations with hospital structures and processes. *Br J Anaesth* 2016; **116** (1): 54–62.

37. The surgeons whose patients were up to 30 times likelier to die: NHS to publish death rates of doctors for the first time. Daily Mail 2015. http://goo.gl/adw8jq (date accessed 4 February 2016).

Debate: The threshold for intervention for abdominal aortic aneurysm should be settled by randomised controlled trials—for the motion

JJ Earnshaw

Introduction

It has been known for a century, since the early post mortem studies, that the risk of rupture of an abdominal aortic aneurysm depends on its size.[1] Modern management of unruptured abdominal aortic aneurysms has evolved based primarily on the seminal study, UKSAT (the UK Small aneurysm trial), which concluded there was no advantage for early surgery over ultrasound surveillance in patients with abdominal aortic aneurysm diameter from 4cm to 5.4cm measured by ultrasound imaging.[2] Around the world, 5.5cm is regarded as the diameter triggering consideration of elective abdominal aortic aneurysm repair. The current situation is more complicated, since new imaging methods have enabled calculations of the stresses and strains in the aneurysmal aortic wall that might predict aneurysm rupture.[3] Studies on growth and rupture risks of small (3–4.4cm) and medium (4.5–5.4cm) abdominal aortic aneurysms have detected some risk factors for early rupture: female sex, smoking and high blood pressure.[4] The issue is important because large numbers of patients are in surveillance programmes for small and medium aneurysms detected either by incidental investigation, or increasingly by population screening.[5] These factors make it worth a re-analysis of whether intervention based solely on size is optimal, or whether decisions about intervention could be individualised, based on other risk factors. Finally, there is also a financial issue; earlier intervention could dramatically increase the number of elective procedures required, and cold, hard economic analysis of any new intervention protocol is fundamental.

UKSAT

This study commenced in 1991. Some 1,090 men and women with abdominal aortic aneurysms 4cm to 5.4cm in diameter (where surgeons had equipoise about intervention) were randomised to early intervention or ultrasound surveillance by trained nurses.[2] Follow-up at 10 years showed death rates were equivalent in the two groups, hence the conclusion that patients with an abdominal aortic aneurysm less than 5.5cm are as safe in surveillance. This was indeed an important study, but even so had some potential confounding factors:

- There were a relatively small number of aneurysms 5cm to 5.4cm compared with 4cm to 5cm.
- The proportion of women was relatively small and they appeared to have a higher risk of rupture, although this was not significant due to small numbers.
- This trial was done in the era of open surgery; in modern times the risk of intervention using endovascular techniques is lower (although risks from open surgery have also fallen in the UK). The CAESAR trial randomised patients with small abdominal aortic aneurysms to surveillance or early endovascular aneurysm repair (EVAR), but unsurprisingly event rates were too low to obtain any significant result.[6]

UKSAT is often misinterpreted as suggesting 5.5cm should be the indication for intervention. It does not, of course, and the size indication for intervention remains unknown; it is to the shame of the vascular community that the Medium Aneurysm Trial was never done (say 5.5cm to 6.4cm diameter). It is illogical to think that an abdominal aortic aneurysm changes from innocent to risky over 1mm in diameter; there must be a gradual increase in risk over 5.5cm.

Screening

A number of ultrasound screening programmes also use 5.5cm as the referral threshold for intervention. The UK National abdominal aortic aneurysm screening programme (NAAASP) and other UK programmes use this threshold, measured using the inner wall to inner wall ultrasound measurement method.[7] Although this method is reliable and reproducible, it measures aortic diameter up to 5mm less than the outer-to-outer diameter method used in UKSAT, which includes aortic wall thickness.[8] Thus abdominal aortic aneurysms referred for treatment from NAAASP at the 5.5cm ultrasound threshold may have aneurysms nearer 6cm in diameter in comparison with UKSAT, and even bigger if measured on computed tomography (CT). Yet this method, which is evidence-based from the previous randomised screening trials,[9,10] does not seem to have increased the risk of aneurysm rupture in surveillance. Ongoing analysis of NAAASP data for men in surveillance will enable calculation of rupture risk during surveillance and may provide reassurance that this is a safe schedule.[11]

Causes of abdominal aortic aneurysm rupture

The mechanisms involved in abdominal aortic aneurysm rupture remain obscure. Size appears the main factor, but analysis of data from collaborative surveillance schedules suggests that female sex, smoking and hypertension are also contributory risk factors, and diabetes may be protective.[4] Rapid growth is also believed to increase the risk of aneurysm rupture and many surgeons would offer elective treatment to a patient with a greater than 1cm growth in one year. A very few of these rapidly expanding aneurysms may be mycotic (infected), but no controlled studies on treatment according to growth rate exist.

Modern imaging

A number of new imaging techniques have shown difference in dynamics and stresses in aortic aneurysm walls. Dynamic CT, magnetic resonance imaging and others showed measurable differences within and between aneurysms, and also between aneurysms that have ruptured compared to intact aneurysms.[3] Apart from the odd case report,[12] there are no prospective studies to confirm whether any of these imaging methods could actually be used to predict aneurysm rupture, but that has not stopped some clinicians using information obtained from these investigations as part of the consent process when discussing elective intervention for non-ruptured aneurysms.

Individualised care for intact aneurysms

It is of course illogical to think that diameter is the only risk factor for aneurysm rupture, and also that the risk of rupture for each aneurysm of similar size is the same. A number of risk factors could be used to create a risk score which might help to make individualised decisions for men with a medium-sized aneurysm. The aneurysm repair decision aid (ARDA) score has been created using data from surveillance trials, but is not yet validated.[13]

The issues

The present method of managing patients with intact medium aneurysms (treatment at 5.5cm in diameter) comes mainly from UKSAT. It has proved an efficient way to process men in aneurysm screening and surveillance programmes, and has shown to be cost-effective. The risk of rupture in surveillance is low; further information may come from analysis of rupture rates in population screening programmes which have large numbers of men in surveillance: there are 10,000 men currently under surveillance in NAAASP.[11] Despite the illogicality of this one-size-fits-all threshold for referral, it has stood the test of time.

For a new individualised system of referral to be adopted, it must be tested against this current standard for both efficacy and cost. A possible randomised trial could include men in surveillance with a 5cm aneurysm, and randomise them to individualised or standard care. The problem is that with such a low risk of rupture in men with a 5cm aneurysm, such a trial would likely have a low event rate, and thus require many thousands of participants. It would also be a challenge to prove that early intervention is cost-effective because of the expense of the intervention procedures. Perhaps the best way to test individualised care would be to randomise low-risk patients with a 5.5cm aneurysm to standard care or delayed intervention. Many vascular surgeons might not have equipoise for this type of trial, and it remains uncertain whether ethics committees would be persuadable that this was a trial in the patient's best interests. It might be possible to commence with a study of elderly patients (say over 80 years) with a 5.5cm aneurysm on ultrasound imaging, where equipoise might exist.

Conclusion

Presently, referral for treatment based on abdominal aortic aneurysm diameter remains the most evidence-based option. A number of new methods for individualised care exist, but the challenge is how to prove that they are more effective and cost-effective than the current method. In the meantime, it is the responsibility of all vascular surgeons to prevent a drift towards unmonitored use of unproven methods to increase the number of elective procedures. It should not be forgotten that elective aneurysm repair is not without risk and increasing the exposure of men to this procedure could cause harm, as well as potential benefit.

Summary

- The standard of care for patients with abdominal aortic aneurysms is to offer treatment once their aortic diameter is greater than 5.4cm.

- This follows UKSAT, where early intervention for aneurysms 4–5.4cm in diameter offered no survival advantage over continued ultrasound surveillance.

- It should not be forgotten that ultrasound imaging and CT may give different diameter measurements for the same aneurysm.

- Instead of using diameter measurement alone, new referral triggers could be developed using computer risk scoring or CT analysis of aortic wall stress.

- Any new method potentially offering personalised indications for intervention must be tested against the current standard of care, and must either save lives or reduce costs.

References

1. Nordon I, Hinchliffe RJ, Loftus IM, Thompson MM. Pathophysiology and epidemiology of abdominal aortic aneurysms. *Nat Rev Cardiol* 2011; **8**: 92–102.
2. UK Small Aneurysm Trial Participants. Final follow-up of surgery *versus* surveillance in the UK small aneurysm trial. *Br J Surg* 2007; **94**: 702–08.
3. Khosla S, Morris DR, Moxon JV, Walker PJ, *et al*. Meta-analysis of peak wall stress in ruptured, symptomatic and intact abdominal aortic aneurysms. *Br J Surg* 2014; **101**: 1350–57.
4. Thompson SG, Brown LC, Sweeting MJ, Bown MJ, *et al*, and the RESCAN Collaborators. Systematic review and meta-analysis of the growth and rupture rates of small abdominal aortic aneurysms: implications for surveillance intervals and their cost effectiveness. *HTA* 2014: **17**: 1–118.
5. Davis M, Harris M, Earnshaw JJ. Implementation of the national Health Service Abdominal Aortic Aneurysm Screening Program in England. *J Vasc Surg* 2013; **57**: 1440–45.
6. Cao P, De Rango P, Verzini F, Parlani G, *et al* on behalf of the CAESAR Trial Group. Comparison of surveillance *versus* aortic endografting for small aneurysm repair (CAESAR): results from a randomised trial. *Eur J Vasc Endovasc Surg* 2011; **41**: 13–25.
7. Hartshorne TC, McCollum CNC, Earnshaw JJ, Morris J, *et al*. Ultrasound measurement of aortic diameter in a national screening programme. *Eur J Vasc Endovasc Surg* 2011; **42**: 195–99.
8. Gurtelschmid M, Bjorck M, Wanhainen A. A comparison of three different ultrasound methods of measuring the abdominal aorta. *Br J Surg* 2014; **101**: 633–36.
9. Thompson SG, Ashton HA, Gao L, Scott RA, MASS Study Group. Screening men for abdominal aortic aneurysm: 10 year mortality and cost effectiveness results from the randomised Multicentre Aneurysm Screening Study. *BMJ* 2009: **338**: b2307.
10. Thompson SG, Ashton HA, Gao L, Buxton MJ, *et al* on behalf of the Multicentre Aneurysm Screening study. Final follow-up of the Multicentre Aneurysm Screening Study randomized trial of abdominal aortic aneurysm screening. *Br J Surg* 2012; **99**: 1649–56.
11. Jacomelli J, Summers L, Stevenson A, Lees T, *et al*. Results of the first five years of the NHS Abdominal Aortic Aneurysm Screening Programme in England *Br J Surg* 2016 (in press).
12. Doyle BJ, McGloughlin TM, Miller K, Powell J, *et al*. Regions of high wall stress can predict the future location of rupture of abdominal aortic aneurysm. *Cardiovasc Intervent Radiol* 2014; **37**: 815–18.
13. Grant SW, Sperrin M, Carlson E, Chinai N, *et al*. Calculating when elective abdominal aortic aneurysm repair improves survival for individual patients: development of the Aneurysm Repair Decision Aid and economic evaluation. *Health Technol Assess* 2015; **19**: 1–154.

Debate: The threshold for intervention for abdominal aortic aneurysm should be settled by randomised controlled trials— against the motion

SW Grant and CN McCollum

Introduction

As most patients with an abdominal aortic aneurysm are asymptomatic in modern clinical practice, the primary aim of aneurysm repair is to improve patient survival by preventing premature death due to aneurysm rupture. The decision of when to perform aneurysm repair should, therefore, balance the risk of premature death due to rupture against the risks of death as a result of repair. Unless there is a prohibitively high surgical risk or significantly limited life expectancy, patients with "large" asymptomatic aneurysms (>5.5cm) are currently offered intervention due to the high risk of rupture in these patients. Unless there is rapid aneurysm growth, patients with asymptomatic "small" aneurysms are offered regular surveillance until the aneurysm reaches 5.5cm in diameter. This threshold for intervention of 5.5cm for asymptomatic aneurysm is widely accepted and appropriately based on data from two randomised controlled trials that completed recruitment over 20 years ago.

In reality, the current threshold for abdominal aortic aneurysm repair at 5.5cm was based predominantly on the opinion of surgeons in the vascular society but then confirmed by randomised controlled trials recruiting a population of patients in a wide age range and with aneurysm between 4cm and 5.5cm. Any such randomised controlled trial is clearly the best way to define policy for populations. However, this approach will inevitably fail to identify the indication for aneurysm repair in individual patients, particularly those outside the age range selected for the trial and/or with excluded comorbidities.

The current threshold

It is generally thought that the current threshold for intervention for abdominal aortic aneurysm is based on data from randomised controlled trials. However, there are actually no randomised data to support intervention for symptomatic aneurysms,

aneurysms that grow >1cm/year, or for a threshold of 5cm in women. These criteria are based on a consensus due to the actual or perceived increased risk of aneurysm rupture under these circumstances. There are data from randomised controlled trials relating to the threshold for intervention for asymptomatic aneurysms, but the current threshold for intervention was actually first decided upon by consensus opinion at meetings of the Vascular Society of Great Britain and Ireland in 1987 and 1988.[1] At these meetings, the size range of abdominal aortic aneurysms that represented the "grey area of indecision" for which the treatment option was not clear was defined as 4–5.5cm. Based on this consensus opinion, two randomised controlled trials were subsequently performed to establish the optimal management strategy for aneurysms in this size range, UKSAT (UK small aneurysm trial) and the ADAM (Aneurysm detection and management) trial.[2,3]

The UKSAT study included 1,090 patients with asymptomatic abdominal aortic aneurysms in the size range of 4cm and 5.5cm aged 60–76 and considered fit for elective aneurysm repair from 93 UK hospitals between 1991 and 1995.[2] These patients were randomly allocated to either ultrasound surveillance or early elective open aneurysm repair. The 30-day mortality in the early repair group was 5.8% meaning survival was initially worse in this group. Survival was subsequently worse in the surveillance group with the survival curves crossing at around three years but there was no significant difference in overall survival between the groups at a mean follow-up of 4.6 years. The overall mean rate of rupture for aneurysms between 4cm and 5.5cm was 1% per year.[2] Over 60% of the group randomised to surveillance underwent aneurysm repair within five years of randomisation. At a final follow-up of 12 years, there remained no difference in survival between the early repair group and the surveillance group.[4]

The ADAM trial included 1,136 patients with asymptomatic abdominal aortic aneurysms in the size range 4cm to 5.4cm, aged 50–79 and considered fit for elective aneurysm repair between 1992 and 1996.[3] As with UKSAT, patients were randomly allocated to either ultrasound surveillance or early elective open aneurysm repair. The 30-day mortality in the early repair group was 2.1%. Unlike UKSAT, the survival curves did not cross during the follow-up period. However, there was still no significant difference in survival between the groups at a mean follow-up of 4.9 years. The rate of aneurysm rupture in the surveillance group was 0.6% per year. The proportions of patients in the group who were randomised to surveillance who subsequently underwent aneurysm repair within five years of randomisation were similar to UKSAT.

A pooled analysis of the UKSAT and ADAM trials confirmed no benefit of early surgery over ultrasound surveillance for asymptomatic aneurysm between 4cm and 5.5cm.[5] This is clearly a valid conclusion from these randomised data. Other valid conclusions from these data include the fact that the overall risk of rupture in asymptomatic patients with an aneurysm between 4cm and 5.5cm is low and that almost 60% of patients with an aneurysm in this size range will undergo repair. However, the threshold at which each individual patient with an asymptomatic aneurysm should be offered intervention to optimise survival cannot be concluded from these population-based data.

Problems with the current threshold

There are a number of problems with basing the threshold for intervention for asymptomatic abdominal aortic aneurysm on data from the UKSAT, ADAM or any future randomised controlled trial. Firstly all randomised controlled trials have inclusion and exclusion criteria that limit the applicability of their findings to the general population. Perhaps the most important exclusion criteria applied in UKSAT was the upper age limit of 76 years. There has been a substantial increase in elective aneurysm repairs performed in patients aged over 75 since 1997,[6] and it is unclear whether the UKSAT findings apply to this increasingly large cohort of patients. Patients who were considered unfit for surgery were also excluded from UKSAT. Although there was no standard definition for this in the study design,[7] it is highly likely that a significant proportion of patients with comorbidities that meant they were excluded from UKSAT would now be considered fit for open surgery or undergo endovascular aneurysm repair (EVAR). Again it is uncertain whether the results of the UKSAT are still applicable to these patients.

Whether the results of UKSAT are applicable to patients excluded from the study is questionable but it is also uncertain whether the results of UKSAT and the ADAM trial are still valid for the cohort of patients that were included. It has now been more than 20 years since the trials completed recruitment and since then, clinical practice has changed significantly. There has been an almost two-fold decrease in deaths from ruptured abdominal aortic aneurysms in men, an increase in admissions for elective aneurysm repair, widespread adoption of screening programmes and a reduction in the operative mortality associated with elective repair.[6]

There have also been reductions in the prevalence of smoking, hypertension and hypercholesterolaemia in the general population along with an increase in the prescription of statins and antihypertensive medications all of which may have decreased the incidence of aneurysm rupture.[6] As both trials represent a five-year snapshot of practice the influence these changes would have on the results of the trial are uncertain. The fast-paced and constant changes in surgery and medicine mean that the relevance of the results of a randomised controlled trial may be outdated even before they are published. This is not a limitation exclusive to UKSAT and the ADAM trial but is in fact a limitation of any randomised controlled trial that has a long-term primary outcome.

A key example of this and undoubtedly the most significant change in practice related to abdominal aortic aneurysms since these trials were conducted has been the introduction and widespread adoption of EVAR. No EVARs were included in either the UKSAT or ADAM trial. As the main benefit of EVAR is a lower risk of postoperative mortality,[8] it was hypothesised that EVAR rather than open repair may demonstrate a survival advantage for aneurysms between 4cm and 5.5cm. To test this hypothesis two randomised controlled trials were conducted that randomised patients to either early intervention with EVAR or surveillance.[9,10] Despite an operative mortality of <1% in both studies there was no survival benefit demonstrated for early intervention by EVAR compared to surveillance. Given the results of these more contemporary trials it is possible that if UKSAT and ADAM were repeated based on contemporary practice the conclusions would be the same. However, perhaps the most important limitation of basing the threshold for intervention for abdominal aortic aneurysms on data from randomised controlled trials such as these is that none are designed to establish the optimum threshold for intervention.

UKSAT and the ADAM trial successfully established that for a population of patients across a range of ages, fitness, comorbidity levels and even gender that there is no benefit derived from early repair over surveillance while the aneurysm is between 4cm and 5.5cm. These trials were not designed to determine whether the threshold for intervention might be different for younger patients or older patients. They were also not designed to determine whether the threshold for intervention should be different for patients with aneurysms at a higher risk of growth and rupture than patients at a low risk of growth and rupture. In reality, this means that the appropriate threshold for repair for most individuals in these population studies is somewhere between 4cm and 5.5cm. There is evidence to support this argument from the subgroup analysis of UKSAT.

In this subgroup analysis, deaths per 100 person years were highest following early surgery in the oldest subgroup and lowest in the youngest subgroup. For smaller aneurysms in the size range 4–4.4cm, the risk of mortality is lower with surveillance than it is with early surgery. However, for larger aneurysms in the size range 4.9–5.5cm, there is a lower risk of death in those patients randomised to early surgery even though this population includes patients of all ages. Although the study was not powered to address differences in outcomes between these subgroups, the results suggest that the optimal threshold for aneurysm repair is different for individuals within the overall study population. There may be a potential benefit of early surgery in younger patients and those with larger aneurysms with a corresponding benefit of surveillance in older patients and those with smaller aneurysms.[2]

Randomised controlled trials can establish a preferred management strategy for a defined population of patients but will never be the appropriate way to define the optimum threshold for intervention for aneurysms for each individual patient. Even if a well-designed randomised controlled trial that came close to achieving this objective started today, the final results would be reported at least 10 years from now and the cost of the trial would be significant. Therefore, a different approach that optimises the threshold for intervention for aneurysms for each individual patient to ensure that the risk of aneurysm-related mortality is as low as possible should be adopted.

Optimising the threshold for individual patients

The primary aim of elective aneurysm repair is to prevent premature death due to rupture; therefore, any threshold for intervention should minimise the risk of aneurysm-related mortality. For each individual patient, the threshold at which the risk of aneurysm-related mortality is lowest will inevitably vary. To base the current threshold for intervention on a single aneurysm diameter across a population is inevitably suboptimal as it does not take into account the following important patient-specific variables which may influence aneurysm-related survival: i) factors that influence aneurysm growth and risk of rupture ii) factors that influence perioperative mortality and iii) factors that influence long-term survival following elective aneurysm repair.

The current threshold for intervention does not consider aneurysm growth unless it is >5–6mm/year but this is clearly a factor that contributes to when a patient should undergo aneurysm repair. Aneurysm growth and risk of rupture have been shown to be dependent on patient specific factors. The RESCAN collaborators performed a meta-analysis of individual patient from over 15,000 patients with small abdominal aortic aneurysms across 18 studies to investigate factors that influenced aneurysm growth and risk of rupture: aneurysm growth rate was found to be increased in smokers and decreased in patients with diabetes with rupture rates higher in women, current smokers and hypertensive patients.[11]

The risk of postoperative mortality following elective aneurysm repair is also known to vary significantly depending on patient comorbidities and type of repair. A number of models have been developed and validated to predict the risk of postoperative mortality following elective repair.[12] Perhaps the most appropriate prediction model currently available was developed using UK national data and included the following risk factors: type of repair, patient age, gender, cardiac disease, American Society of Anesthesiologists (ASA) grade, previous aortic surgery or stent, raised serum creatinine, abnormal white cell count, abnormal sodium level, abnormal ECG and aneurysm diameter.[13] This model has been shown to have good discrimination and calibration for postoperative mortality on external validation with the predicted risk of postoperative mortality ranging from 0% to 44.3% for individual patients.[14] Long-term survival following elective aneurysm repair has also been shown to vary depending on similar patient characteristics. Even as soon as one year after elective aneurysm repair, differences in survival of 66% have been demonstrated between patients, based on easily available preoperative risk factors.[15]

Not considering the influence of these patient-specific risk factors when deciding on the threshold for intervention for abdominal aortic aneurysms is clearly suboptimal. An algorithm that takes into account all of these factors, the aneurysm repair decision aid (ARDA), has been recently developed.[16] This algorithm combines the modelling approaches for each component of the patient pathway into one system using discrete event simulation. It allows multiple data sources and models to be combined to allow a patient with particular baseline characteristics to be simulated forward in time to predict the risk of a range of aneurysm-related outcomes. Advantages of this approach are that the outputs are patient-specific, multiple outcomes can be considered and different intervention thresholds for each individual patient can be simulated to compare the merits (in terms of a range of outcomes) of the various intervention thresholds. Another key advantage of this approach is that ARDA can and should be updated when new data become available for any parts of the patient pathway, for example if the risk of postoperative mortality falls or population life expectancy increases.

An example of the output from ARDA for a 65-year-old man with a 4cm abdominal aortic aneurysm and no significant risk factors for postoperative mortality is shown in Figure 1. Based on the predicted aneurysm growth rate, this 65-year-old man would take a mean of 5.5 years to reach the current threshold for intervention, with a risk of death due to rupture during that interval of just 1%. The median life expectancy remains largely unchanged if the repair is done at any time between 4cm and 4.5cm with little difference up to an aneurysm diameter of 5.5cm. The predicted in-hospital mortality at the time of repair is under 1% at both 4cm and 5.5cm but rises to 2% if surgery is delayed a mean of eight years until the aneurysm reaches 6.5cm. One-, two-, five- and 10-year survival rates for repair at 4cm and 5cm are almost identical. If the patient does not undergo intervention at any stage the median life expectancy is lowest.

Although this model relies on multiple assumptions and the quality of the data available, it uses easily available risk factors that may influence aneurysm-related outcomes and combines them to allow predicted outcomes for different intervention thresholds to be calculated for each individual patient. It can also be quickly

1a

	AAA repair at						No elective repair
	4.0 cm	4.5 cm	5.0 cm	5.5 cm	6.0 cm	6.5 cm	
Median life expectancy	76.92	76.95	76.87	76.83	76.81	76.68	75.50
1 year survival	0.97	0.97	0.97	0.97	0.97	0.97	0.97
5 year survival	0.83	0.83	0.82	0.83	0.83	0.83	0.83
10 year survival	0.60	0.60	0.60	0.60	0.59	0.58	0.51
Other cause death (prior to repair)	0.00	0.08	0.13	0.19	0.24	0.29	0.53
Death due to rupture	0.00	0.00	0.00	0.01	0.01	0.02	0.38
Rupture survival	0.00	0.00	0.00	0.00	0.00	0.01	0.10
Post-op survival	0.99	0.91	0.86	0.79	0.73	0.67	NA
In-hospital mortality	0.01	0.01	0.01	0.01	0.02	0.02	NA
Growth rate at size	0.24	0.30	0.36	0.42	0.48	0.48	NA
Probability of repair	1.00	0.92	0.87	0.81	0.75	0.69	NA
Median age at repair	65.00	68.00	69.00	70.50	71.75	73.00	NA
Median years to reach size	0.00	3.00	4.00	5.50	6.75	8.00	NA

1b

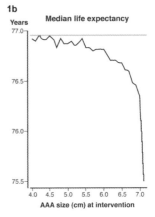

Figure 1: (A) An example of the output from ARDA for a 65-year-old with a 4cm abdominal aortic aneurysm and no significant risk factors for postoperative mortality . Multiple outcomes based on aneurysm repair at different aneurysm diameters or no intervention at all (B) predicted median life expectancy based on intervention at different aneurysm diameters.

adapted to include the most contemporary data from national clinical registries and screening programmes. While an analysis of ARDA suggests that the current threshold for intervention is likely to be appropriate for most patients, particularly those aged over 70 and under 80 years, it will inevitably allow optimisation of the threshold for intervention for a number significant number of patients. At the very least, the ARDA provides the patient and clinician with considerably more patient specific information on aneurysm-related risks and the implications of different management strategies.

Conclusions

The current threshold for intervention for abdominal aortic aneurysm has been largely based on consensus and vascular surgeon opinion, with that judgement confirmed by population studies. Data from randomised controlled trial have established that for a population of patients there is no difference between offering intervention below this threshold over continued surveillance. A single threshold based on aneurysm diameter alone can never be appropriate for individuals of widely ranging age and comorbidities. The threshold for intervention for abdominal aortic aneurysms should be specific for each individual patient and should consider all the relevant risk factors that may influence aneurysm growth rate, risk of rupture and mortality associated with repair. ARDA is one such approach that has significant potential to improve on the current threshold for intervention, particularly for patients who may be excluded from randomised controlled trials. It can also facilitate a patient to reach an informed decision about the threshold for intervention that is most appropriate for them.

Summary

- The current threshold for abdominal aortic aneurysm repair of 5.5cm was initially based on consensus opinion and then confirmed appropriate by data from randomised controlled trials.

- These data are now over 20 years old and an increasing number of patients with abdominal aortic aneurysm now fall outside the original trial inclusion criteria.

- While randomised controlled trials can provide data to support a single threshold for intervention across a wide population, they cannot establish the optimal threshold for individual patients.

- Using contemporary data on individualised risk of surgery, risk or abdominal aortic aneurysm rupture and life expectancy, discrete event simulation modelling can be used to optimise the threshold for intervention for individual patients.

References

1. Powell JT, Greenhalgh RM, Ruckley CV, et al. Prologue to a surgical trial. Lancet 1993; **342**: 1473–74.
2. Powell JT, Brady AR, Brown LC, et al. Mortality results for randomised controlled trial of early elective surgery or ultrasonographic surveillance for small abdominal aortic aneurysms. Lancet 1998; **352** (9141): 1649–55.
3. Lederle FA, Johnson GR, Wilson SE, et al. Immediate repair compared with surveillance of small abdominal aortic aneurysms. N Engl J Med 2002; **346** (19): 1437–44.
4. Powell JT, Brown LC, Forbes JF, et al. Final 12-year follow-up of surgery versus surveillance in the UK small aneurysm trial. Br J Surg, 2007; **94** (6): 702–08.
5. Ballard DJ, Fliardo G, Fowkes G, et al. Surgery for small asymptomatic abdominal aortic aneurysms. Cochrane Database Syst Rev, 2008 (4).
6. Anjum A, von Allmen R, Greenhalgh R, et al. Explaining the decrease in mortality from abdominal aortic aneurysm rupture. Br J Surg, 2012; **99** (5): 637–45.
7. The UK Small Aneurysm Trial Participants. The U.K. small aneurysm trial: Design, methods and progress. Eur J Vasc Endovasc Surg 1995; **9** (1): 42–48.
8. Greenhalgh RM, Brown LC, Epstein D, et al. Endovascular aneurysm repair versus open repair in patients with abdominal aortic aneurysm (EVAR trial 1): randomised controlled trial. Lancet 2005; **365** (9478): 2179–86.
9. Cao P, De Rango P, Verzini F, et al. Comparison of Surveillance Versus Aortic Endografting for Small Aneurysm Repair (CAESAR): Results from a Randomised Trial. Eur J Vasc Endovasc Surg 2011; **41** (1): 13–25.
10. Ouriel K, Clair DG, Kent KC, et al. Endovascular repair compared with surveillance for patients with small abdominal aortic aneurysms. J Vasc Surg 2010; **51**(5): 1081–87.
11. Sweeting MJ, Thompson SG, Brown LC, et al. Meta-analysis of individual patient data to examine factors affecting growth and rupture of small abdominal aortic aneurysms. Br J Surg 2012; **99** (5):655–65.
12. Grant SW, Grayosn AD, Mitchell DC, et al. Evaluation of five risk prediction models for elective abdominal aortic aneurysm repair using the UK National Vascular Database. Br J Surg 2012; **99**(5): 673–79.
13. Grant SW, Hickey GL, Grayson AD, et al. National risk prediction model for elective abdominal aortic aneurysm repair. Br J Surg 2013; **100** (5): 645–53.
14. Grant SW, Hickey GL, Carlson ED, et al. Comparison of Three Contemporary Risk Scores for Mortality Following Elective Abdominal Aortic Aneurysm Repair. Eur J Vasc Endovasc Surg 2014; **48** (1): 38–44.
15. Beck AW, Goodney PP, Nolan BW, et al. Predicting 1-year mortality after elective abdominal aortic aneurysm repair. J Vasc Surg 2009; **49** (4): 838–44.
16. Grant SW, Sperrin M, Carlson E, et al. Calculating when elective abdominal aortic aneurysm repair improves survival for individual patients: development of the Aneurysm Repair Decision Aid and economic evaluation. Health Technol Assess 2015; **19** (32): 1–154.

Abdominal aortic technical challenges

Achieving precise placement, optimal seal and conformability in challenging aortic anatomies

M Shih and R Rhee

Introduction

Endovascular aneurysm repair (EVAR) has revolutionised the care of patients with abdominal aortic aneurysms. Since its introduction by Parodi *et al* in 1991, this disruptive technology has evolved to the point at which the vast majority of aneurysms are now repaired using this approach. The endografts and delivery systems have undergone multiple generations of technological advancement. One of the few remaining challenges that prevents ubiquitous use of this technology is an unfavourable infrarenal aortic neck. In particular, short (<15mm), highly angulated (>60 degrees) necks can threaten long-term exclusion of the aneurysm even with the most modern generation of endografts. Once other facets of a hostile neck are added—for example, calcification, thrombus, or a conical shape—the ability to confidently obtain a proximal seal is greatly decreased.[1–3] However, with the integration of active control technology, namely constrainability and conformability, the boundaries of treating an aneurysm with a hostile neck are continually being pushed.

With constrainable devices, such as the Excluder abdominal aortic aneurysm endoprosthesis with C3 delivery system (Gore) and the Anaconda One-Lok abdominal aortic aneurysm stent graft system (Vascutek), the user has the opportunity to constrain and more importantly, reposition the device after initial deployment. Physician control of the deployment is taken one step further with the new Excluder (Gore) conformable device. This is the first endograft that will allow users to alter the angle of the proximal section of the endoprosthesis and bow the leading edge of the graft to take on the natural angle of the aortic neck.

Constrainability and repositionability

The Excluder endoprosthesis with C3 delivery system and the Anaconda stent graft are unique in the market in that these devices allow the user to constrain and reposition after an initial deployment. This is of utmost benefit in a hostile infrarenal aortic neck where every millimetre of seal is required to achieve favourable long-term results. The precise positioning afforded by this technology allows physicians to more confidently treat aneurysms with less than ideal anatomies.

Most devices on the market mandate a minimum of 10–15mm of normal aorta below the lowest renal artery, and an infrarenal aortic angle to be less than 60 degrees (instructions for use). The short, highly-angulated necks—ones that often fall outside the instructions for use—are where this active control can be most beneficial. Both devices listed have instructions for use that require 15mm of proximal aortic neck. The Excluder is intended for neck angles of less than 60 degrees while the Anaconda has approval for necks of up to 90 degrees.

The C3 Excluder is a third-generation device with a three-step deployment mechanism that allows for up to two repositionings before final deployment[4] (Figure 1) and has demonstrated encouraging early results.[5,6] With the ability to reconstrain and reposition, every millimetre of aorta below the renal arteries can be used for sealing if the device is able to conform to the anatomy. Physicians can be more aggressive in advancing the stent graft cephalad to the ideal position relative to the renal arteries, knowing that an error can be easily corrected.

The European C3 module of the Global Registry for Endovascular Aortic Treatment (GREAT) reported results gathered on 400 real-world patients treated with the C3 Excluder. Seventeen per cent of patients were treated outside the instructions for use, while graft repositioning was performed in 48.1% of the patients.[6] Unplanned use of proximal aortic cuffs was less than 5%, comparing very favourably to previously reported numbers and has been duplicated by other groups.[6–8]

Similar positive results are reported with the Anaconda stent graft. Freyrie *et al* reported on a series of 177 patients treated with the Anaconda system, of which 25% had a neck angle >60 degrees. Repositioning with the constrainable proximal graft was performed in 42% of the patients, with a rate of early and late type Ia endoleak of 1.1%.[9]

Additionally, the ability to reposition and redeploy gives endografts advantages beyond precision at the proximal neck. The repositionable trunks allow for altering the level and orientation of the contralateral gate as well. This can greatly facilitate gate cannulation, especially in large open aneurysm sacs or with very tortuous iliac vessels, or even when these grafts are used as a secondary intervention for treating previously migrated grafts. Lastly, the reconstrainable grafts are ideal in the teaching environment. They provide fellows and residents the opportunity to

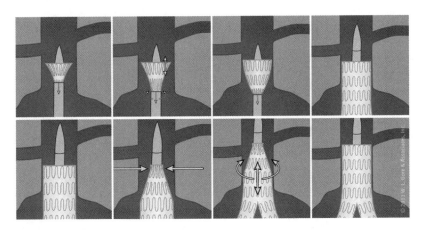

Figure 1: The C3 Excluder can be constrained, repositioned, and redeployed for optimal placement.

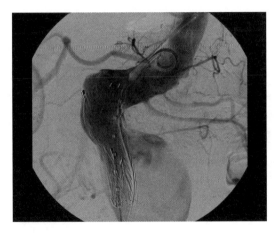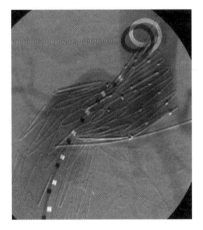

Figure 2: Placement of a standard endograft in a highly angulated aorta can result in poor wall apposition or "bird-beaking".

have the hands-on experience needed to become familiar with the devices, without having to sacrifice patient safety.

Conformability

Current abdominal aortic aneurysm endografts are designed for use in a straight, uniform proximal neck. In highly angulated necks, tight wall apposition is often unattainable with rigid devices (Figure 2). Most devices are approved up to 60 degrees, and a small fraction has US Food and Drug Administration approval for up to 90 degrees. A highly angulated neck translates to high rates of type I endoleaks and secondary interventions[3] to the point where some physicians simply will not offer an endovascular repair. Clearly there are drawbacks to having this form of a hostile neck anatomy, and it is an area open for improvement in endograft technology. Current management of these highly angulated necks include additional ballooning, proximal cuffs, balloon expandable stents, endoanchors, chimney/snorkels, or use of fenestrated grafts. None of the techniques are optimal, and all have individual and very real drawbacks.

The next generation of infrarenal endografts to specifically address these issues should ideally be engineered with the capability of actively angulating and conforming the proximal end of the graft to the native aortic anatomy prior to final deployment. The Excluder conformable abdominal aortic aneurysm endoprosthesis (Figure 3) is the first device designed to conform and adjust to the natural anatomy of the individual patient. Combined with the capabilities of the C3 delivery system, the device can be constrained, repositioned, and angulated to take the natural turns of the aortic neck. This gives the physician the ability to perfectly align the leading edge of the graft perpendicular to the flow lumen. With this orthogonal placement, wall apposition is maximised. In practice, this translates to maximising the seal length and improved fixation, and in turn, the potential for better long-term results. These results will be verified as the device is set to undergo an investigational device exemption clinical trial in the USA and in Japan.

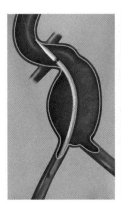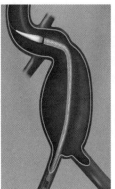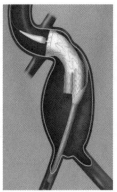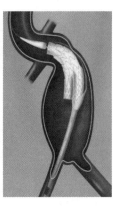

Figure 3: The Excluder conformable device can be manipulated to take on neck angulation for orthogonal placement of the endograft.

Conclusion

Precise deployment of an abdominal aortic endoprosthesis is of the utmost importance in achieving short- and long-term success of aneurysm exclusion. This is particularly true when a hostile neck is encountered. Newer generations of endoprostheses provide options to constrain and reposition, allowing for greater likelihood of maximising the seal zone. The Excluder conformable endoprosthesis now allows the user to actively angulate the device *in situ*, thereby extending the limits of active control technology. These attributes will give physicians the means to maximise the proximal seal zone and therefore more effectively stabilise the infrarenal aortic neck for the best long-term success for EVAR treatment.

Summary

- Reconstrainable devices allow for repositioning of the stent graft if initial deployment is less than perfect.

- Conformable devices allow for angulation of the stent graft to match the aortic neck and deliver the graft in line with the direction of flow.

- These active controls of the deployment of newer generation endografts allow for optimal placement of the devices, particularly in hostile anatomies.

References

1. Antoniou GA, Georgiadis GS, Antoniou SA, *et al*. A meta-analysis of outcomes of endovascular abdominal aortic aneurysm repair in patients with hostile and friendly neck anatomy. *J Vasc Surg* 2013; **57** (2): 527–538.

2. Hager ES, Cho JS, Makaroun MS, *et al*. Endografts with suprarenal fixation do not perform better than those with infrarenal fixation in the treatment of patients with short straight proximal aortic necks. *J Vasc Surg* 2012; **55** (5): 1242–6.

3. Hobo R, Kievit J, Leurs LJ, Buth J; EUROSTAR Collaborators. Influence of severe infrarenal aortic neck angulation on complications at the proximal neck following endovascular AAA repair: a EUROSTAR study. *J Endovasc Ther 2007*; **14** (1): 1–11.

4. Verhoeven EL, Oikonomou K, Mohner B, *et al;* European C3 Global Registry participants. First experience with the new repositionable C3 excluder stent-graft. *J Cardiovasc Surg* 2011; **52** (5): 637–642.

5. Katsargyris A, Botos B, Oikonomou K, *et al*. The new C3 gore excluder stent-graft: single-center experience with 100 patients. *Eur J Vasc Endovasc Surg* 2014; **47** (4): 342–8.
6. Verhoeven EL, Katsargyris A, Bachoo P, *et al;* GREAT European C3 Module Investigators. Real-world performance of the new C3 Gore excluder stent-graft: 1-year results from the European C3 module of the global registry for endovascular aortic treatment (GREAT). *Eur J Vasc Endovasc Surg* 2014; **48** (2): 131–7.
7. AbuRahma AF, Campbell JE, Mousa AY, *et al*. Clinical outcomes for hostile *versus* favorable aortic neck anatomy in endovascular aortic aneurysm repair using modular devices. *J Vasc Surg* 2011; 54(1): 13–21.
8. Smeds MR, Jacobs DL, Peterson GJ, Peterson BG. . Short-term outcomes of the C3 excluder for patients with abdominal aortic aneurysms and unfavorable proximal aortic seal zones. *Ann Vasc Surg* 2013; **27** (1): 8–15.
9. Freyrie A, Gallitto E, Gargiulo M, *et al*. Results of the endovascular abdominal aortic aneurysm repair using the Anaconda aortic endograft. *J Vasc Surg* 2014; **60** (5): 1132–9.

The clinical need for an iliac-branched endoprosthesis

SMM van Sterkenburg, JW Lardenoije, CJ Zeebregts and MMPJ Reijnen

Introduction

Since the introduction of less invasive endovascular treatment options, open repair of abdominal aortic aneurysms has been almost abandoned, especially in straightforward cases.[1] The lower immediate postoperative morbidity and 30-day mortality rates following endovascular aneurysm repair (EVAR)[2] are an inspiration for expanding this technique to more challenging anatomies. One of the challenges is in extending the endograft across side branches, such as visceral and iliac arteries and maintaining patency at the same time. In patients with an ectatic common iliac artery up to 20mm in diameter, a standard EVAR procedure can be performed. Even diameters up to 24mm can be treated with newly designed flared legs, with a low incidence of iliac artery related secondary interventions (5%) at 24-month follow-up.[3]

The incidence of isolated common iliac artery aneurysms of more than 20mm in diameter is rare, but approximately 20–40% of aneurysm cases frequently involve a combination of an abdominal aortic aneurysm and isolated common iliac artery aneurysm.[4,5] Conceptually, two different strategies can be applied to treat a common iliac artery aneurysm using an endovascular approach while maintaining perfusion of the external iliac artery, including (1) coverage and (2) preservation of blood flow to the internal iliac artery. Both strategies have specific advantages and disadvantages in terms of morbidity, reintervention rates, complexity, and costs.

Coverage of the internal iliac artery

Overstenting, and thus covering the orifice, of the internal iliac artery was initially the only way to treat extensive aorto-iliac aneurysmal disease. Nowadays, this technique is only applied to patients with unsuitable distal common iliac artery neck length (<15mm). Two different strategies can be used to cover the internal iliac artery. The easiest way is to overstent the artery through a patent internal iliac artery, without the stent coiling and associated risk of persistent endoleak. Neither Wyers et al[6] nor Stokmans et al[7] experienced endoleaks or reinterventions in a retrospective analysis of their series of patients that were treated with this strategy. In particular, overstenting of the internal iliac artery can be performed safely in patients with adequate sealing zone in the proximal common iliac artery and, therefore, less risk of progressive aortic dilatation due to internal iliac artery type II endoleak. Intentional occlusion of the internal iliac artery, with coils or

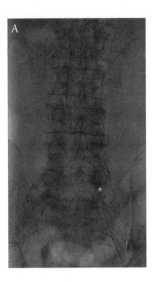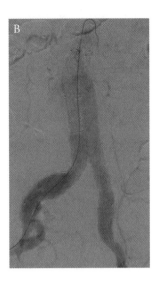

Figure 1: (A) Fluoroscopy and (B) angiography of a patient treated with a right-sided Endurant bell bottom limb (Medtronic).

plugs, is considered a safe method to avoid endoleaks. The positioning of coils or an Amplatzer plug (St Jude Medical) in the primary segmental internal iliac artery is preferred above a more distal placement.[8] The reported complications of covering the artery (especially if both internal iliac arteries are covered) include buttock claudication (with an incidence of 16–55%), erectile dysfunction (with an incidence of 10–46%), and the even more devastating complications colonic or spinal cord ischaemia (with incidence of less than 0.1%).[4,8–11] In a systematic review, buttock claudication was found in 31% of patients who underwent unilateral and in 35% with bilateral embolisation.[9] New onset erectile dysfunction was reported in 17% in the unilateral and 24% in the bilateral embolised patients. Verzini *et al*[9] reported, in a comparative analysis, that the incidence of endoleak and buttock claudication was higher after internal iliac artery embolisation compared with the use of an artery-preserving Zenith iliac branch device (Cook Medical) device (both 19% vs. 4%, respectively).

Internal iliac artery preserving techniques

Several internal iliac artery-preserving techniques have been applied, including open approaches with inclusion of the artery into the distal anastomosis, reimplantation of the artery or the use of an additional bypass to the artery. Hybrid techniques combining an open and endovascular approach may also be used but these techniques are outside the scope of this chapter. Several endovascular internal iliac artery-preserving techniques exist, which will be discussed hereafter.

Bell-bottom technique

In case of an ectatic common iliac artery with a diameter of 18–30mm, complete exclusion of the abdominal aortic aneurysm can be established with preservation of the internal iliac artery when using a bell-bottom limb (Figure 1). By using distal extension grafts with relatively large diameters in the distal common iliac artery, the flow through the internal iliac artery flow can be preserved. An adequate sealing zone of at least 1.5cm just proximal of the origin of the internal iliac artery with a maximum common iliac artery diameter of 24mm is a prerequisite. Kritpacha *et*

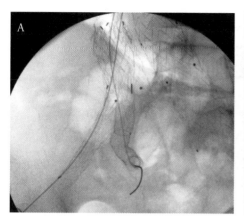
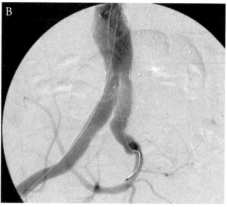

Figure 2: (A) Fluoroscopy and (B) angiography of a patient treated with a trifurcated endograft technique using two Excluder endografts (Gore) on the right side.

al were the first to describe the short-term results of a series of 25 patients treated with the Aneurx graft (n=17) (Medtronic) or the Vanguard graft (n=8) (Boston Scientific).[10] There were no type I endoleaks and the internal iliac artery could be successfully preserved using a flared distal cuff. The three-year results of 21 patients, published by Marcos *et al*, showed no type I endoleaks and an endoleak-free survival and reintervention-free survival comparable with a control group of regular EVAR patients (with the Excluder device, Gore).[11] They concluded that the bell-bottom technique is a feasible and safe alternative for preserving internal iliac artery blood flow, and it does not imply a higher risk of reintervention or endoleak. In a larger series, described by Naughton *et al*, 185 patients with 260 common iliac artery aneurysms were studied. A bell-bottom technique was used in 166 and coil and coverage in the remaining 94 patients. Reinterventions and perioperative complications were significantly higher in the coil and coverage group and, therefore, the authors concluded that the bell bottom technique is preferable.[12] Comparable five-year results were published by the group of Torsello in a subset of patients with moderate-sized common iliac artery <30mm.[13]

Homemade options and outside instructions for use techniques

Different techniques have been described with the use of endografts in an off-label situation, but all were small case series with a short follow-up. Van der Steenhoven *et al* described the upside-down technique using an Excluder iliac limb. After an extracorporeal deployment of the graft, the graft is re-sheathed upside down and deployed in the common iliac artery.[14] Oderich *et al* presented three cases in which a polyester side graft was hand sewn on a standard iliac stent that was re-sheathed in a 20Fr sheath and then used as an iliac branched prosthesis.[15] Minion et al[16] have described the trifurcated endograft technique in which a second bifurcated endoprosthesis is deployed into an iliac limb to create a three-limbed graft. The third limb is then used as the origin for an extension into one hypogastric artery (Figure 2). Another option is the use of parallel or chimney grafts using flexible stent grafts such as the Viabahn (Gore). The iliac leg endografts and the chimney grafts are in a parallel fashion positioned from proximal aortic to distal iliac landing zones, always preserving antegrade flow to at least one internal iliac artery.[17]

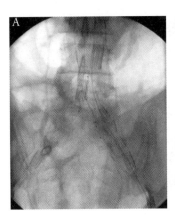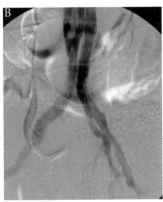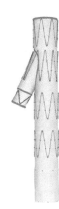

Figure 3: (A) Fluoroscopy and (B) angiography of a patient treated with a Zenith iliac branch device (Cook) on the left side. Still image of the (C) Zenith iliac branch device.

Using another technique, described by Friedman,[18] a Powerlink bifurcated graft (Endologix) was deployed and via the contralateral side a Viabahn was positioned in the internal iliac artery, parallel to the iliac limb in the external iliac artery from the ipsilateral side. Both the internal and external iliac artery limbs were parallel positioned in the iliac branch of the main device. A crossover chimney technique in patients with aorto-iliac aneurysms and especially isolated common iliac artery is also an option with the advantage of only femoral access.[19] As an alternative, a technique has been described wherein a contralateral aorto-uni-iliac device was used in conjunction with a femoral-femoral crossover bypass. The aneurysm was then occluded with a proximal plug in the ipsilateral common iliac artery and flow in the internal iliac artery was preserved through an endograft from the external to the internal iliac artery; a technique referred to as the banana technique.[20]

Endovascular sealing of aneurysm, using the Nellix endovascular aneurysm sealing (EVAS) system (Endologix), is a novel technique for abdominal aortic aneurysm exclusion that could also be applied in common iliac artery aneurysms. The technique consists of balloon-expandable endoframes surrounded by endobags that are filled *in situ* with solidifying polymer, thus sealing the aneurysm. The distal 8mm of the stents are bare and can be positioned across the orifice of the internal iliac artery preserving flow, while the endobag seals the common iliac artery aneurysm.[21]

Branched endografts

In the last two decades, a number of improvements to commercially available endografts have been implemented, not only at the site of the proximal end to accommodate challenging infrarenal aortic necks, but also at the distal site to cope with aneurismal iliac disease. The Zenith iliac side branched device was the first dedicated device to preserve flow through the internal iliac artery (Figure 3). Chuter *et al* were the first to start with a surgeon-modified small standard main body,[22] and the initial results of a commercially available custom-made endograft were published three years later in 2006.[23,24] Initially, the iliac branched device experience was merely based on the Zenith system. The first iliac branched device in the market was a straight side-branch device that had to be pulled into the internal iliac artery. The system was further developed into the Zenith bifurcated

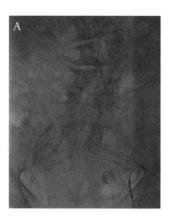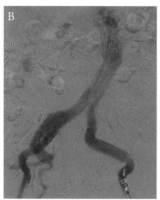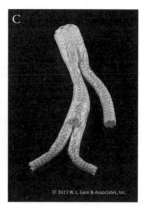

Figure 4: (A) Fluoroscopy and (B) angiography of a patient treated with an Excluder iliac branch endoprosthesis (Gore) on the right side. (C) Still image of the Excluder iliac branch endoprosthesis.

iliac side branch device and the helical branch endograft, which were used in combination with Advanta V12 (Atrium Maquet) or Fluency PLUS (Bard Medical) covered stent-grafts inserted in the internal iliac artery. These two endografts were used in a study published by Parlani et al[25] in which 100 consecutive patients were enrolled in a prospective database. The procedural success rate was 95% and after a median follow-up period of 21 months, two distal type I endoleaks occurred. The estimated patency of internal iliac branch was 91% at one year. Karthikesalingsam et al[26] published a systematic analysis of nine studies including seven series and 196 patients. Technical success varied between 85% and 100%. Occlusion of the treated internal iliac artery occurred immediately after operation in six patients (3.1%), at <30 days in 11 patients (5.6%) and during follow-up in seven patients (3.6%). In these 24 patients, 50% experienced buttock claudication. The reintervention rate was rather low, occurring in only 12 patients (6%). One of the drawbacks in iliac branched device grafting with the Zenith graft is the anatomic criteria to be met. For instance, a proximal common iliac diameter of more than 18mm, excessive tortuosity and severe access stenosis exclude a patient for use of the iliac branched device. Tielliu *et al* observed in a cohort of 52 patients with common iliac artery that only 27 (52%) met the anatomical criteria as listed in the instructions for use.[27] As stated in the latest instructions for use, the iliac/femoral access must be compatible with a 20Fr introduction system. A non-aneurysmal external iliac artery fixation segment distal to the aneurysm is necessary with a length of at least 20mm and with a diameter measured outer wall to outer wall of no greater than 11mm and no less than 8mm. Also, a non-aneurysmal internal iliac artery segment distal to the aneurysm with a length of at least 10mm (with 20–30mm being preferred) is mandatory and with a diameter acceptable for proper sealing.

More recently, the Excluder iliac branch endoprosthesis was introduced, based on the Excluder platform (Figure 4). In contrast to the iliac branched device, in the iliac branch endoprosthesis, a dedicated internal iliac component was added. The low profile of this device (16Fr introducer sheath) offers a good alternative in case of a narrow access but also a tortuous iliac system. The high flexibility of the main body, the possibility of easy repositioning, and the precanulation of the iliac side branch with an indwelling guidewire from the contralateral side, are new in relation to other prostheses. Anatomical limitations (instructions for use) include a common iliac artery diameter of at least 17mm proximal of the implantation zone of the iliac branch endoprosthesis, a diameter range of 6.5–25mm of the external iliac artery and 6.5–13.5mm of the internal iliac artery. A distal sealing zone in the internal iliac artery of 10mm is required, but there is no limitation regarding the length of the common iliac artery. A minimal distance of 165mm between the lowest renal artery and the iliac bifurcation is required.

Initial results with the iliac branch endoprosthesis device were reported by Ferrer *et al* in 2014 in five patients.[28] Technical success and iliac branch patency was 100%. One reintervention was necessary concerning a narrow aortic bifurcation. Schonhofer et al[29] also showed a technical success rate of 100% in 15 patients. During nine months of follow-up, there was a 100% patency, no type I or III endoleaks, and the reintervention rate, buttock claudication rate and pelvic complication rates were 0%. We recently described a retrospective cohort analysis of 46 patients with 51 common iliac artery aneurysms that were treated with the iliac branch endoprosthesis device in 13 sites in The Netherlands.[30] The mean diameter of the treated aneurysm was 41.7±10.6mm. All but one implantations were successful; two type Ib endoleaks were reported, which both spontaneously disappeared <30 days, resulting in a procedural success rate of 93.5%. After a mean follow-up of six months, the mean common iliac artery aneurysm diameter significantly decreased (42.4±7.2mm vs. 38.4±7.5mm; p<0.001). Reinterventions were performed in two patients (7.1%) and the primary patency of the internal component was 94%.

Conclusion

Although the incidence of complications after internal iliac artery coverage may be acceptable, the consequences of buttock claudication and erectile dysfunction may be severe and can have a significant impact on daily life, especially in the young and active patients. Internal iliac artery preservation, therefore, seems to be indicated at least at one side and potentially bilateral in young and active patients. Various techniques are available for preservation of the internal iliac artery. When feasible, the use of a bell-bottom technique is likely to be most cost-effective. As an alternative, commercially-available branched devices can be used with good results. When these are not available or anatomically unsuitable alternative techniques have been successfully applied.

Summary

- The incidence of buttock claudication and erectile dysfunction, due to embolisation and/or overstenting of the internal iliac artery, is underestimated.

- Especially in the young and active elderly patient, preservation of at least one of the internal iliac artery seems to be indicated.

- With the use of new developed dedicated branched endografts, challenging common iliac artery aneurysms can be treated with good results within the instructions for use of the devices.

- In more complex cases, in countries without access to iliac branched devices, or outside instructions for use, techniques can be safely applied.

References

1. Parodi JC, Palmaz JC, Barone HD. Transfemoral intraluminal graft implantation for abdominal aortic aneurysms. *Ann Vasc Surg* 1991; **5**: 491–99.

2. Paravastu SCV, Jayarayasingam R, Cottam R, *et al*. Endovascular repair of abdominal aortic aneurysm. Cochrane Database Syst Rev 2014; **1**: CD004178.

3. Timaran CH, Lipsitz EC, Veith FJ, *et al*. Endovascular aortic aneurysm repair with the Zenith endograft in patients with ectatic iliac arteries. *Ann Vasc Surg* 2005; **19**: 161–66.

4. Richardson JW, Greenfield LJ. Natural history and management of iliac aneurysms. *J Vasc Surg* 1988; **8**; 165–71.

5. Hobo R, Sybrandy JEM, Harris PL, Buth J, on behalf of the EUROSTAR Collaborators. Endovascular repair of abdominal aortic aneurysms with concomitant common iliac artery aneurysm: outcome analysis of the EUROSTAR experience. *J Endovasc Ther* 2008; **15**: 12–22.

6. Wyers MC, Schermerhorn ML, Fillinger MF. Internal iliac occlusion without coil embolization during endovascular abdominal aortic aneurysm repair. *J Vasc Surg* 2002; **36**: 1138–45.

7. Stokmans RA, Willigendael EM, Teijink JA, *et al*. Challenging the evidence for pre-emptive coil embolisation of the internal iliac artery during endovascular aneurysm repair. *Eur J Vasc Endovasc Surg* 2013; **45**: 220–26.

8. Cynamon J, Lerer D, Veith FJ, *et al*. Hypogastric artery coil embolization prior to endoluminal repair of the aneurysms and fistulas: buttock claudication, a recognized but possible preventable complication. *J Vasc Interv Radiol* 2000; **11**: 573–77.

9. Verzini F, Gianbattista P, Romano L, *et al*. Endovascular treatment of iliac aneurysm: Concurrent comparison of side branch endograft *versus* hypogastric exclusion. *J Vasc Surg* 2009; **49**: 1154–61.

10. Kritpacha B, Pigott JP, Russel Todd E, *et al*, Bell-bottom aortoiliac endografts: An alternative that preserves pelvic blood flow.*J Vasc Surg* 2002; **35**: 878–81.

11. Marcos FA, de la Torre AG, Perez MA, *et al*. Use of Aortic Extension Cuffs for Preserving Hypogastric Blood Flow in Endovascular Aneurysm Repair With Aneurysmal Involvement of Common Iliac Arteries. *Ann Vasc Surg* 2013; **27**: 139–45.

12. Naughton PA, Park MS, Kheilrelseid EA, *et al*. A comparative study of the bell-bottom technique vs hypogastric exclusion for the treatment of aneurysmal extension to the iliac bifurcation. *J Vas Surg* 2012; **55**: 956–62.

13. Torsello G, Schonefeld E, Osada N, *et al*. Endovascular treatment of common iliac artery aneurysms using the bell-bottom technique: long-term results. *J Endovasc Ther* 2010; **17**: 504–09.

14. van der Steenhoven TJ, Heyligers JMM, Tielliu IFJ, Zeebregts CJ. The upside-down Gore Excluder contralateral leg without extracorporeal predeployment for aortic or iliac aneurysm exclusion. *J Vasc Surg* 2011; **53**: 1738–41.

15. Oderich GS, Ricotta JJ. Novel surgeon modified hypogastric branch stent graft to preserve pelvic perfusion. *Ann Vasc Surg* 2010; **24**: 278–86.

16. Minion DJ, Xenos E, Sorial E, *et al*. The trifurcated endograft technique for hypogastric preservation during endovascular aneurysm repair. *J Vasc Surg* 2008; **47**: 658–61.

17. Lepidi S, Piazza M, Scrivere P, *et al*. Parallel Endografts in the Treatment of Distal Aortic and Common Iliac Aneurysms. *Eur J Vasc Endovasc Surg* 2014 ; **48**: 29–37.

18. Friedman SG,Wun H. Hypogastric preservation with viabahn stent graft during endovascular aneurysm repair. *J Vasc Surg* 2011; **54**: 504–06.

19. Wu IH, Chou HW, Chang CH. Crossover chimney technique to preserve the internal iliac artery during endovascular repair of iliac or aortoiliac aneurysms: midterm results. *J Endovasc Ther*. 2015; **22**: 388–95.

20. Van Groenendael L, Zeebregts CJ, Verhoeven ELG, *et al*. External-to internal iliac artery endografting for the exclusion of iliac artery aneurysms; an alternative technique with the reservation of pelvic flow. *Cath Cardiovasc Interv* 2009; **73**: 156–60.

21. Ter Mors TG, van Sterkenburg SM, van den Ham LH, *et al*. Common Iliac Artery Aneurysm Repair Using a Sac-Anchoring Endograft to Preserve the Internal Iliac Artery. *J Endovasc Ther* 2015; **22**: 886–88.

22. Abraham CZ, Reilly LM, Schneider DB, *et al*. A modular multibranched system for endovascular repair of bilateral common iliac artery aneurysms. *J Endovasc Ther* 2003; **10**: 203–07.

23. Malina M, Dirven M, Sonesson B, *et al*. Feasibility of a branched stent-graft in common iliac artery aneurysms. *J Endovasc Ther* 2006; **13**: 496–500.

24. Greenberg RK, West K, Pfaff K,et al. Beyond the aortic bifurcation: branched endovascular grafts for thoracoabdominal and aortoiliac aneurysms. *J Vasc Surg* 2006; **43**: 879–86.

25. Parlani G, Verzini F, De Rango, *et al*. Long term results of iliac aneurysm repair with iliac branched endograft: a 5-year experience on 100 consecutive cases. *Eur J Vasc Endovasc Surg* 2012; **3**: 287–92.

26. Karthikesalingsam A, Hinchliffe RJ, Holt PJ, *et al*. Endovascular aneurysm repair with preservation of the internal iliac artery using the iliac branch graft device. *Eur J Vasc Endovasc Surg* 2010; **39**: 285–94.

27. Tielliu IF, Bos WT, Zeebregts CJ, *et al*. The role of branched endografts in preserving internal iliac arteries. *J Cardiovasc Surg* (Torino)2009; **50**: 213–18.

28. Ferrer C, de Creescendo F, Coscarella *et al*. Early experience with the Excluder iliac branch endoprothesis. *J Cardiovasc Surg* 2014; **55**: 679–83.

29. Schönhofer S, Mansour R, Ghotbi R. Initial results of the management of aortoiliac aneurysms with GORE® Excluder® Iliac Branched Endoprosthesis. *J Cardiovasc Surg* 2015; **56**: 883–88.

30. van Sterkenburg, SM, Heyligers JM, Van Bladel M, *et al*. Early experience with the GORE® EXCLUDER® Iliac Branch Endoprosthesis for common iliac artery aneurysms in the Netherlands. *J Vasc Surg*, in press.

Type Ia endoleak and the use of EndoAnchors for the failing endograft

RC Schuurmann and J-PPM de Vries

Introduction

Complications at the proximal aortic neck remain one of the challenges of endovascular aneurysm repair (EVAR). The incidence of intraoperative proximal type I endoleaks, seen at the completion angiogram is quite substantial.[1] During an average of eight years follow-up, about 2.5% of EVAR patients are diagnosed with a type Ia endoleak.[2] Challenging aortic (neck) morphology has often been associated with an increased risk for this type of endoleak, impairing adequate fixation and sealing of the stent graft in the infrarenal neck.

Challenging aortic neck anatomy

Short neck length (<17mm), large diameter (>26mm), mural calcium >2mm in thickness or >180 degrees in circumference, infrarenal neck angulation >60 degrees, large aneurysm sac diameter (>55-65mm), and calcium load >2mm or >180 degrees in circumference, have been associated with neck-related complications, where neck thrombus seems to be protective for sealing failures.[3-9] Recently, Schuurmann and colleagues identified aortic curvature (>21-28m-1), determined over the juxtarenal aortic neck, aneurysm sac and terminal aorta, respectively, as a new risk factor for intraoperative type Ia endoleak.[9]

Morphological characteristics that may cause early sealing problems are likely to be different from neck features that are associated with late failure. The approach route over the iliac arteries, distal aorta and aneurysm itself may account for asymmetrical position, and thus tilt the stent graft, causing intraoperative or early postoperative complications.[3,6,9] Extensive calcification and short neck length may impair adequate fixation of the stent graft in the neck, and may also result in acute problems.[3,4,7,9] In the long term, progressive neck dilatation in combination with initial short or conical necks may increase the risk for migration and for type Ia endoleak.[8,10] It must be argued that sealing failure would lead to repressurisation of the aneurysm, and the risk for aneurysm rupture and death. In other patients, hostile neck characteristics may contraindicate the use of EVAR, which is undesirable in medically compromised patients.

Heli-FX endoanchor system

The Heli-FX endoanchor system (Medtronic) is designed to increase the migration resistance of the endograft in the aortic neck, and may be considered as a prophylactic tool to fixate the endograft in challenging necks, or as a means to treat proximal neck complications.[11] The EndoAnchors are helical wires of a metallic alloy measuring 0.5mm in thickness, 3mm in diameter and 4.5mm in length. The EndoAnchor system consists of two main components: an applier and a steerable sheath. The deflectable tip of the steerable sheath comes in a variety of lengths to facilitate accurate deployment in all anatomies, and in different aortic and endograft diameters. Each EndoAnchor needs to be loaded into the applier before implantation. By applying four to six EndoAnchors in most of the commercially available endografts, the increased migration resistance is similar to that of a hand-sewn anastomosis.[12]

The ANCHOR registry

The ANCHOR registry (aneurysm treatment using the Heli-FX Aortic Securement System global registry) is a prospective, multicentre registry of the real-world use of EndoAnchors in patients undergoing or who have undergone EVAR.[13,14] To date, >600 patients have been included in the ANCHOR trial in >70 trial centres in the USA and Europe. The final goal is to recruit 2,000 patients with five-year follow-up including core-lab analysis. EndoAnchors are also registered for thoracic endovascular aortic repair (TEVAR) and the aim is to include around 200 TEVAR patients in the ANCHOR registry.

In a recent publication, 242 patients (75.9%) had EndoAnchors implantated at time of the initial EVAR procedure as a prophylactic means to avoid potential proximal neck complications or treat acute type Ia endoleaks (primary group). Seventy-seven patients had EndoAnchor treatment for proximal neck complications (type Ia endoleaks and/or migration) during revision surgery (revision group). The primary group was subdivided into patients with hostile proximal neck anatomy (178), patients with intraoperative type Ia endoleaks (60), and patients with extender cuffs after unsatisfactory endograft deployment distally in the neck (4). The revision group was subdivided into patients presenting with type Ia endoleak alone (45), endograft migration alone (11), or a combination of migration and endoleak (21). On average, 5.8±2.1 EndoAnchors were deployed in all patients. Most patients had one or more challenging neck characteristics. The average neck length of all patients included in the ANCHOR registry was 16±13mm, neck diameter 27±4mm, max aneurysm diameter 58±13mm, suprarenal angulation 27±4 degrees and infrarenal angulation 24±15 degrees. Neck thrombus was present in 33.2% of patients, and neck calcification in 40.2% of patients.

Initial technical success in the primary arm was 96.6% for prophylactic use and 98% to treat acute type Ia endoleaks. Figure 1 shows an example of the use of EndoAnchors to treat an acute type IA endoleak in a 76-year-old male patient with a challenging neck (short and angulated). In the revision group, technical success was >90% for all three subgroups. Persistent type Ia endoleaks were seen in a minority of the patients.[13] Interestingly, 75% of patients with persistent type Ia endoleaks in the revision group will not undergo renewed (endovascular) reinterventions, most probably because there are no other bail-out options, or because they are at high risk for surgical conversion. During an average follow-up of 16±5 months, 61 (19.1%) adverse events were reported, resulting in 22 (6.9%) aneurysm-related reinterventions and seven (2%) EndoAnchor-related reinterventions. Out of 202 available imaging follow-up studies, with an average of 7.1±5.6 months follow-up,

19 (10%) reported persistent type Ia endoleaks and none reported migrations. During one-year follow up, sac regression (>5mm) was observed in 39% of the patients and sac enlargement (>5mm) was observed in only 2% of cases. The prophylaxis subgroup showed excellent results: no intraoperative type Ia endoleaks, 4% aneurysm-related reinterventions, no EndoAnchor-related reinterventions, 4% late type IA endoleaks and no endograft migration during follow-up.

Tips and tricks to improve EndoAnchor results

Preoperative planning is crucial for technical success regarding the use of the EndoAnchors. It is important to avoid spicule of thrombus and calcified rims remaining in the aortic wall, as they may hinder adequate penetration. During EndoAnchor implantation, the C-arm should be perpendicular to the tip of the Heli-FX endoguide. Pre-EVAR evaluation of the ideal C-arm angulation can be of help during the procedure. Moreover, the tip of the Heli-FX applier must be pushed towards the endograft to allow apposition of the endograft to the aortic wall, during penetration of the endoanchors. The tip of the Heli-FX endoguide should not be undersized with respect to the diameter of the endograft. Another

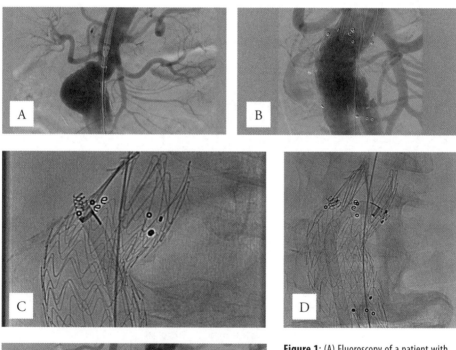

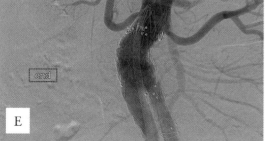

Figure 1: (A) Fluoroscopy of a patient with a short (10mm) and angulated (74 degrees infrarenal angulation) aortic neck. (B) Type Ia endoleak after implantation of a 36mm extender cuff. (C) Targeted implantation of EndoAnchors at the outer curve of the aorta in the proximal part of the cuff. (D) Implantation of EndoAnchors at the contralateral aortic wall to increase migration resistance. (E) Disappearance of the type IA endoleak at the final aniography.

reason not to undersize the endoguide is to avoid any wiggling of the EndoAnchors during deployment. The average learning curve with the device is three to four patients. In case of treatment of a migrated endograft, it is preferred to first secure the primary endograft to the remaining aortic neck before implantation of an extender cuff. If the primary endograft is not secured with endoanchors, the risk of persistent migration and, thus, type III endoleaks, is high.

Conclusion

Hostile neck criteria are associated with substantial early and late aortic neck-related complications, such as migration and type Ia endoleak. The use of endoanchors is a safe and useful adjunct to overcome acute and late type Ia endoleaks. Moreover, the implantation of four to six endoanchors will increase the migration resistance substantially, and can rival a hand-sewn anastomosis. The Heli-FX aortic securement system is intuitive with a short learning curve.

Summary

- Type Ia endoleaks and migration are associated with challenging aortic neck characteristics.

- The Heli-FX aortic securement system can be safely used for treatment of acute and late type Ia endoleaks with high technical success rates

- Implantation of four to six endoanchors rivals the migration resistance of hand-sewn anastomosis.

- Seventy-five per cent of the ANCHOR patients with persistent type Ia endoleaks will not undergo renewed interventions.

- The ANCHOR registry gathers the real word usage of endoanchors in EVAR and TEVAR patients with challenging aortic necks, and will have five years of core-lab follow-up.

References

1. Millen AM, Osman K, Antoniou G a, *et al*. Outcomes of persistent intraoperative type Ia endoleak after standard endovascular aneurysm repair. *J Vasc Surg* 2015; **61**: 1185–91.
2. Brown LC, Powell JT, Thompson SG, *et al*. The UK EndoVascular Aneurysm Repair (EVAR) trials: randomised trials of EVAR *versus* standard therapy. *Health Technol Assess* 2012; **16**: 1–218.
3. Boult M, Babidge W, Maddern G, *et al*. Predictors of success following endovascular aneurysm repair: mid-term results. *Eur J Vasc Endovasc Surg* 2006; **31**: 123–29.
4. Leurs LJ, Kievit J, Dagnelie PC, *et al*. Influence of infrarenal neck length on outcome of endovascular abdominal aortic aneurysm repair. *J Endovasc Ther* 2006; **13**: 640–48.
5. Hobo R, Kievit J, Leurs LJ, *et al*. Influence of severe infrarenal aortic neck angulation on complications at the proximal neck following endovascular AAA repair: a EUROSTAR study. *J Endovasc Ther* 2007; **14**: 1–11.
6. Wyss TR, Dick F, Brown LC, *et al*. The influence of thrombus, calcification, angulation, and tortuosity of attachment sites on the time to the first graft-related complication after endovascular aneurysm repair. *J Vasc Surg* 2011; **54**: 965–71.
7. Bastos Goncalves F, Hoeks SE, Teijink JA, *et al*. Risk factors for proximal neck complications after endovascular aneurysm repair using the endurant stentgraft. *Eur J Vasc Endovasc Surg* 2015; **49**: 156–62.
8. Jordan WD jr, Ouriel K, Mehta M, *et al*. Outcome-based anatomic criteria for defining the hostile aortic neck. *J Vasc Surg* 2015; **61**: 1383–90.
9. Schuurmann RCL, Ouriel K, Muhs BE, *et al*. Aortic Curvature as a Predictor of Intraoperative Type IA Endoleak. *J Vasc Surg* 2015; In Press.

10. Bastos Gonçalves F, Jairam A, Voûte MT, *et al*. Clinical outcome and morphologic analysis after endovascular aneurysm repair using the Excluder endograft. *J Vasc Surg* 2012; **56**: 920–28.
11. De Vries JPPM, Van De Pavoordt HD, Jordan WD jr. Rationale of EndoAnchors in abdominal aortic aneurysms with short or angulated necks. *J Cardiovasc Surg* (Torino) 2014; **55**: 103–7.
12. Melas N, Perdikides T, Saratzis A, *et al*. Helical EndoStaples enhance endograft fixation in an experimental model using human cadaveric aortas. *J Vasc Surg* 2012; **55**: 1726–33.
13. De Vries JPPM, Ouriel K, Mehta M, *et al*. Analysis of EndoAnchors for endovascular aneurysm repair by indications for use. *J Vasc Surg* 2014; **60**: 1460–67.
14. Jordan WD jr, Mehta M, Varnagy D, *et al*. Results of the ANCHOR prospective, multicenter registry of EndoAnchors for type Ia endoleaks and endograft migration in patients with challenging anatomy. *J Vasc Surg* 2014; **60**: 885–892.

EVAR follow-up and avoidance of secondary sac rupture and death

Current treatment of abdominal aortic aneurysm in Germany—outcomes and trends in a five-year follow-up

CA Behrendt, U Marschall, H L'hoest, F Heidemann, T Kölbel and S Debus

Introduction

Clinical registries have gained in importance for medical quality management and health services research. In contrast to randomised controlled trials, which possess the highest evidence basis, clinical registries aim to take large patient populations into consideration. While randomised control trials involve a predetermined, precisely defined patient cohort, clinical registries provide a more realistic sample of the actual medical care situation, without participant restrictions.[1]

In Germany, approximately 450,000 patients with vascular disease are treated annually.[2] Due to the incidence and inhomogeneity of symptoms associated with vascular diseases, systemically ordered data from this large patient cohort do not exist. Despite the usage of larger study populations, randomised trials have not been able to generate reliable evidence for or against specific treatment strategies, for example for abdominal aortic aneurysms. The homogenous study populations that are required in randomised control trials do not reflect the elderly and multimorbid patient clientele in clinical reality. The transferability of trial data into clinical practice is therefore often limited, and critical questions relating to therapeutic strategies remain unanswered.

The Vascular Service Quality Improvement Programme from Great Britain and Ireland shows that a structured record of treatment data in a registry can lead to an improvement in quality of care and, thus, to better treatment results. Treatment standards were successfully derived and implemented based on the structured data collected over multiple years through this registry. This led to the reduction in the mortality associated with elective treatments of abdominal aortic aneurysm from approximately 7.5% in 2008 to 2.4% in 2012.[3]

The establishment of a structured registry to compile data relating to abdominal aortic aneurysm in Germany began at the start of 2013. The registry is based on previously established international vascular registries. It is led under the guidance of the German Society for Vascular Surgery and Vascular Medicine, and was initiated for the purpose of health services research. Structured data for abdominal aortic aneurysm currently exist in the prospective aortic registry from the society.

Larger population-based studies indicate an abdominal aortic aneurysm prevalence between 4% and 7.6% in males over the age of 50, and approximately 1.3% for women in the same age group.[4]

The major risk factors leading to the development of abdominal aortic aneurysms are age, smoking and high blood pressure.[5] The main complication to consider is a rupture; a complete tear in the wall of the aorta. This leads to a life-threatening haemorrhage, with a lethality greater than 53%.[6] The mortality of patients who were operated on during this rupture phase is also very high (50%).[7] In cases where the bleed can be surgically controlled, shock and transfusion-related organ damage (in heart muscle, the intestines, lungs and blood clots) can lead to multiorgan failure. Prolonged and expensive intensive care, high hospital and rehabilitation costs, as well as potentially deadly dismissals from inpatient care, are all onerous consequences of an otherwise symptomless stage of a treatable illness.[7]

Stent implantation via open aortic repair and the minimally-invasive endovascular aneurysm repair (EVAR) are considered to be equivalent treatment methods. The revised guidelines from the American College of Cardiology/ American Heart Association indicate that EVAR, when compared with open aortic repair, possesses a lower lethality percentage.[8] This apparent advantage could not be further supported, however, as no improvement in survival was observed in the long term. The recommendation is, therefore, that the choice between the two treatment options should be based on individual circumstances. Developments in the German register data between 1999 and 2010 show that, at least in the treatment of intact aortic aneurisms, EVAR is the superior operative technique.[9]

This development is motivation to continue the collection of data in the coming years. With this intention, the data from the 2013 abdominal aortic aneurysm registry from the German Society has been published.[10] Currently 76 centres are involved in the German registry. Forty-nine centres provided data for open repair and 32 centres for EVAR. However, not all certified centres provided data for the treatment of abdominal aortic aneurysm for 2013. This illustrates fundamental problems in the national registry: firstly, the partially incomplete and non-population-representative data collection; and, secondly, the mostly non-existent external and internal validation of participating centres.[11] Therefore, the question remains—to which degree does the abdominal aortic aneurysm registry depict the current treatment situation? Does the incomplete participation of certified vascular centres mean, for example, that only cases with fewer complications are represented by the data? The quality of care provided by other specialist disciplines that do not participate in the abdominal aortic aneurysm registry—for example, general surgery or cardiac surgery—also remains unclear.

The degree to which the published registry data depicts the "real world" in treatment in Germany can, however, be investigated through a comparison with administrative data from a large, Germany-wide health insurance company. The routine data from the BARMER GEK can assist with the classification of so far collected data, and help answer the aforementioned questions.

Due to the fact that the available data from the health insurance company includes billing information, the best possible completeness is to be expected and a selection bias due to medical particularities is highly unlikely.

The analyses are based on ambulant and inpatient, anonymised billing data from the approximately 8,600,000 individuals who were insured by BARMER GEK between 2008 and 2013. A total of 7,026 individuals underwent at least one hospital stay between 2008 and 2013 due to the diagnosis and operation of an abdominal aortic aneurysm. In some cases, the patient underwent both an open repair and had a prosthetic stent implanted. These cases are marked as combination cases. These data were compared with the German society register data from 2013.

Results

A total of 7,167 hospital cases that fulfilled the inclusion criteria were identified in the BARMER GEK 2008–2013 data. This cohort includes the patients who, during an inpatient stay, underwent both an open operation and a stent implantation. In the given timeframe, 7,072 patients with intact abdominal aortic aneurysm were operated on. In 704 cases (10.4%), the operation was initiated due to a rupture.

A total of 2,257 patients were included in the German registry in 2013. More than 2,000 patients (90.4%) had an intact abdominal aortic aneurysm, while 216 (9.6 %) had a ruptured aneurysm.

The operated BARMER GEK patients show a similar demographic composition to the patients in the German registry. On average, the BARMER GEK patients are 1–3% older. The proportion of females is also comparable (13–18.3%). A tendency to treat older patients with endovascular stents is observed in both populations. This propensity has increased in recent years, and is, therefore, more pronounced in the data from the year 2013 (German society register), while the data from BARMER GEK also included the larger percentage of open operations from the previous years.

BARMER GEK insures approximately 13% of all public health-insured German residents. The patient sample is therefore similar, in terms of total morbidity, to the population of publicly-insured individuals. Admittedly, however, the proportion of women and the proportion of older patients is higher, which explains the higher average age of operated patients in the BARMER GEK cohort.

Abdominal aortic aneurysm often presents in combination with illnesses, which are associated with particular lifestyle choices and old age. This includes, for example, arterial hypertension, coronary heart disease or type II diabetes mellitus. In both populations, a higher rate of these comorbidities was associated with patients who were treated via EVAR. In light of the higher age bracket of these patients, this is also to be expected.

It is interesting that the comorbidities taken into consideration in the German register are significantly more often documented than they are as main or secondary diagnosis in the BARMER GEK data. This seems paradoxical. Although the BARMER GEK patients are slightly older than the German registry patients, they seem to suffer from less comorbidity.

It is the opinion of the authors that it would be inaccurate to assume, based on this observation, that the registry population is sicker than the BARMER GEK population. This phenomenon typically arises in health services research using routine data, and must be taken into consideration when the results are to be transferred to the clinical setting. Routine data from insurance companies is always associated with billable work. For example, an anamnestically-known, stable coronary heart disease patient will be less frequently billed, if their case requires no expenditure. The billing guidelines stipulate that, most importantly, diagnoses that require a higher expenditure and are revenue-relevant are to be billed. In the case of the German society registry, the aspiration for completeness of medical information is in the foreground, rather than the optimisation of the economic profit. Comorbidities, therefore, appear less frequently in the BARMER GEK routine data, and those that are listed are more serious and are more frequently relevant to the treatment plan.

The collected registry data in Germany between 1999 and 2010, as well as Medicare data from the USA, show that the open aortic repair is being replaced by EVAR. Using 338,278 data records of the invasive treatment of intact abdominal aortic aneurysms, and 69,653 data records of ruptured aneurysms, the development and progress of therapies between 1995 and 2008 was monitored. At the conclusion of the observation period, a significant 77% of the intact abdominal aortic aneurysms (and 31% of those ruptured) were treated using EVAR.[12] The current German register data affirms, with similar values, the increased proportion of EVAR procedures in 2013.

Stent implantation was undertaken in more than 62% of the BARMER GEK patients, while the percentage in the German register (69.3%) was a little higher. Considering that women are less frequently affected, operations are less frequently required in this population. The proportion of women who experienced any operative procedure in the BARMER GEK cohort was 15% over the entire observation period. The proportion in the register data was almost identical, with 14.8% for both procedures.

The following trend was observed during the entire observation period; the older a patient is, the higher the proportion of EVAR procedures they undergo. The percentage of stent implantations has, since 2010, increased from slightly under 40% to over 60%, most notably among those aged 40–60 years. This is yet another indication that this method of treatment is being increasingly implemented. The reasons for this trend, however, can currently only be speculated.

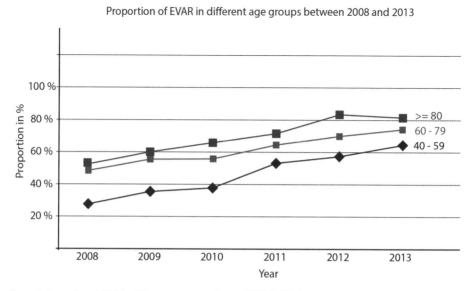

Figure 1: Proportion of EVAR in different age groups. Source: BARMER GEK data 2008–2013.

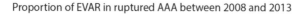

Proportion of EVAR in ruptured AAA between 2008 and 2013

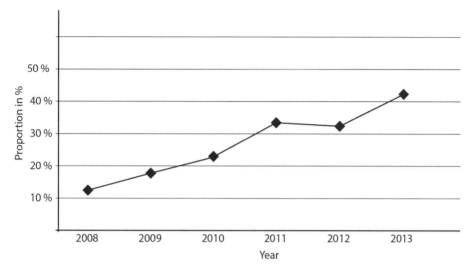

Figure 2: Proportion of EVAR in ruptured AAA. Source: BARMER GEK data 2008–2013.

It is worth noting that this trend can also be observed clearly in ruptured abdominal aortic aneurysms cases. The percentage of EVARs implimented in the treatment of ruptured anuerysms is presented in Figure 2.

Only 15% of ruptured abdominal aortic aneurysms in 2008 were treated via EVAR, in comparison with over 40% in 2013. In the German registry, the percentage of EVAR treatments of ruptured aneurysms was 34.7%.

While the 30-day mortality associated with ruptured abdominal aortic aneurysms treated via open aortic repair in the observation period between 2008 and 2012 remained a stable 35%, the mortality associated with EVAR in the same time period was only 20%. Similarly, the 90-day mortality associated with treatment by EVAR for ruptured aneurysms is significantly lower than that associated with open operations (30% vs. 40%). The 90-day mortality of open repair for ruptured aneurysms shows a decrease.

The 30-day mortality associated with intact abdominal aortic aneurysms treated via open repair during the chosen observation period was, on average, 4%. The EVAR technique, however, presents a mortality of only 1%. The 90-day mortality of an open surgery on an intact aneurysm is, on average, 6%, compared with 4% for EVAR. While the 30-day mortality for females is, in comparison, almost identical between the routine and the registry data, the 30-day mortality for males shows a recognisable disparity. The mortality following EVAR, as well as that following an open repair, is presumably an overestimate, due to the small number of cases included in the register data. The BARMER GEK data show a significantly lower 30-day mortality than the registry data, with 17.6% following EVAR and 33.8% following open repair (27.4% vs. 40.5%, respectively, in the registry data).

When observed in conjunction with international registry data, the notion that EVAR provides better results than open repair is increasingly recognisable. As a comparison, the VASCUNET-data bank gives the hospital mortality flowing the open aortic repair of ruptured abdominal aortic aneurysms as 32.6%, and

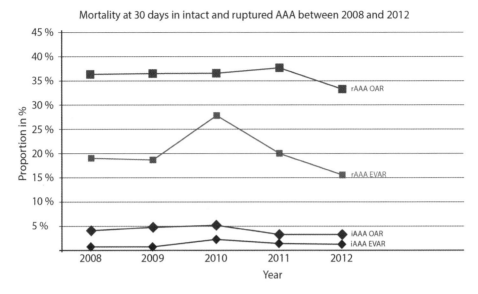

Figure 3: Mortality of EVAR and open aortic repair at 30 days. Source: BARMER GEK data 2008–2013.

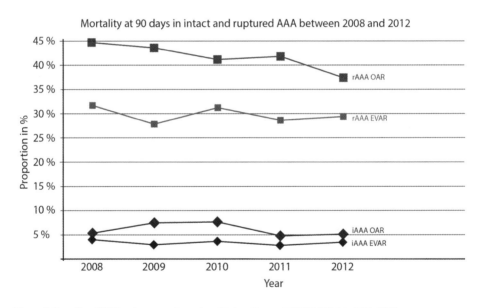

Figure 4: Mortality of EVAR and open aortic repair at 90 days. Source: BARMER GEK data 2008–2013.

only 19.7% following EVAR.[13] These values compare well to the BARMER GEK routine data.

When comparing both the German society registry and the BARMER GEK claims data, one must take both selection bias, and the lack of age and risk adjustment, into consideration. Experience in the respective vascular centres, and the age and gender of the individual being treated, also play a significant role in the interpretation of outcomes, alongside the clinical indications specifically in the case of ruptured abdominal aortic aneurysms.

The data from the German register shows no correlation in the results relating to treatment structure, as currently no comprehensive documentation involving all university medical centres exists. In this regard, the integration of available register data with the routine data collected by health insurance companies is helpful.

The frequency in which a re-operation with a technique swap was required was analysed using the health insurance data. In total, complications associated with the choice of foreign material arose in only 8.1% of open surgeries, compared with 14.1% of cases using EVAR.

These complications arose much less frequently in intact abdominal aortic aneurysms than in ruptured ones. A clear disparity between the open procedure and EVAR also exists here, when excluding the complications which directly relate to the chosen prosthesis. These complications arose in 5.4% of open aortic repair cases and in 6% of EVAR cases.

An additional indication of quality is the number of re-operations required during the initial hospital stay. The data indicate a significant disparity in this regard between open aortic repair and EVAR. During the given observation period, EVAR was associated with a higher rate of consequent operations (4%) than open repair (1.3 %). It is interesting to note that a change in procedure from EVAR to open repair remained throughout the entire observation period uncommon. The swap from an open repair to an EVAR has, however, increased in frequency in the last years. This also supports the observation that the EVAR technique has, with time, become a more valued procedure, seeing as the treatment method is considered as an appropriate alternative when revising therapeutic plans.

A risk adjustment is, however, required, so that the various patient cohorts remain comparable.

Conclusion

The presented analyses show that data sources from health insurances (e.g. BARMER GEK) and the register data from the German Vascular Society are comparable. A recently published study, using the registry data from vascular specialist groups, and the routine data from the third largest health insurance company in Germany, also support this observation.[14] In particular, the rising significance of EVAR as a treatment method for abdominal aortic aneurysms was upheld by both data sources.

The aim of the German Vascular Society to promote the extensive participation, not only of certified vascular centres but also additional doctors with expertise in vascular surgery, leading to the structured documentation of their experiences in a collective registry, is emphasised by these analyses.

Results relating to clinical treatments are particularly important, especially in international comparisons. In particular, the mortality associated with ruptured abdominal aortic aneurysms is highly important, and is a criterion for treatment quality. The mortality, which has proved to be much higher in the German registry than in international data, has been justified by the fact that more patients with a ruptured abdominal aortic aneurysm following hospital admission receive additional treatment in Germany.

The corresponding results from the analysis of the BARMER GEK data show, however, that treatment results in Germany are comparable with other registers on an international scale.

The results analysed thus far from the register data suggest a higher-than-expected mortality rate, presumably due to the small cohort of patients with a ruptured abdominal aortic aneurysm.

The measurement of treatment quality using appropriate assessment parameters is of increasing value to cost bearers. Despite being very comprehensive, the available secondary data on this topic are not always suitable for the assessment of quality indicators and their parameters. When collaborative data entries are sufficiently numerous, comprehensive, and therefore representative of the greater population, a data registry becomes an important contributor to quality management and health services research.

A substantial challenge exists in the procurement of a reliable and permanent source of financial support. Experience from other registries shows that the requisition of participation fees from participants and clinics is counterproductive for the achievement of high participation rates.

A registry in which primary data can concordantly be compared with secondary data would contribute meaningfully to the measurement of quality of care in practical settings. This analysis shows that a significant overlap exists between the two data sources.

Summary

- Registry data from the German Vascular Society and health insurance claims data (BARMER GEK) are comparable for quality improvement purposes.

- Using medical insurance claims data for quality improvement can be a reasonable solution to solve limitations of registry data (e.g. small number of participating centres, not all treating specialist disciplines involved).

- This study confirms the well published fact that EVAR is becoming a more important treatment in the case of both intact and ruptured abdominal aortic aneurysms. More than 40% of ruptured abdominal aortic aneurysms in 2013 were treated by EVAR.

- Mortality following treatment of ruptured abdominal aortic aneurysm in Germany is comparable to that in international registry data.

References

1. Behrendt CA, *et al.* Einführung des GermanVasc. *Gefässchirurgie* 2014; **19**: 403–11.
2. Krankenhausdiagnosestatistik. https://goo.gl/tJMqwM (date accessed 19 February 2016). Gesundheitsberichterstattung des Bundes.
3. Waton S, *et al.* Outcomes after elective repair of infra-renal abdominal aortic aneurysm. *The Royal College of Surgeons of England* 2013.
4. Guirguis-Blake JM, Beil TL, Senger CA, Whitlock EP, *et al.* Ultrasonography screening for abdominal aortic aneurysms: a systematic evidence review for the U.S. Preventive Services Task Force. *Ann Intern Med* 2014; **160**: 321–9.
5. Lederle FA, Johnson GR, Wilson SE, *et al.* The aneurysm detection and management study screening program: validation cohort and final results. Aneurysm Detection and Management Veterans Affairs Cooperative Study Investigators. *Arch Intern Med* 2000; **160**: 1425–30.
6. Karthikesalingam A, Holt PJ, Vidal-Diez A, *et al.* Mortality from ruptured abdominal aortic aneurysms: clinical lessons from a comparison of outcomes in England and the USA. *Lancet* 2014; **383**: 963–9.
7. Torsello G, Can A, Schumacher S. Das Bauchaortenaneurysma. *Gefaesschirurgie* 2005; **10**: 139–53.

8. Rooke TW, Hirsch AT, Misra S, *et al.* 2011 ACCF/AHA focused update of the guideline for the management of patients with peripheral artery disease (updating the 2005 guideline): a report of the American College of Cardiology Foundation/American Heart Association Task Force on Practice Guidelines. *J Am Coll Cardiol* 2011; **58**: 2020–45.
9. Trenner M, *et al.* 12 Jahre "Qualitätssicherung BAA" der DGG. *Gefässchirurgie* 2013; **18**: 206–13.
10. Debus ES, *et al.* Zur Behandlung des abdominellen Aortenaneurysmas in Deutschland. *Gefässchirurgie* 2014; **19**: 412–21.
11. Vikatmaa P, Mitchell D, Jensen LP, *et al.* Variation in clinical practice in carotid surgery in nine countries 2005-2010. Lessons from VASCUNET and recommendations for the future of national clinical audit. *Eur J Vasc Endovasc Surg* 2012; **44**: 11–7.
12. Schermerhorn ML, Bensley RP, Giles KA, *et al.* Changes in abdominal aortic aneurysm rupture and short-term mortality, 1995-2008: a retrospective observational study. *Ann Surg* 2012; **256**: 651–58.
13. Mani K, Lees T, Beiles B, *et al.* Treatment of abdominal aortic aneurysm in nine countries 2005-2009: a vascunet report. *Eur J Vasc Endovasc Surg* 2011; **42**: 598–607.
14. Debus ES, *et al.* Perioperative mortality following repair for abdominal aortic aneurysm in Germany: Comparison of administrative data of the DAK health insurance and clinical registry data of the German Vascular Society. *Chirurg* 2015; **86**: 1041–50.

Randomised controlled trial on effect of aneurysm sac embolisation for endoleak type II prevention

F Grego, M Piazza and M Antonello

Introduction

Type II endoleak represents the most common category of endoleaks recorded after endovascular aneurysm repair (EVAR); treatment is recommended only for cases with significant sac enlargement or suggested in those that are persistent. Type II endoleaks are the cause of reintervention for about 10% of EVAR cases;[1,2] however, the success rate of these secondary procedure is about 45%[3] and multiple access may be required over time.

The extra medical expenses incurred for these additional procedures, as well as the increased exposure of patients to radiation and contrast agents during follow-up, represent a limitation to EVAR and occasionally can lead to a waste of its advantages in terms of costs[4] and clinical success.[5]

In this scenario, prevention of type II endoleak formation could be a valid strategy; previous experiences, with aneurysm sac embolisation during EVAR using variable doses of materials, already demonstrated its efficacy.[6]

In a previous study,[7] we showed a significantly reduced incidence of type II endoleak related complications during mid-term follow-up, with the routine injection of a standard dose of fibrin glue in association with coils into the aneurysmal sac during EVAR compared to those patients who underwent standard EVAR.

However, results obtained from this experience suggested that this procedure may be optimised by the injection of a tapered dose of material based on aneurysm sac dimension rather than a standard dose. Furthermore, in order to reduce costs, its use should not be routine, but limited to those patients "at risk of type II endoleak".

The purpose of this study was to evaluate early and mid-term outcomes of this procedure in a randomised single centre setting comparing standard EVAR *versus* EVAR plus contemporary aneurysm sac embolisation (embo-EVAR) in patients "at risk for type II endoleak". The dose of material injected during embolisation was tapered to the preoperative aneurysm sac-volume dimension. Furthermore, we investigated the effect of embo-EVAR, on aneurysm sac volumetric variation, during follow-up compared to standard EVAR.

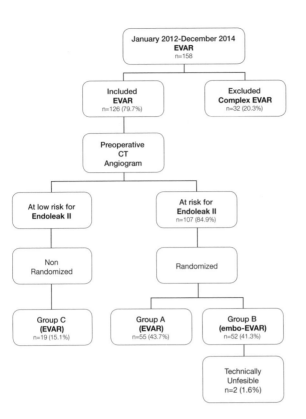

Figure 1: Inclusion and randomisation of patients. (CT: computed tomography; EVAR: endovascular aneurysm repair; embo-EVAR: EVAR with aneurysm sac embolisation).

Methods

Between January 2012 and December 2014, all patients admitted to the Clinic of Vascular and Endovascular Surgery of Padova University who underwent EVAR for infrarenal abdominal aortic aneurysms were prospectively recorded in a dedicated database. This study was approved by the Ethics Committee of our Institution. This is a single centre prospective randomised study designed to evaluate the efficacy of EVAR plus contemporary aneurysm sac embolisation with sac volume-dependent dose of coils and fibrin glue in the prevention of type II endoleak and its complications.

Only patients who underwent elective EVAR were considered. Only patients considered at "risk of endoleak type II" were included in the randomisation and were randomised to standard EVAR (group A) or embo-EVAR (group B). Patients considered at "low risk for type II endoleak" were not randomised; these cases (group C) underwent standard EVAR and received the same follow-up protocol as groups A and B (Figure 1).

The endpoints of the study were to compare type II endoleak rate, freedom from type II endoleak-related reinterventions, and aneurysm sac volume variation during follow-up between patients undergoing the two different interventions.

Treatment of aneurysm sac embolisation in Group B was performed using coils (Tornado, MReye Embolization Coil, Cook Medical) with fibrin glue (Tissucol; Baxter). Based on our previous study,[7] the fibrin glue dose was of 5ml and three coils if the calculated preoperative computed tomography (CT) angiogram aneurysm volume was $\leq 125cm^3$; if the volume was $>125cm^3$ we used 10ml of glue and one additional coil was added every $50cm^3$ of over volume.

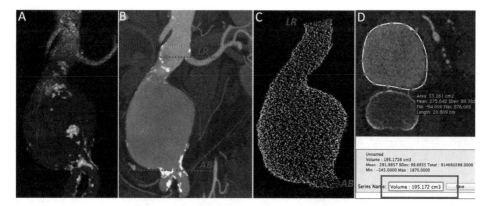

Figure 2: Method for sac volume calculation. (A) 3D CT angiogram reconstruction. (B) Region of interest is calculated from the lowest renal artery to the aortic bifurcation using the Osirix Pro 4.0 software. (C) and (D) Regions of interest of the aneurysm external wall were manually tracked every 8mm axial cuts by an expert operator; subsequently, the software is asked to generate missing regions of interest and compute the entire selected area in volume rendering (values obtained in cubic centimetres).

The definition "risk of type II endoleak" was based on anatomical criteria extracted from the available literature[8,9] and from a preliminary retrospective study conducted at our institution.[7] The anatomic characteristics identified at the preoperative CT angiogram were:

1. Patency of the inferior mesenteric artery, with a luminal diameter at the origin ≥3mm
2. Patency of at least three couples of lumbar arteries, or two couples of lumbar arteries and a sacral artery, or two couples of lumbar arteries and an accessory renal artery, or two couples of lumbar arteries and any diameter (also <3mm) patent inferior mesenteric artery.

Patients who did not match these criteria were considered "at low risk for type II endoleak".

Aneurysm sac volume was calculated (Figure 2). Aneurysm sac volume variation in preoperative and follow-up CT angiograms were measured for all randomised patients in order to evaluate the effect of type II endoleak on sac shrinkage within the two groups. The follow-up was performed in all patients (group A, B and C) by obtaining contrast CT angiogram at approximately three, six, and 12 months, and then yearly after that. Overall average length of follow-up was 16 months (range, one month to 36 months), with a mean follow-up period of 16 months for both group A (15.9±9.9 months) and B (16.4±10.7 months). Indications for type II endoleak-related reintervention were >5mm increase in maximum diameter within two consecutive CT angiograms and persistent type II endoleak (type II endoleak on three or more consecutive CT angiograms during follow-up) with any increase in aneurysm sac diameter. The definition "freedom from reintervention" was applied to those patients who during their follow-up did not have a type II endoleak or had a type II endoleak that did not require additional procedures.

The operative technique of embo-EVAR, has been previously described[7] (Figure 3).

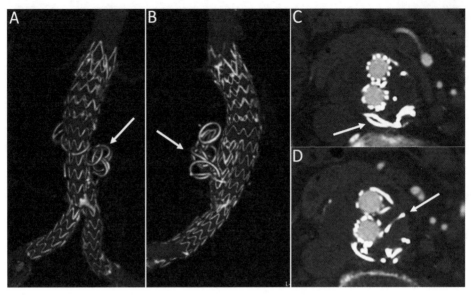

Figure 3: Postoperative CT angiogram of a patient treated with EVAR plus non-selective aneurysm sac embolisation. (A) anterior and (B) lateral 3D reconstruction. (C) and (D) axial CT angiogram images of aortic sac using Tornado MReye coils (white arrows indicate coils.

Intraoperative and postoperative therapy was the same for all patients: 5000 USP heparin units were given by endovenous infusion during the procedure and single antiplatelet therapy were administered from the day after surgery.

Results

No differences were reported between the two groups in terms of major medical or surgical complications within 30 days. Technical success was achieved in 100% of cases in both groups, and no aneurysm ruptures or deaths were reported in this series.

The descriptive analysis of freedom from type II endoleak illustrated in Figure 4 shows that during follow-up the type II endoleak rate was significantly higher in group A compared to group B. Interestingly, group C showed the lowest rate of type II endoleak during the whole follow-up period. Spontaneous type II endoleak resolution occurred in 33% *versus* 30% of patients after six months, 62% *versus* 65% after 12 months, and 66% *versus* 65% after 24 months, respectively in group A and group B (p=0.96). The number of persistent type II endoleaks was eight (14.5%) in group A and three (6%) in group B (p=0.13). During follow-up, there were four cases (7.2%) in group A and three cases (6%) in group B of new-onset type II endoleak (p=0.55) in patients without any previous sign of endoleak at angio-CT scans. The Kaplan-Meier estimates of freedom from type II endoleak-related reinterventions showed a significant higher rate of reintervention in group A compared to group B after 24 months (Figure 5).

At our institution, the cost for a single patient embolisation during EVAR with this technique was calculated to be approximately €600 (US$800), whereas the institutional reimbursement expenses for a secondary reintervention for embolisation with coils of a type II endoleak after EVAR is approximately €9000 (US$11,800). Considering that during follow-up, seven reinterventions were performed in group

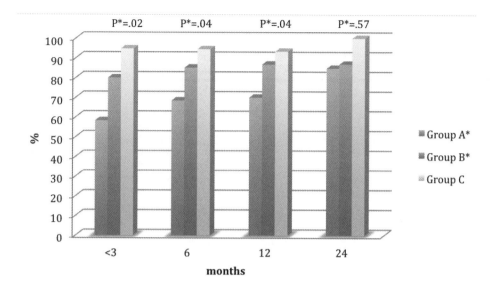

Figure 4: Descriptive analysis of freedom from type II endoleaks during early and midterm follow-up in groups A, B, and C.

A and sac embolisation in all 50 patients and reintervention only in one patient in group B, the total costs were approximately €63,000 (US$70,750) for group A and €39,000 (US$43,800) for group B; expenses were significantly lower overall in group B compared to group A (p=0.0001).

Over time, group A showed a lower shrinkage rate compared to group B and this was significant after six (-2.2±14.2cm3 vs. -10.6 ±17.1cm3; p=0.007), 12 (-2.9±32.2cm3 vs. -18.9±26.6cm3; p=0.02) and 24 months (-4.6±25.9cm3 vs. -27.3±24.7cm3; p=0.008).

The same analysis was performed after stratification for those cases with type II endoleak within the two Groups; in particular even if not statistically significant, the overall sac volume in Group B tended to decrease compared to Group A where the overall sac volume increased both at 12 (-6.1±19.7cm3 vs. +16.8±37.3cm3; p=0.24) and at 24 months (-2.5±10.6cm3 vs. +13.5±37.1cm3; p=0.59).

Discussion

The primary treatment approach for type II endoleak causing sac enlargement is usually endovascular, with selective embolisation of feeding branches. Recently, several authors developed the concept of prevention rather than treatment, using selective embolisation of feeding branches with different methods and materials before EVAR. Even if effective, this approach could be a waste of resources for the patient who needs to undergo two different procedures, as healthcare costs are increased. Muthu *et al* have described routine intraoperative selective inferior mesenteric artery embolisation and thrombin injection into the aneurysm sac just before EVAR.[10] This approach has the advantage of exposing the patient to a single procedure, while on the other side, selective inferior mesenteric artery embolisation, may require longer operative time and higher contrast dose injected compared to standard EVAR.

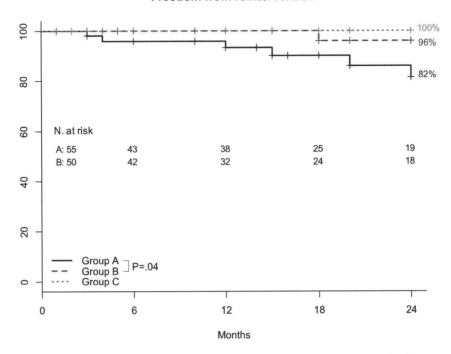

Figure 5: Kaplan-Meier curve for freedom from type II endoleak-related reintervention during early and midterm follow-up in groups A, B, and C. Standard error <10%.

It should be clarified that often the objective of these reported experiences with preventive embolisation is to reduce the incidence of type II endoleak in the patient identified preoperatively as "at high risk", and not to reduce the overall incidence of type II endoleak complication in the EVAR patient-population.

In this regard, we agree with Cieri's[11] conclusion that type II endoleak is an enigmatic and unpredictable marker of worse outcome after EVAR, and any adjunctive preventive procedure to avoid type II endoleak complication in patients "at high risk" maybe over time a waste of resources.

On the other hand, given that type II endoleak complications can be unpredictable, we think that prevention may be effective only if the entire EVAR cohort is routinely exposed to a protocol and the procedure does not have to modify EVAR itself in terms of patient exposure to X-ray and contrast agents, operative time and costs. Furthermore, this procedure needs to be reproducible and standardised.

The technique used at our institution to prevent type II endoleak after EVAR is similar to that reported by Ronsivalle et al,[12] where they used routine non-selective sac embolisation during EVAR with variable doses of fibrin glue in association with coil embolisation; they demonstrated a significant reduction in type II endoleaks compared with standard EVAR (hazard ratio, 0.13; 95% CI, 0.05–0.36; p<0.0001). Subsequently, Pilon et al[6] in 2010, also demonstrated with this approach a comprehensive reduction in healthcare costs.

Our previous experience with this technique[7] however, was performed using a "standard dose" of fibrin glue and coils; the results of this retrospective study in a consecutive series of patients who underwent embo-EVAR compared to those who underwent standard EVAR, demonstrated a significantly lower freedom from related reintervention at 18 months in those who underwent embolisation (93% vs. 99%; p=0.03). It should be emphasised that the use of a standard dose of material was effective up to a sac volume of 125cm^3 (about 5.8cm in diameter), while higher preoperative sac volumes (>125cm^3) were an independent predictor of type II endoleak (odd ratio [OR], 4; 95% confidence interval [CI], 1.5–10.5; p=0.005).

The purpose of this method is to facilitate sac thrombosis after EVAR and not to occlude specific feeding branches. The advantage is that the procedure is easy and fast, with similar operative time (149.4±50.7 minutes vs. 156.8±39.6 minutes; p=0.63) and contrast exposure (83.2±10.9ml vs. 85.4±9.9ml; p=0.28) compared to a standard EVAR procedure. On the other side, routine embolisation may cause an over-treatment in all those EVAR patients that are at really low risk for type II endoleak.

In this scenario, in order to optimise the procedure we applied these concepts: first, is to not only treat those at high risk of type II endoleak, but to exclude from treatment those at low risk of endoleak; second, to taper the dose of material to be injected based on the preoperative sac volume.

This last concept is similar to that of new devices such as the Nellix endograft (Endologix) that employs a volume dependent dose of a polymer injected in endobags surrounding the endograft. In their multicentre retrospective analysis of a consecutive series of 171 patients, they reported a type II endoleak incidence of 2% at 17 months.[13]

Selection criteria included the presence of a patent inferior mesenteric artery plus at least two couples of lumbar arteries. Many of the EVAR patients were included as "at risk", while only those cases with circumferential thrombus and few small collaterals were not treated ("low risk").

In this regard, the selection criteria adopted seems to be effective; in group C, the endoleak rate was the lowest (always <10%) with a progressive spontaneous decrease over time with a 2–3% at 24 months, with no patients in this subgroup needing secondary reintervention at two years. Furthermore, the exclusion of these patients reduced overall costs compared to our previous experience with systematic embolisation (p=0.0001 vs. p=0.90).[7]

During follow-up, a significant lower type II endoleak rate for group B compared to group A up to 12 months (p=0.04) was observed; after that period even if the incidence of type II endoleak was lower in group B, this loses statistically significance (p=0.57). On the other hand, freedom from reintervention at 24 months was significantly higher in group B as compared to group A (96% vs. 82%; p=0.04). Thus, we can assume that even if after one year there was a similar percentage of type II endoleak, those patients who underwent embo-EVAR were more protected from the insidious evolution of type II endoleak with sac expansion or endoleak persistence that usually requires additional intervention; even if not significant (p=0.13), the number of persistent type II endoleak was higher in group A (n=8; 14.5%) than in group B (n=3; 6%).

This consideration is confirmed by the sac volume analysis performed overall within the two groups; this revealed a progressive significant sac volume reduction for group B compared to group A at six (p=0.007), 12 (p=0.02) and 24 months (p=0.008). However, when analysing the same parameter only for those patients with type II endoleak, this difference was maintained but was no longer significant at 12 (-6.1±19.7cm^3 vs. +16.8±37.3cm^3; p=0.24) and 24 months (-2.5±10.6cm^3 vs. +13.5±37.1cm^3; p=0.59); this may be related to the low number of events to be considered in the analysis.

Conclusion

To our knowledge, no other published study has compared in a randomised fashion aneurysm sac embolisation during EVAR for patients at risk of type II endoleak, using a sac volume-dependent dose of fibrin glue and coils with traditional EVAR.

This technique is safe and effective in preventing type II endoleak-related complications during short- and mid-term follow-up after EVAR. Although further confirmatory studies are needed, the faster aneurysm sac volume shrinkage over time in patients who underwent embolisation compared to standard EVAR may be a positive aspect influencing the lower type II endoleak rate also during long term follow-up.

Summary

- Aneurysm sac embolisation during EVAR has already been demonstrated to be effective in the prevention of type II endoleak formation.

- In order to optimise this approach, the dose of material to be injected should be tapered on aneurysm sac dimension; furthermore to reduce costs, its use should not be routinely, but limited to those patients "at risk of type II endoleak".

- We evaluated outcomes of this procedure with a randomised single centre study comparing standard EVAR versus EVAR+ contemporary aneurysm sac embolisation (embo-EVAR) in patients "at risk for type II endoleak". The material used was fibrin glue and coils and the dose of material injected was tapered to the preoperative aneurysm sac-volume.

- Results of this study showed a significative higher freedom from type II endoleak-related reintervention and overall mean difference in aneurysm sac volume shrinkage at 24 months in the embo-EVAR group.

- Sac embolisation during EVAR, using a sac volume-dependent dose of fibrin glue and coils, is a valid method to significantly reduce type II endoleak and its complications during early and midterm follow-up in patients considered at risk. Although further confirmatory studies are needed, the faster aneurysm sac volume shrinkage over time in patients who underwent embolisation compared with standard EVAR may be a positive aspect influencing the lower type II endoleak rate also during long-term follow-up.

References

1. Faries PL, Cadot H, Agarwal G, et al. Management of endoleak after endovascular aneurysm repair: cuffs, coils, and conversion. J Vasc Surg 2003; **37** (6): 1155–61.
2. Laheij RJ, Buth J, Harris PL, et al. Need for secondary interventions after endovascular repair of abdominal aortic aneurysms. Intermediate-term follow-up results of a European collaborative registry (EUROSTAR). Br J Surg 2000; **87** (12): 1666–73.

3. Abularrage CJ, Patel V, Conrad MF, *et al*. Improved results using Onyx glue for the treatment of persistent type 2 endoleak after endovascular aneurysm repair. *J Vasc Surg* 2012; **56** (3): 630–36.
4. Jouhannet C, Alsac JM, Julia P, *et al*. Reinterventions for type 2 endoleaks with enlargement of the aneurismal sac after endovascular treatment of abdominal aortic aneurysms. *Ann Vasc Surg* 2014; **28** (1): 192–200.
5. Antonello M, Menegolo M, Piazza M, *et al*. Outcomes of endovascular aneurysm repair on renal function compared with open repair. *J Vasc Surg* 2013; **58** (4): 886–93.
6. Pilon F, Tosato F, Danieli D, *et al*. Intrasac fibrin glue injection after platinum coils placement: the efficacy of a simple intraoperative procedure in preventing type II endoleak after endovascular aneurysm repair. *Interact Cardiovasc Thorac Surg* 2010; **11** (1): 78–82.
7. Piazza M, Frigatti P, Scrivere P, *et al*. Role of aneurysm sac embolization during endovascular aneurysm repair in the prevention of type II endoleak-related complications. *J Vasc Surg* 2013; **57** (4): 934–41.
8. Abularage CJ, Crawford RS, Conrad MF, *et al*. Preoperative variables predict persistent type 2 endoleak after endovascular aneurysm repair. *J Vasc Surg* 2010; **52**: 19–24.
9. Marchiori A, von Ristow A, Guimaraes M, *et al*. Predictive factors for the development of type II endoleaks. *J Endovasc Ther* 2011; **18**: 299–305.
10. Muthu C, Maani J, Plank LD, *et al*. Strategies to reduce the rate of type II endoleaks: routine intraoperative embolization of the inferior mesenteric artery and thrombin injection into the aneurysm sac. *J Endovasc Ther 2007*; **14** (5): 661–68. 2007
11. Cieri E, De Rango P, Isernia G, *et al*. Type II endoleak is an enigmatic and unpredictable marker of worse outcome after endovascular aneurysm repair. *J Vasc Surg* 2014; **59** (4): 930–37.
12. Ronsivalle S, Faresin F, Franz F, *et al*. Aneurysm sac "thrombization" and stabilization in EVAR: a technique to reduce the risk of type II endoleak. *J Endovasc Ther* 2010; **17** (4): 517–24.
13. Böckler D, Holden A, Thompson M, *et al*. Multicenter Nellix EndoVascular Aneurysm Sealing system experience in aneurysm sac sealing. *J Vasc Surg* 2015; **62** (2): 290–98.

Prevention and management of type Ia endoleaks: EVAR *versus* EVAS

LH van den Ham, R Buijs, CJ Zeebregts
and MMPJ Reijnen

Introduction

Endovascular aneurysm repair (EVAR) has become the preferred treatment for abdominal aortic aneurysms, but the need for a reduction in reintervention rate is ongoing. Endoleak is the major complication of EVAR and the main indication for reinterventions.[1] The EUROSTAR investigators found that endoleak is a predictor for conversion to open repair and secondary rupture. Forty-one per cent of patients without endoleaks remained free from secondary interventions within the first two postoperative years as opposed to 91% in those with endoleaks.[2] Endoleaks are classified in five subtypes based on location and causative mechanics. Proximal endoleak, known as type Ia, is of special interest as it is considered a high pressure endoleak and might have a surgeon and/or graft dependent incidence.[3] In 2013, endovascular aneurysms sealing (EVAS) using the Nellix endoprothesis (Endologix) was introduced. Early results from the EVAS investigational device exemption (IDE) trial and an interim analysis of the EVAS FORWARD Global registry have shown a low overall endoleak rate, but when occurring most are type Ia endoleaks.[4] In the present chapter, we will review literature on type Ia endoleaks after both EVAR and EVAS.

Type Ia endoleak after EVAR

Endoleak is defined as persistent blood flow into the aneurysmal sac despite presumed aneurysm exclusion and can be observed both intraoperatively (Figure 1) and during post-interventional surveillance. A type Ia endoleak shows contrast outside the proximal sealing zone of the endograft filling the aneurysmal lumen. Contrast-enhanced computed tomography (CT) angiography imaging is considered the primary diagnostic (Figure 2), although there is no true consensus.[5] Modalities such as duplex ultrasound and magnetic resonance (MR) angiogram have their value in the diagnostic process, as have the newer options ECG-gated CT and MR angiogram.[6]

Type Ia endoleaks can be related to other endoleaks, specifically types II and V. Especially in combination with a growing aneurysm, a type II endoleak should be evaluated as a "type Ia in disguise", potentially explained by an intermittent inflow.

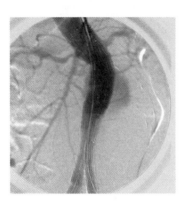

Figure 1: Procedural type Ia endoleak after EVAR as appeared on completion angiography.

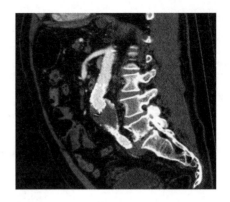

Figure 2: Type Ia endoleak on CTA with proximal contrast extravasation inside the aneurysm sac during the arterial phase.

Type V endoleak is defined as aneurysm growth of uncertain cause that could be the result of previous endoleak that perpetuates its tension on the aneurysm sac. Blackwood *et al* showed that type I endoleak sometimes results in no net inflow of contrast, despite the fact that the aneurysm sac expands. In the absence of net flow into the aneurysm sac, contrast cannot reach outside the endograft in high enough concentrations to visualise its presence.[7]

The occurrence of a type Ia endoleak after EVAR can have various causes, including: 1) patient-specific variables, such as infrarenal aortic neck anatomy; 2) clinician-dependent variables, such as experience with sizing and endovascular technique, and compliance to the instructions for use; and 3) endograft-specific characteristics, such as suprarenal fixation and the presence of hooks or barbs. Early type Ia endoleak, occurring within 30 days after implantation, is often related to pre-operative planning, patient selection and/or technique while a late-type Ia endoleak is more frequently caused by graft migration, infrarenal neck dilatation or kinking of the graft due to severe neck angulation.[8]

Anatomic variations play a key role in the occurrence of type Ia endoleaks and the identification of hostile neck anatomy has led to a better understanding of requirements. This, in turn, has improved endograft design, like the development of endografts with an indication for severe angulation and repositionable endografts. Recently, Jordan *et al* postulated a strong link between the occurrence of type Ia endoleak and the infrarenal neck length, neck diameter, and the presence of mural thrombus, while the other hostile neck characteristics seemed to be less important.[9] In recent years, endografts have been developed to treat aneurysm with a more hostile neck anatomy. The Anaconda endograft (Vascutek) offers a repositionable deployment system, and thus more accurate positioning and as such, potentially less type Ia endoleak. Similar to the Anaconda endograft, the C3 Excluder system (Gore) can be repositioned as well and has proven to succeed in several single centre studies. In these studies, repositioning was applied in 49% of the cases, leading to just two type Ia endoleaks in follow-up.[10] It can be difficult to distinguish whether type Ia endoleak is caused by anatomical factors, technical issues and/or sizing or by a combination of both. Experience is considered important, yet the effect of the clinician's skills has hardly been studied. Some studies have claimed that results were influenced by the learning curve of the department or the clinician.[11,12] No

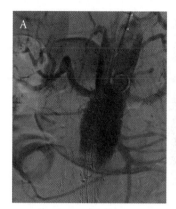
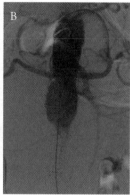

Figure 3: Procedural angiographies of a patient with progressive neck dilation, distal migration and a minor type Ia endoleak repaired using a three-fenestrated cuff.

comparative research has been performed on preoperative sizing techniques, despite the availability of potentially more accurate methods.[13]

The overall incidence of type I endoleak seems to vary between 7.5% and 10.5%.[14] There is a lack of consensus in the outcomes of endoleak type Ia treatment and follow-up. A benign course was described by Millen *et al* who found that only two of 44 type Ia endoleaks persisted beyond the first postoperative CT, following intraoperative treatment of the endoleaks and subsequent watchful waiting. On the other hand, larger studies have shown significantly worse outcomes. In a multicentre study on 2,730 EVAR cases, 22 post-EVAR ruptures were recorded and 73% of them presented in conjunction with a type Ia endoleak. Once type Ia endoleak is found, treatment is usually indicated and several techniques can be applied. When the proximal stent of the device is not fully expanded, an additional ballooning of the stent could complete the seal. If unsuccessful, a proximal cuff could be introduced, although there should be adequate infrarenal aortic neck length for the cuff to land. This technique is chosen to treat a type Ia endoleak that is caused by either misplacement or late migration. Balloon expandable stents can be used in case of folding of the graft material, or an incomplete expanded stent. In an eight-year follow-up study, Rajani *et al* showed a 6% recurrence of type Ia endoleak in cuff-treated patients, and nil in Palmaz stent-treated patients.[15] In case of inadequate infrarenal neck length, a fenestrated cuff could be used (Figure 3). A potential alternative is a proximal cuff in combination with chimney grafts. Chimneys, however, have been related to a high incidence of type Ia endoleak themselves.[16] As an adjunctive, Endoanchors (Aptus Endosystems) can be used to fixate the initial stent graft in case of distal migration and be combined with proximal cuff or can reduce inward folding of graft material (Figure 4).[17]

Should these techniques fail, the option of using embolising agents to close the aneurysm sac opening remains. The introduction of coils and N-butyl cyanoacrylate has shown promising results in the past, but lags behind in recanalisation risk and ease of use. The Onyx system (Covidien), an ethylene vinyl alcohol copolymer, showed excellent applicability in all EVAR devices, low risk of recanalisation, good primary results and acceptable mid-term results up to two years. However, long-term research is required, as the authors only studied the follow-up in one centre and in eight type Ia endoleak patients.[18]

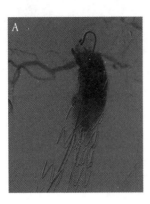
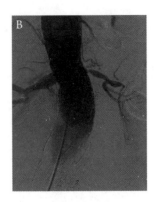
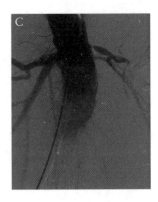

Figure 4: (A) Type Ia endoleak on angiography caused by distal migration of the endograft. (B) Aptus EndoAnchor implantation for fixation of the EVAR device. (C) Additional proximal cuff placement in conjunction with Aptus EndoAnchors to seal the endoleak.

Endovascular aneurysm sealing using the Nellix endograft

The Nellix endovascular aneurysm sealing (EVAS) system (Endologix) was introduced in 2013. The concept differs from EVAR, as endobags surrounding the balloon expandable stents are filled *in situ* with a biocompatible polymer for aneurysmal sealing. The polymer is injected in a liquid state and cures to a solid state at body temperature, thus conforming to the aneurysm shape. This provides stability and seal from the aneurysmal sac and anchoring the stents inside the aneurysm. These polymer-filled endobags reduce the space for endoleaks to occur and could broaden the applicability of treatment of aneurysms.[19]

Procedurally, two Nellix stents are expanded. The endobags are subsequently prefilled with a saline solution in order to expand the endobags, confirm the required filling volume, and to verify the absence of endoleak with the intended 180mmHg pressure in the endobags. In case an endoleak occurs, additional volume is added to increase the pressure by 20mmHg, followed by new angiography to confirm complete seal. Then the saline solution is replaced by the polymer. During polymer curing the Nellix balloons are re-inflated to optimise the flow lumen. When indicated, secondary fill can be performed after removal of the safety wires and primary fill line. Lastly, final angiographies are performed to confirm patency, absence of endoleak, and correct stent positioning. The true incidence of type Ia endoleak after EVAS is unknown. The Nellix system investigational pivotal trial included 150 patients.[4] The mean aneurysm diameter was 58mm and all patients were within the instructions for use. Procedural success was 100% and at 30-days, the core-lab identified nine endoleaks of which eight were type II and one was type Ia. The type Ia endoleak was associated with a procedural stent misalignment and was treated with coil embolisation. In the EVAS FORWARD Global registry, 300 patients were included in 30 sites. Patients were included without prospective screening and only 190 patients were within the instructions for use.[4] There were eight endoleaks within 30 days of which one was type II, one type Ib and six type Ia; all in the cohort within the instructions for use. Four reported endoleaks were treated successfully and two remained present at 30 days. The combined incidence of type Ia endoleak at 30-days after EVAS is 0.4% with an overall early incidence of 1.5%. During longer follow-up, four new type Ia endoleaks occurred that required secondary intervention. One patient suffered from a ruptured aneurysm related to a type Ia endoleak and received secondary open surgery.

Complaint data from the commercial use of Nellix suggests that type Ia endoleaks occur more often during early experience, suggesting that there is a learning curve. For those who reported a type Ia endoleak, the average number of cases until the reported first event was 4.9 cases. The reports of type Ia endoleak submitted within the first 10 cases was 85%, and only 27% submitted more than one type Ia endoleak. Analysis of these endoleaks revealed that they were mostly due to poor stent position and/or alignment. Type Ia endoleaks seem to occur more frequently with new users and new users appear to adapt to the learning curve quickly and improve their technique to eliminate future type Ia endoleaks. Data from this analysis as well as the EVAS FORWARD Global registry have, therefore, suggested that early type Ia endoleaks appear to be related to a learning curve.

Causes of type Ia endoleak after EVAS include incorrect low placement of the endografts, an inadequate filling of the endobags and late migration. Several steps could improve outcome of the procedure. Patient selection is the starting point in preventing type Ia endoleak in the same was as it is with EVAR. Asymmetric shaped and angulated aneurysms, or "stomach-shaped" aneurysms, are deemed to be at risk for type Ia endoleaks, especially in combination with a short infrarenal neck (Figure 5). The increasing volume in the endobags forces the stent lying in the outer curve to move downwards and cause misalignment of the stent. Maintaining proper stent position is crucial at this point and optimally the endobags—located 4mm below the stent—should be positioned immediately infrarenal. When stents tend to dislodge during prefill, inflation of the Nellix balloons during filling will create more stability in the system. The addition of contrast to the prefill solution may also be helpful. During the procedure, angiographies are performed through the nose cones of the devices, but contrast density is lower compared to pigtail angiographies. It is advised to first remove one catheter and replace that with an angiography catheter and make a control angiogram in two directions. This enables the use of a secondary fill from another device, in case a minor endoleak is observed. A lateral view angiogram is important, because endoleaks may occur in the conjunction area of the two endobags, which could be missed on anterior-posterior angiography.

Detection of type Ia endoleaks after EVAS can be challenging because of the presence of the endobags. A type Ia endoleak can be recognised as contrast between the endobags and the aneurysm wall (Figure 6a). This may be subtle and it can

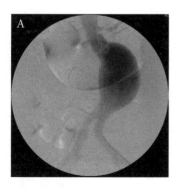
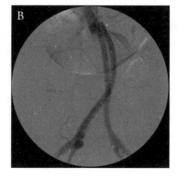

Figure 5: (A) Procedural angiography: "stomach" shaped aneurysm. (B) Two deployed Nellix endografts with misalignment causing a type Ia endoleak.

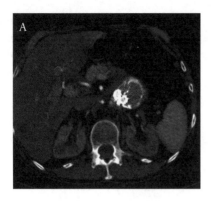
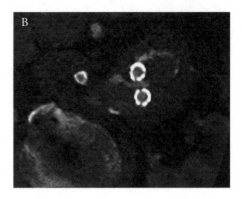

Figure 6: Transversal views of a CTA show contrast between (A) the endobag and the aortic wall, and (B) on a different patient between the endobags.

be difficult to differentiate from calcium or precipitated contrast in the endobag. Another possibility is contrast between the endobags (Figure 6b), while an increasing amount of thrombus between the endobags during follow up can be considered a warning sign. When in doubt, an ECG-gated CT scan can be of additional value in the detection of an endoleak, which can also be visualised on duplex and MR angiogram.[20]

Anecdotal information states that type Ia endoleaks are not benign, and tend to increase over time, potentially causing secondary aneurysm rupture. It is, therefore, advisable to treat type Ia endoleak early. Nevertheless, some type Ia endoleaks

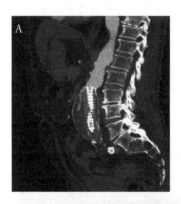
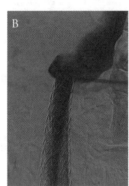

Figure 7: (A) Type Ia endoleak after EVAS on CT angiogram in sagittal view. (B) The endoleak spontaneously resolved on diagnostic angiography three weeks after CT angiogram.

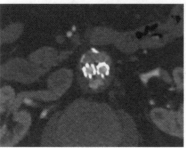
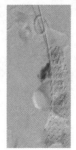
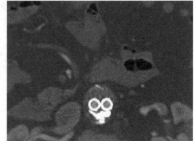

Figure 8: Dorsal type Ia endoleak after EVAS, treated with N-butyl-cyanoacrylate and proximal extension using two balloon expandable covered stents. (Images courtesy of A Holden, Auckland City Hospital, Auckland, New Zealand).

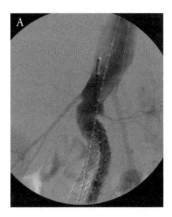
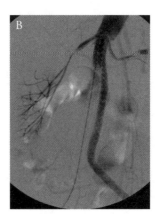

Figure 9: (A) A distally migrated Nellix with a type Ia endoleak, (B) treated by proximal extensions using two new Nellix stents and chimney grafts in the renal arteries.

resolve spontaneously shortly after the procedure (Figure 7). Treatment options include the embolisation with coils in combination N-Butyl-Cyanoacrylate or Onyx treatment or N-Butyl-Cyanoacrylate/Onyx only in minor endoleaks (Figure 8), or the extension of the endograft with another Nellix stent in case of misplacement or distal migration (Figure 9). A comprehensive description of N-Butyl-Cyanoacrylate application in EVAS patients has recently been published by Harvey *et al*.[21] Others have described their experience with transcatheter embolisation of type Ia endoleak after EVAS in seven patients.[22] The mean time from EVAS to embolisation was 136 days. Embolisation was performed with coils and Onyx (Covidien) in six cases and Onyx only in one case and technical success was achieved in all. One patient required a secondary procedure following Onyx reflux into the Nellix endograft. All patients remained free of endoleaks with stable sac size after a mean follow-up of eight months. In case of distal migration during long-term follow-up, proximal extension with another Nellix stent, with or without chimney grafts, appears to be an attractive option, although this technique is still in development. Flaring of the original stent with a 12mm balloon as well as pre-deployment of the endobag before expanding the stents is advisable. The minimum required sealing length is yet to be determined, but seems to be about 2–3cm. Chimney grafts are, therefore, often required.

Summary

- Type Ia endoleaks are an important risk factor for secondary rupture after endovascular treatment of abdominal aortic aneurysms and treatment is usually indicated.

- Conventional CT-angiography is the primary diagnostic method but MR angiogram or ECG-gated CT-angiography can be of additional value.

- Although treatment options for type Ia endoleak are available, the focus should be their prevention by proper patient selection and technique.

- Type Ia endoleak after EVAS seems to be related to a learning curve and early intervention is indicated.

References

1. Moulakakis KG, Dalainas I, Mylonas S, *et al*. Conversion to open repair after endografting for abdominal aortic aneurysm: a review of causes, incidence, results, and surgical techniques of reconstruction. *J Endovasc Ther* 2010; **17** (6): 694.

2. van Marrewijk C, Buth J, Harris PL, *et al.* Significance of endoleaks after endovascular repair of abdominal aortic aneurysms: The EUROSTAR experience. *J Vasc Surg* 2002; **35** (3): 461–73.
3. Schermerhorn ML, O'Malley AJ, Jhaveri A, *et al.* Endovascular vs. open repair of abdominal aortic aneurysms in the Medicare population. *N Engl J Med* 2008; **358** (5): 464–74.
4. Holden A. Nellix Endograft System for EVAS: Key points from the global registry and how to prevent, diagnose and treat type Ia endoleaks. Presented at the 2015 Annual VEITHsymposium, 19 November 2015.
5. Pitton MB, Schweitzer H, Herber S, *et al.* MRI *versus* helical CT for endoleak detection after endovascular aneurysm repair. *AJR Am J Roentgenol* 2005; **185** (5): 1275–81.
6. Koike Y, Ishida K, Hase S, *et al.* Dynamic volumetric CT angiography for the detection and classification of endoleaks: application of cine imaging using a 320-row CT scanner with 16-cm detectors. *J Vasc Interv Radiol* 2014; **25** (8): 1172–80.
7. Blackwood S, Mix D, Chandra A, *et al.* A model to demonstrate that endotension is a nonvisualized type I endoleak. *J Vasc Surg* 2015; DOI: http://dx.doi.org/10.1016/j.jvs.2015.04.422.
8. Mehta M, Sternbach Y, Taggert JB, *et al.* Long-term outcomes of secondary procedures after endovascular aneurysm repair. *J Vasc Surg* 2010; **52** (6): 1442–9.
9. Jordan WD Jr, Ouriel K, Metha M, *et al.* Outcome-based anatomic criteria for defining the hostile aortic neck. Outcome-based anatomic criteria for defining the hostile aortic neck. *J Vasc Surg* 2015; **61** (6): 1383–90.
10. Katsargyris A, Botos B, Oikonomou K, *et al.* The new C3 Gore Excluder stent-graft: single-center experience with 100 patients. *Eur J Vasc Endovasc Surg* 2014; **47** (4): 342–8.
11. Antonopoulos CN, Kakisis JD, Giannakopoulos TG, *et al.* Rupture after endovascular abdominal aortic aneurysm repair: a multicenter study. Vasc Endovascular Surg 2014; **48** (7–8): 476–81.
12. Buth J, van Marrewijk CJ, Harris PL, *et al.* Outcome of endovascular abdominal aortic aneurysm repair in patients with conditions considered unfit for an open procedure: a report on the EUROSTAR experience. *J Vasc Surg* 2002; **35** (2): 211–21.
13. Tielliu IF, Buijs RV, Greuter MJ, *et al.* Circumference as an alternative for diameter measurement in endovascular aneurysm repair. *Med Hypotheses* 2015; **85** (2): 230–3.
14. Franks SC, Sutton AJ, Brown MJ, *et al.* Systematic review and meta-analysis of 12 years of endovascular abdominal aortic aneurysm repair. *Eur J Vasc Endovasc Surg* 2007; **33** (2): 154–71.
15. Rajani RR, Arthurs ZM, Srivastava SD, *et al.* Repairing immediate proximal endoleaks during abdominal aortic aneurysm repair. *J Vasc Surg* 2011; **53** (5): 1174–77.
16. Wilson A, Zhou S, *et al.* Systematic review of chimney and periscope grafts for endovascular aneurysm repair. *Br J Surg* 2013; **100** (12): 1557–64.
17. Donselaar EJ, van der Vijver RJ, van den Ham LH, *et al.* EndoAnchors to resolve persistent type Ia endoleak secondary to proximal cuff with parallel graft placement. *J Endovasc Ther* 2016; **23** (1): 225–8.
18. Eberhardt KM, Sadeghi-Azandaryani M, Worlicek S, *et al.* Treatment of type I endoleaks using transcatheter embolization with onyx. *J Endovasc Ther* 2014; **21** (1): 162–71.
19. Karthikesalingam A, Cobb RJ, Khoury A, *et al.* The morphological applicability of a novel endovascular aneurysm sealing (EVAS) system (Nellix) in patients with abdominal aortic aneurysms. *Eur J Vasc Endovasc Surg* 2013; **46** (4): 440–45.
20. Holden A, Savlovskis J, Winterbottom A, *et al.* Imaging After Nellix Endovascular Aneurysm Sealing: A Consensus Document. *J Endovasc Ther* 2016; **23** (1): 7–20.
21. Ameli-Renani S, Morgan RA. Transcatheter embolisation of proximal type 1 endoleaks following endovascular aneurysm sealing (EVAS) using the Nellix device: Technique and outcomes. Cardiovasc Intervent Radiol 2015; **38** (5): 1137–42.
22. Harvey JJ, Brew S, Hill A, *et al.* Transcatheter embolization of type Ia endoleak after Nellix endovascular aortic aneurysm sealing with N-Butyl-Cyanoacrylate: technique in 3 patients. *J Vasc Interv Radiol* 2015; in press.

The different appearance of endoleaks after endovascular aneurysm sealing

T Martin and A Holden

Introduction

Nellix endovascular aneurysm sealing (EVAS, Endologix) is a novel approach to aneurysmal repair where there is aneurysmal sac exclusion via polymer-filled endobags. As such, the appearance of endoleaks is unique and different to traditional endovascular aneurysm repair (EVAR). Because single Nellix components are usually introduced from each groin, type III endoleaks have been rarely described and type IV and V endoleaks have not been described to date. Type I and II endoleaks have a variable appearance that has been described in recent literature.[1-3] Given that the imaging and natural history of these endoleaks is associated with such a new technology, the imaging protocols for surveillance have not been well established with many centres opting for dual computed tomography (CT)/ ultrasound follow-up to correlate the appearances between the two modalities.

EVAS

EVAS is a very different method of abdominal aortic aneurysm repair when compared to traditional endovascular aneurysm repair (EVAR). It has been previously described in detail with positive results having been reported with a range of aortic anatomical variations.[4,5]

The accepted reference for endoleak classification is based on the source of the endoleak within the stent graft initially described by White *et al* in their 1997 publication[6] and has been subsequently divided into five types.[7,8] With EVAS, IV and V endoleaks have not been described given the presence of endobags that maintain graft integrity. Type III endoleaks can only occur if a graft extension is introduced proximal or distal to the Nellix device.

The EVAS procedure has been previously described in detail.[4,5] Each device consists of a chromium-cobalt balloon-expandable stent covered in expanded polytetrafluoroethylene (ePTFE) and surrounded by a polyurethane endobag. The stent is composed of 4mm long interconnected stent elements, the highest and lowest stent elements are not covered with ePTFE. The stents are mounted on 10mm diameter minimally-compliant angioplasty balloons introduced from each common femoral artery. Prefilling with saline is initially performed to ensure satisfactory aneurysm exclusion. Finally, a hydrogel polymer of polyethylene glycol diacrylate fills the endobags and excludes the aneurysm lumen.

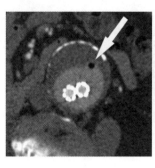
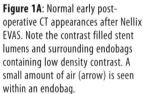
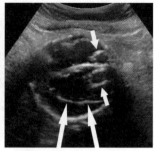
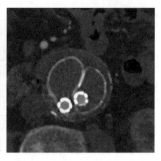

Figure 1A: Normal early post-operative CT appearances after Nellix EVAS. Note the contrast filled stent lumens and surrounding endobags containing low density contrast. A small amount of air (arrow) is seen within an endobag.

Figure 1B: Normal early post-operative ultrasound appearances after Nellix EVAS. Note the Nellix stents (short arrows) with surrounding endobags (long arrows).

Figure 1C: Normal CT appearances one year after Nellix EVAS. Note the density in the endobags has decreased with contrast migrated to the outer surface of the polymer hydrogel.

To date there have been few publications describing imaging after EVAS. These articles are characterised by short-term follow-up and small case numbers.[1–3] The text below is based on a consensus document on the imaging findings after EVAS by Holden *et al* and is based on the collective experience of the sites involved in the Nellix EVAS FORWARD Global registry in addition to the US-based EVAS investigational devices exemption (IDE) trial.[9] The combined experience exceeds 1,000 clinical cases with the longest global follow-up after EVAS.

CT and duplex surveillance following EVAS

The optimal CT protocol following EVAS does not vary significantly when compared to that for conventional EVAR, both non-contrast and arterial-phase imaging is required. The dual phase facilitates the identification of endobags, arterial wall calcification, blood flow within stent lumens and the presence of endoleaks. Dose reduction techniques such as iterative reconstruction are commonly used.

Duplex ultrasound assessment of patients following EVAS involves standard grayscale, colour, spectral and power Doppler studies. Contrast-enhanced studies may be used as an adjunct to standard techniques.

It is important to note some marked differences in follow-up imaging when evaluating EVAS for endoleak. In the immediately post-procedural phase (Figure 1A), the aneurysm is usually the same size or 1–2mm larger. The intraluminal thrombus also may demonstrate a degree of displacement which is secondary to the endobags being inflated above systolic pressure. The endobags are hyperdense compared with non-opacified blood or thrombus due to iodinated contrast within the polymer. It is common to see a small amount of air in the endobags, which is inadvertently introduced during the endobag filling stage. In a minority of cases, air persists to one month but should be resorbed completely by three and six month scans at which point it is replaced by fluid, most probably from the peri-aortic extracellular space.

Early postoperative evaluation with duplex is useful and the same structures identified on CT such as stent, endobags, aortic thrombus and aortic wall are readily identified on ultrasound (Figure 1B). The hydrogel is anechoic and the endobag wall is echogenic. Aortic thrombus is slightly more echogenic than endobag contents and is easily recognised. Flow lumen within the stents can be well interrogated with colour and spectral Doppler. In the early postoperative phase, the air in the endobags and that trapped between endobag and stent may limit stent lumen visualisation.

Late appearances on CT and duplex are important to understand. The radiodensity of the polymer in the endobags decreases over time and eventually reaches a density of 70–80 Hounsfield Units, usually stable at six months (Figure 1C). In addition, contrast migrates to the outer surface of the polymer hydrogel, situated at the inner margin of the endobag. This may be asymmetric in appearance. Iodine ion migration is secondary to a mild osmotic gradient between the blood in the peri-aortic tissues and the polymer hydrogel. Air in the endobag is replaced by fluid, as iodine ions migrate they outline the sites of previous air bubbles and may resemble focal endobag collapse.

In contrast to post-EVAR imaging, the EVAS sac either stays the same size or mildly decreases on long-term follow-up. Decrease in endobag size is secondary to resorption of intraluminal thrombus surrounding the endobags. If the sac wall progresses to abut the endobag, no further shrinkage will occur. Duplex appearances do not significantly alter with time. The endobags remain hypoechoic and the migrated contrast is not sonographically visible.

Magnetic resonance imaging and plain film

The components of EVAS are well seen on magnetic resonance (MR) imaging. The endobags are hypointense on T1-weighted imaging and hyperintense on T2-weighted imaging. On contrast-enhanced MR angiography, some signal loss is demonstrated within the flow lumen. This is due to artefact susceptibility from the adjacent stents, however, a patent lumen can be still visualised.

Plain film imaging easily demonstrates the chromium-cobalt stents. The stents are usually crossed and the upper ends of the stents are aligned. On the images acquired after one month, the migrated contrast provides a visible outline of the endobags. Plain radiographs allow assessment of wireform fractures or stent kinking. The role of plain radiographs in post procedural imaging has not yet been clarified.

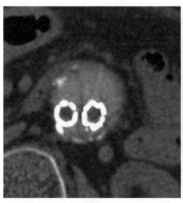 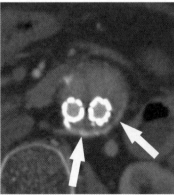

Figure 2: Early small type Ia endoleak after Nellix EVAS. Note the subtle curvilinear contrast rim seen outside the endobags posteriorly (arrows) on the post-contrast CT, not visible on the pre-contrast study.

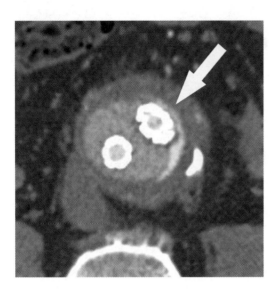

Figure 3: Type Ib endoleak, presenting as curvilinear contrast (arrow) between the endobag and mural thrombus in the distal aneurysm sac.

The appearances of endoleaks after EVAS

Type I and type II endoleaks take on a unique appearance following EVAS. A type I endoleak may be seen both proximally (Ia) and distally (Ib). Most cases of a type Ia endoleak appear to be due to inadequate filling of the endobags or the incorrect low deployment of the device. Type Ib endoleaks are seen if there is inadequate endobag filling or if the device is of inadequate length.

A type I endoleak typically appears as a curvilinear rim of contrast between the endobag and aortic wall or aortic thrombus. A small type Ia endoleak can be very subtle and it can be very challenging to differentiate a small endoleak from calcified atheromatous plaque or contrast within the endobag. It is in this setting that close analysis of both CT phases is of use in resolving the findings (Figure 2). The early natural history of type I endoleaks in the Nellix device suggests that the aneurysmal sac will get larger with time.[9] A unique form of type Ia endoleak involves an endoleak between the endobags. This may be seen as an isolated endoleak or in combination with a typical leak between the aortic wall and the endobags. Type Ib endoleak typically demonstrates contrast around the device in the common iliac artery (Figure 3).

Duplex findings in patients with type I endoleaks include curvilinear flow between the endobag and the aortic wall on colour or power Doppler. Antegrade flow in outflow vessels such as the inferior mesenteric or lumbar arteries is also seen. Spectral imaging demonstrates high-velocity flow within the endoleak with elevated diastolic flow and spectral broadening secondary to associated turbulence.

Type II endoleaks are very uncommon after EVAS.[4] These, by definition, occur in portions of the sac that are not filled by endobag or thrombus and are typically small (Figure 4). Type II endoleaks are perfused in a retrograde direction from patent aortic branches such as inferior mesenteric artery or lumbar arteries. CT imaging confirms sac filling of a nidus from a patent aortic branch artery. Duplex imaging demonstrates low flow retrograde filling of a sac nidus from an aortic branch artery which demonstrates low velocity biphasic flow on spectral Doppler.

Surveillance

The optimum imaging surveillance protocol after EVAS is yet to be established as the longer term natural history of the repair is still being studied. CT is favoured in early follow-up with many centres opting for CT surveillance in the first year post-procedure. Following this, centres are taking on a variable approach with many performing dual ultrasound/CT follow-up to correlate between the two modalities.

Conclusion

EVAS is a novel method for treating aneurysm with unique imaging appearances after repair. In addition, the appearance of the device changes over time, especially on CT. Both type I and type II endoleaks are recognised in EVAS. Complications are uncommon and have distinctive appearances, as detailed above, when compared to conventional EVAR.

Summary

- EVAS with the Endologix Nellix device is a novel approach to aortic aneurysm repair.

- Endobags generally exclude sac inflow and maintain integrity of the graft and as such, Type I and rarely type II and III endoleaks, are the only recognised endoleak complications.

- Type Ia and Ib endoleaks are recognised, the former generally resulting from low deployment or inadequate endobag filling and the latter from inadequate endobag filling or inadequate device length.

- Type I endoleaks appear as a curvilinear rim of contrast between the endobag and the aortic wall or thrombus.

- Type II endoleaks are very uncommon and occur in a portion of sac that is not excluded by endobag or thrombus, these are typically small.

- The Nellix EVAS device has specific imaging appearances that evolve over time, particularly on CT. It is vital that the natural history of imaging appearance is recognised in order to correctly interpret imaging findings.

- Optimum imaging surveillance has yet to be established, most centres use both CT and ultrasound.

References

1. D'Abate F, Harrison SA, Karthikesalingam A, *et al*. Sonographic appearance following endovascular aneurysm repair using the Nellix Endovascular Sealing System. *J Endovasc Ther* 2015; **22**: 182–6.
2. McWilliams RG, Fisher RK, England A, *et al*. Observations on surveillance imaging after endovascular sealing of abdominal aortic aneurysms. *J Endovasc Ther* 2015; **22**: 303–6.
3. Karthikesalingam A, de Bruin JL, Patel SR, *et al*. Appearance of the Nellix Endovascular Aneurysm Sealing System on computed tomography: implications for postoperative imaging surveillance. *J Endovasc Ther* 2015; **22**: 297–302.
4. Bockler D, Holden A, Thompson M, *et al*. Multicenter Nellix EndoVascular Aneurysm Sealing system experience in aneurysm sac sealing. *J Vasc Surg* 2015; **62**: 290–98.
5. Holden A. Endovascular sac sealing concept: will the Endologix Nellix device solve the deficiencies? *J Cardiovasc Surg* (Torino) 2015; **56**: 339–53.

6. White GH, Yu W, May J, *et al.* Endoleak as a complication of endoluminal grafting of abdominal aortic aneurysm: classification, incidence, diagnosis, and management. *J Endovasc Surg* 1997; **4**: 152–68.
7. Chaikof EL, Blankensteijn JD, Harris PL, *et al.* Reporting standards for endovascular aortic aneurysm repair. *J Vasc Surg* 2002; **35**: 1048–60.
8. Veith FJ, Baum RA, Ohki T, *et al.* Nature and significance of   endoleaks and endotension: summary of opinions at an international conference. *J Vasc Surg* 2002; **35**: 1029–35.
9. Holden A, Savlovskis J, Winterbottom A, *et al.* Imaging after Nellix endovascular aneurysm sealing: a consensus document. *J Endovasc Ther* 2016; **23** (1): 7–20.

Infected abdominal aortic aneurysm challenges

EndoVAC—a novel treatment option for infected vascular reconstructions

A Wanhainen, K Thorbjørnsen and M Björck

Introduction

Vascular prosthetic graft infection is a rare yet serious and challenging complication, with high mortality and morbidity, especially in the case of acute bleeding.

The groin represents the most frequent site of vascular graft infection, with an incidence of about 5% and mortality and amputation rates as high as 58% and 79%, respectively.[1-7] The reported incidence of carotid patch infection ranges from 0.5% to 1.8% with high risk of neurological morbidity and mortality.[8-15]

Because of the variable clinical presentations, often small cohorts and the lack of data from comparative studies or randomised controlled trials, there are no clear guidelines for management of infected vascular reconstructions. Nevertheless, the long-established practice in the management of these challenging complications is radical surgical treatment.

Traditional radical surgery includes: 1) debridement, 2) removal of the infected prosthetic graft, and 3) *de novo* revascularisation, by extra-anatomical bypass in non-infected field or by *in-situ* reconstruction, together with long-term antibiotics.[2-5] *In situ* reconstructions using autologous vein grafts, antibiotic or silver-bonded grafts, cryopreserved homograft, or fresh arterial allografts have been reported.[16-19]

Conservative treatment options, such as different muscle flaps and vacuum-assisted wound closure (VAC), may sometimes be an option for high-risk surgical patients due to severe comorbidity.[20-26] The preservation of vascular grafts with muscle flaps has been shown to shorten healing time, decrease wound bacterial counts, augment the delivery of antibiotics, and obliterate dead space to decrease the risk of recurrent infection.[27] VAC-therapy is considered to have several beneficial effects on healing wounds and has been increasingly used for the treatment of vascular surgical site infections, both as a primary wound treatment option or in combination with other treatment modalities.[25,26,28-31] However, bleeding complications from infected and exposed vessels have been reported during VAC therapy,[24-26,28] and if bleeding is already a problem VAC therapy alone is not an option.

Thus, these techniques have their limitations, and in certain circumstances such as adverse anatomy and/or severe comorbidity surgical repair or conservative treatment may be difficult or even not feasible.[19]

Here, we describe a novel hybrid technique for treatment of infected vascular reconstructions, and report our experiences so far.

The EndoVAC hybrid technique

The EndoVAC hybrid technique[32] is a three-step procedure and consists of: 1) relining of the infected reconstruction with a stent graft, preferably self-expanding stent grafts such as Viabahn (Gore) or Fluency (Bard); 2) surgical revision of the infected area with extensive soft tissue debridement followed by removal of the infected vascular prosthesis. The surgical revision is performed without clamping the reconstruction and results in a partial exposure of the stent graft. Muscle flaps are sometimes used to facilitate soft tissue coverage of the exposed stent graft; And 3) VAC therapy, to permit granulation and secondary delayed healing or suture. A continuous topical negative pressure is used during the first 24 hours, followed by intermittent negative pressure of 125mmHg. The VAC sponge is changed every two to four days.

Long-term antibiotic treatment and follow-up are mandatory. We advocate antibiotic treatment for at least three months, or until no sign of infection remains (clinical, laboratory, or radiological).

The Uppsala experience

So far, the Uppsala experience consists of 17 EndoVAC procedures performed in 16 patients between 2007 and 2015.[32] Nine of the cases involved the carotid artery; six infected carotid patches after carotid endarterectomy and three infected neck deviations. Six of the cases involved the femoral artery in the groin; two infected femoropopliteal bypasses, three infected patches after femoral thromboendarterectomy, and one infected vascular access. One case involved an infected large brachial access site.

Five were emergent procedures; three with profuse bleeding from the infected wound, one with a rapid expanding pseudoaneurysm, and one with acute limb ischemia. The remaining procedures performed were subacute.

Wound cultures were positive for coagulase negative *Staphylococci* in 53% of the cases, *Staphylococcus aureus* in 29%, and 18% had negative intraoperative cultures. Twenty nine per cent had polymicrobial infections, including gram-negative organisms.

The duration of VAC treatment was a median of 14 days (range 9–57 days). Supplementary rotated sartorius muscle flaps were used in three patients with infected femoral patches and a sternocleidomastoid flap was used in one patient in the carotid group.

Early complications included one transient stroke and one temporary hypoglossal palsy.

In all patients, the graft infection healed with no recurrence observed after a median of five years of follow-up, neither clinically, nor based on laboratory findings or imaging. Late complications included two asymptomatic occluded bypasses, one asymptomatic moderate carotid stenosis, and one symptomatic stent graft thrombosis. Eight patients died due to severe comorbidities unrelated to the infection or hybrid procedure, one month to seven years after treatment.

Conclusion

The EndoVAC hybrid technique is a promising, less invasive, option for treatment of infected vascular reconstructions in selected cases, when traditional radical surgery is not considered feasible or safe.

Insertion of stent grafts is an attractive option with complete intraluminal sealing of the arteriotomy or vascular anastomosis, allowing safe removal of the infected patch without need of extensive dissection or clamping of the artery and avoiding exposing a suture line (patch or anastomosis) to the infected field.

Implantation of a stent graft in a setting of active infection may be considered controversial and against surgical principles due to the risk of infection of the endoprosthesis. So far, however, we have seen no such complications in the Uppsala experience with up until seven years of follow-up.

Based on these excellent results, EndoVAC has become the procedure of choice at our centre, and fewer graft infections are treated with traditional radical surgery.

Summary

- Vascular prosthetic graft infection is a rare but serious complication.

- Traditional radical surgery consists of debridement, removal of the infected prosthetic graft and *de novo* revascularisation, by extra-anatomical bypass in non-infected field or by *in situ* reconstruction.

- Conservative treatment options, such as different muscle flaps and vacuum-assisted wound closure (VAC), may sometimes be an option for high-risk patient due to severe comorbidities.

- The evidence for this long-established practice is limited.

- The EndoVAC hybrid technique is a less invasive alternative option for treatment of infected vascular reconstructions in selected cases such as adverse anatomy, bleeding and/or severe comorbidity.

- The EndoVAC technique consists of: 1) relining of the infected reconstruction with a stent graft, 2) surgical revision (without clamping the reconstruction), and 3) VAC therapy to permit granulation and secondary delayed healing, followed by long-term antibiotic treatment.

References

1. Exton RJ, Galland RB. Major groin complications following the use of synthetic grafts. *Eur J Vasc Endovasc Surg* 2007; **34**: 188–90
2. Szilagyi DE, Smith RF, Elliott JP, *et al*. Infection in arterial reconstruction with synthetic grafts. *Ann Surg* 1972; **176**: 321–33.
3. Liekweg WG, Greenfield LJ. Vascular prosthetic infections: collected experience and results of treatment. *Surgery* 1977; **81**: 335–42.
4. Yeager RA, McConnell DB, Sasaki TM, Vetto RM. Aortic and peripheral prosthetic graft infection: differential management and causes of mortality. *Am J Surg* 1985; **150**: 36–43.
5. Kikta MJ, Goodson SF, Bishara RA, *et al*. Mortality and limb loss with infected infra- inguinal bypass grafts. *J Vasc Surg* 1987; **5**: 566–71.
6. Calligaro KD, Veith FJ, Schwartz ML, *et al*. Selective preservation of infected prosthetic arterial grafts. Analysis of a 20-year experience with 120 extracavitary-infected grafts. *Ann Surg* 1994; **220**: 461–71.

7. Siracuse JJ, Nandivada P, Giles KA, *et al.* Prosthetic graft infections involving the femoral artery. *J Vasc Surg* 2013; **57**: 700–05.

8. El-Sabrout R, Reul G, Cooley DA. Infected postcarotid endarterectomy pseudoaneurysms: retrospective review of a series. *Ann Vasc Surg* 2000; **14**: 239–47.

9. Rizzo A, Hertzer NR, O'Hara PJ, *et al.* Dacron carotid patch infection: a report of eight cases. *J Vasc Surg* 2000; **32**: 602–06.

10. Naylor AR, Payne D, London NJM, *et al.* Prosthetic patch infection after carotid endarterectomy. *Eur J Vasc Endovasc Surg* 2002; **23**: 11–16.

11. Rockman CB, Su WT, Domenig C, *et al.* Postoperative infection associated with polyester patch angioplasty after carotid endarterectomy. *J Vasc Surg* 2003; **38**: 251–56.

12. Asciutto G, Geier B, Marpe B, *et al.* Dacron patch infection after carotid angioplasty. A report of 6 cases. *Eur J Vasc Endovasc Surg.* 2007; **33**: 55–57.

13. Krishnan S, Clowes AW. Dacron patch infection after carotid endarterectomy: case report and review of the literature. *Ann Vasc Surg* 2006; **20**: 672–77.

14. Knight BC, Tait WF. Dacron patch infection following carotid endarterectomy: a systematic review of the literature. *Eur J Vasc Endovasc Surg* 2009; **37**: 140–48.

15. Mann CD, McCarty M, Nasim A, *et al.* Management and Outcome of Prosthetic Patch Infection after Carotid Endarterectomy: A single-centre Series and Systematic Review of the Literature. *Eur J Vasc Endovasc Surg* 2012; **44**: 20–06.

16. Clagett GP, Bowers BL, Lopez-Viego MA, *et al.* Creation of a neo-aortoiliac system from lower extremity deep and superficial veins. *Ann Surg* 1993; **218**: 239–48.

17. Ehsan O, Gibbons CP. A 10-year experience of using femoropopliteal vein for re-vascularisation in graft and arterial infections. *Eur J Vasc Endovasc Surg* 2009; **38** (2): 172–79.

18. Bandyk DF, Novotney ML, Back MR, *et al.* Expanded application of in situ replacement for prosthetic graft infection. *J Vasc Surg* 2001; **34**: 411–19.

19. Lorentzen JE, Nielsen OM, Arendrup H, *et al:* Vascular graft infection: An analysis of sixty-two graft infections in 2411 consecutively implanned synthetic Vascular grafts. Surgery 1985; **98**: 81–86.

20. Zacharoulis DC, Gupta SK, Seymour P, Landa RA. Use of muscle flap to cover infections of the carotid artery after carotid endarterectomy. *J Vasc Surg* 1997; **25**: 769–73.

21. Colwell AS, Donaldson MC, Belkin M, Orgill DP. Management of early groin vascular bypass graft infections with sartorius and rectus femoris flaps. *Ann Plast Surg* 2004; **52**: 49–53.

22. Morasch MD, Sam AD 2nd, Melina R, Ket al. Early results with use of gracilis muscle flap coverage of infected groin wounds after vascular surgery. *J Vasc Surg* 2004; **39**: 1277–83.

23. Shermak MA, Yee K, Wong L, *et al.* Surgical management of groin lymphatic complications after arterial bypass surgery. *Plast Reconstr Surg* 2005; **115**: 1954–62.

24. Herrera FA, Kohanzadeh S, Nasseri Y, *et al.* Management of vascular graft infections with soft tissue flap coverage: improving limb salvage rates – a veterans affairs experience. *Am Surg* 2009; **75**: 877–81.

25. Nordmyr J, Svensson S, Bjorck M, Acosta S. Vacuum assisted wound closure in patients with lower extremity arterial disease. The experience from two tertiary referral centres. *Int Angiol* 2009; **28**: 26–31.

26. Dosluoglu HH, Loghmanee C, Lall P, *et al.* Management of early (<30 day) vascular groin infections using vacuum-assisted closure alone without muscle flap coverage in a consecutive patient series. *J Vasc Surg* 2010; **51**: 1160–66.

27. Armstrong PA, Back MR, Bandyk DF, *et al.* Selective application of sartorius muscle flaps and aggressive staged surgical debridement can influence long-term outcomes of complex prosthetic graft infections *J Vasc Surg* 2007; **46**: 71–78.

28. Svensson S, Monsen C, Kolbel T, Acosta S. Predictors for outcome after vacuum assisted closure therapy of peri-vascular surgical site infections in the groin. *Eur J Vasc Endovasc Surg* 2008; **36**: 84–89.

29. Acosta S, Monsen S. Outcome after VAC Therapy for infected Bypass Grafts in the Lower Limb. *Eur J Vasc Endovasc Surg* 2012; **44**: 294–99.

30. Mayer D, Hasse B, Koelliker J, *et al.* Long-term results of vascular graft and artery preserving treatment with negative pressure wound therapy in Szilagyi grade III infections justify a paradigm shift. *Ann Surg.* 2011; **254**: 754–59.

31. Monsen C, Wann-Hansson C, Wictorsson C, Acosta S. Vacuum-assisted wound closure *versus* alginate for the treatment of deep perivascular wound infections in the groin after vascular surgery. *J Vasc Surg* 2014; **59**: 145–51.

32. Kragsterman B, Björck M, Wanhainen A. EndoVAC, a Novel Hybrid Technique to Treat Infected Vascular Reconstructions With an Endograft and Vacuum-Assisted Wound Closure. *J Endovasc Ther* 2011; **18**: 666–73.

Ruptured abdominal aortic aneurysm

Benefits of local anaesthesia for ruptured abdominal aortic aneurysm repair

RO Forsythe and RJ Hinchliffe

Introduction

Ruptured abdominal aortic aneurysms represent the 13th commonest cause of death in the UK, with an overall mortality of over 80%.[1] If untreated, a ruptured abdominal aortic aneurysm is almost always fatal and of those patients who survive long enough to reach hospital, 41.6% are too unwell to undergo attempted repair.[2] Moreover, even if a patient reaches the operating theatre, repair using either open or endovascular techniques carries a high mortality that has seen relatively little improvement over the past few decades.

Conversely, the outcomes of elective abdominal aortic aneurysm repair have shown great improvement, with an operative mortality of 4.3% and 1.8% for open repair and endovascular aneurysm repair (EVAR), respectively.[3]

Given that more than 80% of abdominal aortic aneurysm deaths are the result of rupture,[4] new strategies are required to help address the persistently high mortality associated with this condition.

Recent data from the IMPROVE (Immediate management of patients with rupture: open *versus* endovascular repair) trial suggest that perioperative mortality for ruptured abdominal aortic aneurysms remains high and that a strategy of using EVAR where possible (compared with open surgery) does not appear to improve 30-day mortality—36.4% *versus* 40.6% in patients with confirmed rupture.[5] In addition, even though the instructions for use are sometimes relaxed in the context of ruptured aneurysms, only around 65% of aneurysms are deemed morphologically suitable for EVAR according to liberal instructions for use (proximal neck length ≥10mm, diameter ≤32mm and angle <60 degrees),[6] yet the mortality for EVAR-suitable patients (who are intrinsically lower risk) remains high at 20–25% for either open or endovascular repair.[7,8]

Whilst the IMPROVE trial did not suggest a significant perioperative survival advantage for an EVAR strategy compared to open repair, it did highlight an important observation—that patients undergoing EVAR under local anaesthesia may be three to four times more likely to survive than those patients requiring general anaesthesia, even after adjustment for age, sex, Hardman index and other potential confounders.[9]

In the elective setting, general anaesthesia has been demonstrated to be an independent risk factor for operative complications including death (odds ratio [OR]=5.1, 95% confidence interval [CI] 1.9–13.3),[10] whilst the EUROSTAR registry (comprising more than 5,500 patients in 164 centres undergoing EVAR) confirmed that patients appear to benefit from locoregional anaesthesia in elective EVAR to treat infrarenal abdominal aortic aneurysms.[11] EVAR under local anaesthesia may, therefore, represent a potential opportunity to reduce the perioperative mortality in ruptured abdominal aortic aneurysms.

Local anaesthesia *versus* general anaesthesia in elective and emergency surgery

There is increasing awareness of the limitations and potential negative impact on outcomes for surgical patients undergoing general anaesthesia, particularly those that are high-risk or with serious comorbidities. The use of alternatives to general anaesthesia (including local and regional anaesthesia), have been explored in various surgical contexts, particularly in the emergency situation. Two substudies of the Swedish Hernia Registry have demonstrated improved outcomes for local anaesthesia in elective and emergency hernia surgery. A multicentre randomised trial comparing local *versus* regional anaesthesia *versus* general anaesthesia included 10 non-specialised hospitals (616 patients) and demonstrated that local anaesthesia was associated with reduced postoperative pain and nausea when compared to general anaesthesia (mean visual analogue scale scores—1.8 vs. 3.3 for pain and 1.1 vs. 1.7 for nausea; p<0.0001), a reduced frequency of early postoperative complications (15% vs. 44%; p<0.0001) and mean hospital stay (3.1 vs. 6.2 days; p<0.0001).[12] Further analysis of the Swedish Hernia Registry (comprising 237 patients who died within 30 days of elective or emergency hernia surgery) demonstrated that local anaesthesia was used rarely for elective operations (3%) but more commonly for emergency operations (13%). Although used less commonly than either general anaesthesia or regional anaesthesia, local anaesthesia was used less frequently in those who subsequently died perioperatively (13% vs. 17% in elective surgery, p<0.001; 3% vs. 5% in emergency surgery, p=0.02).[13] However, no multivariate analysis was performed in this study; therefore, confounding factors may be undetected.

The use of local anaesthesia in patients undergoing surgery for peripheral vascular disease has been of increasing interest in recent years. A post-hoc substudy analysis of a study investigating the use of an endovascular intervention for acute stroke, the NASA (North American Solitaire stent retriever acute stroke) registry, found that local anaesthesia was associated with good 90-day neurological outcomes (modified Rankin Scale ≤2, p=0.01; OR 1.4 [1.1–1.8]) and that general anaesthesia was associated with mortality in multivariate analysis (OR 3.3 [1.6–7.1]; p=0.001), in 281 patients who underwent mechanical embolectomy using the Solitaire stent-retrieving device.[14] In contrast, in the GALA (General anaesthesia *versus* local anaesthesia for carotid surgery) trial (a multicentre randomised controlled trial of 3,526 patients with carotid stenosis), no definite benefit of local anaesthesia was demonstrated; however, three events (stroke, myocardial infarction or death within 30 days) per 1,000 patients were prevented under local anaesthesia, although this finding failed to reach statistical significance.[15] Carotid endarterectomy under local anaesthesia is common practice in many UK vascular centres—a large prospective cohort study in the UK (published in 2011) demonstrated that roughly half of all operations were performed under local anaesthesia, with a conversion to general anaesthesia rate of 1.4%.[16] This number is likely to have increased in the intervening years—local anaesthesia for carotid endarterectomy is clearly tolerated well by vascular patients, surgeons and anaesthetists and is the best method of intraoperative monitoring of brain function. Therefore, the precedent is set for use in other vascular operations.

Regional anaesthesia (*versus* general anaesthesia) for hip fracture surgery in elderly patients has also been associated with reduced early mortality and fewer postoperative complications such as deep vein thrombosis and acute confusion in at least one large systematic review comprising more than 18,000 patients with hip fractures,[17] although definitive evidence for regional anaesthesia as standard preference to general anaesthesia in hip fracture surgery is limited.

Outcomes of elective EVAR under local anaesthesia

The use of local anaesthesia for elective EVAR has been mooted for over a decade,[18,19] and the benefits of this approach were confirmed in the EUROSTAR registry, where patients undergoing EVAR under local anaesthesia had a shorter operation time (115.7±42.2 minutes vs. 133.3±59.1 minutes, p<0.0001), a shorter hospital stay (3.7±3.1 days vs. 6.2±8.5 days, p=0.007), were less likely to require intensive therapy unit (2% vs. 16.2%, p<0.0001) and had fewer systemic complications (6.6% vs. 13.0%, p=0.0015) than those who underwent EVAR under general anaesthesia,[11] when adjusted for possible confounders. A more recent meta-analysis confirmed that local anaesthesia in elective EVAR is faster than general anaesthesia, associated with reduced postoperative complications but failed to demonstrate a reduction in 30-day mortality.[20] A "local anaesthesia first strategy" may be applied to the majority of patients undergoing elective EVAR and is thought to be feasible in up to 75% of patients with infrarenal abdominal aortic aneurysms, as demonstrated in one observational study of more than 200 patients in a high-volume EVAR centre.[21]

Despite evidence of the feasibility and improved outcomes for elective EVAR under local anaesthesia,[11,20,22] there has not been widespread uptake of the technique, possibly due to the traditional surgical preference for operating under general anaesthesia. Therefore, translating this approach in the setting of ruptured abdominal aortic aneurysms may be arguably more challenging; however, patients with ruptured aneurysms represent the highest risk group who are perhaps more likely to develop complications associated with general anaesthesia. Some highly specialised centres already advocate local anaesthesia for ruptured aneurysms where possible,[23] demonstrating that the majority of their patients have been successfully treated using local anaesthesia, with favourable outcomes.[24] However, there remain no randomised trials to assess the feasibility and effectiveness of EVAR under local anaesthesia for ruptured aneurysms in an unselected population.

Benefits of EVAR under local anaesthesia for ruptured abdominal aortic aneurysms

Observational data suggest that 30-day mortality is reduced for patients who undergo EVAR under local anaesthesia for ruptured abdominal aortic aneurysms, compared with EVAR under general anaesthesia for ruptured aneurysms (13–15%

and 33%, respectively; OR 0.27, 95% CI 0.10–0.70).[9] Local anaesthesia in the elective setting is associated with a reduction in cardiac events (0.8% *versus* 6.4%, p=0.02),[22] and whilst this has not been formally investigated in the setting of ruptured abdominal aortic aneurysms, the use of local anaesthesia in other vascular emergencies (such as endovascular intervention for stroke) has been associated with improved cardiovascular outcomes and survival (as demonstrated by the Solitaire registry).[14]

Local anaesthesia can be offered to the sickest patients who would otherwise be turned down for general anaesthesia, which avoids the inherent risks associated with general anaesthesia including the loss of sympathetic and abdominal wall tone on induction and the cardiorespiratory effects of artificial ventilation, whilst increasing the proportion of patients suitable for attempted repair. Spontaneous ventilation during local anaesthesia procedures improves venous return, decreasing pulmonary morbidity[25] and local anaesthesia allows improved immediate postoperative analgesia. Importantly, in the context of ruptured aneurysms, the use of local anaesthesia potentially allows more rapid aneurysm exclusion (haemorrhage control) and reduces the operative duration, which in turn reduces risks of prolonged metabolic disturbance, thromboembolism and increased venous blood loss. A reduction in hospital stay and requirement for intensive therapy unit stay has also been demonstrated in the setting of elective EVAR.[11]

It is important to note that the use of regional anaesthesia is generally regarded as unsuitable in ruptured abdominal aortic aneurysms due to the potential for loss of sympathetic tone and further cardiovascular collapse in the already compromised patient.

Feasibility, technical considerations and drawbacks of EVAR under local anaesthesia in ruptured abdominal aortic aneurysm

Not all patients are suitable for EVAR under local anaesthesia. Firstly, the aneurysm must be morphologically and technically suitable for a bifurcated endograft. Those who require an aorto-uni-iliac graft and femoro-femoral crossover (to revascularise the contralateral leg) are unsuitable for the local anaesthesia approach; however, this is still a common configuration of stents used in ruptured abdominal aortic aneurysms, especially if the operator is less experienced or the patient particularly unstable—of those patients in the IMPROVE trial who complied with the allocated EVAR-first strategy, 23.3% required an aorto-uni-iliac graft.[5]

The patient must also be suitable for this approach, which necessitates a compliant, conscious and co-operative patient—which may be challenging in ruptured abdominal aortic aneurysms. The patient also needs to be able to lie flat and comply with regular breath-holding instructions; confusion and agitation associated with hypoxia and metabolic disturbance may impede this. The surgeon needs to be comfortable and confident in obtaining vascular access even in the haemodynamically-compromised patient with potentially impalpable femoral pulses. Access vessels must be readily accessed; patient obesity and narrow access vessels can be a barrier to this; however, improved technology (including narrower delivery systems) has gone some way to address these issues.

Preliminary evidence from the National Vascular Registry suggests that 50% of UK vascular centres currently use local anaesthesia for EVAR of ruptured abdominal aortic aneurysms. In order to provide a successful local anaesthesia service, an experienced team is required, with adequate training to address the various drawbacks of local anaesthesia for EVAR in ruptured aneurysms.

In addition, good anaesthesia input will be required throughout the procedure, in order to minimise the pain associated with performing an endovascular intervention without general anaesthesia. If extensive groin dissection is required, the pain of the procedure may not be tolerable or may necessitate heavy sedation. However, percutaneous access and the use of closure devices can overcome this problem.

Some patients may experience ongoing and unacceptable abdominal pain from the expanding haematoma, which may subsequently lead to respiratory insufficiency due to increased intra-abdominal pressure causing restriction of chest wall movements. Pain at the time of stent deployment, in addition to ischaemic leg and buttock pain from prolonged occlusion of access vessels, may be difficult to control.

Movement artefact from an awake patient may compromise image quality, as will insufficient breath-holding. In the case of a complex EVAR leading to a longer operative duration, local anaesthesia may not be tolerated for a prolonged period and the cardiovascular instability associated with ruptured aneurysms may cause anaesthesia difficulties that are difficult to address in an awake patient. Finally, the conversion to general anaesthesia in a high-risk patient previously deemed unsuitable for general anaesthesia raises difficult questions; certainly the benefit of local anaesthesia is not sustained in those patients who start local anaesthesia but require conversion to general anaesthesia.

Future prospects

The IMPROVE trial suggests that EVAR, where possible, is associated with faster recovery and cost-effectiveness; therefore, increasingly more EVAR procedures are likely to be performed for ruptured aneurysms in the future.[26] In addition, recent data demonstrate an increasing prevalence of acute abdominal aortic aneurysm events in the older population (>75 years of age)[27] who may avoid detection during the single screening ultrasound offered at the age of 65 in the UK. We may, therefore, see an increasing number of elderly patients presenting with ruptured aneurysms, who are likely to have significant medical comorbidities that contribute to greater perioperative risk and are perhaps the most likely to benefit from EVAR and a local anaesthesia approach.

Better strategies to reduce the stubbornly high mortality associated with ruptured aneurysm intervention are required. The benefits of local anaesthesia for elective EVAR have been widely documented, and observational data for emergency EVAR in favour of local anaesthesia are emerging.

Local anaesthesia is often used for the sickest patients; therefore, if there is a survival advantage in this selected group (as suggested in recent literature), this may potentially translate to the entire population and could go some way to address the sustained high mortality associated with ruptured aneurysm intervention.

Local anaesthesia may in future be the first choice approach (where possible) for EVAR in ruptured aneurysms; however, further confirmation should be sought from randomised trials, which should be robustly designed, using an intention-to-treat strategy.

Summary

- An EVAR-first strategy for ruptured abdominal aortic aneurysms is commonly performed; however, the mortality rate remains high.

- Local anaesthesia has been associated with improved clinical outcomes (compared to general anaesthesia) for elective EVAR and other elective and emergency operations.

- Recent observational data suggest a significant reduction in 30-day mortality for local anaesthesia in EVAR for ruptured aneurysms, compared to general anaesthesia.

- Other potential benefits of local anaesthesia in EVAR for ruptured aneurysm include shorter operative time, reduced intensive therapy unit and hospital stay, fewer cardiorespiratory complications and improved postoperative analgesia.

- EVAR for ruptured aneurysms is performed under local anaesthesia in approximately half of the UK vascular centres.

- Robust randomised evidence is required to more fully investigate local anaesthesia as a strategy to improve outcomes in ruptured aneurysms.

- The use of local anaesthesia for ruptured aneurysms may increase the proportion of patients offered repair, and may go some way to improve the stubbornly high mortality associated with intervention.

References

1. Ashton HA, Buxton MJ, Day NE, *et al.* Multicentre Aneurysm Screening Study Group. The Multicentre Aneurysm Screening Study (MASS) into the effect of abdominal aortic aneurysm screening on mortality in men: a randomised controlled trial. *Lancet* 2002; **360**: 1531–39.
2. Karthikesalingam A, Holt PJ, Vidal-Diez A, *et al.* Mortality from ruptured abdominal aortic aneurysms: clinical lessons from a comparison of outcomes in England and the USA. *Lancet* 2014; **383** (9921): 963–69.
3. Greenhalgh RM, Brown LC, Powell JT, *et al.* Endovascular *versus* open repair of abdominal aortic aneurysm. *N Engl J Med* 2010; **362** (20): 1863–71.
4. Anjum A, Allmen von R, Greenhalgh R, *et al.* Explaining the decrease in mortality from abdominal aortic aneurysm rupture. *Br J Surg* 2012; **99** (5): 637–45.
5. IMPROVE Trial Investigators, Powell JT, Sweeting MJ, *et al.* Endovascular or open repair strategy for ruptured abdominal aortic aneurysm: 30 day outcomes from IMPROVE randomised trial. *BMJ* 2014; **348** (jan13 2): f7661–f7661.
6. Schanzer A, Greenberg RK, Hevelone N, *et al.* Predictors of abdominal aortic aneurysm sac enlargement after endovascular repair. *Circulation.* 2011; **123** (24): 2848–55.
7. Reimerink JJ, Hoornweg LL, Vahl AC, *et al.* Endovascular repair *versus* open repair of ruptured abdominal aortic aneurysms: a multicenter randomized controlled trial. *Ann Surg* 2013; **258** (2): 248–56.
8. Desgranges P, Kobeiter H, Katsahian S, *et al.* ECAR: Endosvasculaire vs *Chirurgie* dans les Anévrysmes Rompus: A French Randomized Controlled Trial of endovascular *versus* open surgical repair of ruptured aorto-iliac aneurysms. *Eur J Vasc Endovasc Surg* 2015; **50**: 303–10.
9. IMPROVE Trial Investigators, Powell JT, Hinchliffe RJ, *et al.* Observations from the IMPROVE trial concerning the clinical care of patients with ruptured abdominal aortic aneurysm. *Br J Surg* 2014; **101** (3): 216–24.

10. Walschot LH, Laheij RJ, Verbeek AL. Outcomes after endovascular abdominal aortic aneurysm repair: a meta-analysis. *J Endovasc Ther* 2002; **9** (1): 82–89.

11. Ruppert V, Leurs LJ, Steckmeier B, *et al.* Influence of anesthesia type on outcome after endovascular aortic aneurysm repair: An analysis based on EUROSTAR data. *J Vasc Surg* 2006; **44** (1): 16–21.e2.

12. Nordin P, Zetterström H, Gunnarsson U, *et al.* Local, regional, or general anaesthesia in groin hernia repair: multicentre randomised trial. *Lancet* 2003; **362** (9387): 853–58.

13. Nilsson H, Nilsson E, Angerås U, *et al.* Mortality after groin hernia surgery: delay of treatment and cause of death. **Hernia** 2011; **15** (3): 301–07.

14. Abou-Chebl A, Zaidat OO, Castonguay AC, *et al.* North American SOLITAIRE Stent-Retriever Acute Stroke Registry: choice of anesthesia and outcomes. *Stroke* 2014; **45** (5): 1396–1401.

15. GALA Trial Collaborative Group. General anaesthesia *versus* local anaesthesia for carotid surgery (GALA): a multicentre, randomised controlled trial. *The Lancet*. 2008; **372** (9656): 2132–42.

16. Rudarakanchana N, Halliday AW, Kamugasha D, *et al.* Current practice of carotid endarterectomy in the UK. *Br J Surg* 2012; **99** (2): 209–16.

17. Luger TJ, Kammerlander C, Gosch M, *et al.* Neuroaxial *versus* general anaesthesia in geriatric patients for hip fracture surgery: does it matter? Osteoporos Int. 2010; **21** (Suppl 4): S555–72.

18. Verhoeven ELG, Cinà CS, Tielliu IFJ, *et al.* Local anesthesia for endovascular abdominal aortic aneurysm repair. *J Vasc Surg* 2005; **42** (3): 402–09.

19. Sadat U, Cooper DG, Gillard JH, *et al.* Impact of the Type of Anesthesia on Outcome after Elective Endovascular Aortic Aneurysm Repair: Literature Review. *Vascular* 2008; **16** (6): 340–45.

20. Karthikesalingam A, Thrumurthy SG, Young EL, *et al.* Locoregional anesthesia for endovascular aneurysm repair. *J Vasc Surg* 2012; **56** (2): 510–19.

21. Geisbüsch P, Katzen BT, Machado R, *et al.* Local anaesthesia for endovascular repair of infrarenal aortic aneurysms. *Eur J Vasc Endovasc Surg* 2011; **42** (4): 467–73.

22. Bakker EJ, Van de Luijtgaarden KM, van Lier F, *et al.* General Anaesthesia is Associated with Adverse Cardiac Outcome after Endovascular Aneurysm Repair. *Eur J Vasc Endovasc Surg* 2012; **44** (2): 121–25.

23. Lachat ML, Pfammatter T, Witzke HJ, *et al.* Endovascular repair with bifurcated stent-grafts under local anaesthesia to improve outcome of ruptured aortoiliac aneurysms. *Eur J Vasc Endovasc Surg* 2002; **23** (6): 528–36.

24. Mayer D, Pfammatter T, Rancic Z, *et al.* 10 Years of Emergency Endovascular Aneurysm Repair for Ruptured Abdominal Aortoiliac Aneurysms: Lessons Learned. *Ann Surg* 2009; **249** (3): 510–15.

25. Edwards MS, Andrews JS, Edwards AF, *et al.* Results of endovascular aortic aneurysm repair with general, regional, and local/monitored anesthesia care in the American College of *Surgeon*s National Surgical Quality Improvement Program database. *J Vasc Surg* 2011; **54** (5): 1273–82.

26. IMPROVE Trial Investigators. Endovascular strategy or open repair for ruptured abdominal aortic aneurysm: one-year outcomes from the IMPROVE randomized trial. *Eur Heart J* 2015; **36** (31): 2061–69.

27. Howard DPJ, Banerjee A, Fairhead JF, *et al.* Age-specific incidence, risk factors and outcome of acute abdominal aortic aneurysms in a defined population. *Br J Surg* 2015; **102**: 907–15

Increase the number of patients offered intervention for ruptured abdominal aortic aneurysm

A Karthikesalingam and MM Thompson

Introduction

Ruptured abdominal aortic aneurysm is amongst the most severe of surgical emergencies, accounting for the death of at least 45 individuals per 100,000 population.[1] The majority of patients with a ruptured abdominal aortic aneurysm do not survive to presentation at hospital and in those that do, surgical intervention is still associated with high mortality. There is little compelling evidence to suggest that survival has improved over time for patients with ruptured aneurysms,[2–5] reflecting considerable ongoing interest in research to document and improve outcomes for this group of patients. In a number of healthcare settings, mortality has been shown to vary significantly between different hospitals. The fate of patients with abdominal aortic aneurysms has also been shown to vary between countries, with different outcomes published for healthcare systems in the USA, the UK, Western Europe and Australia.[6–8] Such national and international variation in survival suggests that modifiable technical, organisational or process factors can be key determinants of which patients survive ruptured aneurysms, and that closer examination of varying healthcare systems or institutions might shed further light on how best to improve mortality.

Description of topic

Previous national and international studies have documented postoperative survival for patients undergoing ruptured abdominal aortic aneurysm repair in different healthcare settings and reported the association of survival with various presenting factors.[2] However, these studies have focused solely on perioperative care, without documenting the proportion of patients with ruptured aneurysms who were not offered surgical treatment. The proportion of patients with ruptured abdominal aortic aneurysms in the UK who are offered surgery has been stable during the past decade,[1,3] but there has been little focus on international comparisons of ruptured abdominal aortic aneurysms that include an analysis of the proportion of patients offered surgery. Without corrective surgery, survival from ruptured aneurysm is not possible, so the proportion of patients offered intervention is likely to be a key determinant of overall population mortality from this condition.

The present chapter reviews a comparison of the proportion of patients offered intervention for ruptured abdominal aortic aneurysm in two different healthcare settings (England and the USA), shedding light on the impact of this variation on the overall in-hospital mortality from all diagnosed ruptured abdominal aortic aneurysm patients that survived to hospital admission.[4]

Evidence for views

Demographic and in-hospital outcome data were extracted from Hospital Episode Statistics (HES) and the Nationwide Inpatient Sample (NIS) for all patients diagnosed with ruptured abdominal aortic aneurysms between 1 January 2005 and 31 December 2010. The authors compared outcomes in England and the USA, with primary outcome measures of in-hospital mortality for all diagnosed ruptured abdominal aortic aneurysms, mortality after intervention (open or endovascular repair), and the proportion of patients managed by non-corrective treatment for ruptured aneurysms. Non-corrective treatment was defined by the patient having a diagnostic code for ruptured abdominal aortic aneurysm but no procedural code for open surgical or endovascular ruptured aneurysm repair. Secondary outcome measures included the proportion of operated cases managed by endovascular aneurysm repair (EVAR), length of stay, discharge destination, and the proportion of cases managed in teaching hospitals or hospitals of varying bed capacity. Age and gender-matched analyses were constructed to compare English and US outcomes for in-hospital mortality and the decision to offer conservative management.

In total, 11,799 patients in England and 23,838 patients in the USA were admitted to hospital with a ruptured abdominal aortic aneurysm during the study period, with similar demographics seen in both healthcare systems. The key findings of this study were that in-hospital mortality was greater in England (65.90% vs. 53.05%, p<0.001), surgical intervention was offered to a greater proportion of cases in the USA (80.43% vs. 58.56%; p<0.001), and endovascular repair was more common in the USA (20.87% vs. 8.54%; p<0.001), even though operative mortality was similar in both countries when considering only those patients undergoing intervention (41.77% vs. 41.65%; p=0.876). A comparison of age and gender-matched strata demonstrated that overall in-hospital mortality (odds ratio [OR] 1.473, 95% confidence interval [CI] 1.376–1.576; p<0.0001) and the rate of non-corrective treatment (OR 3.193, 95% CI 2.951–3.455; p<0.0001) were significantly greater in England than in the USA (Figures 1 and 2).

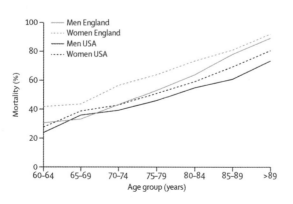

Figure 1: In-hospital mortality for ruptured abdominal aortic aneurysm after stratified matching for sex and five-year age grouping. Reproduced with permission of *The Lancet*.

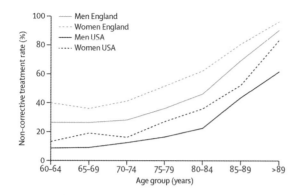

Figure 2: Non-corrective treatment for ruptured abdominal aortic aneurysm after stratified matching for sex and five-year age grouping. Reproduced with permission of *The Lancet*.

Although a similar proportion of hospitals were described as teaching institutions in both countries (15.14% vs. 17.35%; p=0.4951), a greater proportion of ruptured abdominal aortic aneurysms in the USA were treated at teaching institutions (51.53% vs. 29.29%; p<0.0001). Mortality was lower at teaching institutions than non-teaching institutions in both countries (England 56.04% vs. 69·99%, USA 48.43% vs. 58.05%; p<0.0001). The non-corrective treatment rate was also lower in teaching institutions in both countries (England 31.32% vs. 45.63%, USA 14.93% vs. 24.62%; p<0.0001). EVAR was more prevalent in teaching institutions (England 13.12% vs. 6.14%, USA 25.35% vs. 15.54%; p<0.0001). In both countries, mortality and non-corrective treatment rates were better in hospitals with greater annual caseload (volume) for ruptured aneurysms, with greater proportion of intervention by EVAR, with the highest bed capacity, in patients who were transferred, and in patients treated on a weekday rather than a weekend.

The most important finding of this comparison of international practice was that the in-hospital mortality of all patients diagnosed with ruptured abdominal aortic aneurysms was considerably lower in the USA than in England. This was principally because US hospitals were less likely to manage ruptured aneurysms conservatively and performed interventions in a significantly greater proportion of patients. Although procedural mortality rates were similar, patients in the USA were more than twice as likely to be offered EVAR for rupture and were more often managed in a teaching hospital, compared to England.

The proportion of patients offered intervention (EVAR or open repair) in the USA presented a stark difference to England, and provides important context for improving English practice. Previous studies have reported that 68% of Medicare patients with ruptured abdominal aortic aneurysms were offered intervention in the USA[5,6] and although lower than USA estimates from other National Inpatient Sample (NIS) reports,[7] the proportion offered intervention in the USA has been consistently reported to be greater than in England. This represents a significant concern for English practice, because postoperative mortality was similar in both countries. Taken together, the observational data suggest that overall survival from ruptured abdominal aortic aneurysms in England might be improved by offering intervention to a greater proportion of patients (lowering the rate of non-corrective management).

This study had significant limitations, largely relating to the observational and administrative data that were available for comparison. The HES and NIS datasets did not permit examination of 30-day or 90-day mortality, which are immune from the bias potentially relating to clinical discharge from hospital. It should be acknowledged that a greater proportion of patients were discharged to "skilled nursing facilities" rather than to home in the USA compared to England, perhaps raising the possibility that some of these patients would have continued to receive palliative care prior to mortality within 90 days. The proportion of patients that died in this manner, shortly after discharge from the treating hospital, remains unknown and is an important potential confounder of the analysis. Comparisons of in-hospital mortality should be interpreted with a degree of caution but it remains unlikely that the considerable absolute mortality difference between England and the USA could be entirely explained by deaths in secondary care given the stark difference in non-corrective treatment rates.

It is well known that survival from ruptured abdominal aortic aneurysm relates strongly to patient factors such as age, gender and comorbidity; but the present comparison of practice also illustrated the international importance of non-patient-related factors. In both healthcare systems, the best outcomes were obtained in hospitals with highest bed capacity, the greatest annual caseload (volume) of ruptured abdominal aortic aneurysms, and in hospitals in which a larger proportion of ruptured aneurysms were managed by EVAR. Hospital bed size, teaching status, admission on a weekday and ruptured aneurysms caseload might all be regarded as inter-related surrogate markers for the immediacy with which each ruptured aneurysm patient had access to the full range of technology and care by a specialist/experienced aortic team. In the absence of an acceptable alternative, high-risk patients have shown willingness to accept the possibility of considerable perioperative complications;[8] and this should be taken into account when counselling patients and families toward the balance of risk for ruptured abdominal aortic aneurysms. The comparison of international practice suggests strongly that services should be organised to ensure that patients with a ruptured aneurysm are able to promptly access care in a teaching hospital with a high aortic workload, offering both conventional and endovascular repair; where an aggressive approach is taken to offering intervention if this fits with the patient's wishes. Few studies have focused on the proportion of patients turned down for abdominal aortic aneurysm repair,[9,10,11–18] even though these data are required to place perioperative mortality in context and may be subject to considerably greater variation than operative mortality rates.[4] Alongside ongoing initiatives to audit and improve the quality of care for patients undergoing intervention for abdominal aortic aneurysms and/or ruptured aneurysms, the discrepancies seen in international practice suggest that patients might equally benefit from national audits of the proportion of patients being managed by non-corrective intervention.

Summary

- Previous national and international studies have documented the association of postoperative survival for patients undergoing ruptured abdominal aortic aneurysm repair in different healthcare settings, but have largely ignored the proportion of patients not offered intervention.

- A comparison of practice in England and the USA has shown that the poorer outcomes for ruptured aneurysms in England are associated with the tendency to deny patients corrective treatment compared to the USA. In both countries, the best outcomes were obtained in high-caseload specialist centres, where endovascular technology was more often utilised, and where greater bed resources were common.

- The implications for practice are that more patients with ruptured abdominal aortic aneurysms should be offered intervention, that there should be more routine declaration of the proportion managed without intervention, and that service configuration should aim to promptly deliver all patients with ruptured aneurysms to high-caseload specialist centres, with an aggressive policy toward available treatment.

References

1. Anjum A, von Allmen R, Greenhalgh R, Powell JT. Explaining the decrease in mortality from abdominal aortic aneurysm rupture. *Br J Surg* 2012; **99**: 637–45.
2. Mani K, Lees T, Beiles B, Jensen LP, *et al*. Treatment of abdominal aortic aneurysm in nine countries 2005-2009: a vascunet report. *Eur J Vasc Endovasc Surg* 2011; **42**: 598–607.
3. Anjum A and Powell JT. Is the incidence of abdominal aortic aneurysm declining in the 21st century? Mortality and hospital admissions for England & Wales and Scotland. *Eur J Vasc Endovasc Surg* 2012; **43**: 161–66.
4. Karthikesalingam A, Holt PJ, Vidal-Diez A, Ozdemir BA, *et al*. Mortality from ruptured abdominal aortic aneurysms: clinical lessons from a comparison of outcomes in England and the USA. *Lancet* 2014; **383**: 963–9.
5. Schermerhorn ML, Bensley RP, Giles KA, Hurks R, O'Malley A J, Cotterill P, Chaikof E and Landon BE. Changes in abdominal aortic aneurysm rupture and short-term mortality, 1995–2008: a retrospective observational study. *Ann Surg* 2012; **256**: 651–58.
6. Mureebe L, Egorova N, Giacovelli JK, Gelijns A, *et al*. National trends in the repair of ruptured abdominal aortic aneurysms. *J Vasc Surg* 2008; **48**: 1101–07.
7. Park BD, Azefor N, Huang CC, Ricotta JJ. Trends in treatment of ruptured abdominal aortic aneurysm: impact of endovascular repair and implications for future care. *J Am Coll Surg* 2013; 216: 745–54.
8. Cykert S. Risk acceptance and risk aversion: patients' perspectives on lung surgery. *Thorac Surg Clin* 2004; **14**: 287–93.
9. Karthikesalingam A, Nicoli TK, Holt PJ, Hinchliffe RJ, *et al*. The fate of patients referred to a specialist vascular unit with large infra-renal abdominal aortic aneurysms over a two-year period. *Eur J Vasc Endovasc Surg* 2011; **2** (3): 295–301.
10. Szilagyi DE, Smith RF, DeRusso FJ, Elliott JP, *et al*. Contribution of abdominal aortic aneurysmectomy to prolongation of life. *Ann Surg* 1966; **164**: 678–99.
11. Bardram L, Buchardt Hansen HJ and Dahl Hansen AB. Abdominal aortic aneurysms. Early and late results after surgical and non-surgical treatment. *Acta Chir Scand Suppl* 1980; **502**: 85–93.
12. Perko MJ, Schroeder TV, Olsen PS, Jensen LP, *et al*. Natural history of abdominal aortic aneurysm: a survey of 63 patients treated nonoperatively. *Ann Vasc Surg* 1993; **7**: 113–16.
13. Ruberti U, Scorza R, Biasi GM, Odero A. Nineteen year experience on the treatment of aneurysms of the abdominal aorta: a survey of 832 consecutive cases. *J Cardiovasc Surg* (Torino) 1985; **26**: 547–53.
14. Campbell WB, Collin J and Morris PJ. The mortality of abdominal aortic aneurysm. *Ann R Coll Surg Engl* 1986; **68**: 275–78.
15. Woodburn KR, Chant H, Davies JN, Blanshard KS, *et al*. Suitability for endovascular aneurysm repair in an unselected population. *Br J Surg* 2001; **88**: 77–81.

16. Heikkinen M, Salenius J, Zeitlin R, Saarinen J, *et al.* The fate of AAA patients referred electively to vascular surgical unit. *Scand J Surg* 2002; **91**: 345–52.

17. Tambyraja AL, Stuart WP, Sala Tenna A, Murie JA, *et al.* Non-operative management of high-risk patients with abdominal aortic aneurysm. *Eur J Vasc Endovasc Surg* 2003; **26**: 401–4.

18. Tanquilut EM, Veith FJ, Ohki T, Lipsitz EC, *et al.* Nonoperative management with selective delayed surgery for large abdominal aortic aneurysms in patients at high risk. *J Vasc Surg* 2002; **36**: 41–6.

Peripheral arterial challenges

Exercise therapy for claudicants —the guidance from NICE and other healthcare regulators is being ignored

KE Murphy, C Spafford, C Oakley and JD Beard

Introduction

Intermittent claudication is the most common presenting symptom of peripheral arterial disease, and its prevalence ranges from 4.5% of those aged 55–74 to 10% of those older than 70 years. While the natural history of the disease is, in the main, benign (70–80% of patients remain remaining symptomatically unchanged), up to 20% of patients will experience worsening of symptoms and will develop critical limb ischaemia. Additionally, the risk of death from myocardial infarction is up to four times higher in patients with peripheral arterial disease than in those without— about 60% of patients with the disease will have a fatal myocardial infarction and about 10% will have a fatal stroke.[1,2] These patients represent a significant cost burden in terms of primary prevention and subsequent interventions.

In this chapter, we consider why these patients are not receiving the appropriate long-term treatment for their condition. This treatment is exercise therapy, which is recommended by the UK's National Institute for Health and Care Excellence (NICE).[3] Exercise therapy is an inexpensive treatment that requires less manpower and fewer resources than expensive invasive treatments. Typically, improving blood flow to the legs requires open or endovascular surgery. These interventions provide the immediate improvement that is desired by most claudicants, but as well as being expensive, they are associated with a significant complication rate and relatively high rates of morbidity and mortality. Major amputation can cost £50,000 (€70000) in the UK and US$170,000 (€150,000) in the USA, and more than 50% of UK patients die within two years of undergoing a surgical or endovascular intervention.

If a patient with peripheral arterial disease does have an adverse vascular event (eg. non-fatal stroke or myocardial infarction), they require risk-factor (such as smoking) modification and antiplatelet and statin therapies to reduce their otherwise high risk of morbidity and mortality. But these interventions rarely improve intermittent claudication. However, exercise therapy is not only an important therapy, it is also important for improving cardiovascular health. Given the concomitant nature of ischaemic heart disease, respiratory disease (particularly chronic obstructive pulmonary disease), and peripheral arterial disease, exercise therapy can be used for the management of all three with obvious cost advantage.

Data for the efficacy of exercise therapy are plentiful; supervised physical exercise for peripheral arterial disease is endorsed (with class 1 recommendations) by both the American Heart Association (AHA) and the American College of Cardiology (ACC).[4] This is reinforced by Williams et al's[5] observation: "The presentation of a patient with intermitted claudication should, therefore, be considered a golden opportunity to embark on a package of care that will reduce their risk of cardiovascular death, and improve their walking rather than simply an indication to dilate or bypass their arterial disease."

Supervised exercise programmes

Despite being recommended by NICE guidance, as well as being associated with lower costs and less of a need for further intervention, supervised exercise therapy is only available for 25% of eligible patients in the UK.[3,6,7] Coupled with appropriate medical therapy, supervised exercise therapy may be the solution for most patients.

The reasons for this lack of provision are multifactorial, but inter-specialty rivalry between vascular surgeons and interventional radiologists may be a factor. The requirement to perform a minimum number of interventions to be revalidated, or to remain significant in the surgical community, may encourage the practitioner to choose an interventional rather than a non-interventional approach. Bradbury et al note that: "Asking vascular surgeons and interventional radiologists to embrace the NICE CG 147 guidelines on intermittent claudication may be akin to asking turkeys to vote for Christmas!"[8]

The geographical dispersion of hospitals and patients will also be a factor. Patients with peripheral arterial disease located in metropolitan areas will have access to arterial intervention from major teaching hospitals, whereas patients from smaller towns and rural areas will have to rely upon local hospitals and local councils for their provision. Coordination of this different and dispersed provision is also an issue. When medical services are delivered by hub and spoke hospital structure, patients may have to travel significant distances for clinical review. This travel factor has an impact upon the uptake and use of exercise programmes, which is currently poor. There is also strong evidence that telling patients to "go home and walk" is ineffective, as patients rarely comply due to lack of support and motivation.[9,10]

NICE recommends that all claudicants should be offered at least two hours of supervised exercise a week for three months, but patients may struggle with accessing such programmes (or the costs involved) and compliance may be as low as 34%.[11] Not all patients are suitable candidates for exercise programmes. However, when used for the correct group, with good quality regular clinical follow up, supervised exercise has been shown to be as clinically effective as percutaneous transluminal angioplasty at one year.[12]

Funding difficulties

The funding model that we have in place currently in the UK for supervised exercise programmes is a complex mess and another contributory factor. This is partly a result of the half-hearted support that clinicians, patients and—perhaps more significantly—the Department of Health have given the funding of treatment for peripheral arterial disease. For despite the cost burden of these patients over time, they remain profoundly "unfashionable"—heart attacks and cancer attract funding but peripheral arterial disease does not.

In funding terms, the coding tariff for intervention is highly rewarded, but that for exercise is not. Indeed there is a strong feeling in the vascular community that peripheral arterial disease is both ignored and neglected compared with other conditions. For example, the supervised exercise programme funded by Sheffield Council includes patients with coronary artery disease, diabetes, stress, depression, obesity and hypertension; but despite the concomitance of some of these conditions, nowhere is peripheral arterial disease mentioned in its own right. The distribution of the national health budget between primary and secondary care within the NHS and also to local government creates a minefield for treatments, such as exercise, that fall between "specialties" and "administrative systems". Interventions by contrast are more easily located to centres and administrative systems and hence the NICE guidance is set aside because it is too difficult to implement. The first hurdle in the NICE algorithm (Figure 1) is removed, clearing the way for intervention.

Other factors for the lack of availability of supervised exercise programmes include a lack of specific data—less than 2% of all clinical trials in the last 10 years were focused on peripheral arterial disease, and these largely are focused on technological advancements rather than novel treatments.[13] These trials reinforce the preference for intervention over exercise or to it put another way, for a reactive response rather than a proactive preventative one.

Overall spending

The percentage of the UK's gross domestic product that is spent on healthcare (about 7%) is much lower than it is in other countries—i.e. behind France, Germany, Sweden, Denmark, Belgium, Austria, Italy, Portugal and the Netherlands. There are fewer practising physicians in the UK per head of population than in France, and Germany has almost twice as many physicians per head than the UK.

When it comes to the UK's outlook on healthcare, on disease prevention and public health in general, the country is light years behind the curve and is simply

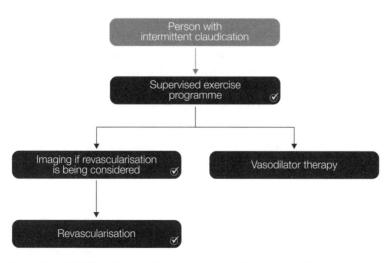

Figure 1: Adapted from NICE CG 147- Schematic for management of stable intermitted claudication.

burying it head in the sand about this. Arguments about raising the level of public spending on healthcare will continue, but the proverbial stable door needs to be closed before the horse bolts when it comes to ensuring adequate preventative healthcare strategies and national engagement with public health. The cost of a supervised exercise programme per one quality adjusted life year (QALY) is about £700–£1,600. The cost of angioplasty, stenting and follow up may be upwards of 10 times that amount.[14] With an ageing population and increasing prevalence of obesity and diabetes, coupled with real-term reductions in the budget of the NHS, with ever increasing strains on both inpatients and outpatient work, ignoring the benefits that can be accrued from supervised exercise programmes would be grossly negligent. Additionally, there is evidence that patients with peripheral arterial disease are less aggressively treated in terms of atherosclerotic risk factor modification than patients with isolated ischaemic heart disease.[15]

The seven leading risk factors for death in the UK are poor diet, high blood pressure, smoking, obesity or elevated body mass index, hyperglycaemia, hypercholesterolaemia and low physical activity.[16] With a single intervention, such as supervised exercise therapy, we can address many of these conditions; however, we are encountering inertia and a serious lack of focus and imagination. The National Cardiovascular Health Intelligence Network, which is coordinated by Public Health England (PHE), is a step in the right direction. It is an attempt to coordinate multiple bodies to focus on improvements in delivery of cardiovascular health. But, there a heavy bias towards ischaemic heart disease with peripheral arterial disease remaining the poor relation. While government intervention in healthcare rarely provides clarity of clinical direction and a national policy for exercise would be expensive to set up and tricky to implement, the reduction in the health burden would be significant in the long term.

Motivating patients

The response of patients to exercise therapy is a very significant issue since without their acceptance of the treatment, there will be no improvement either in health terms or in the willingness of clinicians to promote it. Therefore motivation of the patients to accept and participate in the treatment is crucial. This motivation in turn must be accompanied by education of the patients about the precise nature of the treatment as well as its advantages for them. The patients need to be informed that improvement is incremental and that compliance needs to be good for successful outcomes. Sessions of supervised exercise additionally need to be coupled with improvement in other lifestyle factors and smoking cessation. The patients need to be made aware that they will encounter pain and that continuing to exercise when this happens will not result in adverse outcomes.

Human nature plays its part as most people do not believe that they will suffer significant harm as a result of their own actions or lifestyle, and perhaps take too lightly a doctor telling them to exercise. Added to this notion, if they fail to see rapid improvement with an intervention that may be inaccessible and causing them pain, it is hardly a surprise that uptake is low. By comparison, being brought to and from hospital for a day-case angioplasty under local anaesthetic may seem much more preferable to weeks of travelling to a supervised exercise programme clinic where they will be repeatedly criticised for failing to quit smoking or lose weight.

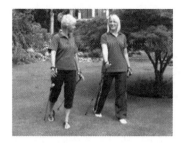

Figure 2: Use of Nordic walking poles (Courtesy of STEPS Physiotherapy).

While the clinician may view an increase in the walking distance as a successful outcome, this is not mirrored in studies looking at quality of life as an independent outcome measure. Although a Cochrane review showed statistically significant improvements in maximal treadmill walking distance with supervised exercise programme, no improvement in quality of life was observed.[17] Another study has shown improvement in quality of life when a supervised exercise programme was combined with percutaneous angioplasty.[18] However, concerns about the merits of supervised exercise therapy alone exist, fuelling uncertainty and inhibiting NHS Commissioners from investing in non-interventional treatments for intermittent claudication.

Several small-centre studies have shown that the addition of Nordic walking poles (Figure 2) to a traditional supervised exercise therapy has a statistically significant impact on walking distance. At one-year follow-up, compliance was much better than previously predicted: 94% of the Nordic walking pole group and 78% of the standard group were still walking. A subsequent quality of life study on another cohort of 20 patients has demonstrated that all Walking Impairment Questionnaire and generic EQ-5D health scores increased significantly. The actual health scores improved by 12%, and the perceived health scores increased by 79%, confirming the "feel-good factor" engendered by using Nordic Poles.[15,19,20]

Conclusion

Frans Moll suggests there are three pillars for the treatment of intermittent claudication: smoking cessation, supervised exercise, and best medical practice. Few countries are reliably achieving any one of these—and certainly not all three. Early and aggressive primary prevention is crucial, but so often we find ourselves playing catch-up for patients whose risk factors are out of control by the time they reach a threshold for treatment. Vascular surgeons need to embrace physical and medical therapy for peripheral arterial disease, and fight for funding. The fight is not likely to be easy, but unless we face the growing problem of sedentary lifestyle, obesity, diabetes and cardiovascular disease, we are going to fall further into a healthcare crisis with catastrophic consequences.

Summary

- Supervised exercise therapy has broad-ranging health benefits.

- The costs of primary prevention and exercise are significantly lower than the costs of intervention (percutaneous transluminal angioplasty, surgical bypass and major amputation).

- Access to exercise therapy is poor, as well as uptake for a number of key reasons: poor use by surgeons and radiologists as a first-line treatment; issues relating to commissioning services and who foots the bill for exercise (the clinical commissioning groups, hospital trusts or the local authorities); low uptake and commitment from patients; and low satisfaction and quality of life scores associated with supervised exercise programmes.

- Nordic walking poles used with supervised exercise may provide a realistic improvement in quality of life and improvement in walking distance.

References

1. Smith GD, Shipley MJ, Roase G. Intermittent Claudication, heart disease risk factors and Mortality: The Whitehall Consensus. *Circulation* 1990; **82**: 1925–31.
2. Criqui MH, Langer RD, Fronek A, Feigelson HS, *et al* Mortality over a period of 10 years in patients with peripheral arterial disease, *N Engl J Med* 1992; **326**: 381–86
3. National Institute for Health and Care Excellence. Lower limb peripheral arterial disease: diagnosis and management. (Clinical guideline 147); 2012 http://www.nice.org.uk/guidance/CG147 (date accessed 26 January 2016)
4. Hirsch AT, Haskal ZJ, Hertzer NR, *et al.* ACC/AHA 2005 Practice Guidelines for the management of patients with peripheral arterial disease (lower extremity, renal, mesenteric, and abdominal aortic). *Circulation* 2006;113:e463-e654(PMID:16549646)
5. Williams G, Shearman CP, Supervised Exercise, smoking cessation and best medical treatment should precede intervention. in Greenhalgh RM (ed). Vascular and endovascular consensus update. London: BIBA publishing; 2014. p217–25
6. Yost M. Cost-benefit analysis of critical limb ischaemia in the era of the Affordable care act. The Sage Group; 2014. http://bit.ly/1nMQsIY CG147 (date accessed 26 January 2016).
7. Shalhoub J, Hamish M, Davies AH. Supervised exercise for intermittent claudication—an under-utilised tool. *Ann R Coll Surg Eng* 2009; **91**: 473–76.
8. Popplewell MA, Bradbury AW. Why Do Health Systems Not Fund Supervised Exercise Programmes for Intermittent Claudication? *Eur J Vasc Endovasc Surg* 2014; **48**: 608–10.
9. Van Asselt AD, Nicolaï SP, Joore MA, *et al*, Group ETiPADS. Cost-effectiveness of exercise therapy in patients with intermittent claudication: supervised exercise therapy *versus* a 'go home and walk' advice. *Eur J Vasc Endovasc Surg* 2011; **41**: 97–103.
10. Wind J, Koelemay MJ. Exercise therapy and the additional effect of supervision on exercise therapy in patients with intermittent claudication. Systemic review of randomised controlled trials. *Eur J Vasc Endovasc Surg* 2007; **34**: 1–9.
11. Layden J, Michaels J, Bermingham S, Higgins B, Group GD. Diagnosis and management of lower limb peripheral arterial disease: summary of NICE guidance. *BMJ* 2012; **345**: e 4947.
12. Mazari FAK, Khan J A, Carradice D, Samuel N *et al.* Randomized clinical trial of percutaneous transluminal angioplasty, supervised exercise and combined treatment for intermittent claudication due to femoropopliteal arterial disease. *Br J Surg* 2012; **99**: 39–48.
13. Subherwals, PatelMR, Chiswell K, Tiderman-Miller BA, *et al.* Clinical Trial in peripheral vascular disease:pipeline and trial designs:an evaluation of the ClinicalTrials.gov database. *Circulation* 2014; **130**: 1812–19
14. Bermingham SL, Sparrow K, Mullis R, et al.The cost-effectiveness of supervised exercise for the treatment of intermittent claudication *Eur J Vasc Endovasc Surg* 2013; **46** (6): 707–14.
15. Pereg D, Neuman Y, Elis A, *et al.* Comparison of lipid control in patients with coronary *versus* peripheral artery disease following the first vascular intervention. *Am J Cardiol* 2012; **110**: 1266–69.

16. Murray CJ, Richards MA, Newton JN, *et al.* UK health performance: findings of the Global Burden of Disease Study 2010. *Lancet* 2013; **381**(9871): 997–1020

17. Lane R, Ellis B, Watson L, Leng GC. Exercise for intermittent claudication. Cochrane Database Syst Rev 2014; 7: CD000990.

18. Greenhalgh RM1, Belch JJ, Brown LC, *et al.* The adjuvant benefit of angioplasty in patients with mild to moderate intermittent claudication (MIMIC) managed by supervised exercise, smoking cessation advice and best medical therapy: results from two randomised trials for stenotic femoropopliteal and aortoiliac arterial disease. *Eur J Vasc Endovasc Surg* 2008; **36** (6): 680–88

19. Oakley C, Zwierska I, Tew G, *et al.* Nordic poles immediately improve walking distance in patients with intermittent claudication. *Eur J Vasc Endovasc Surg* 2008; **36**: 689–94.

20. Spafford C, Oakley C, Beard JD. Randomised clinical trial comparing Nordic pole walking and a standard home exercise programme in patients with intermittent claudication. *Br J Surg* 2014; **101**: 760–67.

Wearable activity tracker improves intermittent claudication

P Normahani, C Bicknell, L Allen, R Kwasnicki,
M Jenkins, R Gibbs, N Cheshire, A Darzi and C Riga

Introduction

Intermittent claudication is highly prevalent, affecting 3% of patients aged older than 40 years and 6% of patients aged older than 60 years.[1] Patients with intermittent claudication have a significant walking impairment and a reduced quality of life.[1,2] Furthermore, the socio-economic impact of claudication is likely to be considerable.[3]

The management of patients with peripheral arterial disease aims to reduce mortality and morbidity from disease progression and associated systemic cardiovascular disease. The mainstay of treatment for mild-to-moderate disease is the provision of a supervised exercise programme and management of cardiovascular risk factors.[4] Although supervised exercise programmes have been shown to improve walking distances and quality of life,[4] patient compliance has been documented to be as low as 34%.[5] Patients also often fail to maintain exercise levels following completion of the programme. This highlights the challenge of encouraging positive exercise habits in this group of patients who have a reduced level of overall physical activity compared with the rest of the population.[6] The gained benefits of supervised exercise programmes are also quickly lost if exercise levels are not maintained.[7] Clearly, a more sustainable solution to patient engagement and behavioural change is necessary.

Furthermore, supervised exercise programmes are expensive and survey studies suggest that only one third of vascular surgeons have access to a supervised exercise programme for their patients.[8,9] The clinical challenge is to develop a system that minimises the use of healthcare resources whilst maximising patient motivation.

Structured, home-based or community exercise programmes have been suggested to be a feasible alternative to costly supervised exercise programmes.[9] These programmes vary widely, but in general incorporate activity logging with daily goals. They are designed to increase daily activity congruent with patients' everyday schedules, which is more convenient and, therefore, more likely to lead to habitual activity. However, there is a lack of quality long-term evidence to support this approach. Wearable activity trackers may have a role to play in augmenting supervised or unsupervised exercise programmes to better engage patients and promote physical activity.

Wearable technology

Consumer wearable devices are a popular and growing market, and are estimated to be worth approximately US$20.6 billion by 2018.[10] Subsets of wearable devices used for monitoring physical activity are referred to as "activity trackers" or "fitness trackers". Other wearable devices, such as smart watches, also allow for monitoring of physical activity.

Wearable activity trackers are sensors that are worn on the body with a built-in accelerometer for motion quantification and an accessible interface that allows the user to monitor their own activity levels; thereby, engaging them to modify their health behaviours (Figure 1A). They also allow for personalised goal setting and give real-time feedback regarding goal progression; such as walking a target number of steps or expending a target number of calories per day. They also offer interactive behaviour change tools via the graphical interface of the band, a paired mobile device or computer (Figure 1B). These include reminders to keep active, interactive graphs of activity, activity statistics and comparison of activity with one's peers or a broader community of users.

The commercial use of wearable activity trackers has risen as they have become more affordable, discrete and interactive. Commercially available wearable activity trackers currently on the market include Fitbit, Jawbone, and Pebble among many others.

Implications for intermittent claudication

Traditional pedometers have been shown to significantly increase physical activity in adults in a systematic review by Bravata *et al* (26 studies, 2,767 participants).[11] They showed that the use of pedometers improved physical activity by over 2,000 steps per day, which was combined with improvements in body mass index and blood pressure. This was particularly seen if pedometers were used with a target number of steps per day, highlighting the importance of goal setting in behavioural change.

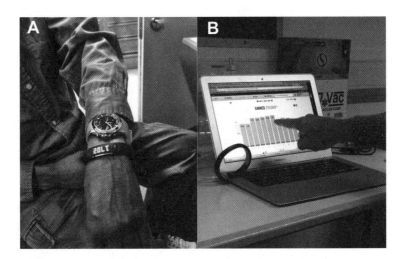

Figure 1: (A) Wrist-worn activity monitor (Nike+ FuelBand, Nike) displaying the number of earned "fuel points" (metric of energy expenditure); row of lights on the band give real-time feedback regarding progression towards daily "goal". (B) Graph demonstrating monthly activity trend for patient.

The use of pedometers in combination with individual planning and tracking or virtual coaching interventions have also been shown to be more effective in promoting physical activity than the use of pedometers alone.[12,13] Coaching is increasingly recognised as an important component in the management of chronic conditions in the promotion of healthy behaviours.[14] It appears, therefore, that the ideal intervention should incorporate activity monitoring and goal setting with an online coaching platform.

Modern wearable activity trackers incorporate goal setting, feedback on performance, self-monitoring and reviewing behavioural goals.[15] They are also more precise than pedometers, which are limited in their accuracy when used in older adults who have slow walking speeds and gait disorders.[16]

Although wearable devices have been predominantly used recreationally by healthy adults, they have also been shown to encourage self-monitoring and physical activity in patients.[17–19] Despite the lack of patients with peripheral arterial disease in these small number of studies, the potential benefits of using wearable activity trackers to promote exercise habit are encouraging.

Study

Our group has conducted the first single-centre, randomised-controlled study to determine whether the use of a wearable activity tracker (Nike+ FuelBand, Nike) is more effective at improving walking distances and quality of life than standard conservative therapy alone.

We randomised 37 short-distance claudicants to either the tracker device (n=20) or to no device (control; n=17). Data were analysed for 18 patients in the tracker group and for 13 patients in the control group. All patients followed a standard clinical pathway, which included routine information on maintaining physical activity, best medical therapy and advice to attend our supervised exercise programme. Additionally, patients in the tracker group were given a band and asked to wear it daily—daily targets were programmed into their band and feedback regarding exercise habit was given at each follow up.

Treadmill-maximum walking distance, claudication distance, patient reported walking distance and quality of life (VascuQol questionnaire) were measured at baseline, three months, six months and 12 months. The two groups were well matched for age, sex, smoking status and supervised exercise programme enrolment (10.5% for the tracker group vs. 30% for the control group; p=0.32).

Our six-month follow-up results demonstrated that the tracker group made significant improvements in maximum walking distance over six months (178m at six months vs. 80m at baseline; p<0.001), and had greater improvements than the control group (82m vs. -5m, respectively; p=0.01). Additionally, patients in the tracker made significant improvements in median claudication distance (115m vs. 40m at baseline; p<0.001) and also had significantly greater improvements than the control group (63m vs. 10m, respectively; p=0.002). In terms of quality of life, the results also showed that patients in the tracker group made significant improvements in VascuQol score across six months (4.7 vs. 5.6 at baseline; p=0.001). As with the previous outcome measures, these improvements were higher than those seen in the control group (p=0.031 for the difference).

While implementation of activity monitor-based programmes looks promising, few centres have adequately used this technology. In an international survey of

379 vascular surgeons, 67% said they would support the use of an online coaching platform to monitor physical activity if a supervised exercise programme was not available—suggesting that implementation of new technology would be welcomed by the vascular community.[9]

Using the web as a platform to promote physical activity may also be extended to optimise vascular risk factors. Goessens *et al* evaluated a nurse led web-based vascular risk factor intervention programme and demonstrated that patients liked it and it was effective at risk factor reduction.[20] Web-based interventions such as this empower patients to enhance self-management needed for long lasting changes in lifestyle.

Conclusion

With increasing burden of vascular disease, it is clear that an affordable population-based strategy with a broad sustained impact is required. Supervised exercise programmes are expensive and disliked by patients. Wearable activity trackers are accessible, inexpensive and may provide a scalable solution to promoting physical activity. Early results suggest that the use of wearable activity tracker technology is effective in improving walking distances and quality of life in patients suffering from intermittent claudication. This approach may be valuable in the management of intermittent claudication in the community. Further work is required to establish efficacy in a larger group of patients. With further technological advancements wearable technology may be also used in combination with an online coaching platform to optimise cardiovascular risk factors.

Summary

- Supervised exercise programmes are limited by poor patient compliance and limited availability. There is a need to develop a system that minimises the use of healthcare resources while maximising patient motivation.

- Wearable activity trackers are sensors that are worn on the body with a built-in accelerometer for motion quantification. They allow for monitoring of activity levels, personalised goal setting and give real-time feedback regarding goal progression.

- Early results suggest that the use of wearable activity tracker technology is effective in improving walking distances and quality of life in patients suffering from intermittent claudication. This approach may be valuable in the management of intermittent claudication in the community.

References

1. Norgren L, Hiatt WR, Dormandy JA, *et al*. Inter-Society Consensus for the Management of Peripheral Arterial Disease (TASC II). *Eur J Vasc Endovasc Surg* 2007; **33** Suppl 1(1): S1–75.
2. Spronk S, White J V, Bosch JL, Hunink MGM. Impact of claudication and its treatment on quality of life. *Semin Vasc Surg* 2007; **20** (1): 3–9.
3. Cassar K. Intermittent claudication. *BMJ* 2006; **333** (7576): 1002–05.
4. Watson L, Ellis B, Leng GC. Exercise for intermittent claudication. Cochrane database Syst Rev 2008;(4): CD000990.

5. Gardner AW, Parker DE, Montgomery PS, *et al*. Efficacy of quantified home-based exercise and supervised exercise in patients with intermittent claudication: a randomized controlled trial. *Circulation* 2011; **123** (5): 491–98.

6. McDermott MM, Liu K, O'Brien E, Guralnik JM, Criqui MH, Martin GJ, *et al*. Measuring physical activity in peripheral arterial disease: a comparison of two physical activity questionnaires with an accelerometer. *Angiology* 2000; **51** (2): 91–100.

7. Menard JR, Smith HE, Riebe D, *et al*. Long-term results of peripheral arterial disease rehabilitation. *J Vasc Surg* 2004; **39** (6): 1186–92.

8. Shalhoub J, Hamish M, Davies AH. Supervised exercise for intermittent claudication - an under-utilised tool. *Ann R Coll Surg Engl* 2009; **91** (6): 473–76.

9. Makris GC, Lattimer CR, Lavida A, Geroulakos G. Availability of supervised exercise programs and the role of structured home-based exercise in peripheral arterial disease. *Eur J Vasc Endovasc Surg* 2012; **44** (6): 569–75; discussion 576.

10. Mindtree.com. Wearables – Is the future as bright as it seems? http://bit.ly/1Qq6u4U (date accessed: 26 January 2016).

11. Bravata DM, Smith-Spangler C, Sundaram V, *et al*. Using pedometers to increase physical activity and improve health: a systematic review. *JAMA* 2007; **298** (19): 2296–304.

12. Reid RD, Morrin LI, Beaton LJ, *et al*. Randomized trial of an internet-based computer-tailored expert system for physical activity in patients with heart disease. *Eur J Prev Cardiol* 2012; **19** (6): 1357–64.

13. Watson A, Bickmore T, Cange A, *et al*. An internet-based virtual coach to promote physical activity adherence in overweight adults: randomized controlled trial. *J Med Internet Res* 2012; **14** (1): e1.

14. Jelinek M, Vale MJ, Liew D, *et al*. The COACH program produces sustained improvements in cardiovascular risk factors and adherence to recommended medications-two years follow-up. *Heart Lung Circ* 2009; **18** (6): 388–92.

15. Evenson KR, Goto MM, Furberg RD. Systematic review of the validity and reliability of consumer-wearable activity trackers. *Int J Behav Nutr Phys Act* 2015; **12** (1): 159.

16. Cyarto EV, Myers AM, Tudor-Locke C. Pedometer accuracy in nursing home and community-dwelling older adults. *Med Sci Sports Exerc* 2004; **36** (2): 205–09.

17. Cadmus-Bertram L, Marcus BH, Patterson RE, *et al*. Use of the Fitbit to Measure Adherence to a Physical Activity Intervention Among Overweight or Obese, Postmenopausal Women: Self-Monitoring Trajectory During 16 Weeks. *JMIR* 2015; **3** (4): e96.

18. Wang JB, Cadmus-Bertram LA, Natarajan L, *et al*. Wearable Sensor/Device (Fitbit One) and SMS Text-Messaging Prompts to Increase Physical Activity in Overweight and Obese Adults: A Randomized Controlled Trial. *Telemed J E Health* 2015; **21** (10): 782–92.

19. Cadmus-Bertram LA, Marcus BH, Patterson RE, *et al*. Randomized trial of a Fitbit-based physical activity intervention for women. *Am J Prev Med* 2015; **49** (3): 414–18.

20. Goessens BMB, Visseren FLJ, de Nooijer J, *et al*. A pilot-study to identify the feasibility of an Internet-based coaching programme for changing the vascular risk profile of high-risk patients. *Patient Educ Couns* 2008; **73** (1): 67–72.

Endovascular debulking technique using rotational thrombectomy: A review of published literature

M Lichtenberg

Introduction

Acute and subacute ischaemia of the lower extremity is still a common reason for amputation. The treatment of this condition includes the well-known procedure of local thrombolysis, surgical thrombectomy and, in recent times, percutaneous mechanical thrombectomy procedures such as rotational thrombectomy. However, in randomised studies, Fogarty's procedure of surgical thrombectomy was associated with a high rate of perioperative complications and, in part, low technical success rates. On the other hand, local thrombolysis is associated with haemorrhage as well as high costs because of measures requiring substantial resources, such as intensive care monitoring or repeat angiographies. In several studies, the endovascular therapy options Rotarex and Aspirex (both Straub Medical), both products of technical advancements in the field, were shown to be successful in terms of amputation-free survival. Their use was also associated with low complication rates. The majority of studies were focused on arterial blood flow in the femur. In the present chapter, the current study-based value of rotational thrombectomy in the arterial system is reviewed.

Overview of acute and subacute ischaemia of the extremity

Acute and subacute ischaemia of the extremity is caused by impaired arterial perfusion. The reason, in most cases, is local arterial thrombosis or embolism. Cardiac embolism is the most common cause. An acute arterial perfusion disorder of an extremity may, in addition to involving the risk of irreversible damage to or loss of the extremity, cause life-threatening complications. Due to the anaerobic local and eventually systemic metabolic situation secondary to hypoperfusion, organs such as the heart and kidney are directly involved in the process. The management of patients includes, as well as general intensive-care measures, the decision to perform an adequate revascularisation procedure. An acute embolic arterial occlusion can very frequently occur in a peripheral vascular system with no previous haemodynamic impairment, and with the collateral compensation required for this condition. This results in a much more severe clinical ischaemic situation (so-called white ischaemia) accompanied by characteristic pain and neurological

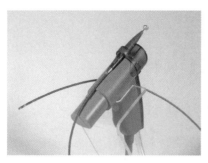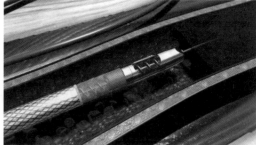

Figure 1 and 2: Motor unit and Rotarex catheter.

abnormalities in the affected extremity. On the other hand, the formation of a local arterial thrombus, such as one due to rupture of a plaque in the presence of pre-existing peripheral arterial occlusive disease, causes fewer and less severe symptoms because of compensatory collateral circulation.[1] Differentiating between an arterial occlusion of embolic or local thrombotic origin may be aided by the patient's medical history, such as the presence of heart disease, atrial fibrillation, cardiac valve defect, or a known peripheral arterial occlusive disease treated several times by various interventions. In cases of suspected acute ischaemia of the extremity, the location of an acute arterial occlusion must be determined rapidly with the aid of contemporary ultrasound procedures and, if necessary, computed tomography (CT) or magnetic resonance (MR) angiography. According to current international guidelines in keeping with the consensus agreement (TASC II guidelines), acute ischaemia of the extremity is graded in categories I to III.[2] In particular, the vitally threatened extremity of category II calls for immediate diagnostic investigation and therapy (Table 1). According to the current TASC II guidelines, the consensus that applies today is that acute ischaemia of the extremity must be treated by an interventional procedure (local thrombolysis, interventional embolectomy) or surgery (embolectomy). Since the TASC II guidelines are entirely based on studies and experience prior to 2007, they do not conform to the current level of study-based development. The intervention of percutaneous mechanical thrombectomy, employing the principle of rotational thrombectomy, has achieved impressive results in the last few years, as observed in single-centre and multicentre studies focusing on various aetiologies and locations of acute ischaemia of the extremity. This has led to a paradigm shift in favour of less invasive therapy. The general advantage of a percutaneous mechanical thrombectomy device is its rapid use without major preparations (such as preparation for anaesthesia and the presence of various specialists), which permits rapid reperfusion of a hypoperfused extremity. The use of any new therapy option should be amenable to, and should demonstrate a significant advantage for, comparison with established measures. In comparative studies concerning local thrombolysis and surgical embolectomy, the following criteria were used for direct comparison of therapeutic measures:[3–6]

- Technical success rates
- Reintervention measures/re-occlusion
- Preservation rate of the extremity
- Death
- Peripheral embolism as a complication

- Duration of the intervention
- Haemorrhage.

Technique of rotational thrombectomy

The Rotarex thrombectomy system (Figures 1 and 2) functions on the basis of the Archimedes' screw principle. This consists of a spiral rotating at a speed of about 40,000 rotations per minute. The system consists of three individual components, which can be assembled in a few minutes by a practised team. It is driven by a motor that also serves as an electronic control unit and displays information about the functionality of the rotating helix. The conveyor helix connected to the motor through a magnetic coupling operates within the catheter. Rapid rotation of the helix creates a persistent vacuum inside the catheter, which causes thrombotic material in the target lesion to be suctioned and conveyed into a collection bag at the end of the catheter. The difference between the Aspirex catheter system, used in the venous system, and the Rotarex system, mainly used in the arterial system, is the configuration of the catheter head. The Rotarex system allows occlusive (thrombotic and organised) material to become detached and be removed. In contrast, the Aspirex catheter (indicated for the thin-walled venous system) serves to aspirate and remove thrombotic material. Depending on the size of the system used (Rotarex 6–8Fr, Aspirex 6–10Fr), aspiration rates of 1.5ml/sec can be achieved with the 8Fr Rotarex system. Larger systems are used in the pelvic and femoral flow region. In cases of thrombotic occlusions at these locations, a larger quantity of thrombotic material has to be removed because of the large vessel diameter. Depending on the size of the target vessel, the 6Fr system permits thrombectomy well into the lower leg. After performing a diagnostic angiography, one should use a 6Fr or 8Fr Rotarex system, depending on the diameter of the vessel. It may be necessary to switch to an 8Fr catheter. When using the roadmap or overlay technique, a 0.018inch guidewire is introduced into the target lesion and guided in distal direction. Through this guidewire, the respective Rotarex system is inserted to a point a few centimetres above the occlusion and then activated. Passage of the occlusion should be performed slowly. Particularly in cases of subacute occlusions with partly organised material, one should proceed slowly to avoid peripheral embolism. Depending on morphological conditions after the achievement of

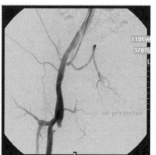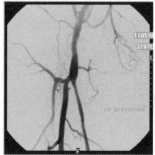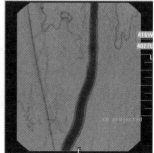

Figure 3–5: Closed femoropopliteal P1 bypass on the right side, before and after rotational thrombectomy with a Rotarex 8Fr catheter and implantation of a nitinol stent in the distal aspect in a patient with a high-grade stenosis of the bypass at the point of insertion.

re-flow, one should perform an angioplasty with or without stent implantation, according to current recommendations. In my department's experience, a stent is required in the large majority of treated lesions because dissection or relevant haemodynamic stenosis are quite common in the region of intervention. This may have to be followed by guideline-based antithrombotic combination therapy consisting of acetylsalicylic acid and clopidogrel.

Indications for rotational thrombectomy

Recent studies and case reports mention very high technical success rates for primary re-opening of an infra-aortic vessel;[3–6] these are generally well above 90%. The crossover system has been available since 2003. Catheter shaft lengths of 85cm may be used for antegrade application. Technical advancements have resulted in highly flexible encasing shaft material. The most recent version appears to markedly reduce the risk of helix breakage in crossover use. In this context, the use of wire-reinforced crossover sheaths is considered mandatory and effective anticoagulation is recommended. At our department, the crossover system is used for the distal portion of the external iliac artery and the common femoral artery, and the proximal portion of the superficial femoral artery. The 8Fr system should be used for vessel sizes to 4mm in the distal region and is not suitable for the lower leg because the risk of vessel perforation or dissection is markedly higher in this setting. Using the 6Fr Rotarex system, depending on anatomical conditions, we have been able to perform interventions well into the lower leg. A vessel diameter of 3mm in the crural region is sufficient.

The risk of vessel perforation or dissection is mainly dependent on the safe intravascular position of the guidewire. Wissgott reported a perforation rate of 1% (3/265) in his patients while Zeller mentions 9%. Bérczi *et al*[7] registered perforation

	Category	Prognosis	Report		Doppler signal	
			Loss of Sensitivity	Muscle weakness	Arterial	Venous
I Viable		No immediate threat	None	None	Audible	Audible
II Vitality is endangered						
	A	Favourable prognosis in cases of immediate treatment	Minimal	None	Often no evidence	Audible
	B	Extremity can be preserved when revascularisation is performed immediately	Pain at rest	Moderate	No evidence	Audible
III Irreversible		Marked tissue necrosis	Anaesthesia	Paralysis	No evidence	No evidence

Table 1: Categories of acute ischaemia in the extremity.

in two of 19 interventions, which occurred in markedly calcified arteries. The risk of perforation is especially high in calcified arteries. This phenomenon is attributed to the fact that hard calcified plaque is suctioned and becomes entangled at the inlet of the helix. The rotating helix may exert a strong pulling force on the wall of the artery, thus leading to perforation. The motor unit may show signs of this condition because the velocity of the rotating helix will be reduced in this setting and displayed by light-emitting diodes on the motor unit. A crucial step to avoid severe injury to vessels and/or dissection is to ensure correct positioning of the wire. After successful removal of thrombotic/embolic material, in many cases one needs to perform balloon angioplasty or stent implantation. This is probably the reason for low long-term patency rates after re-opening, which is a point of criticism for this technique. In the patients followed-up by Zeller et al, balloon dilatation or additional stent implantation was required in every second patient. This was confirmed by our data. Particularly in patients with pre-existing arteriosclerosis, a culprit lesion requiring intervention was commonly found after thrombectomy. Wissgot et al[3] refer to the necessity of subsequent balloon angioplasty in 72%, whereas Duc[8] performed an additional percutaneous transluminal angioplasty in just two of 38 patients and stent implantation in five patients. Bérczi et al[7] performed balloon angioplasty or stent implantation in 17 of 19 extremities. A direct prospective comparison of thrombolysis, rotational thrombectomy and the established procedure of local thrombolysis has not been performed thus far. A direct and scientific comparison of therapy options is rendered difficult by this fact. However, one can compare efficacy on the basis of endpoint criteria, amputation-free survival after 12 months, and re-intervention rates. This comparison shows a clear benefit of the mechanical thrombectomy over local lytic therapy in terms of efficiency (thrombus removal) and safety (bleeding complication).[3,6,9,10] On direct comparison of the various therapy studies, amputation-free survival at 12 months after rotational thrombectomy was markedly higher than it was after local thrombolysis or a vascular surgery-based thrombectomy manoeuvre.

Rotational thrombectomy is an effective therapy option for acute or subacute occlusion of a femoropopliteal bypass as well. In a recently published study performed by our group,[11] the use of rotational thrombectomy for the treatment of acute and subacute occlusion of a femoropopliteal bypass was associated with a high rate of technical success by way of effective thrombectomy in terms of haemodynamics. In this follow-up study, 14 patients (nine male) with acute occlusions of a femoropopliteal bypass (eight venous bypasses and six polytetrafluoroethylene bypasses) were treated at our clinic with the Rotarex system from June 2009 to June 2010. In these patients, only P1 bypasses were treated by intervention and then evaluated. Clinically, eight patients had stage I and six patients stage IIa disease in accordance with the TASC classification of acute ischaemia of the extremity (Figures 3–5). In several cases, the cause of femoropopliteal occlusion was a high-grade and haemodynamically relevant stenosis at the point of insertion, which was treated by an intervention in the same session. In the follow-up period of six months, our patients developed no renewed bypass occlusion or haemodynamically relevant restenosis. The ankle-brachial index (ABI) value after six months was 0.81±0.1. Our data are in agreement with those reported by Wissgott et al,[4,12] who followed their patients for 12 months. The authors registered a primary patency rate of 66% and a secondary patency rate of 86%.

Conclusion

Rotational thrombectomy is an effective and reliable means of performing thrombectomy in the arteries as well as veins. Sufficient validated data are available for the use of the Rotarex system in arteries of the lower extremity. Thus, it may be regarded as a safe and effective method of treatment. Whether rotational thrombectomy can be used for specific situations and indications, such as acute arterial occlusion of the lower extremity, thrombotic occlusions of mesenteric vessels or aortic prostheses, must be analysed in larger studies and registries.

Summary

- Acute and subacute ischemia of the limbs are frequent and could be severe.

- Different therapy options are available.

- Rotational thrombectomy is a pure mechanical approach for debulking therapy.

References

1. Kasirajan K, Marek JM, Longsfeld M. Mechanical thrombectomy as a first-line treatment for arterial occlusion. *Semin Vasc Surg* 2001; **14** (2): 123–31.

2. Norgren L, Hiatt WR, Dormandy JA, *et al* on behalf of the TASC II Working Group. Inter-society consensus for the management of peripheral arterial disease (TASCII). *Eur J Vasc Endovasc Surg* 2007; 45 Suppl S:S5–67.

3. Wissgott C, Kamusella P, Richter A, *et al*. Rotationsthrombektomie zur Behandlung von akuten und subakuten Okklusionen der femoropoplitealen Arterien: Retrospektive Auswertung der Ergebnisse von 1999–2005. *Fortschr Röntgenstr* 2008; **180**: 1–7.

4. Wissgott C, Kamusella P, Richter A, *et al*. Behandlung akuter Okklusionen von femoropoplitealen Bypässen: Vergleich der mechanischen Rotationsthrombektomie mit der ultraschallgestützten Lyse. *Fortschr Röntgenstr* 2008; **180**: 547–52.

5. Zeller T, Frank U, Bürgelin K, *et al*. Early experience with a rotational thrombectomy device for treatment of acute and subacute infra-aortic arterial occlusions. *J Endovasc Ther* 2003; **10**: 322–31.

6. Zeller T, Frank U, Bürgelin K, *et al*. Langzeitergebnisse nach Rekanalisation akuter und subakuter thrombotischer arterieller Verschlüsse der unteren Extremitäten mit einem Rotations-Thrombektomiekatheter. *Fortschr Röntgenstr* 2002; **174**: 1559–65.

7. Bérczi V, Deutschmann HA, Schedlbauer P, *et al*. Early experience and midterm follow-up results with a new, rotational thrombectomy catheter. *Cardiovasc Intervent Radiol* 2002; **25** (4): 275–81.

8. Duc SR, Schoch E, Pfyffer M *et al*. Recanalisation of acute and subacute femoropopliteal artery occlusions with the Rotarex catheter: one-year follow-up, single-centre experience. *Cardiovasc Intervent Radiol* 2005; **28**: 603–10.

9. Ouriel K, Veith FJ, Sasahara AA for the Thrombolysis or Peripheral Arterial Surgery (TOPAS) investigators. A comparison of recombinant urokinase with vascular surgery as initial treatment for acute arterial occlusion of the legs. *N Eng J Med* 1998; **338** (16): 1105–11.

10. The STILE Trial: results of a prospective randomized trial evaluating surgery *versus* thrombolysis for ischemia of the lower extremity. *Ann Surg* 1994; **220** (3): 251–66.

11. M Lichtenberg, M Käunicke, B Hailer. Rotationsthrombektomie als therapeutische Option bei akuten thrombotischen Verschlüssen von femoropoplitealen *Bypässen*. *Z Gefäßmed* 2011; **8** (4): 5–10.

12. Wissgott C, Kamusella P, Richter A, *et al*. Mechanical rotational thrombectomy for treatment thrombolysis in acute and subacute occlusion of femoropopliteal arteries: retrospective analysis of the results from 1999 to 2005. *Fortschr Röntgenstr* 2008; **180**: 1–7.

Superficial femoral artery

IN.PACT SFA two-year results— drug-coated balloon use in women and in diabetics

C Richards and PA Schneider

Introduction

Drug-coated balloon angioplasty in the femoropopliteal region offers the hope of improved patency with fewer complications than stent placement.[1-3] In the femoropopliteal region, stents have better long-term patency than plain old balloon angioplasty but complications from stent placement—including stent fracture and in-stent restenosis—are difficult to manage.[4-7] While there is variability in the estimated occurrence of stent fracture and in-stent restenosis, both seem to be more common with longer segments of stenting and when multiple stents are used.[8-11] As the use of femoropopliteal drug-coated balloons expands, diabetics and women deserve special attention. These groups make up significant portions of studied vascular populations and have distinctive responses to endovascular interventions, but they often do not receive subgroup analysis. Therefore, the question evaluated in this chapter is: Is there a benefit to drug-coated balloon angioplasty in diabetics and women?

Drug-coated balloon angioplasty in the femoropopliteal region

Drugs delivered by drug-coated balloons inhibit the immune response via cytotoxic mechanisms. Inhibition of neointimal hyperplasia—the pathological healing process—limits restenosis. While the drug is only temporarily in the patient's circulation, it has been found to remain in the tissue for months.[12] The use of excipients permit up to 17% of the drug to be taken up by the arterial wall.[13] The drug most commonly used is paclitaxel, while sirolimus and rapamycin have also been discussed. Paclitaxel acts by inhibiting arterial smooth muscle cell proliferation without a long incubation time. Concern that this mechanism may lead to delayed healing has prompted some interest in the alternative agents mentioned above as well as others.[14-16] Paclitaxel is excellent at inhibiting unwanted cell proliferation, but it has a poor dissolution rate, probably in part due to its lipophilic nature.[17] Additionally, different dosages of paclitaxel have been studied with a dose-dependent relationship up to 2–4µg/mm^2.[18] Successive generations of drug-coated balloons have been created with improved tissue uptake—although in light of the technology's novelty, long-term data are only now starting to emerge.[19]

Drug-coated balloon angioplasty trials

To study the specific effect of the medication, drug-coated balloons have mostly been tested against plain old balloon angioplasty. In the late 2000s, pilot studies from Europe demonstrated reductions in late lumen loss with drug-coated balloon angioplasty. The trials listed in Table 1 generally had paclitaxel concentrations of $3\mu g/mm^2$ and mean lesion lengths from 6.3cm to 8.9cm. Enrolled patients had Rutherford 2–5 ischaemia.[20] The THUNDER (Local taxan with short time contact for reduction of restenosis in distal arteries) study (2008) randomly assigned 154 patients to drug-coated balloons with paclitaxel, uncoated balloons with paclitaxel dissolved in contrast medium, or uncoated balloons. At six months, paclitaxel-coated balloons resulted in significantly less late lumen loss and target lesion revascularisation than the other two groups.[21] In 2012, the PACIFIER (Paclitaxel-coated balloons in femoral indication to defeat restenosis) study showed a significant reduction in late lumen loss with drug-coated balloons compared with plain balloon angioplasty. The study size was small (85 patients) and the timeframe was limited (six-month primary endpoint).[3] The LEVANT I (Lutonix paclitaxel-coated balloon for the prevention of femoropopliteal restenosis) trial (2014) used a concentration of $2\mu g/mm^2$ paclitaxel. At six months, the drug-coated balloon group showed significantly less late lumen loss than the plain old balloon angioplasty group. The authors noted that a larger than expected number of patients had drug-coated balloon devices that did not appropriately deploy. In these patients, the target lesion

Study	Year	Study Size	Location	Outcome(s)	Follow-up Time	Results			
						Outcome	POBA	DCB	P Value
THUNDER	2008	154	Germany	LLL and TLR	6 Months	LLL	1.7mm	0.4mm	<0.001
						TLR	37%	4%	<0.001
Werk et al	2008	87	Germany	LLL and TLR	6 Months	LLL	0.8mm	0.3mm	0.031
						TLR	50%	13%	0.001
LEVANT I	2014	101	Primarily Germany and Belgium	LLL	6 Months	LLL	1.09mm	0.46mm	0.016
LEVANT II	2015	476	US and Europe	PP and TLR	12 Months	PP	52.6%	65.2%	0.02
						TLR	16.8%	12.3%	0.21
						PP (US)	56.5%	69.9%	not given
						PP (Non-US)	46%	69.1%	not given
PACIFIER	2015	85	Germany	LLL and TLR	12 Months	LLL	0.65mm	0.1mm	0.001
						TLR	27.90%	7.10%	0.02
IN.PACT SFA	2015	331	US and Europe	PP and CD-TLR	24 Months	PP	50.10%	78.9%	<0.001
						CD-TLR	28.30%	9.10%	<0.001

Table 1 DCB Trials

POBA: Plain old balloon angioplasty; **DCB:** Drug-coated balloon; **LLL:** Late lumen loss; **TLR:** Target lesion revascularisation; **CD-TLR:** Clinically driven target lesion revascularisation; **PP:** Primary patency

revascularisation rates and late lumen loss were 63% and 0.71mm, respectively, compared with 20% and 0.39mm for the successfully deployed drug-coated balloon group. This is especially pertinent when compared with the uncoated balloon group at 33% and 1.09mm.[9] The LEVANT II trial was subsequently conducted at 54 sites in Europe and the USA with 476 participants and showed significantly improved primary patency and non-significantly decreased target lesion revascularisation with drug-coated balloon *versus* plain old balloon angioplasty. Primary patency in the drug-coated balloon arm was 65.2% and 52.6% in the control arm at one year.[22] The IN.PACT SFA trial (2015) was performed in Europe and the USA. Primary patency in the drug-coated balloon group was 82.2% at one year *versus* 52.4% in the plain old balloon angioplasty group. At two years, the difference in primary patency between the groups was stable (78.9% vs. 50.1%). Both groups showed similar functional improvement at two years, but the plain old balloon angioplasty group underwent 58% more procedures.[1-2] In 2015, the THUNDER trial published five-year follow-up results from approximately 80% of originally enrolled patients. Target lesion revascularisation rates at five years remained significantly lower in the drug-coated balloon group (21%) *versus* the plain old balloon angioplasty group (56%).[23] The next questions to ask include whether drug-coated balloon is superior to stenting and what to do with longer lesions. Several studies are focusing on these issues. The RAPID (Randomised trial of legflow paclitaxel eluting balloon and stenting *versus* standard percutaneous transluminal angioplasty and stenting for the treatment of intermediate and long lesions of the superficial femoral artery) trial plans to compare drug-coated balloon and stenting *versus* plain old balloon angioplasty and stenting for intermediate length femoropopliteal lesions.[24] With the results of this trial, and the other ongoing studies, the role for drug-coated balloons should be better defined.

Why study female patients?

Patient populations in large vascular studies are typically comprised of a majority of men, although women are better represented in more recent studies. Questions remain regarding the effect that gender has on the disease process, interventions, and long-term outcomes.[25-26] This is especially relevant since women are more likely to have femoropopliteal disease than men when presenting with critical limb ischaemia, and are also more likely to present with diffuse atherosclerotic disease.[27] The DURABILITY II (The US study for evaluating endovascular treatments of lesions in the superficial femoral artery and proximal popliteal by using the Protégé Everflex nitinol stent system II) trial evaluated outcomes of femoropopliteal stenting in women and found equivalent responses to endovascular treatment as men at two years but diminished at three years.[28] This is a similar timeframe to what Pulli *et al* found with women having an equivalent response to men early after endovascular intervention, but with diminished patency at three years.[29] Stavroulakis *et al* evaluated 517 patients, including 184 women, undergoing primary femoropopliteal stenting and followed patients for five years. Findings included: women were more likely to present with critical limb ischaemia; stenting of femoropopliteal lesions in women resulted in poor secondary patency rates *versus* men, and women had a higher rate of restenosis in TASC C/D lesions. Despite this, there was no difference in limb salvage or survival between the genders.[30] It is unclear why women respond differently to treatment. A suggested mechanism is

Table 2 DCB Trials with Gender Subgroup Analysis							
Study	Outcome(s)	Follow-up Time		POBA	DCB	Absolute Difference (DCB-POBA)	P Value
THUNDER	TLR rates	5 Years					
			MALE	71%	17%	-54%	not given
			FEMALE	52%	38%	-14%	not given
LEVANT II	PP	12 Months					
			MALE	48.4%	70.6%	22.2%	not given
			FEMALE	61.4%	56.4%	-5%	not given
PACIFIER	LLL	12 Months					
			MALE	0.53mm	-0.23mm	-0.76mm	0.003
			FEMALE	0.85mm	0.36mm	-0.49mm	0.13
IN.PACT SFA	PP	24 Months					
			MALE	53.7%	80.2%	26.5%	<0.001
			FEMALE	42.3%	76.7%	34.40%	<0.001

POBA: Plain old balloon angioplasty; DCB: Drug-coated balloon;
LLL: Late lumen loss; TLR: Target lesion revascularisation;

the anatomical differences between genders with interventions better suited to the larger arteries found in men.[31] Additionally, as described above, women develop different lesion configurations and morphology than men do.[27] All of this calls for more information on how women respond to new technologies.

Subgroup analysis of drug-coated balloons in women

While there are no specific trials addressing drug-coated balloons in women and diabetic patients, there are mounting data from subgroup analysis in recently conducted trials. Several trials that compare drug-coated balloons and plain old balloon angioplasty also contain gender subgroup analysis: IN.PACT SFA, PACIFIER, LEVANT II and THUNDER (Table 2). The PACIFIER trial found a significant difference in men between drug-coated balloon *versus* plain old balloon angioplasty with a lower target lesion revascularisation rate and lower late lumen loss. In women, however, there was no difference between the two groups. The study was small, with 35 women (including both treatment arms) out of 91 total patients.[3] Conversely, the IN.PACT study found no difference between women and men at 24 months. Women had a primary patency rate of 76.7% with drug-coated balloons *versus* 42.3% with plain old balloon angioplasty. Very similarly, men had a primary patency rate of 80.2% with drug-coated balloon and 53.7% with plain old balloon angioplasty at 24 months. Of 331 total trial patients (with a 2:1 ratio of drug-coated balloon to plain old balloon angioplasty), 113 were female, three times as many as the PACIFIER trial.[1–2] In the THUNDER trial, 10 of 20 women in the control arm and six of 17 women in the drug-coated balloon arm were followed to five years. They found a significantly higher target lesion revascularisation rate in women *versus* men at two years but no difference between them at five years.[23] The LEVANT II trial included 176 women from Europe and the USA. When evaluated by geography, US women in the drug-coated balloon group had a 19.7% lower primary patency rate (50.7% at one year) than the plain old balloon angioplasty group (70.4%). Conversely, non-US women in the drug-coated balloon group had a primary patency rate of 70%, 22.9% higher than the plain old balloon angioplasty group at 47.1% and compared very similarly to their male counterparts (US and non-US combined). Men combined had a primary patency rate of 70.6% in the drug-coated balloon group and 48.4% in the plain old balloon angioplasty group. US men had a patency rate of 71.9% with drug-coated balloon and 50% with plain old balloon angioplasty. Non-US men had a patency rate of 68.7% with drug-coated balloon and 45.5% with plain old balloon angioplasty. Hence, US men did nearly 10% points better with drug-coated balloon than non-US men, but both US and non-US men did significantly better with drug-coated balloon angioplasty *versus* plain old balloon angioplasty. One possible explanation is that in the US women drug-coated balloon group, there was a higher proportion of smaller reference diameters and popliteal lesions and there may have been under dilation with utilisation of drug-coated balloons.[32]

There is a trend suggesting that women benefit from drug-coated balloon angioplasty of the femoropopliteal arteries, as much as men. As mentioned above, women tend to present at an older age with worse lesions but with fewer comorbidities, separating them from their male cohorts both anatomically as well as clinically.[26] Risk-factor adjusted analysis of a large group of women would be an appropriate next step.

Why study diabetic patients?

Diabetic patients comprise a significant portion of any vascular service but remain somewhat unpredictable in their responsiveness to different treatment modalities. Both open and endovascular treatment modalities are effective with diabetic patients but specific and direct comparisons between diabetic patients and non-diabetic patients are infrequent.[33–34] There are differences within the diabetic population including: insulin *versus* non-insulin dependence; well-controlled *versus* poorly controlled; new diagnosis *versus* long-term patient; HgbA1C levels; other diabetic complications (such as renal impairment or symptomatic coronary artery disease); and others. Diabetic patients are also more likely to undergo amputation and to

Table 3 DCB Trial(s) with Diabetes Subgroup Analysis							
Study	Outcome	Follow-up Time		POBA	DCB	Absolute Difference (DCB-POBA)	P Value
IN.PACT SFA	PP	24 Months					
			Diabetic	45.80%	73.3%	27.5%	<0.001
			Non-Diabetic	54.5%	82.5%	28%	<0.001

present with longer segments of occlusion (≥10cm) in this region.[35–37] Diabetic patients have higher reintervention rates than non-diabetic patients but can have similar short-term secondary patency.[38] Long-term limb salvage appears to be poorer in diabetics, even with close follow-up and reintervention. This is possibly due to worse clinical status at presentation and worse runoff.[39] More information is needed, however, to make better clinical prescriptions and predictions regarding treatment in this this subgroup of patients.

Subgroup analysis of drug-coated balloons in diabetics patients

The IN.PACT trial was the only drug-coated balloon *versus* plain old balloon angioplasty study to include a subgroup analysis of diabetic *versus* non-diabetic patients (Table 3). Diabetic patients had equivalent outcomes with drug-coated balloon *versus* plain old balloon angioplasty when compared to non-diabetic patients at two years. Both diabetics and non-diabetics had an approximately 28% better primary patency in the drug-coated balloon group with 73.3% and 82.5%, respectively, in the drug-coated balloon group *versus* 45.8% and 54.5% in the plain old balloon angioplasty group. However, diabetic patients in both plain old balloon angioplasty and drug-coated balloon groups experienced approximately 10 absolute percentage points lower success than their non-diabetic cohorts.[1–2] Although there is certainly a dearth of data, based on the trial described above, it is possible that drug-coated balloon angioplasty offers equal benefit to diabetic and non-diabetic patients. It is also possible that, like women, diabetic patients start to differ from their non-diabetic cohorts only after a longer period of study. Drug-coated balloon angioplasty appears to be a reasonable option in diabetics with femoropopliteal occlusive disease.

Conclusion

Drug-coated balloon angioplasty of the femoropopliteal arteries is a promising endovascular technique and appears to be broadly applicable, including both women and diabetics. Without knowing exactly why these two populations do not respond as well to certain vascular techniques as their male and non-diabetic cohorts, it is difficult to make prognostications. It is imperative, however, to analyse these subgroups going forward. The next step is treatment of longer superficial femoral artery lesions with drug-coated balloon angioplasty, as both women and diabetic patients are more likely to present with more diffuse lesions. This analysis in particular will help to define the optimal treatment pathway in these populations.

Summary

- Drug-coated balloon angioplasty in the femoropopliteal region offers a promising alternative to stenting.

- Drugs delivered via drug-coated balloons inhibit neointimal hyperplasia thus limiting restenosis.

- Multiple large-scale European and US trials have shown benefits with drug-coated balloons *versus* plain old balloon angioplasty.

- Both female and diabetic patients tend to present with different vascular disease than male and non-diabetic patients do. They also react differently to interventions with varied long-term results.

- Multiple drug-coated balloon trials have studied women while only a few have looked at diabetic patients specifically.

- Women seem to respond as well as their male cohorts to drug-coated balloons but more long-term follow-up is needed.

- Diabetic patients had the same effect with drug-coated balloons as non-diabetic patients, but diabetic patients as a whole did worse than non-diabetic patients. More long-term follow-up is needed.

References

1. Tepe G, Laird J, Schneider P, *et al.* Drug-coated balloon *versus* standard percutaneous transluminal angioplasty for the treatment of superficial femoral and popliteal peripheral artery disease: 12-month results from the IN.PACT SFA randomized trial. *Circulation* 2015; **131** (5): 495–502.

2. Laird JR, Schneider PA, Tepe G, *et al.* Durability of treatment effect using a drug-coated balloon for femoropopliteal lesions: 24-month results of IN.PACT SFA. *J Am Coll Cardiol* 2015; **66** (21): 2329–38.

3. Werk M, Albrecht T, Meyer DR, *et al.* Paclitaxel-coated balloons reduce restenosis after femoropopliteal angioplasty: evidence from the randomized PACIFIER trial. *Circ Cardiovasc Interv* 2012; **5** (6): 831–40.

4. Laird JR, Katzen BT, Scheinert D, *et al.* Nitinol stent implantation *versus* balloon angioplasty for lesions in the superficial femoral artery and proximal popliteal artery: twelve-month results from the RESILIENT randomized trial. *Circ Cardiovasc Interv* 2010; **3** (3): 267–76.

5. Laird JR, Katzen BT, Scheinert D, *et al.* Nitinol stent implantation vs. balloon angioplasty for lesions in the superficial femoral and proximal popliteal arteries of patients with claudication: three-year follow-up from the RESILIENT randomized trial. *J Endovasc Ther* 2012; **19** (1): 1–9.

6. Dake MD, Ansel GM, Jaff MR, *et al.* Paclitaxel eluting stents show superiority to balloon angioplasty and bare metal stents in femoropopliteal disease: twelve-month Zilver PTX randomized study results. *Circ Cardiovasc Interv* 2011; **4** (5): 495–504.

7. Schillinger M, Sabeti S, Loewe C, *et al.* Balloon angioplasty vs. implantation of nitinol stents in the superficial femoral artery. *N Engl J Med* 2006; **354** (18): 1879–88.

8. Iida O, Nanto S, Uematsu M, *et al.* Influence of stent fracture on the long-term patency in the femoropopliteal artery: experience of four years. *JACC Cardiovasc Interv* 2009; **2** (7): 665–71.

9. Scheinert D, Duda S, Zeller T, *et al.* The LEVANT I (Lutonix paclitaxel-coated balloon for the prevention of femoropopliteal restenosis) trial for femoropopliteal revascularization: first-in-human randomized trial of low-dose drug-coated balloon *versus* uncoated balloon angioplasty. *JACC Cardiovasc Interv* 2014; **7** (1): 10–9.

10. Armstrong EJ, Singh S, Singh GD, *et al.* Angiographic characteristics of femoropopliteal in-stent restenosis: association with long-term outcomes after endovascular intervention. *Catheter Cardiovasc Interv* 2013; **82** (7): 1168–74.

11. Peidro J, Boufi M, Loundou Dieudonne A, *et al.* Atheromatous occlusive lesions of the popliteal artery treated with stent grafts: predictive factors of midterm patency. *Ann Vasc Surg* 2015; **29** (4): 708–15.

12. Gongora CA, Shibuya M, Wessler JD, et al. Impact of paclitaxel dose on tissue pharmacokinetics and vascular healing: a comparative drug-coated balloon study in the familial hypercholesterolemic swine model of superficial femoral in-stent restenosis. JACC Cardiovasc Interv 2015; **8** (8): 1115–23.

13. Kempin W, Kaule S, Reske T, et al. In vitro evaluation of paclitaxel coatings for delivery via drug-coated balloons. Eur J Pharm Biopharm 2015; **96**: 322–28.

14. Axel DI, Kunert W, Goggelmann C, et al. Paclitaxel inhibits arterial smooth muscle cell proliferation and migration in vitro and in vivo using local drug delivery. Circulation 1997; **96** (2): 636–45.

15. Finn AV, John M, Nakazawa G, et al. Differential healing after sirolimus, paclitaxel, and bare metal stent placement in combination with peroxisome proliferator-activator receptor gamma agonists: requirement for mTOR/Akt2 in PPARgamma activation. Circ Res 2009; **105** (10): 1003–12.

16. Schmehl J, von der Ruhr J, Dobratz M, et al. Balloon coating with rapamycin using an on-site coating device. Cardiovasc Intervent Radiol 2013; **36** (3): 756–63.

17. Moes J, Koolen S, Huitema A, et al. Development of an oral solid dispersion formulation for use in low-dose metronomic chemotherapy of paclitaxel. Eur J Pharm Biopharm 2013; **83** (1): 87–94.

18. Milewski K, Afari ME, Tellez A, et al. Evaluation of efficacy and dose response of different paclitaxel-coated balloon formulations in a novel swine model of iliofemoral in-stent restenosis. JACC Cardiovasc Interv 2012; **5** (10): 1081–88.

19. Buszman PP, Tellez A, Afari ME, et al. Tissue uptake, distribution, and healing response after delivery of paclitaxel via second-generation iopromide-based balloon coating: a comparison with the first-generation technology in the iliofemoral porcine model. JACC Cardiovasc Interv 2013; **6** (8): 883–90.

20. Werk M, Langner S, Reinkensmeier B, et al. Inhibition of restenosis in femoropopliteal arteries: paclitaxel-coated vs. uncoated balloon: femoral paclitaxel randomized pilot trial. Circulation 2008; **118** (13): 1358–65.

21. Tepe G, Zeller T, Albrecht T, et al. Local delivery of paclitaxel to inhibit restenosis during angioplasty of the leg. N Engl J Med 2008; **358** (7): 689–99.

22. Rosenfield K, Jaff MR, White CJ, et al. Trial of a paclitaxel-coated balloon for femoropopliteal artery disease. N Engl J Med 2015; **373** (2): 145–53.

23. Tepe G, Schnorr B, Albrecht T, et al. Angioplasty of femoralpopliteal arteries with drug-coated balloons: five-year follow-up of the THUNDER trial. JACC Cardiovasc Interv 2015; **8** (1 Pt A): 102–08.

24. Karimi A, de Boer SW, van den Heuvel DA, et al. Randomized trial of Legflow paclitaxel eluting balloon and stenting vs. standard percutaneous transluminal angioplasty and stenting for the treatment of intermediate and long lesions of the superficial femoral artery (RAPID trial): study protocol for a randomized controlled trial. Trials 2013; 14: 87, 6215–14–87.

25. Chung C, Tadros R, Torres M, et al. Evolution of gender-related differences in outcomes from two decades of endovascular aneurysm repair. J Vasc Surg 2015; **61** (4): 843–52.

26. DeRubertis BG, Vouyouka A, Rhee SJ, et al. Percutaneous intervention for infrainguinal occlusive disease in women: equivalent outcomes despite increased severity of disease compared with men. J Vasc Surg 2008; **48** (1):150–57.

27. Ortmann J, Nuesch E, Traupe T, et al. Gender is an independent risk factor for distribution pattern and lesion morphology in chronic critical limb ischaemia. J Vasc Surg 2012; **55** (1): 98–104.

28. Han DK, Faries PL, Chung C, et al. Intermediate outcomes of femoropopliteal stenting in women: three-year results of the DURABILITY II Trial. Ann Vasc Surg 2016; **30**: 110–17.

29. Pulli R, Dorigo W, Pratesi G, et al. Gender-related outcomes in the endovascular treatment of infrainguinal arterial obstructive disease. J Vasc Surg 2012; **55** (1): 105–12.

30. Stavroulakis K, Donas KP, Torsello G, et al. Gender-related long-term outcome of primary femoropopliteal stent placement for peripheral artery disease. J Endovasc Ther 2015; **22** (1): 31–37.

31. Sandgren T, Sonesson B, Ahlgren R, Lanne T. The diameter of the common femoral artery in healthy human: influence of sex, age, and body size. J Vasc Surg 1999; **29** (3): 503–10.

32. Circulatory System Devices Advisory Panel. FDA Executive Summary P130024 Bard LUTONIX® 035 Drug Coated Balloon PTA Catheter. Department of Health and Human Services; Public Health Service; Food and Drug Administration; 2014.

33. Hertzer NR, Bena JF, Karafa MT. A personal experience with the influence of diabetes and other factors on the outcome of infrainguinal bypass grafts for occlusive disease. J Vasc Surg. 2007; **46** (2): 271–79.

34. Faglia E, Clerici G, Clerissi J, et al. Angioplasty for diabetic patients with failing bypass graft or residual critical ischaemia after bypass graft. Eur J Vasc Endovasc Surg 2008; **36** (3): 331–38.

35. Jude EB, Oyibo SO, Chalmers N, Boulton AJ. Peripheral arterial disease in diabetic and non-diabetic patients: a comparison of severity and outcome. Diabetes Care 2001; **24** (8): 1433–37.

36. Tan M, Pua U, Wong DE, et al. Critical limb ischaemia in a diabetic population from an Asian Centre: angiographic pattern of disease and three-year limb salvage rate with percutaneous angioplasty as first line of treatment. Biomed Imaging Interv J 2010; **6**(4): e33.

37. Faglia E, Mantero M, Caminiti M, *et al.* Extensive use of peripheral angioplasty, particularly infrapopliteal, in the treatment of ischaemic diabetic foot ulcers: clinical results of a multicentric study of 221 consecutive diabetic subjects. *J Intern Med* 2002; **252** (3): 225–32.

38. DeRubertis BG, Pierce M, Ryer EJ, *et al.* Reduced primary patency rate in diabetic patients after percutaneous intervention results from more frequent presentation with limb-threatening ischemia. *J Vasc Surg* 2008; **47** (1): 101–08.

39. Abularrage CJ, Conrad MF, Hackney LA, *et al.* Long-term outcomes of diabetic patients undergoing endovascular infrainguinal interventions. *J Vasc Surg* 2010; **52**(2): 314,22.e1–4.

An update on the ILLUMENATE Global study and ILLUMENATE clinical programme

T Zeller

Introduction

Despite an initial technical success rate of more than 95% for percutaneous transluminal angioplasty to recanalise the femoropopliteal artery using dedicated crossing and re-entry devices,[1,2] recanalisation procedures are limited by restenosis rates of 20% to 65% of the treated segments after six to 12 months.[3,4] Recently published pilot and pivotal studies investigating drug-coated balloons have shown a substantial improvement of durability of endovascular treatment.[5-13]

Appropriate drug coating of a balloon catheter surface still remains a challenge. On the one hand, due to its lipophilic nature, paclitaxel does not penetrate into the vessel wall sufficiently without a co-drug, a so called spacer or excipient. On the other hand, (1) both drugs have to be fixed effectively on top of the balloon surface in order to avoid significant drug loss prior to balloon expansion and (2) a sufficient—under optimal conditions, 100%—drug release into the vessel wall during balloon expansion has to be guaranteed. In both terms, current drug-coated balloon coatings are still imperfect. Whereas crystalline coatings result in a higher vessel wall persistence and as a result in a more effective suppression of neointima hyperproliferation, amorphous coatings are more stable on the surface of the balloon catheter with a significant lower loss of drug during balloon insertion into and through the sheath.

Researchers are investigating potential excipients in order to optimise drug transfer into the vessel wall as well as drug persistence in the vessel wall in order to optimise the biological efficacy of drug-coated balloons and to potentially reduce the dose of the antiproliferative drug. The ILLUMINATE clinical programme is one of the most recently established drug-coated balloon programmes with promising two-year patency and freedom from target lesion revascularisation outcomes of the first in-man trial published just recently.[14]

The ILLUMINATE Global study design

The ILLUMINATE Global study was designed to evaluate the safety and performance of the Stellarex drug-coated balloon (Spectranetics) in a broad patient population. It is a prospective, single-arm, multicentre study that enrolled 371 patients at 37 centres in Europe, Australia and New Zealand. All patients enrolled were treated with the Stellarex drug-coated balloon and will be followed for three years. The Stellarex drug-coated balloon is a 0.035inch guide wire compatible angioplasty catheter coated with paclitaxel ($2\mu g/mm^2$ balloon surface) and polyethylene glycol, an excipient that facilitates the transfer of the paclitaxel into the vessel wall.

Key inclusion criteria:
- Rutherford clinical category 2–4
- Target limb has at least one patent (<50% stenosis) run-off vessel to the foot
- Patient has one or two target lesions in the femoropopliteal artery with a cumulative length ≤20cm.

Key exclusion criteria:
- In-stent restenosis
- Severe calcification that precludes adequate percutaneous transluminal angioplasty treatment
- Lesions that would require adjunctive therapies such as atherectomy catheters or scoring balloons.

Study endpoints:
- The primary safety endpoint is freedom from device and procedure-related death through 30 days post-procedure and freedom from target limb major amputation and clinically-driven target lesion revascularisation through 12 months
- The primary effectiveness endpoint is primary patency at 12 months. Primary patency is defined as the absence of restenosis per duplex ultrasound peak systolic velocity ≤2.5 and freedom from clinically-driven target lesion revascularisation.

Interim 12-month data are being presented at the Charing Cross Symposium 2016, but were not ready for publication during the writing of this chapter.

The ILLUMINATE clinical programme

The ILLUMENATE Global study is one of five studies in the ILLUMENATE series. In total, 1,103 patients are enrolled across these studies, 929 of whom were treated with the Stellarex drug-coated balloon. All of these studies are being conducted with rigorous measures such as independent angiographic and duplex ultrasound core laboratories and clinical events committees to ensure unbiased review and adjudication of key endpoints such as patency and clinically-driven target lesion revascularisation. This large pool of robust data will facilitate a thorough evaluation of the safety and effectiveness of this second generation drug-coated balloon within the studied population. It will also enable the detection of rare adverse events.
The four additional studies include:
- The ILLUMENATE European randomised controlled trial enrolled 327 patients with symptoms of claudication or rest pain at 18 sites in the European Union. Patients were randomised to treatment with the Stellarex drug-coated balloon or a bare percutaneous transluminal angioplasty balloon catheter for *de novo* or restenotic lesions in the superficial femoral artery and/or popliteal arteries. Patients will be followed for five years.

- The ILLUMENATE pivotal randomised clinical trial is being conducted at 43 centres in the USA and the European Union. It is a prospective, randomised, multicentre, single-blinded study. It includes 300 claudicant or rest-pain patients with follow-up through five years.
- The ILLUMENATE pharmacokinetic study is a prospective, non-randomised, single-arm, multicentre, pharmacokinetic study that is currently ongoing in New Zealand. Twenty-five patients were enrolled and all were treated with the Stellarex drug-coated balloon and had periodic blood draws to measure the paclitaxel in their bloodstream.
- The recently completed ILLUMENATE first in-human study.

The ILLUMINATE first-in-human study

The ILLUMENATE first-in-human study was designed to assess the safety and effectiveness of the Stellarex drug-coated balloon to inhibit restenosis in the superficial femoral and/or popliteal artery. This was a prospective, single-arm, multicentre study with independent adjudication by angiographic and duplex ultrasound core laboratories. The study was comprised of two sequentially enrolled patient cohorts. In the first 50-patient cohort, lesions were treated with traditional pre-dilatation with an uncoated angioplasty balloon prior to inflation of the drug-coated balloon. In the second 30-patient cohort, lesions were treated by direct drug-coated balloon inflation, without pre-dilation.

In the first cohort (the pre-dilatation group, n=58 lesions), the mean lesion length was 7.2cm and baseline stenosis was 75.1%. Calcification was present in 62.1% of lesions and 12.1% were occluded. Kaplan-Meier estimate of primary patency, as determined by the duplex ultrasound core laboratory, was 89.5% at 12 months and 80.3% at 24 months while freedom from clinically-driven target lesion revascularisation was 90.0% at 12 months and 85.8% at 24 months. Additionally, there were no amputations or cardiovascular deaths reported through 24 months.

Twenty-eight patients, with 37 lesions, were included in the direct cohort analysis; two patients were excluded because they were pre-dilatated. The mean lesion length was 6.4cm and calcification was present in 48.6% of lesions. The primary patency rate was 86.2% at 12 months and 78.2% at 24 months, similar to the rates observed in the pre-dilatation cohort. The freedom from clinically-driven target lesion revascularisation rate, per Kaplan-Meier estimate, was 85.4% at 12 months and 81.7% at 24-months.

It is noteworthy that the rates of post-dilatation (35.1% vs. 12.1%) and stent placement (8.1% vs. 5.2%) were higher in the direct cohort as compared with the pre-dilatation cohort. These findings suggest a role for pre-dilatation in potentially improving outcomes and lowering the need for permanent implants thus, supporting the value proposition of drug-coated balloons.

Initial results are promising for this second generation drug-coated balloon technology and much more will be learned in 2016 as the steady cadence of robust clinical study results are generated.

Summary

- The ILLUMINATE study programme explores the clinical performance of the Stellarex drug-coated balloon, which is a 0.035inch guide wire compatible angioplasty catheter coated with paclitaxel ($2\mu g/mm^2$ balloon surface) and the excipient polyethylene glycol.

- The ILLUMENATE first-in-human study was a prospective, single-arm, multicentre study. It was comprised of two sequentially enrolled patient cohorts. In the first 50-patient cohort, lesions were treated with traditional pre-dilatation with an uncoated angioplasty balloon prior to inflation of the drug-coated balloon. In the second 30-patient cohort, lesions were treated by direct drug-coated balloon inflation, without pre-dilation.

- In the ILLUMENATE first-in-human study, Kaplan-Meier estimate of primary patency in the pre-dilatation cohort was 89.5% at 12 months and 80.3% at 24 months, respectively, while freedom from clinically-driven target lesion revascularisation was 90% at 12 months and 85.8% at 24 months, respectively.

- In the direct drug-coated balloon cohort outcomes were similar (primary patency rate 86.2% at 12 months and 78.2% at 24 months, and freedom from clinically-driven target lesion revascularisation rate 85.4% at 12 months and 81.7% at 24 months).

- The ILLUMENATE European randomised controlled trial enrolled 327 patients at 18 sites in the European Union, first data are expected to be presented by the end of 2016.

- The prospective, randomised, multicentre, single-blinded ILLUMENATE pivotal clinical trial is being conducted at 43 centres in the USA and the European Union; it includes 300 claudicant or rest-pain patients with follow-up through five years.

- The ILLUMENATE global study is a prospective, single-arm, multicentre study that enrolled 371 patients at 37 centres in Europe, Australia and New Zealand. All subjects enrolled will be followed for three years. First data will be presented at the Charing Cross Symposium 2016 in London.

References

1. Norgren L, Hiatt WR, Dormandy JA, *et al.* Inter-society consensus for the management of peripheral arterial disease. *Int Angiol* 2007; **26**: 81–157.
2. Beschorner U, Sixt S, Schwarzwälder U, *et al.* Recanalization of chronic occlusions of the superficial femoral artery using the Outback re-entry catheter: A single centre experience. *Cath Cardiovasc Intervent* 2009; **74**: 934–938.
3. Johnston KW. Femoral and popliteal arteries: reanalysis of results of balloon angioplasty. *Radiology* 1992; **183**: 767–771.
4. Schillinger M, Sabeti S, Loewe C, *et al.* Balloon angioplasty *versus* implantation of nitinol stents in the superficial femoral artery. *N Engl J Med* 2006; **354**: 1879–1888.
5. Tepe G, Zeller T, Albrecht T, *et al.* Local delivery of paclitaxel to inhibit restenosis during angioplasty of the leg. *N Engl J Med* 2008; **358**: 689–699.
6. Werk M, Langner S, Reinkensmeier B, *et al.* Inhibition of restenosis in femoropopliteal arteries: paclitaxel-coated *versus* uncoated balloon: femoral paclitaxel randomized pilot trial. *Circulation* 2008; **118**: 1358–1365.

7. Werk M, Albrecht T, Meyer DR, *et al.* Paclitaxel-coated balloons reduce restenosis after femoropopliteal angioplasty: evidence from the randomized PACIFIER trial. *Circ Cardiovasc Interv* 2012; **5**: 831–40.

8. Scheinert D, Duda S, Zeller T, *et al.* The LEVANT I (Lutonix paclitaxel-coated balloon for the prevention of femoropopliteal restenosis) trial for femoropopliteal revascularization: First in-human randomized trial of low-dose drug-coated balloon *versus* uncoated balloon angioplasty. *JACC Cardiovasc Interv* 2014; **7**: 10–9.

9. Scheinert D, Schulte KL, Zeller T, *et al.* Novel paclitaxel releasing balloon in femoropopliteal lesions: 12-month evidence from the BIOLUX P-I randomized trial. *JEVT* 2015; **22**: 14–21.

10. Micari A, Cioppa A, Vadalà G, *et al.* Clinical evaluation of a paclitaxel-eluting balloon for treatment of femoropopliteal arterial disease: 12-month results from a multicenter Italian registry. *JACC Cardiovasc Interv* 2012; 5: 331–338.

11. Tepe G, Laird J, Schneider P, *et al* for the IN.PACT SFA trial investigators. Drug-Coated balloon *versus* standard percutaneous transluminal angioplasty for the treatment of superficial femoral and/or popliteal peripheral artery disease: 12-month results from the IN.PACT SFA randomized trial. *Circulation* 2015; **131** (5): 495–502.

12. Laird JR, Schneider P, Tepe G, *et al.* Sustained durability of treatment effect using a drug-coated balloon for femoropopliteal lesions: twenty-four month results of the IN.PACT SFA randomized trial. *JACC* 2015; **66** (21): 2329–2338.

13. Rosenfield K, Jaff MR, White CJ, *et al.* Trial of paclitaxel-coated balloon for femoropopliteal artery disease. *N Eng J Med* 2015; **373**: 145–153.

14. Schroeder H, Meyer DR, Lux B, *et al.* Two-year results of a low-dose drug-coated balloon for revascularization of the femoropopliteal artery: outcomes from the ILLUMENATE First-in-Human study. *Catheter Cardiovasc Interv* 2015; **86** (2): 278–86.

Swirling flow is the aim for durable results

PA Gaines

Introduction

Endovascular techniques have revolutionised our approach to treating patients suffering from peripheral arterial disease. The treatment of iliac artery disease using either simple angioplasty for stenoses or stents for occlusions is now the standard of care for all but the most complex pattern of disease. The best approach to the management of infra-inguinal disease remains controversial because the relatively high morbidity and mortality following open surgery are considered by some to be balanced by the high rates of re-occlusion and re-intervention following endovascular intervention.

The importance of reocclusion and reintervention

There are good data that show patients suffer when the site of endovascular intervention fails, both from recurrence of symptoms and the risks of re-intervention.[1,2] In addition, health economic analysis has demonstrated that the main driver of endovascular costs is re-intervention.[3] Unfortunately, simple angioplasty, when used to treat all but the simplest pattern of disease in the superficial femoral artery, has unacceptably high restenosis rates. A review of the outcome from the angioplasty control arm of three femoropopliteal stenting studies reveals 12-month patency of only 28%.[4]

The initial attempts to improve patency using non-dedicated stents proved futile.[5,6] Engineering developments over the subsequent years have been hugely important. That the development of the early generation of dedicated straight nitinol stents were supported by high quality randomised controlled trials showing better outcomes than simple angioplasty, demonstrated conclusively that stent design matters.[7,8] And because stent design matters, engineers are capable of optimising the characteristics of new stent designs to affect outcome. The latest generation of stents has taken stent design into a new area by learning lessons from the characteristics of normal blood flow, in particular by acknowledging that normal healthy arterial flow is swirling flow. That ability to utilise nature's patterns and strategies, as defined by the Biomimicry Institute, is what defines the new generation of biomimetic stents.

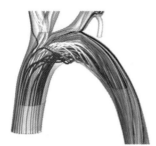

Figure 1: Swirling flow in the aorta (computational fluid dynamics model, courtesy of Imperial College London).

The potential value of swirling flow

We are all taught that normal human arterial blood flow is laminar. Whilst that is true, there is also a rotational element to the blood flow, induced by the non-planar curvature of the vessels, resulting in what is referred to as swirling flow (Figure 1).

The flow of blood, by virtue of its viscosity, results in a frictional force on the vessel wall that is known as wall shear stress. Swirling flow, when compared with simple laminar flow in a straight vessel, increases the velocity of blood against the artery wall and therefore increases the wall shear stress.

High wall shear has a number of desirable effects. Caro showed in 1969 that high wall shear is protective against the development of atheroma, and others have confirmed this observation.[9,10] The precise mechanisms for this effect are complex, have not yet been precisely defined, and are beyond the scope of this chapter.

Wall shear also has an effect on the development of restenosis after arterial intervention. The implantation of arterial stents, among other effects, changes the curvature leading to changes in the wall shear stress. In animal models, it has been convincingly demonstrated that increasing the wall shear stress significantly reduces the amount of in-stent restenosis.[11]

Within human coronary arteries, neointimal hyperplasia can be predicted to build at sites of low wall shear.[12]

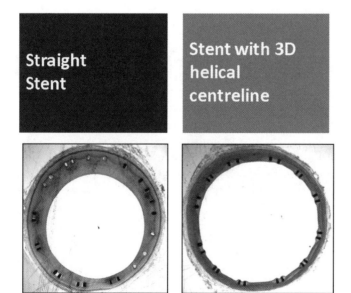

Figure 2: 30-day histology from pre-clinical study in which stents identical in all respects except for their centreline (either straight or 3D helical) were implanted, resulting in a 45% reduction in neointimal thickness at 30 days (p<0.001) in the stent with the 3D helical centreline.

A clear solution to the development of neointima following intervention is favourably to affect the haemodynamics through the stent. A helical stent has been demonstrated in an animal model to (i) be capable of deforming the centreline of the artery, (ii) elevate the wall shear stress, and (iii) reduce the degree of neointimal hyperplasia when compared to a straight stent (Figure 2).[13–15]

Can a helical stent that induces swirling flow improve outcomes in the human superficial femoral artery?

As previously mentioned, local haemodynamics, including the ability to generate swirling flow, are strongly affected by the arterial morphology. Wall shear stress of greater than 1.5Pa appears to be protective against atheroma and restenosis while low wall shear stress (<0.5Pa) is related to the development of atherosclerosis and restenosis (Figure 3A).[10,11]

The superficial femoral artery naturally experiences low wall shear stress.[16] All conventional straight stents will not only induce neointimal hyperplasia but will also straighten the artery. This reduction of normal curvature may reduce any naturally occurring swirling flow, and further lower the wall shear stress to pathological levels possibly leading to increased neo-intima deposition (Figure 3B).

The BioMimics 3D stent (Veryan Medical) has been specifically designed to impart a helical centreline to the native artery with the intention of developing an improved haemodynamic environment (Figure 4). Computational fluid dynamics have demonstrated that the helical arterial centreline imparts swirling flow that may elevate wall shear stress.

The potential clinical advantages of this biomimetic stent were tested in the Mimics Trial—a multicentre, core-lab controlled, prospective, randomised controlled trial in which the BioMimics 3D stent was compared to a conventional straight stent (primarily the LifeStent, Bard; 24/26 patients) in 76 patients with symptomatic occlusive disease of the superficial femoral artery. Conventional radiographs and angiography confirmed via core-lab analysis that the stent imparts curvature to the diseased artery. Unlike drug elution from stents and balloons, the imposition of curvature is not transient and could be anticipated to have

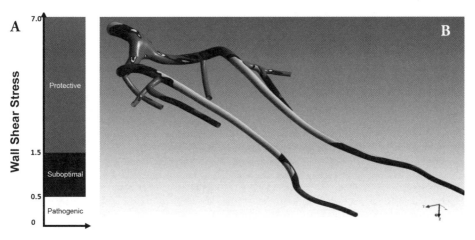

Figure 3: (A) Malek AM, *et al. JAMA* 1999; (B) Computational fluid dynamic idealised model illustrating areas of protective and pathogenic wall shear stress in the lower extremity arteries.

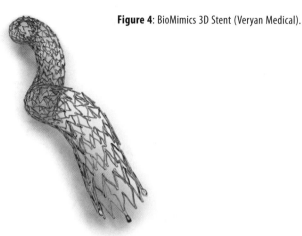

Figure 4: BioMimics 3D Stent (Veryan Medical).

benefit over restenosis and atherosclerosis in the long term. Compared with the control arm, the BioMimics 3D stent had significantly better freedom from loss of primary patency through two years (p=0.049) and significantly better freedom from clinically driven target lesion revascularisation between one and two years (p=0.0263).[17]

Summary

- The design of a stent affects its performance.

- Biomimetic stents harness nature's patterns to improve outcomes.

- Swirling flow has been demonstrated to increase wall shear, which in turn is protective against the development of atherosclerosis and in-stent restenosis.

- A helical stent can deform the arterial centreline and increase wall shear.

- The BioMimics 3D stent, a new generation biomimetic stent, has improved long-term outcomes when compared to conventional straight stents.

References

1. Dick F, Diehm N, Galimanis A, *et al*. Surgical or endovascular revascularization in patients with critical limb ischemia: Influence of diabetes mellitus on clinical outcome. *J Vasc Surg* 2007; **45**: 751–61.

2. Karch LA, Mattos MA, Henretta JP, *et al*. Clinical failure after percutaneous transluminal angioplasty of the superficial femoral and popliteal arteries. *J Vasc Surg* 2000; **31**: 880–87.

3. Kearns BC, Michaels JA, Stevenson MD, Thomas SM. Cost-effectiveness analysis of enhancements to angioplasty for infrainguinal arterial disease. *Br J Surg* 2013; **100**: 1180–88.

4. Rocha-Singh KJ, Jaff M, Crabtree TR, *et al*, Physicians OBOVIVA. Performance goals and endpoint assessments for clinical trials of femoropopliteal bare nitinol stents in patients with symptomatic peripheral arterial disease. *Catheter Cardiovasc Interv* 2007; **69**: 910–19.

5. Chalmers N, Walker PT, Belli AM, *et al*. Randomized trial of the SMART stent *versus* balloon angioplasty in long superficial femoral artery lesions: the SUPER study. *Cardiovasc Intervent Radiol* 2013; **36**: 353–61.

6. Krankenberg H, Schluter M, Steinkamp HJ *et al*. Nitinol stent implantation *versus* percutaneous transluminal angioplasty in superficial femoral artery lesions up to 10 cm in length: the femoral artery stenting trial (FAST). *Circulation* 2007; **116**: 285–92.

7. Laird JR, Katzen BT, Scheinert D, *et al*. Nitinol stent implantation *versus* balloon angioplasty for lesions in the superficial femoral artery and proximal popliteal artery: twelve-month results from the RESILIENT randomized trial. *Circ Cardiovasc Interv* 2010; **3**: 267–76.

8. Schillinger M, Sabeti S, Loewe C, *et al*. Balloon Angioplasty *versus* Implantation of nitinol stents in the superficial femoral artery. *N Engl J Med* 2006; **354**: 1879–88.

9. Caro CG, Fitz-Gerald JM, Schroter RC. Arterial wall shear and distribution of early atheroma in man. *Nature* 1969; **223**: 1159–60.

10. Malek AM, Alper SL, Izumo S. Hemodynamic shear stress and its role in atherosclerosis. *JAMA* 1999; **282:** 2035–42.

11. Carlier SG, van Damme LC, Blommerde CP, *et al*. Augmentation of wall shear stress inhibits neointimal hyperplasia after stent implantation: inhibition through reduction of inflammation? *Circulation* 2003; **107**: 2741–46.

12. Thury A, Wentzel JJ, Vinke RV, *et al*. Images in cardiovascular medicine. Focal in-stent restenosis near step-up: roles of low and oscillating shear stress? *Circulation* 2002; **105** :e185–77.

13. Coppola G, Caro C. Arterial geometry, flow pattern, wall shear and mass transport: potential physiological significance. *J R Soc Interface* 2009; **6**: 519–28.

14. Shinke T, Robinson K, Burke MG, *et al*. Novel helical stent design elicits swirling blood flow pattern and inhibits neointima formation in porcine carotid arteries. *Circulation* 2008; **118**: S1054.

15. Caro CG, Seneviratne A, Heraty KB, *et al*. Intimal hyperplasia following implantation of helical-centreline and straight-centreline stents in common carotid arteries in healthy pigs: influence of intraluminal flow. *J R Soc Interface* 2013; **10**: 20130578.

16. Wood NB, Zhao SZ, Zambanini A, *et al*. Curvature and tortuosity of the superficial femoral artery: a possible risk factor for peripheral arterial disease. *J Appl Physiol (1985)* 2006; **101**: 1412–18.

17. Zeller T. BioMimics 3D - advanced stent design: concept to randomised controlled trial. LINC Congress 2014.

Latest generation of conforming dual component stent

F Thaveau, V Méteyer, A Lejay and N Chakfé

Introduction

Over the last decade, the use of bare metal stents for the endovascular management of peripheral arterial occlusive disease has become widely adopted for the treatment of TASC A and B lesions, whereas TASC C and D lesions remain in the realm of open surgery, despite the great progress in endovascular techniques.[1] The first-generation nitinol stents had interconnected stent struts resulting in a stiffer endoprosthesis with limited radial strength. Second-generation nitinol stents took a helical approach for strut interconnections, which resulted in a significant step forward in terms of flexibility, radial strength and number of stent fractures.

The majority of these stents became well accepted for the treatment of the superficial femoral artery and the proximal popliteal artery. However, stenting of the popliteal artery remained a controversial topic, resulting in a lack of broad acceptance for the technique. This can be mainly attributed to the fear of stent fractures and possible subsequent restenosis in this vascular location, with its high biomechanical stress next to the knee joint.[2-5]

Despite a good rate of primary technical success with stents, mechanical bending due to knee joint flexion can limit long term patency in the femoropopliteal segment. These biomechanical forces have to be considered in assessing the influence of new stent design.[6] First- and second-generation nitinol stents have typically been manufactured from nitinol slotted tubes. Recently, so-called third-generation nitinol stents have been introduced and these focus more on conformability of the nitinol stent to the native vessel, with the intention of producing a better response to the biomechanical forces (extension, compression, flexion and torsion) applied to the distal superficial femoral and popliteal artery (P2–P3) during movement of the knee.[7-9] Consequently, the third generation of nitinol stents were designed with better flexibility and conformability.[10] In 2012, Gore introduced a novel dual component stent that uses a combination of both nitinol and polytetrafluoroethylene (ePTFE) interconnections.

Description of topic

Technical device features

The Tigris (Gore) stent consists of a continuous nitinol wire with interconnections using an e-PTFE lattice, which is also coated with heparin surface (Carmeda BioActive surface) (Figure 1).

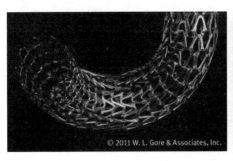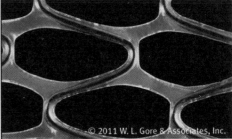

Figure 1: Photographs of Tigris vascular stent. On the right, a magnified view of dual component continuous nitinol stent with interconnections of ePTFE, coated with heparin surface.

The combination of the two materials and the absence of interconnecting stent struts results in a high flexibility and a stent platform that conforms well to the anatomy and does not straighten the vessel compared with previous generation stents. Additionally, the ePTFE connections make it almost impossible to have stent elongation but still allow for axial compression (Figure 2).

There are, however, some points that could be improved upon moving forward. One of the main points would be the range of stent lengths available, currently available up to 100mm. For treatment of longer lesions, a longer stent length would be preferred to avoid having to overlap devices as this could impair outcomes. Another limitation of the current version of the stent is the absence of radiopaque markers on the endoprosthesis resulting in limited visibility. This is again amplified by the fact that in comparison to other nitinol stents, there is less metal present that contributes to the lower visibility. This can be addressed by using a higher magnification, but is definitely a limitation compared with competitive devices.

On the other hand, since there are no nitinol interconnections, data in fact indicate that the stent does not behave the same as a faraday cage on magnetic resonance angiography and allows artefact-free in-stent lumen visualisation, enabling intra-stent contrast flow measurement and evaluation of stent restenosis.[11]

Evidence for views

Evidence to date

Currently, a limited number of publications are available. Piorkowski *et al* were the first to share their real-world experiences. They evaluated 32 consecutive patients for the treatment of femoropopliteal occlusive lesions. Besides the typical comorbidities, lesions treated had an average lesion length of 4.3cm and 5% total occlusions. It is, however, important to highlight that 25% of the patients were treated for symptoms of critical limb ischaemia. The one-year primary patency, according to Kaplan-Meyer, was 85.5% for these short lesions.[12]

Following this, was Parthipun *et al's* evaluation[11] that focused on longer popliteal artery lesions. A total of 50 lesions were treated with an average stented length of 11.4cm with 70% of patients treated for critical limb ischaemia and 74% of lesions treated were chronic total occlusions. After 12 months, the primary patency was 69.5% and with a 86.1% freedom from target lesion revascularisation. These data are promising considering the complexity of lesions treated.

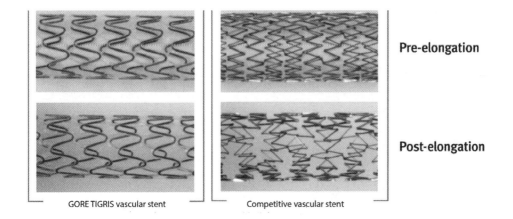

Figure 2: Gore Tigris vascular stent and a competitive stent under mechanical stress forces showing that the Tigris stent behaviour is resistant to traction forces with absence of dual component structure deformation.

Parthipun *et al* further describe a review of studies exclusively addressing stenting treatment options of the popliteal artery to make a comparison between recently published data for stenting in the popliteal artery.

Scheinert et al[13] in their retrospective single-centre study using the Supera stent (Abbott Vascular) evaluated 101 cases. Of the patients treated, 22.8% were critical limb ischaemia patients with a mean stented length of 5.8cm and chronic total occlusions in 47.5% of cases. One-year primary patency was 87.7% and freedom from target lesion revascularisation was 90%, which are similar reintervention rates for less complex pathology treated compared with that seen in Parthipun *et al's* evaluation.

In a single, multicentre, controlled trial, Rastan *et al* randomised 246 patients between primary nitinol stenting or plain balloon angioplasty of the popliteal artery. Patients allocated to primary nitinol popliteal stenting had an average lesion length of 4.1cm and 32.8% of chronic total occlusions at baseline. Primary patency at one year was 67.4% and freedom from target lesion revascularisation was 85.1%.[14]

The results from the nitinol stent arm of this randomised controlled trial correlate very well with the outcomes reported by Parthipun *et al* in their popliteal Tigris experience. Keeping in mind that the study by Rastan had a much smaller critical limb ischaemia patient population (20.7%) and popliteal chronic total occlusion (32.8%) compared with those described by Parthipun *et al* (70% and 74%, respectively).

Our experience with the Tigris stent is close to that of Parthipun *et al*.[11] In terms of severity of patient clinical outcomes and lesions, since 2013, we have treated 98 patients; 61.2% of whom had peripheral arterial disease at the stage of critical limb ischaemia. The Tigris stent was used to treat 60.2% of chronic total occlusions and 39.8% of stenoses for infrainguinal lesions. The stented area was only the superficial femoral artery in 53.1% of cases and included the popliteal segment in 46.9% of patients, with an average lesion length of 9.2cm. The stented area was only the superficial femoral artery in 53.1% of cases, and included the popliteal artery in 46.9% of cases. The morbidity and mortality rates within 30 days were 1% and 3.1% respectively. The average follow-up duration was 19.4±21 months.

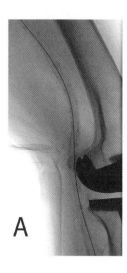
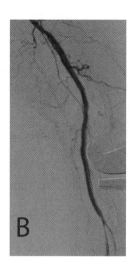

Figure 3: (A) Example of preoperative control radiography of two Tigris stents of 6x100mm and 5x100mm respectively, implanted after a right popliteal artery recanalisation by a 83 year-old woman with right critical limb ischaemia. (B) Perioperative angiogram shows the successful deployment of both stents with a good runoff.

The survival rate was 77.4% and 66.2% at one and two years, respectively. Primary patency was 90.5%, 72.4% and 55.6% at six months, one year and two years, respectively. The secondary patency was 100%, 92% and 92% at six months, one year and two years, respectively. An increase in the walking distance was observed in 84.2% of claudication patients, and wound healing or the disappearance of rest pain was observed in 73.8% of patients with critical ischaemia. Despite the challenges posed by the severity of lesions and advanced clinical stage, these results are promising, although long-term follow-up is expected.

Concerning popliteal stenting with second-generation nitinol stents, the results published to date are still scarce. The fracture rates remain important and are often correlated with loss of patency.[15]

The increased flexibility and conformability of third-generation stents are expected to respond better to the external biomechanical forces applied to the popliteal artery, encouraging vascular teams to use this type of stent to treat risky arterial segment with the aim of decreasing the rate of restenosis and thrombosis over time.

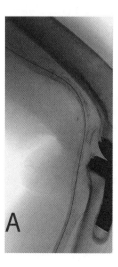
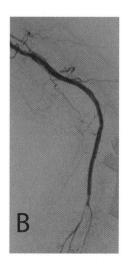

Figure 4: (A) The same operative case as Figure 3 with a radiography and (B) a perioperative angiogram during dynamic knee flexion (lateral projection), showing a good conformability of two overlapping stents.

Technical experience

Experience of Tigris deployment after more than 200 implantations shows that poor stent visibility is not a limitation of current use if a correct analysis of the distal landing zone and correct length choice are made preoperatively using standard imaging techniques. Indeed, the combination of two radiopaque markers located on the delivery catheter at each end of compressed stent provides a good visualisation of the devices crossing the target lesion.

Original secure deployment is ensured by slight expansion of a compressed endoprosthesis after unlocking the device, from the tip of the delivery catheter toward the hub. If a minimal distal advance of the stent is observed during unlocking, the device should be placed at its final position under fluoroscopy guidance at the end of this process. In our experience, neither jump nor elongation of the endoprosthesis were observed and deployment was successful in all cases.

For popliteal segment treatment, a lateral projection of the control angiogram allows us to check the conformability of the devices during bending stresses (Figures 3 and 4).

As mentioned in the instructions for use,[16] chosen devices should respect an overlapping zone of at least 1cm and should not differ by more than 1mm in diameter. Considering that the popliteal segment up to the patella (P1–P2) is the most subject to the external forces, we suggest placing the overlap at a different location (P2–P3). The diameter of the stent should be approximately 5–20% larger than the healthy vessel diameter immediately proximal and distal to the lesion, although our current practice is to avoid oversizing the diameter of the device, especially in cases of recanalisation of chronic total occlusion. The decision on the right diameter of endoprosthesis is done preoperatively via computed tomography (CT) in our practice.

The Tigris stent is contraindicated in patients with known hypersensitivity to heparin, including those patients who have had a previous incidence of heparin-induced thrombocytopenia type II. However, we did not observe adverse events related to this in our cohort of patients. All of them were treated immediately after the procedure with dual antiplatelet therapy for one month.

Summary

- The hybrid design of stents introduces a new generation of self-expandable stents with a novel concept for post-angioplasty scaffolding of artery exposed to biomechanical external forces.

- The new dual component heparin-bonded Tigris stent with a combination of both nitinol and ePTFE interconnections is one of the third-generation of self-expandable stents, producing promising results for threatening severe lesions of femoropopliteal and popliteal arteries.

- The expected behaviour is better conformability and a decreased rate of restenosis and fractures.

- Improving clinical outcomes are expected especially for the critical limb ischaemia where arterial lesions are severe at the femoropopliteal and popliteal level.

- Progress in stent design with this latest generation of conforming dual component stents should extend endovascular indication to TASC C and D infrainguinal lesions.

References

1. Norgren L, Hiatt WR, Dormandy JA, *et al.* Inter-society consensus for the management of peripheral arterial disease (TASC II). *J Vasc Surg* 2007; **45**: (Suppl S): S5–67.
2. Babalik E, Gülbaran M, Gürmen T, *et al.* Fracture of popliteal artery stents. *Circ J* 2003; **67**: 643–45.
3. Nikanorov A, Smouse HB, Osman K, *et al.* Fracture of self-expanding nitinol stents stressed in vitro under simulated intravascular conditions. *J Vasc Surg* 2008; **48**: 435–40.
4. Kröger K, Santosa F, Goyen M. Biomechanical incompatibility of popliteal stent placement. *J Endovasc Ther* 2004; **11**: 686–94.
5. Scheinert D, Scheinert S, Sax J, *et al.* Prevalence and clinical impact of stent fractures after femoropopliteal stenting. *J Am Coll Cardiol* 2005; **45**: 312–15.
6. Kröger K, Santosa F, Goyen M. Biomechanical incompability of popliteal stent placement. *J Endovasc Ther* 2004; **11** (6): 686–94.
7. Hoffmann U, Vetter J, Rainoni L, *et al.* Popliteal artery compression and force of active plantar flexion in young healthy volunteers. *J Vasc Surg* 1997; **26** (2): 281–87.
8. Kroger K, Santosa F, Goyen M. Biomechanical incompability of popliteal stent placement. *J Endovasc Ther* 2004; **11** (6): 686–94.
9. Piorkowski M, *et al.* The use of the Gore Tigris vascular stent with dual component design in the superficial femoral and popliteal arteries at 6 months. *J Cardiovasc Surg* (Torino) 2013; **54** (4): 447–53.
10. Diamantopoulos A, Katsanos K. Treating femoropopliteal disease: established and emerging technologies. *Semin Intervent Radiol* 2014; **31** (4): 345–52.
11. Parthipun A, *et al.* Use of a New Hybrid Heparin-Bonded Nitinol Ring Stent in the Popliteal Artery: Procedural and Mid-term Clinical and Anatomical Outcomes. *Cardiovasc Intervent Radiol* 2015; **38** (4): 846–54.
12. Piorkowski M, Freitas B, Steiner S, *et al.* Twelve-month experience with the GORE® TIGRIS® Vascular Stent in the superficial femoral and popliteal arteries. *J Cardiovasc Surg* (Torino) 2014; **56**: 89.
13. Scheinert D, Grummt L, Piorkowski M, *et al.* A novel self-expanding interwoven nitinol stent for complex femoropopliteal lesions: 24-month results of the SUPERA SFA registry. *J Endovasc Ther* 2011; **18** (6): 745–52.
14. Rastan A, Krankenberg H, Baumgartner I, *et al.* Stent placement *versus* balloon angioplasty for the treatment of obstructive lesions of the popliteal artery: a prospective, multicenter, randomized trial. *Circulation* 2013; **127** (25): 2535–41.
15. Chang IS, Chee HK, Park SW, *et al.* The primary patency and fracture rates of self-expandable nitinol stents placed in the popliteal arteries, especially in the P2 and P3 segments, in Korean patients. *Korean Journal Radiol* 2011; **12** (2): 203–09.
16. Mechanical properties of the Gore Tigris vascular stent. Available at: http://www.goremedical.com/resources/dam/assets/AR0092-EU2.pdf. Accessed April 2015.

Atherectomy and drug-coated balloon angioplasty for long and calcified femoropopliteal lesions: The DEFINITIVE AR trial

T Zeller, A Rastan, R Macharzina, U Beschorner and E Noory

Introduction

Despite an initial technical success rate of more than 95% for percutaneous transluminal angioplasty to recanalise the superficial femoral artery using dedicated interventional devices[1,2] and improved durability with drug-coated technologies including drug-eluting stents[3] and drug-coated balloons,[4] recanalisation procedures of long and calcified femoropopliteal lesions are still limited by significant acute and chronic failure rates.[5,8] However, both modalities have their specific limitations, drug-coated balloons in particular have the same limitations as plain old balloon angioplasty, specifically acute recoil, including undilatable calcified lesions and severe dissections requiring provisional bare metal stenting.[9] Preparation of the vessel bed might improve the acute treatment outcome of drug-coated balloon angioplasty and might in addition improve the biological effect of the antiproliferative drug. On the other hand, reduced patency has been seen with increasing lesion length for almost all treatment modalities. These considerations represent the background of the DEFINITVE AR (Atherectomy and drug-coated balloon angioplasty for long and calcified femoropopliteal lesions) trial. Recently published and presented studies investigating either directional atherectomy alone in calcified lesions[10] or directional atherectomy in combination with drug-coated balloon have shown substantial improvements in acute outcomes and durability of endovascular treatment.[11,12]

The main goal of the treatment of patients with claudication is a sustained relief from their lifestyle-limiting claudication without the frequent need of reintervention, and not to prevent amputation. Thus, the treatment applied must be safe, durable and cheap, in other words cost effective.

The impact of calcification on treatment outcome following drug-coated balloon angioplasty of femoropopliteal arteries

After drug-coated balloon angioplasty only 15% to 20% of paclitaxel transfers from the balloon surface into the vessel wall.[13] Intimal intraluminal calcification

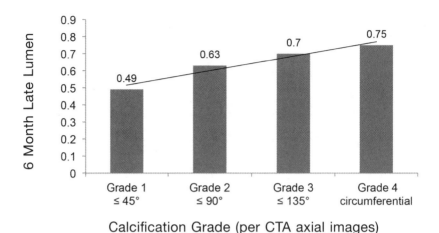

P = 0.03 (0.49) vs. 073)

Figure 1: Increase in late lumen loss at six months after drug-coated balloon angioplasty of femoropopliteal lesions with increasing degree of calcification.[7]

can increase the loss of antiproliferative drug when advancing the coated balloon into the lesion, in particular if the lesion is insufficiently predilated and can impair uptake.[14] The role of medial calcification type Mönckeberg (a common manifestation in patients with diabetes and end-stage renal insufficiency)[15] on the biological efficacy of drug-coated balloons is still unknown.[5,6] Fanelli *et al*[7] reported a significant drop in primary patency and increase in late lumen loss following drug-coated balloon angioplasty of femoropopliteal lesions with concentric calcification (Figure 1).

Atherectomy mechanically recanalises the vessel without overstretch, removes the perfusion barrier for a subsequent antirestenotic therapy with a drug-coated balloon, and reduces the likelihood of bailout stenting even in calcified lesions and as a result preserves the native vessel. The DEFINITIVE Ca++ single-arm trial demonstrated that calcified disease can be treated effectively with directional atherectomy using an embolic protection device.[10] Directional atherectomy-related

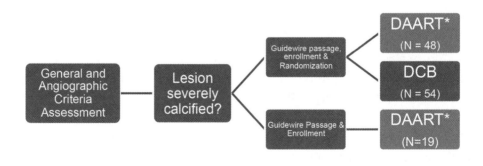

Figure 2: Study inclusion flow chart (DAART = directional atherectomy and antirestenotic therapy, DCB = drug-coated balloon angioplasty)

lumen gain was 2.2mm, the bailout stent rate was as low as 4.1%, and flow-limiting dissections were found in 1.5% of patients.

However, even after atherectomy, loss of patency ranges from 20% to 40% due to neointima hyperproliferation, in particular if the external elastic lamina is damaged during the atherectomy procedure. Thus, supplementing atherectomy with drug-coated balloon angioplasty is an attractive approach to preserve the acute lumen gain achieved with atherectomy.

In a retrospective analysis, we examined the impact of drug-coated balloon angioplasty following directional atherectomy in restenotic femoropopliteal lesions.[11] In this retrospective study, restenotic lesions of the femoropopliteal arteries were treated with directed atherectomy in 89 lesions of consecutive patients. All patients received adjunctive treatment with conventional balloon percutaneous angioplasty (n=60) or drug-coated balloon angioplasty (n=29). Lesion location was either in the stent or in native restenotic vessels. The one-year Kaplan-Meier freedom from restenosis estimates in the drug-coated balloon and percutaneous transluminal atherectomy groups were 84.7% and 43.8%, respectively. In a multivariable Cox model for restenosis, drug-coated balloon treatment had a hazard ratio of 0.28 (p=0.0036) compared with the percutaneous transluminal atherectomy group. Thus, the combination of directed atherectomy with adjunctive drug-coated balloon angioplasty is associated with a better event-free survival at 12 months of follow-up compared with percutaneous transluminal atherectomy after directed atherectomy in the treatment of femoropopliteal restenosis (native vessel and in-stent restenosis).

In a prospective, single-centre study including 30 patients suffering from peripheral vascular disease Rutherford categories 3–6, heavily calcified femoropopliteal lesions, defined as fluoroscopic calcification on both sides of a vessel wall longer than 1cm in length, were treated with directional atherectomy.[12] All procedures included distal protection with the SpiderFX filter (Coividen) and IVUS-guided atherectomy with the TurboHawk peripheral plaque excision system (Coividen). Once a <30% residual stenosis was achieved, confirmed by IVUS and angiography, a drug-coated balloon was used for post-dilation. A <30% residual stenosis was achieved in all cases without procedure-related adverse events; the bail out stenting rate was 6.5%. After one year, the duplex-derived primary patency rate

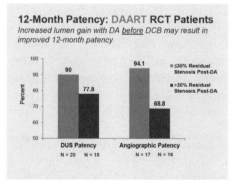

Figure 3: Impact of post-procedural residual stenosis on 12-month duplex ultrasound and angiographic patency showing trends towards better outcome for a residual stenosis of <30%.

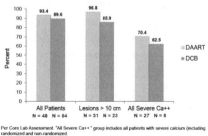

Figure 4: Duplex ultrasound 12-month patency of the entire study cohort and stratified to lesions >10cm in length and severely calcified lesions (DAART = directional atherectomy and antirestenotic treatment, DCB = drug-coated balloon).

was 90% (27/30) and freedom from major adverse events 87% (26/30). The authors concluded that directional atherectomy and drug-coated balloon angioplasty may represent a potential alternative strategy for the treatment of severely calcified femoropopliteal lesions. These very promising data and the considered hypothesis have to be confirmed in a multicentre randomised trial.

The DEFINITIVE AR trial

The purpose of the investigator-initiated DEFINITVE AR (Directional atherectomy followed by a paclitaxel-coated balloon to inhibit restenosis and maintain vessel patency: a pilot study of anti-restenosis treatment) trial is to assess and estimate the effect of treating a vessel with directional atherectomy followed by drug-coated balloon angioplasty, compared to treatment with drug-coated balloon alone. The randomised study arm was supplemented by a registry arm treating severely calcified lesions with the combination therapy using the Turbohawk atherectomy catheter in conjunction with a distal protection filter. Overall, 121 patients were enrolled at 10 centres in Europe—102 patients in the randomised study arm and 19 patients into the calcium registry (Figure 2). The study is independently controlled by a clinical events committee, a data safety monitoring board and a steering committee. Angiographic and duplex core laboratory analyses will be performed. The study was funded by Covidien. The key study inclusion and exclusion criteria are summarised below.

Key study inclusion criteria:
- Rutherford category 2–4
- Target lesion 7–15cm in length
- Reference vessel diameter 4–7mm
- Baseline stenosis ≥70%.

Key study exclusion criteria:
- In-stent restenosis
- Aneurysmal target vessel
- Two or more lesions that require treatment in the target limb.

The primary study endpoint is per cent diameter determined by quantitative angiography at one year. Follow-up assessments are planned predischarge, after 30 days, six months, and one year. Table 2 summarises the baseline patient demographics of the randomised study cohort. No statistical significant differences were observed between the study cohorts. Table 3 summarises the core lab adjudicated baseline lesion characteristics, mean lesion length was approximately 10cm in both study arms.

Acute and 30-day results: The technical success defined as ≤30% residual stenosis following the protocol-defined treatment at the target lesion as determined by the angiographic core laboratory was achieved in 89.6% of patients in the combination therapy cohort as compared to 64.2% in the drug-coated balloon angioplasty cohort (p=0.004). Post-protocol defined treatment adjunctive therapies are summarised in Table 4; no patient in the combination therapy cohort received a stent.

	DAART (N=48)	DCB (N = 54)	P Value*
Age	70.1 ± 9.7	69.0 ± 8.2	0.4383
Male	64.6%	68.5%	0.6807
History and Risk Factors			
Angina	4.2%	9.3%	0.4425
Diabetes	27.1%	35.2%	0.4014
Hypertension	87.5%	81.5%	0.4300
Hyperlidemia	70.8%	68.5%	0.8323
Renal Insufficiency	12.5%	14.8%	0.7807
Current/Previous Smoker	50.0%	63.0%	0.3076
Rutherford Clinical Category			
2	27.1%	24.0%	
3	70.8%	74.1%	
4	2.1%	1.9%	

Table 2: Baseline patient demographics randomised patient cohort (DAART = directional atherectomy and anti-restenotic therapy; DCB = drug-coated balloon angioplasty)

	DAART (N=48)	DCB (N = 54)	P Value*
Lesion Length (cm)	10.6	9.7	0.3034
Diameter Stenosis	82%	85%	0.3468
Reference vessel diameter (mm)	4.9	4.9	0.4794
Minimum lumen diameter (mm)	1.0	0.8	0.3372
Calcification	70.8%	74.1%	0.4758

Table 3: Baseline lesion characteristics randomised study cohort (DAART = directional atherectomy & anti-restenotic therapy; DCB = drug-coated balloon angioplasty)

	DAART (N=48)	DCB (N = 54)	P Value*
Adjunctive Therapy			
PTA (post-dil)	6.3% (3/48)	33.3% (18/54)	0.0011
Bail-out Stent	0	3.7% (2/54)	0.4968

Table 4: Adjunctive therapies following index procedure (DAART = directional atherectomy and anti-restenotic therapy; DCB = drug-coated balloon angioplasty)

The residual diameter stenosis post-protocol defined therapy and post-adjunctive therapy was significantly lower in the combination treatment cohort (18% vs. 28%, p=0.0002).

As a result of debulking the lesion prior to drug-coated balloon angioplasty, the combination therapy cohort achieved a significantly higher acute lumen gain compared to the plain drug-coated balloon cohort (minimal lumen diameter 4.27mm vs. 3.78mm, p=0.045).

Periprocedural complications as verified by the clinical events committee occurred in 12% of the combination therapy cohort and in 19% of the drug-coated balloon angioplasty cohort (Table 5).

	DAART (N=48)	DCB (N = 54)	P Value*
Distal Embolization	6% (3/48)	0/54	0.101
No Intervention	1	0	
Surgical Intervention	0	0	
Endovascular Intervention	2	0	
Dissection (flow-limiting, Grade C/D)	2% (1/48)	19% (10/54)	0.009
No Intervention	1	6	
Surgical Intervention	0	0	
Endovascular Intervention	0	4	
Perforation	4% (2/48)	0/54	0.219
No Intervention	0	0	
Surgical Intervention	0	0	
Endovascular Intervention	2	0	

Table 5: Periprocedural complications (DAART = directional atherectomy and anti-restenotic therapy; DCB = drug-coated balloon angioplasty)

One-year results: due to the limited sample size at one year, none of the predefined endpoints reached statistical significance. Most interesting findings were trends favouring the dual treatment strategy with regard to better patency outcomes if post-procedural residual stenosis was less than 30% (Figure 3), when lesions were calcified, and in lesions longer than 10cm (Figure 4).

In summary, acute results of combining directional atherectomy with drug-coated balloon angioplasty treatment show a significantly higher acute technical success rate and acceptable periprocedural complications. One-year outcomes do not show a significant difference for any technical endpoint. However, trends are seen for higher patency rates, in particular in the subgroups of lesions longer than 10cm and with severe calcification, for the combination of directional atherectomy and drug-coated balloon angioplasty. Long-term data, from a sufficiently powered randomised study with focus on the differential indications (identified in the DEFINITIVE AR study) that are most likely to be associated with a benefit from the combination therapy, are mandatory, including a cost-effectiveness analysis.

Summary

- Drug-coated balloons have improved patency rates of femoropopliteal lesions compared to plain balloon angioplasty.

- However, drug-coated balloons have the same technical limitations as plain balloon angioplasty, specifically undilatable lesions due to concentric calcification, early elastic recoil and dissection.

- Atherectomy removes the plaque reducing balloon dilatation specific limitations. However, atherectomy results in a large, potentially thrombotic surface and may destroy the internal elastic lamina potentially resulting in overwhelming neointima proliferation and delayed restenosis development due to the initial lumen gain following plaque removal.

- Atherectomy prior to drug-coated balloon angioplasty may improve drug penetration into the vessel wall layers and as such improve the biological efficacy of paclitaxel. Furthermore, it improves the acute luminal gain and reduces acute recoil.

- The DEFINITIVE AR trial is the first randomised controlled pilot trial investigating the effect of upfront directional atherectomy prior to drug-coated balloon angioplasty compared to drug-coated balloon angioplasty alone.

- Early 30-day results confirmed the assumption of a higher initial lumen gain of the dual interventional approach without significant acute risks.

- One-year outcome data, however, did not show any significant technical benefit for the combined therapy due to an insufficient sample size of the study. Trends for superior primary one-year patency rates have been found for the most challenging lesions included in the study, the longer lesion cohort and the severely calcified vessels.

- A sufficiently powered global study is needed to confirm those trends in particularly in relation to cost-effectiveness reasons.

- Two-year clinical data are expected to be available first quarter 2016.

References

1. Norgren L, Hiatt WR, Dormandy JA, et al. Inter-society consensus for the management of peripheral arterial disease. *Int Angiol* 2007; **26**: 81–157.
2. Beschorner U, Sixt S, Schwarzwälder U, et al. Recanalization of Chronic Occlusions of the Superficial Femoral Artery Using the Outback™ Re-Entry Catheter: A Single Centre Experience. *Cath Cardiovasc Intervent* 2009; **74**: 934–38.
3. Dake M, Ansel GM, Jaff MR, et al. Sustained safety and effectiveness of paclitaxel-eluting stents for femoropopliteal lesions: two-year follow-up from the Zilver PTX randomized and single-arm clinical studies. *J Am Coll Cardiol.* 2013; **61** (24): 2417–27.
4. Laird JR, Schneider P, Tepe G, et al. Sustained Durability of Treatment Effect Using a Drug-Coated Balloon for Femoropopliteal Lesions: Twenty-Four Month Results of the IN.PACT SFA Randomized Trial. *JACC* 2015; **66** (21): 2329–38.
5. Rocha-Singh KJ, Zeller T, Jaff MR. Peripheral Arterial Calcification: Prevalence, Detection and Clinical Implications. *Cath Cardiovasc Intervent* 2013, in revision.
6. Lanzer P, Böhm M, Sorribas V, et al. Mönckeberg's media sclerosis; a non-inflammatory vascular calcification disorder. *EHJ* 2013, in revision.

7. Fanelli F, Cannavale A, Gazzetti M, *et al*. Calcium burden assessment and impact on drug-eluting balloons in peripheral arterial disease. *Cardiovasc Intervent Radiol* 2014; **37** (4): 898–907.

8. Tepe G, Beschorner U, Ruether C, *et al*. Predictors of outcomes of drug-eluting balloon therapy for femoropopliteal arterial disease with a special emphasis on calcium. *J Endovasc Ther* 2015; **22** (5): 727–33.

9. Werk M, Albrecht T, Meyer DR, *et al*. Paclitaxel-coated balloons reduce restenosis after femoro-popliteal angioplasty: evidence from the randomized PACIFIER trial. *Circ Cardiovasc Interv* 2012; **5** (6): 831–40.

10. Clair DG, Roberts DK. Treatment of Severely Calcified Femoropopliteal Lesions with Plaque Excision and Embolic Protection- DEFINITIVE Ca++. *J Vasc Interv Radiol* 2011; **22**: 1785.e2.

11. Sixt S, Carpio-Cancino G, Treszl A *et al*. Drug Coated Balloon Angioplasty after Directional Atherectomy Improves Outcome in Restenotic Femoropopliteal Arteries. *J Vasc Surg* 2013; **58**: 682–86.

12. Cioppa A, Stabile E, Popusoi G, *et al*. Combined treatment of heavy calcified femoro-popliteal lesions using directional atherectomy and a paclitaxel coated balloon: One-year single centre clinical results. *Cardiovasc Revasc Med* 2012; **13**: 219–23

13. Schnorr B, Kelsch B, Cremers B, *et al*. Paclitaxel-coated balloons - Survey of preclinical data. *Minerva Cardioangiol* 2010; **58** (5): 567–82.

14. Schnorr B, Albrecht T. Drug-coated balloons and their place in treating peripheral arterial disease. *Expert Rev Med Devices* 2013; **10** (1): 105–14.

15. Jude EB, Eleftheriadou I, Tentolouris N. Peripheral arterial disease in diabetes–a review. *Diabet Med* 2010; **27** (1): 4–14.

Patterns are different for bare metal stent and drug-eluting stent which affect ease of management

G Ansel and P Harnish

Introduction

Technological advancements for the percutaneous treatment of peripheral arterial disease have led to better outcomes and widespread use. The use of stand-alone balloon angioplasty is increasingly being replaced by newer technologies that address shortcomings including acute vessel recoil, dissections, and intimal hyperplasia. The one-year restenosis rate for balloon angioplasty of lesions greater than 70% in 4–15cm lesions[1,2] and randomised trials have demonstrated superior outcomes with bare metal stents, stent grafts, drug-eluting stents, and drug-coated balloons.[3,4,5,6,7] However, longer term effectiveness is still problematic due to the complexity of in-stent restenosis, the rate of which appears to be related to lesion length, edge restenosis in stent grafts, a continued decline in patency in drug-coated balloons and the frequent need for adjunctive stenting in longer lesions. Surveillance during follow-up may be necessary since there is a discrepancy between the duplex definition of restenosis and recurrence of clinical symptoms. This lack of symptoms is most clearly represented in patients that have undergone bypass grafting and often will not have a significant drop in resting ankle-brachial index or recurrent symptoms until the focal anastomotic stenosis progresses to graft closure. Flow rates can be 50% higher in focal lesions *versus* diffuse disease.

Evidence

Emerging data demonstrates variable outcomes of repeat intervention depending on the restenosis pattern that is initially treated. The importance of surveillance and treatment of restenotic venous bypasses is well documented. Freedom from a recurrent restenosis when treated with balloon angioplasty or open surgical techniques for patent but stenotic lesions is reported to be 43–61.2% at two years, while the treatment of venous bypass total occlusion leads to the need for retreatment in 78.8%–84.5%.[8]

A similar effect on outcome has been noted when treating bare metal stents with balloon angioplasty. The largest study to date with bare metal stent restenosis and purposed classification scheme has recently been published by Tosaka *et al.*[9] Their multicentre, Japan-based, retrospective, observational study included patients from 2000 to 2009. A total of 133 restenotic lesions that had undergone femoropopliteal artery stenting were classified by angiographic pattern using a visual estimation: class I included focal lesions (<50mm in length); class II included diffuse lesions (>50mm in length); and class III included totally occluded in-stent restenosis. All patients were treated by balloon angioplasty. Recurrent in-stent restenosis or occlusion was defined by duplex peak systolic velocity ratio or ≥50% stenosis on angiography. A class I pattern was found in 29% of the limbs, class II in 38%, and class III in 33%. Mean follow-up period was 24±17 months. Death had occurred in 14 patients; bypass surgery was performed in 11 limbs, and major amputation was performed in one limb during follow-up. Kaplan-Meier survival curves showed that the rate of recurrent in-stent restenosis at two years was 84.8% in class III patients compared with 49.9% in class I patients (p<0.0001) and 53.3% in class II patients (p<0.0003), and the rate of recurrent occlusion at two years was 64.6% in class III patients compared with 15.9% in class I patients (p<0.0001) and 18.9% in class II patients (p<0.0001). Though the Tosaka scheme clearly demonstrates the outcomes with in-stent restenosis with balloon angioplasty, its capacity for generalisation may be limited due to its purity of device and homogeneous population. The population treated was all of Japanese nationality and no excimer laser, atherectomy, stents, covered stents, or drug-eluting devices were utilised. Laird and his group retrospectively applied the Tosaka classification to 75 patients who underwent endovascular treatment for in-stent restenosis using a more multimodality approach at their institution. Adjunctive devices that had been previously utilised included laser atherectomy, excisional atherectomy, and repeat stenting. Despite the use of these adjunctive therapies in the majority of cases, rates of repeat restenosis treatment at two years were 39% for class I, 67% for class II, and 72% for class III in-stent restenosis. Class III in-stent restenosis was also associated with significantly increased rates of recurrent occlusion (hazards ratio [HR] 5.8, 95% confidence interval [CI] 1.8–19.0) compared to the other angiographic categories. These results confirmed the independent association of class III in-stent restenosis with recurrent total occlusion and suggests that the addition of other currently available (non-drug-coated) and expensive adjunctive devices may not be associated with significantly improved long-term outcomes compared to balloon angioplasty alone.[10]

More systematic evaluations of adjunctive therapy have been recently completed utilising newer excimer laser technology and stent grafts. The EXCITE (Excimer laser randomized controlled study for treatment of femoropopliteal in-stent restenosis) trial that utilised a more effective excimer laser system demonstrated superiority to plain balloon angioplasty for in-stent restenosis at six months.[11]

The SALVAGE (A prospective, multicentre trial to evaluate the safety and performance of Spectranetics laser with adjunct PTA and Gore Viabahn endoprosthesis with heparin bioactive surface for the treatment of SFA in-stent restenosis) trial evaluated the combined use of excimer laser debulking and non-contoured edge stent graft coverage for long in-stent restenosis lesions. The patency results appear to be suboptimal with a restenosis rate of 48% but the need for repeat procedures was surprisingly low at 17.4% and may have been due to the focal nature of the edge restenosis characteristic of stent graft usage.[12] The larger multicentre RELINE (Gore Viabahn *versus* plain old balloon angioplasty for superficial femoral artery in-stent restenosis) trial utilising the heparin coated and contoured edge stent graft demonstrated a significantly improved patency at one year of almost 75%.[13]

More promising results have started to be seen with the emergence of drug-coated technology. Though currently no data exists for these technologies using Tosaka classification, the overall results appear to be more promising for the treatment of in-stent restenosis. The first drug-eluting stent Zilver PTX, available in the USA has demonstrated reasonable outcomes. A subset analysis of a large outside US study, which included 108 patients with in-stent restenosis, is available. In this group, 31% of the lesions were stent occlusions. At 12 months the duplex defined primary patency was 78.8% and freedom from clinically driven target lesion revascularisation at 12 and 24 months was 81% and 60.8%, respectively.[14]

In an effort to move to a "leave nothing behind" philosophy, drug-coated balloon delivery of paclitaxel locally has emerged. Paclitaxel inhibits microtubule formation, thereby limiting recoil and smooth muscle cell proliferation. The ability to deliver an antirestenotic agent locally without leaving behind additional scaffolding is attractive and of particular interest in the treatment of stent restenosis. The homogenous tissue also seems particularly well suited to this technology. The first published report of drug-coated balloons for the treatment of in-stent restenosis was a single centre registry of 39 patients.[15] The mean lesion was 83mm with approximately one fifth of the stented lesions occluded. The one-year primary patency rate was 92.1%. Interestingly, a post-hoc analysis did not demonstrate an association of total occlusion and recurrent restenosis.

The DEBATE-ISR (Drug-eluting balloon in peripheral intervention for in-stent restenosis) trial recently reported outcomes of drug-coated balloon angioplasty for treatment among patients with diabetes.[16] The cohort included 44 consecutive patients who were compared to historical controls. Over half the patients had stent occlusion. The one-year primary patency rate was 80.5%, with only 13.6% of patients treated for recurrent restenosis.

A small retrospective study compared excisional atherectomy in patients with restenosis treated with bare *versus* drug-coated balloons. With an overall lesion length of 171mm, one-year restenosis rates were 15.3% for drug-coated balloon *versus* 56.2% for plain balloon angioplasty. Additionally, in a multivariable cox model for restenosis, drug-coated balloon treatment had a hazard ratio of 0.28 (95% confidence interval, 0.12–0.66; p=0.0036) compared with the plain balloon group, suggesting superior patency rates when excisional atherectomy and drug-coated balloons are combined.[17]

Conclusion

The pattern of restenosis for venous bypass and bare metal stents appears to be similar in that the treatment of total occlusion is associated with a higher need for repeated treatment. Treatment of bare metal stent restenosis with stent grafts and drug-based technology appears to be improving outcomes with a possible further benefit of debulking. The pattern of restenosis and most effective treatment options for drug-eluting stents and drug-coated balloon restenosis are yet to be defined.

Summary

- Advances in the endovascular treatment of superficial femoral artery disease have improved outcomes.

- Data are present that support prevention of venous bypass and bare metal stenting from going on to total occlusion.

- Restenosis patterns can affect the return of symptoms.

- Restenosis patterns can help predict the need for repeat procedures in bare metal stents.

- Restenosis patterns have yet to be defined for drug based technologies.

References

1. Rocha-Singh KJ, Jaff MR, Crabtree TR, *et al.* VIVA Physicians, Inc. Performance goals and endpoint assessments for clinical trials of femoropopliteal bare nitinol stents in patients with symptomatic peripheral arterial disease. *Catheter Cardiovasc Interv* 2007; **69**: 910–19.

2. Norgen L, Hiatt WR, Dormandy JA, *et al.* Inter- Society Consensus for the Management of Peripheral Arterial Disease (TASC II). *J Vasc Surg* 2007; **45**: 55–67

3. Schillinger M, Sabeti S, Loewe C, *et al.* Balloon angioplasty *versus* implantation of nitinol stents in the superficial femoral artery. *N Engl J Med* 2006; **354**: 1879–88.

4. Laird JR, Katzen BT, for the RESILIENT Investigators. Nitinol stent implantation *versus* balloon angioplasty for lesions in the superficial femoral artery and proximal popliteal artery: twelve-month results from the RESILIENT randomized trial. *Circ Cardiovasc Interv* 2010; **3**: 267–76.

5. Hartung O, *et al.* Efficacy of Hemobahn in the treatment of superficial femoral artery lesions in patients with acute or critical ischemia: a comparative study with claudicants. *Eur J Vasc Endovasc Surg* 2005; **30**: 300–06.

6. Werk M, Langner S, Reinkensmeier B, *et al.* Inhibition of restenosis in femoropopliteal arteries: paclitaxel-coated *versus* uncoated balloons: femoral paclitaxel randomized pilot trial. *Circulation.* 2008; **118**: 1358–65.

7. Dake MD, Ansel GM, Jaff MR, *et al.* Paclitaxel-eluting stents show superiority to balloon angioplasty and bare metal stents in femoropopliteal disease: twelve-month Zilver PTX randomized study results. *Circ Cardiovasc Interv* 2011; **4**: 495–504

8. Nguyen LL, Conte MS, Menard MT, *et al.* Infrainguinal vein bypass graft revision: factors affecting long-term outcome. *J Vasc Surg* 2004; **40**: 916–23.

9. Tosaka A, Soga Y, Iida O, *et al.* Classification and clinical impact of restenosis after femoropopliteal stenting. *J Am Coll Cardiol* 2012; **59**: 16–23.

10. Armstrong EJ, Singh S, Singh GD, Yeo KK, et.al. Angiographic characteristics of femoropopliteal in-stent restenosis: association with long-term outcomes after endovascular intervention. *Catheter Cardiovasc Interv.* 2013; **82**: 1168-74

11. Dippel EJ, Makam P, Kovach R, *et al;* EXCITE ISR Investigators. Randomized controlled study of excimer laser atherectomy for treatment of femoropopliteal in-stent restenosis: initial results from the EXCITE ISR trial (EXCImer Laser Randomized Controlled Study for Treatment of FemoropopliTEal In-Stent Restenosis). *JACC Cardiovasc Interv* 2015; **8**: 92–101.

12. Laird JR, Jr., Yeo KK, Rocha-Singh K, *et al.* Excimer laser with adjunctive balloon angioplasty and heparin-coated self-expanding stent grafts for the treatment of femoropopliteal artery in-stent restenosis: Twelve-month results from the SALVAGE study. *Catheter Cardiovasc Interv* 2012; **80**: 852–59

13. Bosiers M, Deloose K, Callaert J, *et al.* Superiority of stent-grafts for in-stent restenosis in the superficial femoral artery: twelve-month results from a multicenter randomized trial. *J Endovasc Ther* 2015; **22**: 1–10.

14. Dake MD, Scheinert D, Tepe G, *et al.* Nitinol stents with polymer-free paclitaxel coating for lesions in the superficial femoral and popliteal arteries above the knee: Twelve-month safety and effectiveness results from the Zilver PTX single-arm clinical study. *J Endovasc Ther* 2011; **18**: 613–23.

15. Stabile E, Virga V, Salemme L, Cioppa A, *et al.* Drug-eluting balloon for treatment of superficial femoral artery in-stent restenosis. *J Am Coll Cardiol* 2012; **60**: 1739–42.

16. Liistro F, Angioli P, Porto I, *et al.* Paclitaxel-eluting balloon vs. standard angioplasty to reduce recurrent restenosis in diabetic patients with in-stent restenosis of the superficial femoral and proximal popliteal arteries: The DEBATE-ISR Study. *J Endovasc Ther* 2014; **21**: 1–8.

17. Sixt S, Cancino O, Treszl A, *et al.* Drug-coated balloon angioplasty after directional atherectomy improves outcomes in restenotic femoro- popliteal arteries. *J Vasc Surg* 2013; **58**: 682–86.

Treatment of iliac in-stent restenosis with laser debulking and covered stents

JC van den Berg

Introduction

The occurrence of in-stent restenosis after endovascular treatment of iliac artery stenosis with (uncovered) stents is less frequent than after superficial femoral artery stenting, but can pose a significant clinical problem. As with the treatment of in-stent restenosis in other territories, treatment with conventional balloon angioplasty has limited durability. Therefore, alternative therapies have been used to improve long-term outcomes after re-intervention. This chapter will describe the initial experience with excimer laser ablation followed by covered stents in the treatment of in-stent restenosis of the iliac artery.

Technique

Either an ipsilateral, retrograde approach or a retrograde, contralateral approach with crossover (and antegrade crossing) can be used. The initial approach is always through an ipsilateral retrograde access, and only when it is impossible to enter the stent distally, or to cross the entire length of the stent occlusion with the guide wire (inability to create the "loop", with the guidewire exiting the stent struts) an antegrade recanalisation is attempted (preferably using a contralateral crossover technique; alternatively a brachial access can be obtained), with "snaring" of the wire from below. The laser debulking is always performed through the ipsilateral retrograde approach, especially to address situations in which a flush occlusion of a stent in the common iliac artery is present (the steep angle of the bifurcation will prohibit proper debulking when working in a crossover fashion). After obtaining arterial access, a 4Fr introducer sheath is placed, and a diagnostic angiography of the aorto-iliac segment is obtained. After successfully crossing the lesion with a hydrophilic guidewire (Glidewire, Terumo), a diagnostic catheter is advanced and contrast injected proximally (or distally in case of an antegrade crossing) from the lesion to confirm intraluminal position. In case of a total occlusion, the lesion should preferably be crossed with the guidewire looped to avoid exiting of the wire through the struts of the stent in a subintimal fashion, and to be sure that the wire has crossed intraluminally. The 4Fr introducer sheath can then be exchanged for a 6Fr or 7Fr sheath (depending on the size of the laser catheter that is to be used), while maintaining the guidewire in a position with its tip proximally from the lesion. Then the hydrophilic guidewire should be exchanged for a 0.014inch guidewire or a 0.018inch guidewire, again this is depending on which type of laser catheter is used.

For smaller diameter vessels (up to 6mm), a Turbo-Elite (Spectranetics) laser catheter (with a diameter of at least 2mm) is subsequently introduced, while applying continuous saline flush on both the introducer sheath and through the laser catheter. The laser catheter is then slowly advanced through the lesion under fluoroscopic control (speed <1mm/sec). It is recommended to perform two passages with the laser catheter. Fluence and pulse repetition rate settings for the first passage should be intermediate, which will allow for more efficacious ablation of any soft (thrombotic) material present, thus minimising the risk of distal embolisation. The second passage will be performed using the maximum fluence and frequency (as set by the manufacturer). At maximum settings, the vapour bubble that is typically formed around the tip of the laser catheter (and that is contributing significantly to the ablative effect) is larger, and thus the debulking will be more efficient. After removal of the laser catheter, a control angiography is performed. This is followed by placement of a balloon-expandable covered stent.

For larger vessel diameters (>7mm), the Turbo-Tandem system (Spectranetics) can be used for debulking. The Turbo Tandem requires a 7Fr sheath, and consists of a guiding catheter with a ramp and a pre-mounted laser catheter that can be advanced onto the ramp allowing for an off-centre position of the laser catheter during ablation. This technique allows the operator to obtain a larger luminal gain. The Turbo Tandem catheter can only be used after creating a so-called pilot channel in the occlusion (the minimum diameter required is 2mm). The pilot channel can be obtained by using a small size Turbo Elite catheter, or predilation of the occlusion with an angioplasty balloon of at least 2mm. After the first pass of the Turbo Tandem through the occlusion, the laser catheter is retracted off the ramp, the whole system is withdrawn, and a new pass is performed. A total of four quadrant passes (at 0, 90, 180 and 270 degrees) is recommended. The subsequent steps are identical as when using the standard laser catheter as described above.

Case series

A cohort of nine consecutive patients (six female, three male; mean age 63 years (range 44–74 years) with symptomatic iliac artery in–stent restenosis or occlusion were evaluated. A total of 10 vessel segments were treated (one patient with a bilateral common iliac occlusion; nine patients with unilateral disease). In most cases, the lesion was limited to the common iliac artery (n=9), with all lesions except one limited to the stented segment (in one patient there was an extension of the occlusion 1cm distally from the occluded stent). One lesion involved both the common and external iliac artery (common iliac artery in-stent occlusion, external iliac artery *de novo* lesion). One lesion was a high-grade stenosis, the remaining nine were total occlusions. The mean lesion length was 57mm (range 26–110mm) the mean vessel diameter was 8.1mm (range 7–10mm). A total of 12 covered stents was used (Advanta V12 [Maquet] n=7; Be-graft [Bentley Medical] n=5). In the patient that demonstrated an extension of the occlusion beyond the stent (until the iliac bifurcation), a non-covered balloon-expandable stent was placed distally from the covered stent in order not to compromise the patency of the internal iliac artery. In the patient with a concomitant *de novo* external iliac artery stenosis, a bare metal self-expanding stent was placed. All patients became fully asymptomatic after the procedure. No patients were lost to follow-up. During a mean follow-up of 25.9 months (range 5–71 months) one case of symptomatic in-stent restenosis was seen six months after the re-intervention (this was the patient with a non-covered balloon-expandable stent distal from covered stent, restenosis was found within the non-covered stent; given the young age of the patient (44 years) it was decided to perform an aorto-femoral bypass). Re-occlusion of the treated segment was seen in one case, seven months after the debulking and covered stent procedure. This occlusion was treated with thrombolysis. After thrombolysis, a stenosis distal to the covered stent was revealed that was treated with a bare metal balloon expandable stent. At three year follow-up, this patient was asymptomatic with patency of the iliac axis. One patient demonstrated a symptomatic stenosis in the common iliac artery distal from the covered stent that was treated with a covered stent. The primary patency was thus 80% (8/10), and the primary assisted patency and secondary patency was 90%.

Discussion

The endovascular treatment of iliac artery stenosis with (uncovered) stents shows patency rates that are better than those typically seen after stenting of the superficial

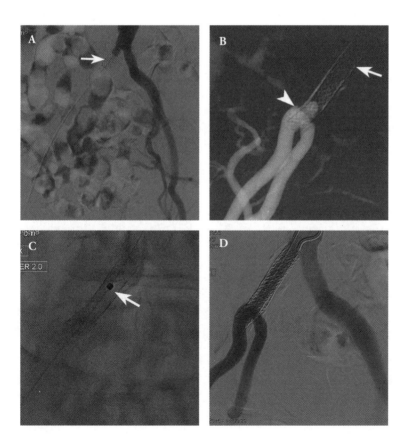

Figure 1: (A) Digital subtraction angiography and (B) roadmap image demonstrating occlusion of a stent in the right common iliac artery (arrow), note the patent distal end of the stent extending into the external iliac artery with patency of the internal iliac artery (arrowhead); (C) fluoroscopic image of 2mm Turbo Elite laser catheter (arrow); (D) control angiography after covered stent placement demonstrating complete restoration of flow.

femoral artery. The Dutch iliac stent trial, which randomised 279 patients with iliac artery disease (stenosis and occlusion) to undergo primary stent placement (143 patients) or percutaneous transluminal angioplasty with selective stent placement, showed an iliac patency that decreased from 97% (122 of 126 patients) at three months after treatment to 83% (90 of 109 patients) at the final follow-up (six–eight years after treatment) in the patients with primary stent placement.[1] Similar results were seen in other, non-randomised studies: Gandini evaluated 138 patients with iliac artery occlusions, and found a primary patency of 90%, 85%, 80%, and 68% at three, five, seven, and 10 years respectively,[2] while Scheinert *et al* described a primary patency rate of 84% at one year, 81% at two years, 78% at three years, and 76% at four years in a cohort of 212 patients with iliac artery occlusions.[3] The last study that needs to be mentioned here is the COBEST (Covered vs. balloon expandable stent) trial.[4] In this study, a randomised comparison was made of bare metal stents and covered stents for the treatment of iliac artery stenosis, and demonstrated a significantly lower rate of binary restenosis in the covered stent group for TASC lesions.

The histopathology of in-stent restenosis in the iliac arteries is similar to that seen in the superficial femoral artery. Evaluation of directional atherectomy specimens demonstrated typical myointimal hyperplasia. In addition to this, areas of intimal fibrosis, atheroma and small foci of amorphous oeosinophilic material consistent with thrombus were seen, but all were not representing the major part of the lesion,[5] the majority of the volume being extra-cellular matrix. Due to this unique morphology, in-stent restenotic lesions tend to feel "spongy" and recoil quickly. The extracellular matrix accounts for 50% of the total volume of neointimal restenotic lesions, and explains why balloon angioplasty alone does not work in restenotic lesions.[6] These histological findings have important implications for the optimal treatment of iliac in-stent restenosis.

Relatively little is published on the treatment of iliac in-stent restenosis/occlusion with percutaneous transluminal angioplasty or other techniques, and most reports deal with the treatment of restenotic lesions. One study analysed 68 patients, with a total of 84 procedures (percutaneous transluminal angioplastyand percutaneous transluminal angioplasty with stenting).[7] The majority of the lesions were of stenotic origin (n=61; 75%) while the remaining 25% presented with an occlusion. Technical success was 100%. In 86% of the cases, percutaneous transluminal atherectomy was performed as a stand-alone procedure, while 14% of the procedures required placement of a stent. During follow-up, 28 re-interventions were performed (12 surgical conversions; 16 re-do endovascular), with a primary clinical patency at one, three and five years of 88%, 62%, 38% respectively. No subgroup analysis was performed, and, therefore, it is not known whether there was a difference in outcome between the occlusive and stenotic lesions. Another paper reported on 41 lesions in 24 patients who underwent endovascular intervention for iliac in-stent restenosis.[8] Most lesions were unilateral and involved the common iliac artery (66%). The mean lesion length was 30.1mm with type I (focal) and II (diffuse) in-stent restenosis occurring with the greatest frequency (34% and 39%, respectively). The remaining 27% presented with totally occluded stents. All patients underwent balloon angioplasty and additional stenting was performed in 66% of the lesions. Type II lesions more frequently required stenting. The six and 12-month primary patency rates were 96% and 82% respectively. The 12-month

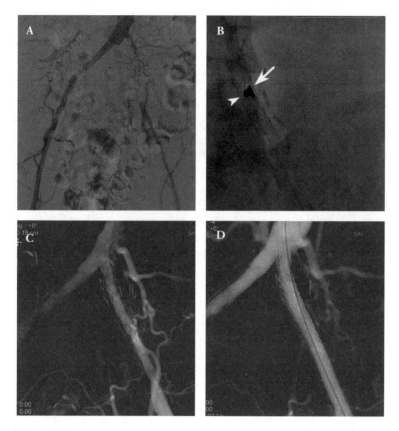

Figure 2: (A) Digital subtraction angiography demonstrating occlusion of a stent in the left common iliac artery (arrow); (B) fluoroscopic image demonstrating 90-degree position of Turbo Tandem catheter with ramp (arrow) and laser tip (arrowhead) clearly visible (prior to the use of the Turbo Tandem catheter a balloon angioplasty with a 2.5 x 80 mm balloon was performed (not shown); (C) roadmap image after four passages with Turbo Tandem laser catheter demonstrating significant debulking with almost complete restoration of the lumen; (D) roadmap image after covered stent placement demonstrating complete restoration of flow.

primary-assisted patency rate was 90% with clinically driven target lesion revascularisation in three patients.

As an alternative to plain balloon angioplasty several treatment modalities have been described and include directional atherectomy, cutting balloon angioplasty and the use of covered stents.

The results of directional atherectomy in 12 patients with 14 lesions (of which 13 were treated) have been described by Ettles *et al.*[5] A total of four occlusions and nine stenoses were treated (mean lesion length not specified). All occluded lesions were pre-treated with overnight thrombolysis. Nine patients (one occlusion, eight stenoses) remained symptom free with unlimited walking distance, normal femoral pulses, and normal common femoral duplex ultrasound examinations at a mean of 10.5 months (range 3–24 months) following initial atherectomy. Although this represents a small series, the results indicate that the treatment of in-stent occlusion is more cumbersome than that of re-stenotic lesions.

Cutting-balloon angioplasty was performed in a series of 14 cases of haemodynamically significant iliac artery in-stent restenosis, either primarily or after failed conventional balloon angioplasty.[9] The mean length of in-stent restenosis was

11.9 mm (range 2–48mm), and the average stenosis was 75.4% (no total occlusions were treated). In one case, a contained rupture occurred that was treated with a covered stent. In the remainder of the cases, the cutting balloons allowed successful treatment without further stent implantation. During a mean follow-up of 23.6 months (range 12-60 months), no patient showed clinical deterioration, and no recurrent in-stent restenosis was detected with colour duplex.

The use of covered stents has also been proposed as treatment for iliac in–stent restenosis.[10] In a subgroup of 46 patients (46 lesions, 54.3% stenosis, 45.7% occlusion) treated with polytetrafluoroethylene-covered balloon-expandable stents, the primary patency at one, two, and four years was 77.9%, 72.1%, and 53%, respectively. This was significantly lower than the patency in primary lesion treatment with covered stents in the same study. An explanation for the differences noted was not provided by the authors.

Recently the use of drug-coated balloons has been described, mainly in patients with in-stent stenosis, and the results of two published studies are not equivocal. One paper describes the results of the treatment of six patients with iliac in-stent restenosis with drug-coated balloons.[11] The mean lesion length was 61.7mm (range, 40–80mm), no total occlusions were treated. Technical success was achieved in all cases. During follow-up with a mean duration of 15.5 months (range, 3–30 months), healing of the lesions/relief of symptoms was obtained in five of six cases (83.3%). The authors estimated the two–year rate of overall patency and limb salvage at 100% (probably using Kaplan-Meier analysis, although this is not clear from the paper). Completely different results were found in another study, involving a larger group of patients that showed less favourable results of treatment with drug-coated balloons. Data for 18 patients treated with drug-coated balloons for iliac in-stent restenosis were retrospectively evaluated and compared with a control group of 22 patients treated with standard balloon angioplasty.[12] The mean length of the lesions in the drug-coated balloon group was 27.1mm *versus* 20mm, while the grade of restenosis was 70.4% and 64%, respectively. No occlusions were treated. The primary patency rates were 90.5% *versus* 85.7% at six months and 71.4% *versus* 75.6% at 12 months for drug-coated *versus* conventional balloon angioplasty respectively (not statistically significant), while the target lesion restenosis rate was 28.6% and 20% respectively. In the drug-coated group two patients (9.5%) required adjunctive stenting.

The (assisted) primary patency in the series presented in this chapter treated with debulking and covered stents is equivalent or superior to the above mentioned treatment modalities. Especially considering the longer lesion length and the high number of total occlusions, the results are remarkable. It is known from several studies in the superficial femoral artery territory that in-stent occlusions tend to perform worse as compared with in-stent stenotic lesions, both after plain balloon angioplasty and drug-coated balloon angioplasty[13, 14,] and the above mentioned review of the literature indicates that this is most probably also true for iliac in-stent restenosis. In the case of iliac in-stent occlusion, the significant amount of neo-intimal hyperplasia and the large diameter of the vessel may be a limiting factor when using drug-coated balloons (until recently the maximum diameter available was 7mm), or additional (drug-eluting) stents. Repeat (non-covered) stent placement, especially without prior debulking will over-expand the arterial wall and potentially cause a further neointimal response. The good results seen with cutting-balloon angioplasty are probably related to the superiority of this technique in extruding neointimal plaque outside the stent, and in decreasing plaque volume through compression.[9] This benefit is probably limited to short, stenotic lesions. Laser debulking, such as directional atherectomy allows for significant reduction of the plaque burden, and this is especially of importance in vessels larger than 8mm, but will not be sufficient as a stand-alone technique. Combination with covered stent placement allows reduction of embolic risk during the procedure and will allow exclusion of residual plaque and endothelium, potentially mitigating late luminal loss by halting migration and proliferation of vascular smooth muscle cells and inflammatory cells through open stent struts, as is indicated by the good mid-term results described herein. Combination of laser debulking with the currently available larger diameter drug-coated balloons is another treatment option that still needs to be explored.

Conclusion

The occurrence of iliac in-stent restenosis and occlusion is relatively infrequent, and the treatment with conventional balloon angioplasty leads to disappointing long-term results. Combination of debulking and covered stent treatment of iliac occlusive in-stent restenosis is safe with good mid-to long-term results.

Summary

- The occurrence of iliac in-stent restenosis and occlusion is relatively infrequent.

- The treatment with conventional balloon angioplasty of iliac in-stent restenosis has disappointing long-term results.

- The role of drug-eluting balloon technology for iliac in-stent restenosis is not well established.

- Combination of debulking and covered stent treatment of iliac occlusive in-stent restenosis is safe with good mid-to long-term results.

References

1. Klein WM, van der Graaf Y, Seegers J, Spithoven JH, et al. Dutch iliac stent trial: long-term results in patients randomized for primary or selective stent placement. *Radiology* 2006; **238** (2): 734–44.
2. Gandini R, Fabiano S, Chiocchi M, et al. Percutaneous treatment in iliac artery occlusion: long-term results. *Cardiovasc Intervent Radiol* 2008; **31** (6): 1069–76.
3. Scheinert D, Schroder M, Ludwig J, et al. Stent-supported recanalization of chronic iliac artery occlusions. *Am J Med* 2001; **110** (9): 708–15.
4. Mwipatayi BP, Thomas S, Wong J, et al. A comparison of covered vs bare expandable stents for the treatment of aortoiliac occlusive disease. *J Vasc Surg* 2011; **54** (6): 1561–70.
5. Ettles DF, MacDonald AW, Burgess PA, et al. Directional atherectomy in iliac stent failure: clinical technique and histopathologic correlation. *Cardiovasc Intervent Radiol* 1998; **21** (6): 475–80.
6. Farb A, Virmani R, Atkinson JB, Kolodgie FD. Plaque morphology and pathologic changes in arteries from patients dying after coronary balloon angioplasty. *J Am Coll Cardiol* 1990; **16**(6): 1421–29.
7. Kropman RH, Bemelman M, Vos JA, et al. Long-term results of percutaneous transluminal angioplasty for symptomatic iliac in-stent stenosis. *Eur J Vasc Endovasc Surg* 2006; **32**(6) : 634–38.

8. Javed U, Balwanz CR, Armstrong EJ, *et al.* Mid-term outcomes following endovascular re-intervention for iliac artery ISR. *Catheter Cardiovasc Interv* 2013; **82** (7): 1176–84.

9. Tsetis D, Belli AM, Morgan R, *et al.* Preliminary experience with cutting balloon angioplasty for iliac artery ISR. *J Endovasc Ther* 2008; **15** (2): 193–202.

10. Grimme FA, Spithoven JH, Zeebregts CJ, *et al.* Midterm outcome of balloon-expandable polytetrafluoroethylene-covered stents in the treatment of iliac artery chronic occlusive disease. *J Endovasc Ther* 2012; **19** (6): 797–804.

11. Troisi N, Ercolini L, Peretti E, *et al.* Drug-eluting balloons to treat iliac ISR. *Ann Vasc Surg* 2015; **29** (6): 1315–16.

12. Stahlhoff S, Donas KP, Torsello G, *et al.* Drug-Eluting vs Standard Balloon Angioplasty for Iliac Stent Restenosis: Midterm Results. *J Endovasc Ther* 2015; **22** (3): 314–18.

13. Tosaka A, Soga Y, Lida O, *et al.* Classification and clinical impact of restenosis after femoropopliteal stenting. *J Am Coll Cardiol* 2012; **59** (1): 16-23.

14. Virga V, Stabile E, Biamino G, *et al.* Drug-eluting balloons for the treatment of the superficial femoral artery ISR: 2-year follow-up. *JACC Cardiovasc Interv* 2014; **7** (4): 411–15.

Angioplasty alone or drug-coated balloon or laser debulking/drug-coated balloon for in-stent restenosis

E Ducasse, C Caradu and D Midy

Introduction

Peripheral arterial disease affects more than 27 million people throughout the world and its impact will continue to grow when the ageing population and the increasing incidence of diabetes is considered. Endovascular treatment is now the first-line strategy, but results of plain old balloon angioplasty in the superficial femoral artery are limited by dissection, elastic recoil and restenosis, which led to the use of self-expanding stents, with a clear advantage over plain old balloon angioplasty in randomised controlled trials. However, long-term outcomes are hindered by up to 60% of in-stent restenosis, with lack of sustained clinical benefit,[1] even with drug-eluting stents. Since longer lesions are treated daily, with higher restenosis rates, the number of patients needing in-stent restenosis treatment will increase dramatically. Several treatment modalities have become available to pursue an endovascular approach but recommendations for the optimal strategy have not yet been established.

In-stent restenosis mechanisms

In-stent restenosis lesions constitute a unique disease state compared with atherosclerosis (Figure 1). Stent implantation, stent fractures and malapposed stent struts in calcified lesions induce deep vessel injury, damaging the internal elastic lamina, and result in endothelial cell loss, leading to platelet fibrin thrombus formation around the struts, which serves as extracellular matrix for subsequent cellular repair. Within the first three days, monocytes differentiate into macrophages and release cytokines as an initial acute inflammatory response. Smooth muscle cells turn from a contractile phenotype to a secreting phenotype, proliferate and migrate into the intima. Proteoglycans, hyaluronan and type III collagen secretion creates a thin hydrophilic extracellular matrix, which will be digested by metallo-proteinases and replaced by a more structured extracellular matrix with type I collagen. These steps are called neointimal proliferation and occur as a normal healing phenomenon.

In-stent restenosis is defined as an exaggerated response that results in >75% cross-sectional luminal narrowing by neointimal hyperplasia, 80% of the restenotic

449

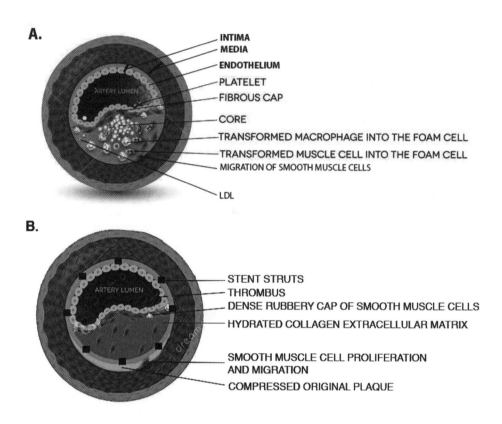

Figure 1: Schematic representations of the differences between atherosclerosis and in-stent restenosis. (A) Atherosclerosis. (B) In-stent restenosis.

volume being highly-compliant, soft and aqueous extracellular matrix, and occurs when these pro-inflammatory regenerative processes do not get counter-balanced within four weeks.

Moreover, the superficial femoral artery, popliteal and tibial arteries are muscular arteries and present with fewer elastic fibres and more smooth muscle cells than do elastic arteries, leading to higher restenosis rates. The superficial femoral artery also undergoes complex deformations leading to decreased wall shear stress. Yet, neotintimal hyperplasia is prominent at sites of low wall shear stress and acute elevations in spatial wall shear stress gradients, which are mostly located within the proximal and distal transition zones of stented segments.[2] Diabetic patients are also at higher risk due to endothelial dysfunction and enhanced platelet activity, as well as female gender, dialysis and active inflammatory states.

Plain old balloon angioplasty and cutting balloons

Tosaka *et al* published a classification of in-stent restenosis angiographical patterns (Figure 2),[3] along with the results of a retrospective study of 133 patients with femoropopliteal in-stent restenosis lesions treated by plain old balloon angioplasty, showing acceptable immediate procedural success. However, two-year restenosis and reocclusion rates were extremely high, especially in Tosaka class II or III lesions (84.8% in class III vs. 49.9% in class I [p<0.0001] and 53.3% in class II [p=0.0003] lesions; and 64.6% in class III vs. 15.9% in class I [p<0.0001] and 18.9% in class II lesions [p<0.0001], respectively). These disappointing results might be explained by the fact that balloon inflation squeezes water content out of the aqueous extracellular matrix and upon deflation the lesion acts like a sponge and rehydrates within 100 minutes leading to acute recoil.[4]

Cutting balloons were thought to offer more effective dilation with less balloon slippage. However, they failed to prove superiority over plain old balloon angioplasty in a pilot study.[4]

Drug-coated balloons

Currently available drug-coated balloons deliver paclitaxel locally to inhibit microtubule formation, thereby limiting smooth muscle cell proliferation, without inhibition of endothelial cell proliferation and results in prevention of restenosis without stopping reendothelialisation, with a recommended inflation time of 45 seconds.

The first published study included 39 patients with 48.7% of diabetics (mean lesion length 82.9±78.9mm, 20.5% Tosaka class III).[5] After predilation, patients were treated with a median of two drug-coated balloons (IN.PACT, Medtronic) to avoid geographic miss. Bail out stenting was necessary in 10%. Primary patency rates were 92.1% at one year and 70.3% at two years; two year freedom from target lesion revascularisation was 78.4%.[6] Tosaka class II and III lesions were associated with an increased rate of recurrent in-stent restenosis at two years compared with class I lesions (33.3 % and 36.3 % vs. 12.5%; p=0.05).

The DEBATE-ISR (Drug-eluting balloon in peripheral intervention for in-stent restenosis) trial reported the outcomes of 44 patients with diabetes (64% with critical limb ischaemia, mean lesion length 132±86mm; 51% Tosaka class III) compared with historical plain old balloon angioplasty controls.[7] Recurrent in-stent restenosis occurred in 19.5% *versus* 71.8% (p<0.001) and clinically driven target lesion revascularisation was performed in 13.6% *versus* 31.0% (p=0.045), showing significantly better results with drug-coated balloons. However, this superiority was not sustained at three years (target lesion revascularisation 40% vs. 43%; p=0.8) and Tosaka class III lesions were associated with worse outcome in both groups (p=0.004).[8]

FAIR (Femoral artery in-stent restenosis) was the first prospective multicentre randomised controlled trial to assess the efficacy of drug-coated balloons for in-stent restenosis. Patients were randomised to drug-coated balloon (n=62, mean lesion length 82.2±68.4mm, 28.6% Tosaka class III) or to plain old balloon

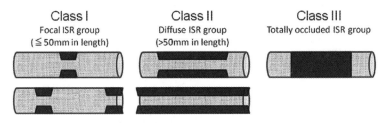

Figure 2: Femoropopliteal in-stent restenosis classification scheme. Lesions are classified based on visual estimate: Class I: focal (<50mm) ISR within the stent body, stent edge, or a combination of the two. Class II: diffuse lesions (>50mm) within the stent body and / or stent edge. Class III: total occlusion within the stent. (Source: Tosaka *et al*).

angioplasty (n=57).[9] At six and 12 months, results showed a significant decrease in recurrent in-stent restenosis (15.4% vs. 44.7% [p=0.002] and 30% vs. 63% [p=0.004]) and superior freedom from target lesion revascularisation (96.4% vs. 81.0% [p=0.0117] and 90.8% vs. 52.6% [p<0.0001]). Clinical improvement by ≥1 Rutherford category without the need for target lesion revascularisation was observed in 77.8% *versus* 52.3% (p=0.015). No major amputation was needed.

Hence, drug-coated balloons seem safe and efficient with significantly lower recurrent in-stent restenosis and target lesion revascularisation up to one year. However, there seems to be a late catch-up phenomenon of recurrent restenosis. Moreover, this approach suffers the same technical limitations as plain old balloon angioplasty in terms of elastic recoil or flow-limiting dissection—not to mention that questions about how drug-coated balloons deal with highly calcified lesions and subintimal recanalisation are still unanswered.

Mechanical excisional atherectomy

Results of directional atherectomy with the SilverHawk (Covidien), showed more favourable outcomes in primary lesions than in in-stent restenosis, due to its soft and aqueous structure making the catheter "spin in the mud".[10] This technique remains off-label, the promise of minimising barotrauma to limit dissection fell short and it is burdened by high embolisation rates and low patency rates, which may be caused by the aggressive mechanical excision of the neointima, inducing an inflammatory response resulting in recurrent in-stent restenosis.

Excimer laser atherectomy

The lasing medium of excimer laser atherectomy (xenon gas and hydrogen chloride) bombarded with high voltage generates ultraviolet light energy photons (308nm), which are absorbed by the aqueous extracellular matrix, smooth muscle cells, collagen and thrombus, vaporising material without mechanical components to reduce embolic potential. This "cold-tipped" laser results in a dose-dependent "stunned platelet" phenomenon, which enhances thrombus dissolution.[11]

Two laser catheters are used in actual studies, the Turbo-Elite and Turbo-Tandem (Spectranetics). A continuous saline infusion to flush contrast and blood is mandatory and a two passages "step-by-step" technique (1mm/sec) is recommended.

The PATENT prospective multicentre trial enrolled 90 patients (mean lesion length 123±95.9mm, 34.4% Tosaka class III).[12] A pilot channel was created in 96.7% of lesions and adjunctive plain old balloon angioplasty was performed in 87.8%. Procedure success was 98.9% with the preservation of stent integrity. The mean percentage stenosis improved from 87% to 32.3% after excimer laser atherectomy and 7.4% after final treatment. Distal embolisation occurred in 10%. At six and 12 months, freedom from target lesion revascularisation was 87.8% and 64.4% and primary patency rates were 64.1% and 37.8% (54.5% for Tosaka class I lesions, 27.6% for class II and 24% for class III). Only a history of prior intervention for in-stent restenosis (p<0.01) was a predictor of target lesion revascularisation.

Similarly, Shammas *et al* reported freedom from target lesion revascularisation in 51% at one year despite longer (210mm) and more Tosaka class III (48%) lesions.[13]

EXCITE ISR (Excimer laser randomised controlled study for treatment of femoropopliteal in-stent restenosis) stopped enrolment at 169 excimer laser atherectomy plus plain old balloon angioplasty patients (mean lesion length 196±120mm; 30.5% Tosaka class III lesions) and 81 plain old balloon angioplasty patients (mean lesion length 193±119mm; 36.8% Tosaka class III lesions) due to early efficacy demonstrated at the six month interim analysis.[14] Excimer laser atherectomy with adjunctive plain old balloon angioplasty showed clear superiority in terms of procedural success (93.5% vs. 82.7%; p=0.01) with significantly fewer complications (30-day major adverse event rates 5.8% vs. 20.5%; p<0.001). Freedom from target lesion revascularisation was 73.5% *versus* 51.8% (p<0.005), with a 52% reduction in target lesion revascularisation.

Combined technique

Vessel preparation is essential to ensure maximum efficacy in drug delivery, especially in Tosaka class III lesions or reocclusions due to the large amount of non-cellular material and thrombus that needs to be dealt with to allow the cytotoxic effect of the paclitaxel to reach the cellular layer. A combined technique may have the advantage of acute debulking from atherectomy plus the enhanced anti-restenotic effect of a drug-coated balloon.

The first indication that the outcome of combining excimer laser atherectomy and drug-coated balloon angioplasty was better came from an initial study on 10 patients (50% with critical limb ischaemia, mean lesion length 115mm, 80% Tosaka class III) with two cases of distal embolisation treated successfully by aspiration thrombectomy and seven- and 16-month primary patency rates of 70%,[15] and 50%; only one target lesion revascularisation occurred at 36 months.[16] Another recently published randomised controlled trial reported patency rates at six and 12 months of 91.7% and 66.7% *versus* 58.3% and 37.5%, respectively (p=0.01) and 12-month target lesion revascularisation rates of 16.7% *versus* 50% (p=0.01) in critical limb ischaemia patients (100% Tosaka class III) treated by excimer laser atherectomy plus drug-coated balloon (n=24, mean lesion length 224±9.4mm) *versus* drug-coated balloon alone (n=24, mean lesion length 259±87mm).[17] Importantly, major amputation rates were also significantly lower with excimer laser atherectomy plus drug-coated balloon (8% vs. 46%, p=0.003) and ulcer healing was better. The combination of excimer laser atherectomy and drug-coated balloon angioplasty emerges as a promising approach with better outcomes compared to drug-coated balloon alone, especially for challenging patients and the ongoing PHOTOPAC (Photoablative atherectomy followed by a paclitaxel-coated balloon to inhibit restenosis in in stent femoro-popliteal obstructions) randomised controlled trial will further evaluate this approach.[18]

Discussion

There are increasing indications that treatment of Tosaka class III lesions tends to be related to worse mid- and long-term outcomes.[3] Armstrong *et al* reported the results of 75 patients who underwent multimodality endovascular treatment, including excimer laser atherectomy, mechanical excisional atherectomy, and repeat-stenting.[19] Rates of recurrent restenosis at two years were 39% for class I, 67% for class II and 72% for class III in-stent restenosis (Figure 3). Class III in-stent restenosis was also

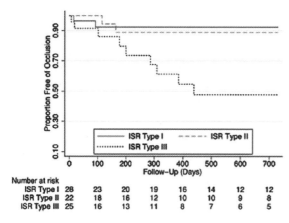

Figure 3: Outcomes of in-stent restenosis treatment stratified by angiographic Tosaka classification. Patients with type III in-stent restenosis were significantly more likely to develop recurrent occlusion than patients with type I or II in-stent restenosis. (Source: Armstrong *et al*).

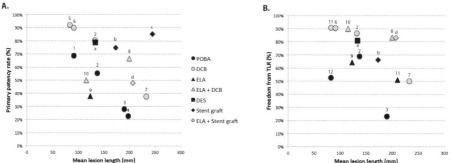

Figure 4: Results of the principal trials on in-stent restenosis with at least 12 months follow-up. (A) Patency rate depending on mean lesion length. (B) Freedom from target lesion revascularisation rate depending on mean lesion length.

associated with significantly increased rates of recurrent reocclusion (hazard ratio [HR]: 5.8, 95% confidence interval [CI]: 1.8–19), confirming the independent association of class III in-stent restenosis with recurrent reocclusion. Hence, more extensive treatment may not be associated with significantly improved long-term outcomes for such lesions (Figure 4).

Therefore, before implementing these new and more costly therapies in a broader patient population, randomised controlled trials with Tosaka class stratification and cost-effectiveness evaluation are necessary to help decide upon optimal treatment modality for each specific type of lesion. A new multicentre randomised controlled trial, INTACT, is now enrolling and should enrol 246 patients divided into three arms, plain old balloon angioplasty, drug-coated balloon and excimer laser atherectomy followed by drug-coated balloon, with an 18-month clinical and economical follow-up evaluation in order to help clarify those questions.[20]

Even though many operators advocate avoiding repeat-stenting, flow-limiting dissections occur in a subset of patients and it remains an alternative solution. Recently, Zeller *et al* showed that treatment of femoropopliteal in-stent restenosis with paclitaxel drug-eluting stents (Zilver-PTX, Cook Medical) resulted in favourable acute and long-term outcomes in 108 patients (mean lesion length 133±91.7mm, 31% Tosaka class III).[21] At six and 12 months, primary patency was 95.7% and 78.8% and freedom from clinically driven target lesion revascularisation was 96.2% and 81%, and 60.8% at 24 months. Fracture rate of stents used in in-stent restenosis lesions was 1.2% at 12 months and a multivariate analysis did not identify any significant predictors of recurrent stenosis. These are encouraging results but further studies will be necessary to compare drug-eluting stents to other technologies.

Moreover, stent grafts such as the Viabahn (Gore) have the potential advantage of excluding the neointima, thereby minimising the likelihood of restenosis within the stented region.[22] In a single-centre series of 27 patients (52% Tosaka class III), the one-year primary patency rate was up to 85.1%.[23] All restenosis events occurred at the stent graft edge, emphasising the importance of avoiding post-dilation outside the edges of the graft and proper sizing to the reference vessel. Moreover, the study did not include the newer version of the Viabahn device with proximal contoured edge to reduce the potential for proximal edge restenosis.

Following those encouraging results, especially when considering the long lesion lengths treated, the RELINE prospective multicentre randomised controlled trial enrolled 39 patients to heparin-bonded Viabahn grafting and 44 patients to plain old balloon angioplasty.[24] Technical success was 100% *versus* 81.8% (bail out stenting 20.5%; p=0.002). The 12-month primary patency rates were 74.8% *versus* 28% (p<0.001). At 24 months, primary patency rates were 58.4% *versus* 11.6% (p<0.001) and freedom from target lesion revascularisation rates were 66.3% *versus* 23% (p<0.001), proving that even in the long run, a mechanical barrier is a promising tool for treatment of in-stent restenosis.[25]

However, in the SALVAGE trial, in which 27 patients (74% with critical limb ischaemia) were treated by excimer laser atherectomy assisted angioplasty and heparin-coated Viabhan stent grafts, the one-year primary patency rate was disappointing (48%, with a majority of edge restenosis) even though there was only a 17% need for target lesion revascularisation and all patients had substantial clinical improvement.[26]

Summary

- In-stent restenosis is a challenging problem.

- Plain old balloon angioplasty may be an acceptable choice for focal, class I in-stent restenosis, but results are suboptimal.

- Drug-coated balloon studies show significantly fewer recurrent in-stent restenosis and target lesion revascularisation up to one year.

- There seems to be a late catch-up phenomenon of recurrent restenosis and this approach is limited in case of elastic recoil or flow-limiting dissection.

- Vessel preparation is the key, even if there is insufficient evidence for now to support routine use of excimer laser atherectomy.

- Adding drug-coated balloon angioplasty to excimer laser atherectomy debulking is a very promising approach.

- Stent grafting could represent another attractive solution, especially in Tosaka class III lesions and long-term randomised controlled trial follow-up are eagerly awaited to further define the role of each approach in the treatment of in-stent restenosis.

References

1. Iida O, *et al.* Long-term outcomes and risk stratification of patency following nitinol stenting in the femoropopliteal segment: retrospective multicenter analysis. *J Endovasc Ther* 2011; **18** (6): 753–61.

2. LaDisa JF, *et al.* Alterations in wall shear stress predict sites of neointimal hyperplasia after stent implantation in rabbit iliac arteries. *Am J Physiol Heart Circ Physiol* 2005; **288** (5): H2465–75.

3. Tosaka A, Soga Y, Iida O, *et al.* Classification and clinical impact of restenosis after femoropopliteal stenting. *J Am Coll Cardiol* 2012; **59** (1): 16–23.

4. Dick P, *et al.* Conventional balloon angioplasty *versus* peripheral cutting balloon angioplasty for treatment of femoropopliteal artery in-stent restenosis: initial experience. *Radiology* 2008; **248** (1): 297–302.

5. Stabile E, *et al.* Drug-eluting balloon for treatment of superficial femoral artery in-stent restenosis. *J Am Coll Cardiol* 2012; **60** (18): 1739–42.

6. Virga V, *et al.* Drug-eluting balloons for the treatment of the superficial femoral artery in-stent restenosis: 2-year follow-up. *JACC Cardiovasc Interv* 2014; **7** (4): 411–15.

7. Liistro F, A, *et al.* Paclitaxel-eluting balloon vs. standard angioplasty to reduce recurrent restenosis in diabetic patients with in-stent restenosis of the superficial femoral and proximal popliteal arteries: the DEBATE-ISR study. *J Endovasc Ther* 2014; **21** (1): 1–8.

8. Grotti S, *et al.* Paclitaxel-eluting balloon vs. standard angioplasty to reduce restenosis in diabetic patients with in-stent restenosis of the superficial femoral and proximal popliteal arteries: Three-year results of the DEBATE-ISR study. *J Endovasc Ther* 2015; **21** (1): 1–8.

9. Krankenberg H, *et al.* Drug-coated balloon *versus* standard balloon for superficial femoral artery in-stent restenosis: The randomized femoral artery in-stent restenosis (FAIR) trial. *Circulation* 2015; **132** (23): 2230–36.

10. Zeller T, Rastan A, Sixt S, *et al.* Long-term results after directional atherectomy of femoro-popliteal lesions. *J Am Coll Cardiol* 2006; **48** (8): 1573–78.

11. Topaz O, *et al.* Alterations of platelet aggregation kinetics with ultraviolet laser emission: the "stunned platelet" phenomenon. *Thromb Haemost* 2001; **86** (4): 1087–93.

12. Schmidt A, *et al.* Photoablation using the turbo-booster and excimer laser for in-stent restenosis treatment: twelve-month results from the PATENT study. *J Endovasc Ther* 2014; **21** (1): 52–60.

13. Shammas NW, S *et al.* Safety and one-year revascularization outcome of excimer laser ablation therapy in treating in-stent restenosis of femoropopliteal arteries: A retrospective review from a single center. *Cardiovasc Revascularization Med Mol Interv* 2012; **13** (6): 341–44.

14. Dippel EJ, *et al.* Randomized controlled study of excimer laser atherectomy for treatment of femoropopliteal in-stent restenosis: initial results from the EXCITE ISR trial. *JACC Cardiovasc Interv* 2015; **8**: 92–101.

15. Van Den Berg JC, *et al.* Endovascular treatment of in-stent restenosis using excimer laser angioplasty and drug eluting balloons. *J Cardiovasc Surg* (Torino) 2012; **53** (2): 215–22.

16. Van den Berg JC. Commentary: laser debulking and drug-eluting balloons for in-stent restenosis: a light at the end of the tunnel? *J Endovasc Ther Off J Int Soc Endovasc Spec* 2013; **20** (6): 815–18.

17. Gandini R, *et al.* Treatment of chronic SFA in-stent occlusion with combined laser atherectomy and drug-eluting balloon angioplasty in patients with critical limb ischemia: a single-center, prospective, randomized study. *J Endovasc Ther* 2013; **20** (6): 805–14.

18. Zeller, T. Photoablative atherectomy followed by a paclitaxel-coated balloon to inhibit restenosis in in stent femoro-popliteal obstructions (PHOTOPAC). ClinicalTrials.gov Identifier: NCT01298947

19. Armstrong EJ, *et al.* Angiographic characteristics of femoropopliteal in-stent restenosis: association with long-term outcomes after endovascular intervention. *Catheter Cardiovasc Interv* 2013; **82** (7): 1168–74.

20. Comparison of angioplasty/drug coated balloon/laser + drug coated balloon for femoropopliteal artery in-stent restenosis (INTACT). ClinicalTrials.gov Identifier: NCT02599389.

21. Zeller T, Dake MD, Tepe G, *et al.* Treatment of femoropopliteal in-stent restenosis with paclitaxel-eluting stents. *JACC Cardiovasc Interv* 2013; **6** (3): 274–81.

22. Doomernik DE, Golchehr B, Lensvelt MMA, *et al.* The role of superficial femoral artery endoluminal bypass in long de novo lesions and in-stent restenosis. *J Cardiovasc Surg* (Torino) 2012; **53** (4): 447–57.

23. Al Shammeri O, *et al.* Viabahn for femoropopliteal in-stent restenosis. *Ann Saudi Med* 2012; **32** (6): 572–82.

24. Bosiers M, Deloose K, Callaert J, *et al.* Superiority of stent-grafts for in-stent restenosis in the superficial femoral artery: twelve-month results from a multicenter randomized trial. *J Endovasc Ther* 2015; **22** (1): 1–10.

25. Deloose K. RELINE-trial : 24 months results with the Viabahn vs PTA for in-stent restenosis. Presented at LINC 2015

26. Laird JR, *et al.* Excimer laser with adjunctive balloon angioplasty and heparin-coated self-expanding stent grafts for the treatment of femoropopliteal artery in-stent restenosis: twelve-month results from the SALVAGE study. *Catheter Cardiovasc Interv* 2012; **80** (5): 852–9.

27. Gouëffic Y. Pacilitaxel eluting balloon application in SFA in-stent restenosis: PLAISIR registry. Presented at LINC 2015

The heparin bonding makes a difference on PTFE femoropopliteal bypass grafts

T Schmitz-Rixen and K Mayer

Introduction

Despite advances in endovascular techniques, vascular surgeons and endovascular specialists acknowledge that the infrainguinal bypass still plays a role in limb salvage. While greater saphenous vein is the best replacement material, the value of alternative autogenous venous conduits for treating critical limb ischaemia with infragenicular bypass surgery is well established.[1] It has been shown that a conduit derived from arm vein is a reasonable alternative in lower-limb bypass surgery.[2] Another alternative to greater saphenous vein is spliced vein consisting of short segments of greater saphenous vein, lesser saphenous vein, arm vein, and at least one anastomosis. The vein must be greater than 2.5mm, and preferably greater than 3mm, as measured by duplex scanning. If greater saphenous vein or alternative vein conduits are not available, prosthetic grafts must be considered. In the femoropopliteal or even crural position, polytetrafluoroethylene (PTFE) is the material of choice. Despite this graft material displaying a long history of good clinical performance above the knee, there is room for improvement. Failure is due to thrombus deposition, poor outflow and anastomotic intimal hyperplasia. One strategy to reduce thrombogenicity is to bind heparin to the prosthetic graft surface. Different heparin coatings are available, based upon different heparin binding modalities. Graft manufacturers claim that their bindings lead to a better "bioactive surface" and better graft performance.[3]

Outcome is based on graft or endovascular treatment patency, limb salvage, infection status, complication rate, life expectancy and quality of life. Short-term patency is an outcome parameter reflecting technical considerations as well as acute graft thrombosis.[4] The ultimate treatment decision to ensure long-term graft patency entails considerations about life quality and shared decision-making. Other issues to consider include site of distal anastomosis, runoff, cardiac performance, renal performance, diabetes, postoperative care of the patient and postoperative wound care.[5]

Faced with a critical limb, the surgeon must ensure pulsatile blood flow to the foot, regardless of which artery is available and the decision to employ a prosthetic graft or vein should be evidence-based. Since heparin-bonded PTFE grafts have shown improved performance over PTFE grafts without heparin, heparinised grafts could possibly be used instead of spliced veins. However, data to evaluate whether heparin-bonded PTFE grafts are viable substitutes for spliced vein grafts is sparse.

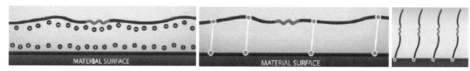

Courtesy of WL Gore & Associates

Figure 1: Types of heparin bonding: (A) Ionic bonding: considered unstable with early wash out. (B) Covalent multi-point bonding: considered to have limited bioactivity. (C) Endpoint covalent bonding: considered stable with long-term bioactivity. Data comparing the three types of bonding are not available.

Heparin-bonded grafts

A variety of different technologies for attaching heparin to a graft inner surface have been developed. Some grafts allow heparin to elute as a soluble drug, while others keep heparin surface bound (see Figure 1). According to the manufacturer, endpoint covalent bonding maintains heparin's anticoagulant activity best and longest, and comparative biochemical data are available. Experimental data have convincingly shown better thromboresistance and sustained heparin activity over six months.[5] In experimental models, heparin also inhibits intimal hyperplasia, possibly explaining part of its mode of action.[6]

Using an ionic bonding graft, investigators were able to achieve significantly better patency with heparin-bonded Dacron grafts over PTFE grafts in 209 femoropopliteal bypass grafts after three years. In this randomised controlled trial, the difference was no longer apparent after five years.[7]

In Scandinavia, a large, independent prospective randomised controlled demonstrated significantly enhanced patency of an endpoint covalent heparin-bonded PTFE graft (Carmeda BioActive Surface technology PTFE graft or CBAS-PTFE graft) over a standard PTFE graft. The greatest benefit was to patients with critical limb ischaemia, and occurred only after six months and sustained over the study period.[8] These findings have led the authors to focus on CBAS-PTFE grafts (Figure 2) in clinical practice and in this report.

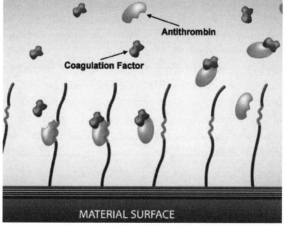

Courtesy of WL Gore & Associates

Figure 2: Possible mechanism of action of the CBAS-PTFE graft: Heparin´s anticoagulatory action requires antithrombin to bind to an active sequence within the heparin molecule. Heparin binding to antithrombin greatly accelerates the antithrombin neutralisation of coagulant factors. Heparin, due to the stable covalent bonding, is neither consumed nor destroyed, remaining available for the next reaction on the graft surface.

Results

An evaluation of overall primary patency rates[9,10] has revealed that the CBAS-PTFE graft has a one-year primary patency of 76%, falling between non-heparin-bonded PTFE grafts (60%) and vein grafts (79%). The CBAS-PTFE graft continues to perform better than the non-heparin-bonded PTFE graft, but worse than the vein graft at two, three and four years. It is clear that heparin-bonded grafts perform better than non-heparin-bonded grafts. Whether the better performance is due to the anticoagulatory effect of heparin or to diminished intimal hyperplasia is not clear. The question remains as to whether these grafts perform better than arm veins or spliced veins, which perform better than non-heparin-bonded grafts.

An arm vein is considered the last autogenous option for infrainguinal bypass surgery. In 2007, investigators examined the efficacy of arm vein as a last autogenous option before use of a synthetic conduit in a prospective database to identify infrainguinal arm vein bypasses performed between 1997 and 2005. The investigators identified 37 arm vein bypasses and determined patency, limb salvage and survival data. No perioperative deaths were found in the cohort. The 30-day primary patency rate was 89%, secondary patency was 95% and limb salvage was 95%. At 12 months, the primary patency was 56%, secondary patency was 79% and limb salvage was 91%. Five-year primary patency was 37%, secondary patency was 76% and limb salvage was 91%. The investigators reported no significant patency advantage for primary *versus* "redo" grafts, single vessel *versus* spliced conduits, or popliteal *versus* tibial outflow. The patients had a 92% survival rate at one year and a 65% survival rate at five years. Lower-limb bypasses using arm vein were found to have favourable patency and limb salvage when compared to synthetic conduits.[2] The investigators noted, however, that arm vein bypasses frequently required secondary intervention to maintain patency.[2]

An additional study evaluated 30-day patency of all conduit configurations used for infrapopliteal bypass.[4] The investigators examined all primary infrapopliteal bypasses from the American College of Surgeons' National Surgical Quality Improvement Program database between 2005 and 2010 (n=5,375). Patients from the database were divided into six groups: 1) great saphenous vein (75%); 2) prosthetic conduit (17%); 3) prosthetic conduit with a distal anastomotic venous adjunct (2%); 4) composite graft of prosthetic and vein segments (2%); 5) spliced autogenous vein (3%); and 6) arm vein (2%). No differences in demographics and comorbidities were found among the groups and perioperative mortality rates were similar for the different conduits. Adjusted for age, sex, weight, race and previous cardiac surgery, it was found that the bypass conduit had a significant independent association with 30-day graft patency (p=0.006). No significant difference in the 30-day failure rate between spliced vein (5.6%) or arm vein (4.3%) conduits, compared to greater saphenous vein (7.5%), was found. Prosthetic grafts had a significantly higher 30-day failure rate than greater saphenous vein (10.5%, p=0.004). No significant difference in graft patency between alternative venous conduits and prosthetic plus anastomotic venous cuff was apparent. The investigators concluded that vein conduits (great saphenous vein, spliced vein and arm vein) together deliver the best 30-day patency for infrapopliteal bypasses.[4] In contrast, prosthetic grafts had a higher 30-day failure rate. The researchers also suggested that composite grafts be abandoned since early patency is not superior to that of pure prosthetic grafts.[4]

A long-term follow-up (median of 58 months) of 38 infrainguinal bypass surgeries performed using arm vein found that the surgery was safe with favourable patency and high rates of limb salvage.[11] At 12 months, the investigators reported 52% primary patency, 73% assisted primary patency and 76% secondary patency. The investigators also pointed out that vigilant surveillance is important in this patient population, and that secondary interventions are commonly required to maintain patency.[11]

A direct comparison of arm vein *versus* prosthetic graft for infrapopliteal bypasses for critical limb ischaemia showed that even when spliced, arm vein conduits were superior to prosthetic grafts with regard to midterm assisted primary patency, secondary patency and limb salvage.[12] Patients were evaluated for a median of 35 months. The two patient groups (arm vein and prosthetic graft) were similar, except that cerebrovascular disease was more common in the prosthetic group.[12] Prior to that, the group had published their experience with a polyester mesh facilitating the use of non-optimal vein grafts.[13] This multicentre study reported that the mesh was a safe and feasible adjunct to peripheral revascularisation and resulted in acceptable short-term patency. The investigators suggest that external scaffolding of infrainguinal vein grafts may be a promising innovation.[13]

Peripheral arterial disease treatment policy

When all data are analysed, it appears that there is a role for the CBAS-PTFE graft in treating claudication and non-infected critical limb ischaemia. With claudication, the CBAS-PTFE graft is indicated when endovascular treatment is not feasible or has failed. It is also indicated if there is no ipsilateral vein for above-knee bypass and a minimum of two-vessel runoff. With critical limb ischaemia, the CBAS-PTFE graft is likewise indicated when endovascular intervention is not feasible or has failed. The CBAS-PTFE graft is also indicated for patients with no ipsilateral vein, no contralateral vein and no lesser saphenous vein or arm vein. Patients who are under dual anti-aggregation therapy and have more than one vessel runoff are also candidates for the CBAS-PTFE graft, due to lesser harvest trauma.[14] Patients with critical limb ischaemia and a foot or limb infection should not receive an endpoint covalent bonded heparin PTFE graft.

Comparative series

Our group performed a retrospective analysis of patients who received surgical bypass as a treatment for peripheral arterial disease between January 2011 and July 2014. The surgical bypasses were performed in a tertiary referral centre by six vascular surgeons, experienced in open surgery and endovascular procedures (five surgeons were fellows-in-training). Patients were followed for three years. There were 324 thromboendarterectomies with patch angioplasty. The series included 264 bypasses over three years with the majority (n=141) performed with a vein conduit. Only a small number of patients had good-quality greater saphenous vein. Sixteen patients received alternative autologous veins and 107 patients received prosthetic grafts. Of these patients, 80 received the CBAS-PTFE graft. Within this group of patients, the CBAS-PTFE graft was implanted above-knee (n=5), below-knee popliteal artery (n=21), femoral-crural bypass (n=51), popliteal-pedal (n=1), popliteal 1–3 (n=1) and bypass-interposition (n=1). There were more redo

Bonding Technology	Graft Material	Brand Name
Ionic	Polyester + Collagen	MAQUET INTERGARD Heparin
Covalent	PTFE	PEROUSE POLYMAILLE® Flow Plus Heparin
Covalent	PTFE	JOTEC FLOWLINE BIPORE® Heparin
Covalent	PTFE/PET	MAQUET FUSION BIOLINE Heparin
End-point Covalent	PTFE	GORE® PROPATEN® Vascular Graft

Table: Bonding technology of different graft materials.

(n=38) than primary bypasses (n=34). Many primary bypasses were performed following failed endovascular procedures. The CBAS-PTFE graft was used for two different indications: claudication (n=8) and non-infected critical limb ischaemia (n=67). Five additional patients were treated for acute ischaemia. There were several common comorbidities: diabetes (67%), severe cardiac problems (44%) and dialysis (22%). Postoperatively, patients were prescribed dual anti-aggregation therapy (acetylsalicylic acid and clopidogrel) for at least six months. All patients had already received anticoagulatory therapy for other reasons.

During the study period, there were 25 failed grafts in the below-knee popliteal artery and femoral-crural groups, including three infected grafts requiring explant. There were no problems with the other grafts. Graft failure resulted in 10 major amputations. A closer examination of overall below-knee bypasses revealed one and two-year patency of 69% and 65%, respectively. Thus, most failures occurred during the first year. Patients who received alternative veins had an 81% patency rate in the first year and a 75% patency rate in the second year. Complication rates were low for both groups. There were no differences in wound-healing complications and cardiac complications between patients who received the CBAS-PTFE graft and those who received spliced vein. However, there was one death in the CBAS-PTFE graft group related to graft infection.

Conclusion

Our goal is to facilitate personalised medicine for patients with peripheral arterial disease. Patients with non-infected claudication are treated with endovascular therapy whenever possible. Long occlusions and ultimately failed endovascular therapy are treated with bypass surgery. Patients with critical limb ischaemia who have an infection are primarily treated with endovascular therapy and secondarily with biologic surgical intervention. The treatment approach used at our facility delivers results falling within the expected range and is consistent with published data. The next step is to extend the analysis of peripheral arterial disease treatment policy to a nationwide registry.

Summary

- Experimental data and several non-randomised trials indicate that heparin-bonded grafts are superior to standard grafts in terms of patency.

- A single prospective, independent randomised controlled trial showed superiority of CBAS-PTFE graft over standard PTFE graft.

- Results with CBAS-PTFE grafts equal results with spliced or arm vein grafts and could serve as an alternative in peripheral arterial disease treatment.

- Autologous greater saphenous vein remains the gold standard in peripheral bypass grafting.

References

1. Brochado Neto F, Sandri GA, Kalaf MJ, *et al*. Arm vein as an alternative autogenous conduit for infragenicular bypass in the treatment of critical limb ischaemia: a 15 year experience. *Eur J Vasc Endovasc Surg* 2014; **47** (6): 609–14.

2. Varcoe RL, Chee W, Subramaniam P, *et al*. Arm vein as a last autogenous option for infrainguinal bypass surgery: it is worth the effort. *Eur J Vasc Endovasc Surg* 2007; **33** (6): 737–41.

3. Begovac PC, Thomson RC, Fisher JL, *et al*. Improvements in GORE-TEX Vascular Graft Performance by Carmeda BioActive Surface Heparin Immobilization. *Eur J Vasc Endovasc Surg* 2003; **25**: 432–37.

4. Nguyen BN, Neville RF, Abugideiri M, *et al*. The effect of graft configuration on 30-day failure of infrapopliteal bypasses. *J Vasc Surg* 2014; **59** (4): 1003–08.

5. Najafian A, Selvarajah S, Schneider EB *et al*. Thirty-day readmission after lower extremity bypass in diabetic patients. *J Surg Res* 2016; **200** (1): 356–64.

6. Lin PH1, Chen C, Bush RL *et al*. Small-caliber heparin-coated ePTFE grafts reduce platelet deposition and neointimal hyperplasia in a baboon model. *J Vasc Surg* 2004; **39** (6): 1322–28.

7. Devine C, McCollum C. North West femoro-popliteal trial participants heparin-bonded Dacron or polytetrafluoroethylene for femoropopliteal bypass: five-year results of a prospective randomized multicenter clinical trial. *J Vasc Surg* 2004; **40** (5): 924–31.

8. Lindholt JS, Gottschalksen B, Johannesen N, *et al*. The Scandinavian Propaten trial - 1-year patency of PTFE vascular prostheses with heparin-bonded luminal surfaces compared to ordinary pure PTFE vascular prostheses - a randomised clinical controlled multi-centre trial. *Eur J Vasc Endovasc Surg* 2011; **41** (5): 668–73.

9. Ten years of experience with the heparin-bonded ePTFE graft - the newest advancement in vascular surgery. *Vascular Disease Management* 2010; **7** (9) Supplement: 3–27.

10. Neville R, Recknor J. Bound to perform: GORE PROPATEN Vascular Graft and CBAS heparin surface technology. *Endovascular Today* 2014; **13** (6) Supplement: 3–6.

11. Robinson DR, Varcoe RL, Chee W, *et al*. Long-term follow-up of last autogenous option arm vein bypass. *ANZ J Surg* 2013; **83** (10): 769–73.

12. Arvela E, Soderstrom M, Alback A, *et al*. Arm vein conduit vs prosthetic graft in infrainguinal revascularization for critical leg ischemia. *J Vasc Surg* 2010; **52** (3): 616–23.

13. Arvela E, Kauhanen P, Alback A, *et al*. Initial experience with a new method of external polyester scaffolding for infrainguinal vein grafts. *Eur J Vasc Endovasc Surg* 2009; **38** (4): 456–62.

14. Avgerinos ED, Sachdev U, Naddaf A *et al*. Autologous alternative veins may not provide better outcomes than prosthetic conduits for below-knee bypass when great saphenous vein is unavailable. *J Vasc Surg* 2015; **62** (2): 385–91.

Popliteal aneurysm

Popliteal aneurysm sac volume shrinkage after stent graft

M Antonello, M Menegolo and M Piazza

Introduction

Popliteal artery aneurysm is the most frequent peripheral aneurysm.[1] Typically, it is asymptomatic, but when symptoms arise, the risk of limb loss can be as high as 40%.[2] Surgery is indicated when aneurysm diameter is more than 20mm; otherwise, a symptomatic aneurysm must be repaired regardless of its size.[3] Open repair is still considered the gold standard;[4] however, advantages of a mini-invasive approach have led to a significant increase in the amount of endovascular popliteal artery aneurysm repairs. In the US Medicare population, endovascular popliteal artery aneurysm repair rose significantly between 2005 and 2007, from 11.7% to 23.6% (p<0.0001). Moreover different experiences comparing endovascular popliteal artery aneurysm repair *versus* open repair, including a randomised study, demonstrated comparable outcomes in terms of patency and limb salvage rate.[5] Early and mid-term outcomes of endovascular popliteal artery aneurysm repair have been well described,[6–8] but there are still few data regarding long-term results. In a tabular review, Tsilimparis *et al*[9] reported 87% average (range 67–100%) three-year primary assisted patency and 85% (range 82–100%) secondary patency. Similarly, Pulli *et al*,[8] in a multicentre study of 134 endovascular popliteal artery aneurysm repair patients, reported a primary patency of 73.4% at 48-month follow-up and a secondary patency of 85% with a long-term primary patency at five years of 76% and a primary assisted and secondary patency of 79% and 82%, respectively. Moreover, it is not clear which is the real incidence of endoleak and which is the fate of the aneurismal sac after the endovascular exclusion. Some studies have described residual patent branches mimicking type II endoleak after open surgical repair;[10] none have evaluated the impact of endovascular popliteal artery aneurysm repair in relation to exclusion efficacy. Knowing if the popliteal artery aneurysm sac shrank after exclusion, just as an abdominal aortic aneurysm does after repair, or if it continued to exert compression in the limited popliteal fossa space even after the aneurysm has been perfectly excluded is a controversial and extremely relevant point that may influence the future of endovascular popliteal artery aneurysm repair.

Description

The aim of this retrospective study was to report on the long-term outcomes of endovascular popliteal artery aneurysm repair focusing on patency and limb salvage rates, and also to identify predictors of patency. Long-term sac volume shrinkage was analysed to assess durability and efficacy of endovascular popliteal artery aneurysm repair in aneurysmal exclusion. A retrospective review of all patients admitted to the

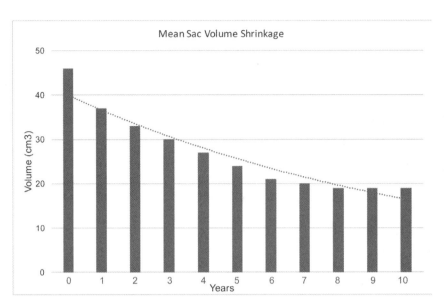

Figure 1: Mean sac volume shrinkage during the follow-up period.

Vascular and Endovascular Surgery Clinic of Padua who underwent endovascular popliteal artery aneurysm repair between January 2006 and December 2015 was carried out. Demographic information, preoperative characteristics, perioperative outcomes, and follow-up data including all medical records and invasive and non-invasive diagnostic procedures were reviewed. Popliteal aneurysm sac volume was estimated in all cases from a 1mm computed tomography (CT) angiogram using a dedicated software (Osirix Pro 4s). To standardise volume computation ensuring homogeneous measurements, the calculation was performed, starting from the beginning to the end of the dilatation without considering the proximal and the distal landing zone. A three-dimensional volume change of 5% or more was considered significant following Society of Vascular Surgery standards.[11] The overall sac volume shrinkage during follow-up was evaluated as the mean of values. The efficacy of the exclusion was calculated as the time needed for 50% sac shrinkage during the follow-up in four groups stratified on the basis of preoperative mean volume (<30mL; 30–60mL; 60–90mL; >90mL).

Inclusion criteria:

- All asymptomatic popliteal artery aneurysms with a diameter ≥2cm on the CT angiogram
- At least one patent tibial artery or a distal run-off score of <8 according to the Society for Vascular Surgery/International Society for Cardiovascular Surgery[12]
- A proximal and distal landing zone with a length of >1.5cm.

Exclusion criteria:

- Age <50 years old
- History of thrombophilia
- Contraindication to antiplatelet, anticoagulant, or thrombolytic therapy.

Operative technique

Stent length and diameter were measured on the preoperative CT angiogram; an oversizing of about 10–15% maximum was performed to ensure an adequate sealing of the endograft. The coverage length was confirmed at the intraoperative angiogram; the landing zones were always above the upper margin of the patella and well below to the level of the knee joint to avoid any bending between the endograft and artery especially during leg flexion. If multiple stent grafts were required to seal the popliteal artery aneurysm, the endografts were made to overlap by at least 1.5cm. No more than three grafts were deployed with a diameter discrepancy between them of maximum 2mm (e.g. 8mm endograft inside a 6mm). The endograft was deployed using an antegrade access from the common femoral artery. Post-procedural digital subtraction angiography in anterior and lateral projection with a knee flexion >120 degrees were always performed to confirm popliteal artery aneurysm exclusion the conformability of the endograft and to identify any signs of kinking or endoleak. The endograft used in all cases was the Viabahn (Gore); from 2010 to date, the new heparin bonded-Viabahn was adopted.

The postoperative therapy includes a double antiplatelet therapy with aspirin (100mg daily) and clopidogrel (75mg daily) for three months; thereafter, patients were prescribed aspirin alone indefinitely.

The mean follow-up was 46±31 months (range 3–120 months); four patients were lost after a follow-up period of respectively of 12, 18, 30, 48 months. All patients underwent a duplex ultrasound and ankle-brachial index measurement the day before discharge. Follow-up appointments included a complete physical examination, a duplex ultrasound and ankle-brachial index measurements at one, six, and 12 months during the first year and annually thereafter. All patients underwent CT angiogram with early and delayed phase and plain radiograph of the knee joint with forced leg flexion (>120 degrees) to evaluate patency, stent skeleton integrity, flexibility, and sac volume once a year. Long-term patency and limb salvage were determined in concordance with the Society for Vascular Surgery/International Society for Cardiovascular Surgery guidelines.[12]

Statistical analysis

The mean and standard deviation of sac volume, thrombus volumes, and diameters before and after surgery were compared using a two-sample T-test. The Kaplan-Meier life-table method was used to calculate patency and survival. The predictive value of the different variables was assessed using the multivariate Cox proportional hazards model. A p value <0.05 was considered statistically significant.

Results

Thirty-four patients underwent endovascular popliteal artery aneurysm repair; two of these were bilateral, so a total of 36 limbs were treated. The mean maximum preoperative aneurysm sac diameter was 3.4±0.68cm, while the mean aneurysm sac volume was 45.6±3.7mL with a range from 28mL to 133mL. There was a 100% technical success rate. In five of 10 cases in whom the covered length was >20cm and the distal landing zone was in the middle of the below-knee popliteal artery, the final intraoperative angiogram with knee flexion showed a bending between the endograft and the artery. In all cases, an adjunctive stent-graft was successfully deployed within 1cm of the anterior tibial artery origin solving the problem. No perioperative deaths were reported. There was one early occlusion that was treated successfully after thrombolysis and a percutaneous transluminal angioplasty of the posterior tibial artery. At 30 days, there was a 97% primary patency rate with a 100% of secondary patency and limb salvage rate.

The Kaplan-Meier analysis showed a primary patency at five years of 78%, while the secondary patency was 88% respectively. The long-term overall survival rate was 89%, while limb salvage was 98%. Two patients were identified and treated before occlusion during the follow-up period: one was asymptomatic and developed 80% stenosis in the distal landing zone discovered during a duplex ultrasound examination, the other one had a severe proximal restenosis; both were succesfully treated with percutaneous transluminal angioplasty. A stent fracture without loss of patency was found in one case (3%) on plain radiograph of the knee joint after two-year follow-up. The multivariate analysis for patency after endovascular popliteal artery aneurysm repair showed that the only negative predictors for patency was a covered artery length >20cm (hazard ratio [HR] 2.7; 95% confidence interval [CI] 0.2; ratio limit of 8.2; p=0.032); distal landing zone site close to the origin of the anterior tibial artery appear to be a positive predictor of patency only at the univariate analysis. Stent graft diameter and aneurysm sac size (diameter and volume) did not appear to be related to long-term primary patency. Overall, aneurysm sac volume shrank from 45.6±3.7mL to 22.5±4.8mL during the follow-up period (Figure 1); the shrinkage was significant (p<0.001) with a 25.9±5.6mL (95% confidence interval [CI] 18.1–22.9) difference between the means. In five cases, there was no shrinkage over time (14%). Sac shrinkage, as shown in Figure 2 was faster for small aneurysms (<30cm³) and reaches a plateau after seven years.

There were three endoleaks (8%): two type II and one type I. The type II endoleak resolved spontaneously within six and 12 months of surgery; the type I endoleak, presenting 12 months after endovascular popliteal artery aneurysm repair due to a distal upward stent dislodgement, was treated by deploying a distal extension of

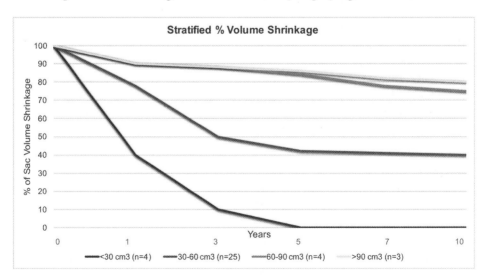

Figure 2: Rate of sac volume shrinkage during the follow-up period.

the endograft close to the origin of the anterior tibial artery. Endoleak appears not to affect sac volume shrinkage rate; as well the percentage of thrombus volume in the aneurysm sac.

Conclusion

Endovascular popliteal artery aneurysm repair in asymptomatic selected popliteal artery aneurysms appears to be a valid alternative to open repair with comparable patency and limb salvage rate even during the long run. Type II endoleak was an uncommon finding after the endograft deployment with a rate of about 5% and it disappeared spontaneously without suspending the antiplatelet therapy. Moreover they do not seem to affect sac shrinkage (p=0.877). The only case with sac growth in this group of patients was one with a type Ib endoleak, which occurred after 12 months. These findings are consistent with those of Midy *et al*,[13] who described six endoleaks in a sample of 57 (10.5%) treated limbs, all type I and III, and all as a consequence of stent malfunctioning. The results of this study confirm the optimal performance of endovascular popliteal artery aneurysm repair not only in terms of patency and limb salvage rate, but also in favouring sac volume shrinkage. In fact, five years after endovascular popliteal artery aneurysm repair, a reduction of 25.9±5.6mL (95% CI 18.1–22.9) in mean popliteal artery aneurysm volume was observed. This study has some limitations that are worthy of mention. This was a retrospective, non-randomised study with a small cohort of patients. Nevertheless, all patients were accurately selected with a careful and complete follow-up comprehensive of adequate imaging, allowing robust and exhaustive assessment of patency and sac volume shrinkage in the long term.

Summary

- Endovascular popliteal artery aneurysm repair is a valid, mini-invasive alternative to open repair with the great saphenous vein in the treatment of asymptomatic selected popliteal artery aneurysms.

- Results are comparable in terms of patency and limb salvage rate.

- Incidence of endoleak is relatively rare with a rate of about 5% for type II, which always disappear spontaneously within one year.

- Shrinkage of the popliteal artery aneurysm sac after endovascular exclusion is a continuous and effective phenomenon that reaches a plateau after seven years.

- Type II endoleak seems not to affect aneurysmal sac shrinkage.

References

1. Johnson, ON 3rd, Slidell, MB, Macsata, RA, *et al.* Outcomes of surgical management for popliteal artery aneurysms: an analysis of 583 cases. *J Vasc Surg* 2008; **48**: 845–51.
2. Mahmood, A, Salaman, R, Sintler, M, *et al.* Surgery of popliteal artery aneurysms: a 12-year experience. *J Vasc Surg* 2003; **37**: 586–93.
3. Lowell, RC, Gloviczki, P, Hallett, JW Jr, *et al.* Popliteal artery aneurysms: the risk of nonoperative management. *Ann Vasc Surg* 1994; **8**: 14–23.

4. Huang, Y, Gloviczki, P, Noel, AA, *et al*. Early complications and long-term outcome after open surgical treatment of popliteal artery aneurysms: is exclusion with saphenous vein bypass still the gold standard? *J Vasc Surg* 2007; **45**: 706–13.

5. Antonello, M, Frigatti, P, Battocchio, P, *et al*. Open repair *versus* endovascular treatment for asymptomatic popliteal artery aneurysm: results of a prospective randomized study. *J Vasc Surg* 2005; **42**: 185–93.

6. Antonello, M, Frigatti, P, Battocchio, P, *et al*. Endovascular treatment of asymptomatic popliteal aneurysms: 8-year concurrent comparison with open repair. *J Cardiovasc Surg* (Torino) 2007; **48**: 267–74.

7. Garg, K, Rockman, CB, Kim, BJ, *et al*. Outcome of endovascular repair of popliteal artery aneurysm using the Viabahn endoprosthesis. *J Vasc Surg* 2012; **55**: 1647–53.

8. Pulli, R, Dorigo, W, Castelli, P, *et al*. A multicentric experience with open surgical repair and endovascular exclusion of popliteal artery aneurysms. *Eur J Vasc Endovasc Surg* 2013; 45: 357–63.

9. Tsilimparis, N, Dayama, A, and Ricotta, JJ 2nd. Open and endovascular repair of popliteal artery aneurysms: tabular review of the literature. *Ann Vasc Surg* 2013; **27**: 259–65.

10. Mehta, M, Champagne, B, Darling, RC 3rd, *et al*. Outcome of popliteal artery aneurysms after exclusion and bypass: significance of residual patent branches mimicking type II endoleaks. *J Vasc Surg* 2004; 40: 886–90.

11. Johnston, KW, Rutherford, RB, Tilson, MD, *et al*. Suggested standards for reporting on arterial aneurysms. Subcommittee on reporting standards for arterial aneurysms, Ad Hoc Committee on reporting standards, SVS/ISCVS. *J Vasc Surg* 1991; **13**: 452–58.

12. Rutherford, RB, Baker, JD, Ernst, C, *et al*. Recommended standards for reports dealing with lower extremity ischemia: revised version. *J Vasc Surg* 1997; **26**: 517–38.

13. Midy, D, Berard, X, Ferdani, M, *et al*. A retrospective multicenter study of endovascular treatment of popliteal artery aneurysm. *J Vasc Surg* 2010; **51**: 850–06.

Below the knee

The angiosome concept in the treatment of critical limb ischaemia

M Venermo, K Spillerova and N Settembre

Introduction

The ultimate aim of revascularisation of a critically ischaemic foot with a tissue lesion is to increase arterial circulation and perfusion pressure, thereby enhancing the wound healing capacity. Multiple studies in the vascular literature support the primary idea that, without pulsatile flow into the ischaemic region in the foot, the wound does not heal. Indeed, as many as 10–18% of ischaemic wounds fail to heal despite good bypass patency or successful endovascular treatment, leading to frustrating major amputations.[1–5] The question of defining the optimal region of the foot that should be revascularised has become a topic of discussion, and the so-called angiosome theory has gained popularity, but also resistance, among vascular surgeons.

In 1987, Taylor defined the angiosome principles in his landmark anatomy study in the field of reconstructive plastic surgery. He divided the body into three-dimensional anatomic units of tissue—"arteriosomes"—which were supplied by a specific source of arteries.[6] In 2006, Attinger, in turn, divided the foot into six angiosome regions supplied by the three main crural arteries and their branches.[7] In vascular surgery, the presented angiosome concept targets the revascularisation onto the site of the tissue lesion to improve healing.[8,9] This entails that direct revascularisation of an artery feeding the area of the foot affected by an ischaemic tissue lesion is expected to have a better chance of clinical success than revascularisation of any other artery not directly feeding the affected anatomical area. Recently, several retrospective studies comparing angiosome-targeted *versus* non-angiosome-targeted endovascular revascularisation have been carried out, showing promising results in terms of wound healing and limb salvage in favour of targeted revascularisation, especially in the diabetic foot.

Review of the literature

The majority of the patients in the studies on the angiosome concept have been treated with endovascular revascularisation, and the studies with patients who have undergone surgical bypass are few. A systematic review and meta-analysis of angiosome-targeted lower limb revascularisation, published in 2013, included nine studies with a total of 715 legs treated by direct revascularisation according to the angiosome principle and 575 legs treated by indirect revascularisation. Two of the

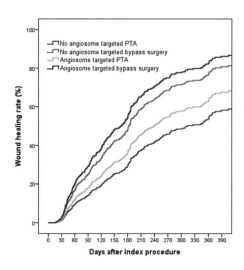

Figure 1: Adjusted Cox proportional hazards estimates of wound healing according to treatment method and angiosome targeted revascularisation (p<0.0001) (Published by permission of Elsevier. Original publication: Spillerova K *et al.* Differential Impact of Bypass Surgery and Angioplasty on Angiosome-Targeted Infrapopliteal Revascularization. *Eur J Vasc Endovasc Surg* 2015; **49** (4): 412–9.)

studies, with a combined 140 patients, included both surgical and endovascular revascularisations, four studies included only endovascular patients with a total of 874 procedures, and two studies included only surgical bypasses with a total of 276 limbs. No randomised controlled studies were available. Both wound healing (four studies included, hazard ratio [HR] 0.64 for unhealed wound, favouring direct revascularisation) and leg salvage (eight studies included, HR for major amputation 0.44, favouring direct revascularisation) were significantly better after direct than indirect revascularisation. The pooled limb salvage rates after direct and indirect revascularisations were 86.2% *versus* 77.8% at one year and 84.9% *versus* 70.1% at two years, respectively. The analysis of three studies reporting only on patients with diabetes confirmed the benefit of direct revascularisation in terms of limb salvage (HR 0.48, 95% confidence interval [CI] 0.31–0.75).

One of the few studies on surgical revascularisations is by Azuma *et al* (2012),[11] including 228 patients (81% being diabetics and 49% having end-stage renal disease) and 249 consecutive limbs with critical limb ischaemia and tissue loss. Bypasses were performed on the crural artery in 57% and on the pedal artery in 43% of the cases. Complete healing of ischaemic wounds was achieved in 85% of the cases. The strongest negative predictors for wound healing were end-stage renal disease, diabetes and Rutherford category 6 with a heel ulcer/gangrene. After adjustment with propensity score analysis, the healing rates of the direct and indirect groups were similar, but wound healing was slower in the indirect group. The authors concluded that, in the field of bypass surgery, the angiosome concept seems unimportant, at least in non-end-stage renal disease cases. The location and extent of ischaemic wounds as well as comorbidities may be more relevant than the angiosome in terms of wound healing.

Indeed, in the light of published retrospective studies, there may be some differences between endovascular and surgical revascularisation in the importance of an angiosome-targeted approach. The largest study comparing direct with indirect revascularisation is from Helsinki University Hospital published in 2015, including 744 consecutive patients who underwent infrapopliteal endovascular (n=502) or surgical revascularisation (n=242).[12] We compared wound healing and leg salvage as well as survival and amputation-free survival between 408 patients who underwent targeted revascularisation (265 endovascular, 143 surgical

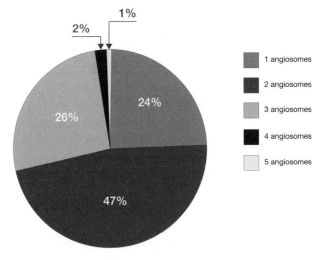

1%

2%

24%

26%

47%

- 1 angiosomes
- 2 angiosomes
- 3 angiosomes
- 4 angiosomes
- 5 angiosomes

Figure 2: The number of angiosomes affected by tissue lesion in legs with critical limb ischaemia. Original publication: Spillerova K. The Feasibility of Angiosome-Targeted Endovascular Treatment in Patients with Critical Limb Ischemia and Foot Ulcer. *Ann Vasc Surg* 2016; **30**: 270–76.

bypasses) and 336 patients who underwent non-targeted revascularisation (237 endovascular and 99 surgical) due to critical limb ischaemia and a tissue lesion. The differences between the study groups (targeted vs. non-targeted) were adjusted by estimating a propensity score. In Cox proportional hazards analysis, we found angiosome-targeted revascularisation, C-reactive protein ≤10mg/dL, and the number of affected angiosomes to be independent predictors of wound healing. Interestingly, there was a positive impact of angiosome-targeted bypass surgery on wound healing when compared with angiosome-targeted angioplasty. Furthermore, non-angiosome-targeted bypass surgery achieved better wound healing rates than angioplasty independently of the angiosome-oriented strategy (Figure 1). In Cox analysis regarding leg salvage, an increasing number of affected angiosomes, atrial fibrillation, C-reactive protein >10mg/dL, chronic kidney disease class 5, and non-angiosome-targeted revascularisation were independent predictors of major amputation. When the differences between the four subgroups were analysed using a regression model, non-angiosome-targeted angioplasty was associated with the highest risk of major amputation. After matching of the baseline and operative characteristics using a propensity score between patients who underwent angiosome-targeted *versus* non-targeted revascularisation, we were able to analyse 252 pairs forming two similar groups. When these groups were compared, angiosome-targeted revascularisation was associated with significantly better leg salvage and a trend towards improved wound healing. When adjusted for propensity score and treatment method (bypass surgery vs. angioplasty), angiosome-targeted revascularisation was associated with a significantly higher wound healing rate. When treatment strategy (i.e. bypass surgery vs. angioplasty) was included in this regression model, bypass surgery yielded a lower risk of major amputation. If only patients who underwent angiosome-targeted revascularisation were included in the analysis, the propensity score-adjusted analysis revealed that bypass surgery was associated with a significantly better rate of wound healing. However, angioplasty and bypass surgery achieved similar leg salvage rates.

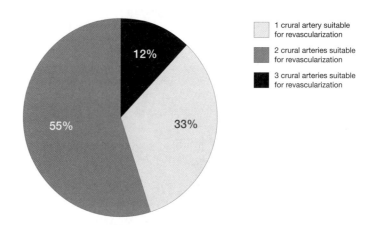

1 crural artery suitable for revascularization

2 crural arteries suitable for revascularization

3 crural arteries suitable for revascularization

Figure 3: Feasibility of the angiosome concept. Number of crural vessels suitable for revascularisation in patients with ischaemic tissue lesion and crural peripheral arterial occlusive disease.

Feasibility of the angiosome concept

Although current literature suggests that angiosome-targeted revascularisation leads to a better clinical outcome, the feasibility of this tactic has not been clear. Critical limb ischaemia patients usually have widespread atherosclerosis with long occlusions in several crural vessels. In most of the cases, there are not many arteries to choose from for the revascularisation. Furthermore, the wound may span several angiosomes. We performed a retrospective study to answer the following questions: in how many cases is angiosome-targeted revascularisation really possible? How often can the target vessel be chosen? And in how many cases does the wound spread over several angiosomes? To answer these questions, a feasibility study was set up aiming to determine the wound location according to the angiosome concept and to investigate the feasibility and success of angiosome-based revascularisation in below-the-knee arteries. We reviewed 161 legs with ischaemic ulcers and found that the wound(s) interfered with one angiosome in only 24% of the cases (Figure 2).[13] If the ulceration was limited to one or two angiosomes, targeted revascularisation was possible in 80% of the cases; when four angiosomes were affected, the rate dropped to 25%; and if the ulceration extended over five angiosomes, revascularisation was not possible. In one third of the legs, there was only one crural artery that was suitable to revascularisation (Figure 3). Angiosome-targeted revascularisation was not performed, although it was possible in 31 cases. In 14/31 legs, it was attempted without success and in 11/31 legs it was deemed to be too long occlusion (more suitable for bypass), resulting in another vessel being revascularised. In the end, direct flow into the affected angiosomes was successfully achieved in 98 (60.9%) cases.

Ongoing study

We have received some interesting preliminary data for our prospective study at Helsinki University Hospital. We are prospectively collecting data on patients who undergo either surgical or endovascular revascularisation of a crural vessel due to critical limb ischaemia and a tissue lesion. The details of the wounds are recorded, including photography at each follow-up visit and wound healing details as well as angiograms and all revascularisation procedures. Furthermore, we are measuring the tissue perfusion before and after revascularisation in each angiosome using indocyanine green fluorescence imaging. The analysis of the data for 34 patients shows that the increase in perfusion in the angiosomes that have been revascularised directly is higher in comparison to those that have been revascularised indirectly. The increase after the revascularisation is poorest in the angiosomes that have been revascularised indirectly with an endovascular procedure. The preliminary results are in line with the wound healing results from our retrospective study.

Conclusion

The results of the studies available strongly suggest that there is benefit to be gained from opting for angiosome-targeted revascularisation as opposed to a non-targeted approach. However, the studies are retrospective and mainly do not consider the role of significant collaterals to the wound area nor the wound classification. Furthermore, most of the studies include endovascular procedures only or both without a separate analysis of endovascular compared to surgical revascularisation. Most of the studies define the approach as targeted revascularisation if at least one of the angiosomal arteries is open after angioplasty, without paying attention to which of the arteries is the major source for the affected area. In the light of current knowledge, the angiosome concept is promising in the treatment of critical limb ischaemia with a tissue lesion.

Summary

- When treating critical limb ischaemia with tissue lesion, the potential application of the presented angiosome model is targeting the revascularisation on the site of the tissue lesion to improve healing.

- Studies that have been published so far on the angiosome concept are mostly retrospective and majority of the included patients have been treated with endovascular procedure.

- The results of these studies show that there is benefit to be gained from opting for angiosome-targeted revascularisation. However, the studies mainly do not consider the role of significant collaterals to the wound area. Furthermore, the wound classification is limited and the depth of the tissue lesion has not been analysed.

- One large retrospective study, which included the treatment method to the analysis, suggests that the angiosome concept may not be as important in surgical bypass than as in endovascular revascularisation.

- A randomised trial would be unethical, but a well-planned prospective study with a measurement of circulation in different angiosomes before and after the procedure is the next step to gain more information.

References

1. Lepäntalo M, Biancari F, Tukiainen E. Never amputate without consultation of a vascular surgeon. *Diabetes Metab Res Rev* 2000; **16**: Suppl 1: S27–32.

2. Söderström M, Aho PS, Lepäntalo M, Albäck A. The influence of the characteristics of ischemic tissue lesions on ulcer healing time after infrainguinal bypass for critical leg ischemia. *J Vasc Surg* 2009; **49** (4): 932–37.

3. Blevins WA, Schneider PA. Endovascular management of critical limb ischemia. *Eur J Vasc Endovasc Surg* 2010; **39**: 756–61.

4. Markose G, Bolia A. Below the knee angioplasty among diabetic patients. *J Cardiovasc Surg* (Torino) 2009; **50** (3): 323–29.

5. Khan MU, Lall P, Harriss LM, *et al.* Predictors of limb loss despite a patent endovascular-treated arterial segment. *J Vasc Surg* 2009; **49** (6): 1445–46.

6. Taylor GI, Palmer JH. The vascular territories (angiosomes) of the body: experimental studies and clinical applications. Br J Plast Surg 1987; **40**: 113–41.

7. Attinger CE, Evans KK, Mesbahi A. Angiosomes of the foot and angiosome-dependent healing. In: Diabetic foot, lower extremity arterial disease and limb salvage. Philadelphia, Lippincott Williams & Wilkins, 2006: 341–50.

8. Alexandrescu V. Anatomical evaluation of distal leg arteries; the angiosome concept and its eventual application in critical limb ischemia revascularization. In: Endovascular below the knee revascularization. MEET combo 2011: 21–30.

9. Neville RF, Attinger CE, Bulan EJ, *et al.* Revascularization of a specific angiosome for limb salvage: does the target artery matter? *Ann Vasc Surg* 2009; **23** (3): 367–73.

10. Biancari F, Juvonen T. Angiosome-targeted lower limb revascularization for ischemic foot wounds: systematic review and meta-analysis. *Eur J Vasc Endovasc Surg* 2014; **47** (5): 517–22.

11. N Azuma, H Uchida, T Kokubo, *et al.* Factors influencing wound healing of critical ischaemic foot after bypass surgery: is the angiosome important in selecting bypass target artery? *Eur J Vasc Endovasc Surg* 2012; **43**: 322–28.

12. Spillerova K, Biancari F, Leppäniemi A, *et al.* Differential Impact of Bypass Surgery and Angioplasty on Angiosome-Targeted Infrapopliteal Revascularization. *Eur J Vasc Endovasc Surg* 2015; **49** (4): 412–9.

13. Špillerová K, Sörderström M, Albäck A, Venermo M. The Feasibility of Angiosome-Targeted Endovascular Treatment in Patients with Critical Limb Ischemia and Foot Ulcer. *Ann Vasc Surg* 2016; **30**: 270–6.

14. Terasaki H, Inoue Y, Sugano N *et al.* A quantitative method for evaluating local perfusion using indocyanine green fluorescence imaging. *Ann Vasc Surg* 2013; **27** (8): 1154–61.

Ten-year results of pedal bypass surgery

A Albäck, E Saarinen, P Kauhanen and M Venermo

Introduction

Critical limb ischaemia is caused by peripheral arterial disease, largely affecting the crural arteries, especially in patients with diabetes and in those of an advanced age.[1] With the ageing population and an increasing incidence of diabetes, the number of patients with critical limb ischaemia requiring extensive revascularisations will increase in the future. The pattern of atherosclerosis is unique in patients with diabetes; despite excessive occlusive disease in the crural arteries, the foot arteries are often preserved,[2,3] allowing an inframalleolar bypass in cases of limb-threatening ischaemia.

Infrapopliteal bypass down to the crural or pedal arteries is an established method for the treatment of critical limb ischaemia. Mid- and long-term results of pedal and plantar or tarsal bypasses have already been reported (more than 10 years ago). In published series, the secondary patency rates at three to five years have ranged from 39% to 89% and leg salvage rates from 46% to 87%, respectively.[4–10] In a large series published in 2003, Pomposelli and colleagues included a total of 1,032 patients with pedal bypasses performed over a 10-year period.[8] The majority of the patients (92%) were diabetics, and the mean age was 67 years. The authors reported a long-term outcome of 42% secondary patency and 58% leg salvage rate at 10 years. The long-term survival in this cohort was poor as only 24% of the patients were alive at 10 years.

Endovascular revascularisation has challenged bypass surgery in the treatment of critical limb ischaemia and is considered the first-line treatment in most centres worldwide. This is mainly due to its less-invasive nature and subsequent favourable short-term survival rates, especially in elderly patients.[11,12] Excellent technical success rates as well as short- and mid-term outcomes have been reported for the endovascular revascularisation of crural arteries.[13] A good technical success rate in the endovascular revascularisation of foot arteries has also been described.[14] However, long-term data for these procedures are lacking. According to one propensity-score-matched study, the haemodynamic result after the endovascular revascularisation of long distal lesions may be inferior to that of bypass surgery as the cumulative wound healing rates have been shown to be lower and amputation rates higher, with the importance of angiosome-directed procedures in endovascular treatment being more pronounced.[15]

Patient selection and techniques of pedal bypass

Despite the rapidly evolving endovascular techniques, there are still selected patients with multilevel infrainguinal disease and long calcified occlusions of crural arteries that, in the authors' opinion, will benefit from pedal bypass surgery. A good life expectancy and low operative risk certainly improve both the short- and the long-term outcome of femorodistal bypass surgery.[16] Another important determinant of bypass surgery outcome is vein graft quality, which should be evaluated prior to the decision on treatment strategy.[17] Unsuccessful endovascular revascularisation or repetitive occlusions of the crural arteries after endovascular revascularisation are also indications for bypass to the pedal or plantar arteries. Furthermore, even after successful endovascular revascularisation, legs with a large tissue lesion may not show sufficient healing tendency. These patients with extensive tissue loss need rapid and maximal reperfusion of the foot and may, therefore, benefit from surgical revascularisation of the foot arteries. One special indication for pedal or plantar bypass, in highly selected and mostly young diabetic patients, is the need for simultaneous microvascular flap coverage of a large ischaemic lesion that would otherwise lead to major amputation.[18]

At our institution, the treatment policy for critical limb ischaemia has traditionally been aggressive, and revascularisation is considered for all patients unless they are bedridden, in permanent institutional care or suffering from severe dementia, which seems to be an increasing population of patients at a high age. Despite a marked increase in the number of patients undergoing endovascular treatment for critical limb ischaemia, there has been only a minor decrease in the number of infrapopliteal bypasses performed over the years (Figure 1).

The suitability of the inflow and outflow arterial anatomy for bypass is routinely investigated with magnetic resonance angiography, the foot vessels being further evaluated by conventional digital subtraction angiography and duplex scanning when necessary. Duplex is used for marking the site of pedal anastomosis in order to minimise surgical exploration and enhance the wound healing of this critical

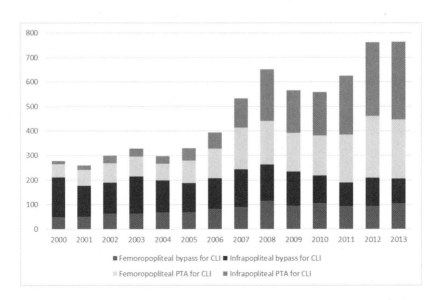

Figure 1: The development of treatment for critical limb ischaemia at the Helsinki University Hospital 2000–2013.

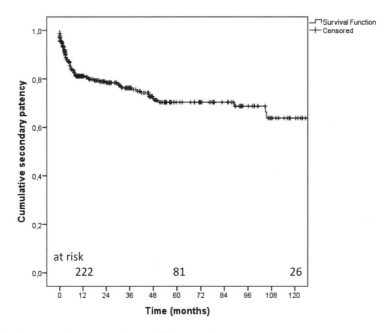

Figure 2: Cumulative secondary patency of 352 pedal bypass grafts.

surgical incision. Autologous vein grafts are exclusively preferred. The size and quality of the vein graft material is evaluated preoperatively with a high-frequency ultrasound transducer to aid decision-making, and the veins to be used are marked prior to surgery for minimal surgical preparation of the graft through small bridged incisions. The ipsilateral greater saphenous vein is the graft of choice. There is no conclusive evidence in the literature to support the use of the *in situ* technique over other configurations.[19] For optimal vein quality and the size-matching of anastomosed vessels, as well as to avoid wound complications from multiple pedal incisions for vein harvesting and arterial exposition, the grafts are used in a translocated non-reversed fashion. Thus, the contralateral greater saphenous vein can equally be used as a conduit, unless the donor limb is evidently ischaemic. Arm veins or the lesser saphenous vein are used if a viable great saphenous vein is absent. When a single-segment vein graft is not available, a spliced vein graft with two or more segments can be applied. However, endovascular treatment of the superficial femoral artery to enable a shorter bypass is an important alternative to a long femoropedal bypass. A hybrid endovascular and open reconstruction is an alternative, but as the vascular access can be obtained outside the surgical field, the endovascular treatment can also be done prior to surgery. As the vein graft is mapped and completely explored during harvesting, the only routine intraoperative evaluation method used in our department is transit-time flowmetry, with intraoperative duplex scanning or angiography in cases of unexpected graft or outflow problems, respectively, being carried out as required.

Long-term results of pedal bypasses performed in 2002–2013

Demographic changes in the population of patients who are candidates for pedal bypass as well as the strong shift towards endovascular treatment over the past two

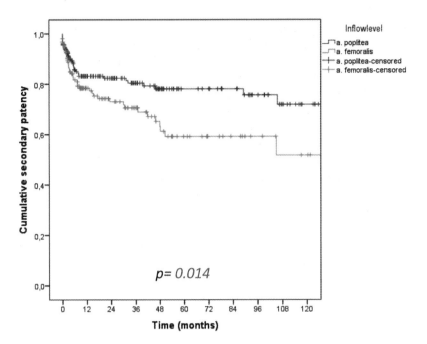

Figure 3: Cumulative secondary patency of bypasses originating from the popliteal artery (n=194) and bypasses originating from the femoral artery (n=158).

decades may influence the outcome for those patients who are referred to pedal bypass surgery. A retrospective study was carried out with the aim of critically evaluating the recent long-term results of inframalleolar bypasses at the Department of Vascular Surgery at Helsinki University Hospital. Furthermore, we aimed to compare the results of these bypasses between diabetics and non-diabetics, and to assess the role of inflow and outflow arteries in these ultradistal bypasses.[20]

A total of 352 patients underwent inframalleolar bypass between January 2002 and December 2013. Demographic data, procedural details, postoperative outcome and follow-up data were retrieved from the prospectively collected institutional vascular and endovascular database and scrutinised retrospectively from the patients' case records. The duplex-based surveillance protocol included follow-up visits at one, six, 12 and 24 months postoperatively, and in cases of graft revision, the protocol started again from the beginning. The dates of death and amputations were crosschecked and, if missing, retrieved from the national Population Register Centre and the amputation register, respectively.

The median follow-up time was 29 months (range 1–163 months). The median age of the study population was 73 years, and 67% of the patients were male. The incidence of diabetes was 69%. In the majority of cases (82%), the indication for bypass surgery was an ulcer or gangrene. The majority of the vein grafts (n=241) were single-segment greater saphenous vein grafts. There were 24 alternative autologous vein grafts, and 82 bypasses were performed using spliced vein grafts.

At the end of the study period, 83 patients were alive and had not undergone an amputation. Of these patients, 42 had attended a recent control visit and routine duplex control, and the patency of their graft was documented in their patient records. The remaining 41 patients with uncertain graft patency were invited to visit the outpatient clinic for duplex scanning.

The respective primary, assisted primary and secondary patency rates were 71.2%, 76.8% and 81.1%; 58.5%, 68.5% and 70.3%; and 45.3%, 54.4% and 63.8% at one, five and 10 years, respectively (Figure 2). The popliteal artery as the inflow artery (n=194) was associated with significantly superior patency rates when compared with bypasses originating from the femoral artery (n=158) (Figure 3). The recipient artery did not affect patency; pedal bypasses (n=281) had equal patency in comparison to plantar bypasses (n=71). The leg salvage rate of the overall study population at one, five and 10 years was 78.6%, 72% and 67.2%, respectively (Figure 4). Leg salvage was equal in patients with and without diabetes. The respective survival rates at one, five and 10 years were 70.3%, 37.4% and 15.9%.

These results compare well with the earlier study reporting on 10-year outcome,[8] the secondary patency in the recent study being somewhat superior but the overall survival poorer. A probable reason for the inferior survival is the higher median age of the patients and the high incidence of coronary artery disease in the recent study. This reflects the fact that there were two types of patients undergoing inframalleolar bypass—younger diabetics with distal peripheral artery disease and elderly patients with multilevel disease. The latter group has several comorbid conditions and can be considered high-risk patients.

The patency and leg salvage rates of bypasses originating from the popliteal artery seem to be superior to those originating from the femoral artery. The leg salvage rate of these short bypasses remained more than 70% at 10 years. The patients undergoing a femoral-to-pedal/plantar bypass are probably those suffering from the most serious form of peripheral artery disease, whereas those undergoing a

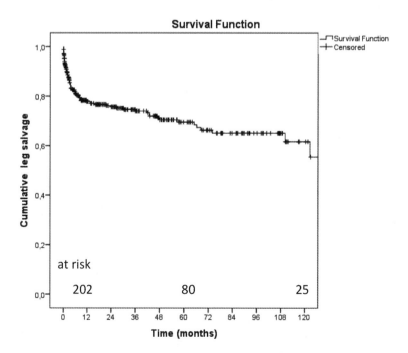

Figure 4: Cumulative leg salvage after pedal bypass surgery.

popliteo-pedal/plantar bypass have more restricted disease. A shorter bypass enables the use of an optimal size and quality of vein graft, which also seems to enhance patency rates. Both the pattern of the atherosclerotic disease with more distal occlusions in the ageing population[1] and the better outcome in the endovascular treatment of the superficial femoral artery will increase the possibilities of performing short pedal bypasses. Further research on this topic is certainly needed.

The revascularisation of long crural artery occlusions is often the last option in regard to limb salvage. In the light of the two studies reporting excellent long-term durability of pedal bypass, it seems reasonable that patients with good technical requisites and life expectancy should be offered pedal bypass for critical limb ischaemia with major tissue loss. As endovascular techniques and pedal bypass are complementary options for limb salvage, pedal bypass should also be offered after failed or inadequate endovascular revascularisation; the data concerning the effect of previous failed endovascular treatment on bypass outcome is contradictory.[21,22]

Conclusion

According to two large studies with 10-year follow-up, pedal bypass is associated with excellent long-term patency and leg salvage rates in the treatment of severe critical limb ischaemia. However, patient survival is poor as only one in five patients are alive after 10 years. Patient selection for this treatment is therefore of paramount importance. Despite the strong development in endovascular treatment, patients with good life expectancy and technical requisites may benefit from primary pedal bypass. Further studies focusing on the haemodynamic results of the different modes of revascularisation as well as the application of outcome measures describing wound healing and ambulation will specify the indication for pedal bypass in the future.

Summary

- Pedal bypass is an established technique for the revascularisation of severe ischaemia of the foot with the long-term, even 10-year, outcome being excellent.

- Patients with good life expectancy, good-quality vein graft material and a pattern of the atherosclerotic disease enabling a short pedal bypass, originating in the superficial femoral or popliteal artery, will benefit the most from this technique.

- A comprehensive workup with ultrasound marking and a meticulous surgical technique are mandatory for a good outcome.

- It is our position that duplex-based follow-up is important and graft stenosis should be treated promptly.

References

1. Diehm N, Shang A, Silvestro A, et al. Association of cardiovascular risk factors with pattern of lower limb atherosclerosis in 2659 patients undergoing angioplasty. *Eur J Vasc Endovasc Surg* 2006; **31**: 59–63.
2. Strandness Jr DE, Priest RE, Gibbons GE. A combined clinical and pathological study of non-diabetic and diabetic vascular disease. *Diabetes* 1964; **13**: 366–72.

3. Conrad MC. Large and small artery occlusion in diabetics and nondiabetics with severe vascular disease. *Circulation* 1967; **36**: 83–91.

4. Tordoir JH, van der Plas JP, Jacobs MJ, Kitslaar PJ. Factors determining the outcome of crural and pedal revascularisation for critical limb ischaemia. *Eur J Vasc Surg* 1993; **7**: 82–86.

5. Biancari F, Albäck A, Kantonen I, *et al*. Predictive factors for adverse outcome of pedal bypasses. *Eur J Vasc Endovasc Surg* 1999; **18**: 138–43.

6. Dorweiler B, Neufang A, Schmiedt W, Oelert H. Pedal arterial bypass for limb salvage in patients with diabetes mellitus. *Eur J Vasc Endovasc Surg* 2002; **24**: 309–313.

7. Frankini AD and Pezzella MV. Foot revascularization in patients with critical limb ischemia. *Rev Port Cir Cardiotorac Vasc* 2003; **10**: 75–81.

8. Pomposelli FB, Kansal N, Hamdan AD, *et al*. A decade of experience with dorsalis pedis artery bypass: analysis of outcome of in more than 1000 cases. *J Vasc Surg* 2003; **37**: 207–14.

9. Hughes K, Domenig CM, Hamdan AD, *et al*. Bypass to plantar and tarsal arteries: an acceptable approach to limb salvage. *J Vasc Surg* 2004; **40**: 1149–56.

10. Staffa R, Leypold J, Kríz Z. Pedal bypass for limb salvage. *Acta Chir Belg* 2005; **105**: 491–6.

11. Doslouglu HH, Lall P, Cherr GS, *et al*. Superior limb salvage with endovascular therapy in octogenarians with critical limb ischemia. *J Vasc Surg* 2009; **50**: 305–15.

12. Arvela E, Venermo M, Söderström M, *et al*. Infrainguinal percutaneous transluminal angioplasty or bypass surgery in patients aged 80 years and older with critical limb ischemia. *Br J Surg* 2011; **98**: 518–26.

13. Ferraresi R, Centola M, Ferlini M, *et al*. Long-term outcomes after angioplasty of isolated, below-the-knee arteries in diabetic patients with critical limb ischaemia. *Eur J Vasc Endovasc Surg* 2009; **37**: 226–342.

14. Manzi M, Fusaro M, Cecacci T, *et al*. Clinical results of below-the-knee intervention using pedal-plantar loop technique for the revascularization of foot arteries. *J Cardiovasc Surg* 2009; **50**: 331–37.

15. Spillerova K, Biancari F, Leppäniemi A, *et al*. Differential impact of bypass surgery and angioplasty on angiosome-targeted infrapopliteal revascularization. *Eur J Vasc Endovasc Surg* 2015; **49**: 412–19.

16. Adam DJ, Beard JD, Cleveland T, *et al*, BASIL Trial participants. Bypass *versus* angioplasty in severe ischemia of the leg (BASIL): multicentre, randomised, controlled trial. *Lancet* 2005; **366:** 1925–34.

17. Arvela E, Venermo M, Söderström M, *et al*. Outcome of infrainguinal single- segment great saphenous vein bypass for critical limb ischemia is superior to alternative autologous vein bypass especially in patients with high operative risk. *Ann Vasc Surg* 2012; **26**: 396–403.

18. Kallio M, Vikatmaa P, Kantonen I, *et al*. Strategies for Free Flap Transfer and revascularization with long- term outcome in the treatment of large diabetic foot lesions. *Eur J Vasc Endovasc Surg* 2015; **50**: 223–30.

19. Watelet J, Soury P, Menard JF, *et al*. Femoropopliteal bypass: in situ or reversed vein grafts? Ten-year results of a randomized prospective study. *Ann Vasc Surg* 1997; **11**: 510–19.

20. Saarinen E, Kauhanen P, Albäck A, Venermo M. Long term results of inframalleolar bypass for critical limb ischaemia. Abstract 29th Annual meeting of the European Society for Vascular, Porto 23-25.9.2015.

21. Uhl C, Hock C, Betz T, *et al*. Pedal bypass surgery after crural endovascular intervention. *J Vasc Surg* 2014; **59**: 1583–7.

22. Nolan B, De Martino R, Stone D, *et al*. Prior failed ipsilateral percutaneous endovascular intervention in patients with critical limb ischemia predicts poor outcome after lower extremity bypass. *J Vasc Surg* 2011; **54:** 730–36.

Wound healing

Early detection of ulceration in diabetic feet—an intelligent telemedicine system

CEVB Hazenberg, JJ van Netten and JG van Baal

Introduction

Foot complications in diabetes are a worldwide major medical, social and economic problem. The lifetime risk of developing a foot ulcer has been estimated to be as high as 15–25%,[1] with the most devastating and costly outcome being a lower limb amputation, which is nearly always preceded by a foot ulcer. Healthcare expenditure on diabetic foot care adds up to one third of total expenditure on diabetes care,[2,3] and the direct costs of a foot ulcer that results in amputation may be on average US$40,000.[4] The prevention of these lower limb complications of diabetes would have major positive impact on morbidity, mortality, and patient wellbeing, and would lead to significant savings on healthcare expenditure.

Frequent inspection of the foot is an important cornerstone of prevention. Guidelines recommend that patients are screened at least once every one to six months.[5] However, foot ulcers mostly occur in-between clinic visits when the patient is at home. Patient self-monitoring is needed to timely identify signs of foot disease and to contribute to a sense of self-efficacy in the prevention of foot ulceration. Once an ulcer has developed, monitoring of the ulcer is important to assess treatment efficacy, to predict healing, and to respond swiftly in case a complication, such as a foot infection, develops. Patients are often seen every week or every other week at the outpatient foot clinic for ulcer monitoring. This places a burden on the patient and healthcare system, while at the same time rapidly developing foot infections may still not be detected in time. Patient self-monitoring of an ulcer would be a valuable addition to treatment. Self-monitoring is, however, not easy and may be hampered when patients are physically limited because of limited joint mobility, visual impairment, or obesity, or when they lack sufficient knowledge about the disease.[6–8] Foot inspection by a relative may be troublesome as well, since many patients live alone and relatives may also be limited in their ability to inspect the patient's foot.

The development of an intelligent telemedicine system that can effectively contribute to monitoring the patient's foot health status may be a great asset for diabetic foot management. Because of rapid developments in telecommunication technology and the widespread availability of internet, telemedicine has become increasingly popular in monitoring and treating patients. Although telemedicine still has to be proven to be cost-effective in a large number of applications,[9] it is used to improve efficiency and effectiveness of care and patient's well-being and autonomy in a world with rapidly changing socio-economic perspectives in healthcare.[10] Several applications have been developed for the diabetic foot. This includes the use of mobile phone and video interaction to support foot care,[11–14] imaging devices,[15–21] and dermal thermography[22–24] for monitoring a foot ulcer and for diagnosing foot disease. Nevertheless, very few applications seem to be implemented in diabetic foot care. In this chapter, we focus on current insights in available and potential home-monitoring applications in the diabetic foot with respect to the assessment, monitoring, prevention, and management of the diabetic foot.

Dermal thermography

In the literature, most papers on telemedicine and home-monitoring applications for the diabetic foot are on dermal thermography (infrared thermography and liquid-christal thermography) and deal with the prediction and prevention of neuropathic foot ulceration.

Three randomised controlled trials showed that home monitoring of foot temperatures using infrared thermography can contribute significantly to reducing the incidence of diabetic foot ulcers.[22–24] One recent small randomised controlled trial did not confirm these findings by showing no significant difference between temperature measuring group and standard therapy group, but this study was clearly underpowered.[25] A recent systematic review and meta-analysis suggests that the use of at-home temperature-monitoring is an effective way to predict and prevent diabetic foot ulceration.[26] Effect sizes found were large, among the largest of any intervention that aims to prevent foot ulcers in diabetes.[1] It is, therefore, remarkable and rather disappointing to observe that such monitoring is hardly adopted in clinical practice. There may be some issues regarding the usability and applicability of such at-home daily foot temperature monitoring, with one randomised controlled trial reporting reasons for withdrawal from the study (highest in the intervention group) with "too much to do" being the main reason.[22] Diagnostic accuracy may also be questioned, with a case series by van Netten *et al* showing the most optimal cut-off infrared temperature to detect diabetic foot complications (2.2 degrees Celsius) to be only 76% sensitive and 40% specific.[27] Furthermore, in several settings, reimbursement issues remain unresolved. Except local cost calculations of foot complications,[28] no data have been published on the cost-effectiveness of the approach. Confirmation of the positive outcomes of these studies on at-home dermal thermography through well-designed trials in other settings is needed, together with proof of the usability and cost-effectiveness of the approach in order to improve the widespread acceptance and use in diabetic foot care.

Liquid-crystal thermography may be a promising tool for the prediction of diabetic foot ulceration.[29,30] Liquid-crystal thermography is easy to use and is low cost. However, the thermometers used in published studies were quite large, while smaller thermometers exist. Future studies should assess the effectiveness of the approach in the home setting.

Hyperspectral imaging

Most studies on hyperspectral imaging in foot disease showed that this technique can accurately predict the healing of diabetic foot ulcers and therefore seems promising in the treatment of foot disease.[31–36] These studies used hyperspectral imaging to assess tissue oxygenation at or near the ulcer according to measured oxyhaemoglobin and deoxyhaemoglobin levels. From these levels, a healing index was calculated to determine the potential for healing. However, most studies included only a small number of ulcers, and treatment/follow-up strategies (influencing ulcer healing and outcome) were not reported.[31,32,34,35] One study assessed the value of hyperspectral imaging in predicting foot ulceration.[37]

Although hyperspectral imaging seems a promising tool for an intelligent telemedicine system, well-designed clinical effectiveness studies are needed to support this. Furthermore, hyperspectral imaging is currently still an experimental and expensive technique, only suitable in a clinical setting to support treatment of foot ulcers in diabetes patients. Applications for the home environment are far from being developed, and first must be proven cost-effective to be implemented in foot care for high-risk diabetic patients.

Photographic imaging

Photographic imaging of the foot has been mainly used for the diagnosis of ulcers and pre-ulcerative lesions, and to measure ulcer area.[15–18,20,21,38–41] Most papers report on the accuracy with which the ulcer area is measured using digital photography as compared with live assessments,[20,38–41] or with a scanner using specially developed software.[21] Two photographic imaging devices have been designed to monitor the diabetic foot in the home environment: Bus *et al* showed that using a photographic foot imaging device, a good compromise between live and photographic assessment, repeated photographic assessments could be obtained for diagnosis of different (pre-) signs of ulceration.[15] This was further elaborated on by Hazenberg *et al* who showed assessments from photographs to be in good agreement with live assessment for the presence of ulcers (kappa 0.87), abundant callus (kappa 0.61), and for absence of any sign of diabetic foot disease (kappa 0.83). Outcomes were also reliable between repeated photographic assessments (kappa 0.70–1.00).[18] Interobserver agreement for photographic assessments was good for ulcer and for absence of any signs, and moderate for abundant callus.[18] In another study by the same group, Hazenberg *et al* showed a good feasibility of using the photographic foot imaging device in the home environment: patient adherence was high, referrals based on photographic assessment justified, and perceived usability was good.[19] Furthermore, the same authors showed in another paper that diagnosis of foot infection is valid and reliable using photographic imaging in combination with infrared thermography, taking clinical diagnosis as gold standard (sensitivity >60%, specificity >79%), and better than when using each modality alone.[42] Foltynski *et al* report on a feasibility analysis of at-home usage of the TelediaFos system with respect to the total number of assessed wound pictures, the length of the monitoring period, and change in ulcer area after four and 12 weeks follow-up (descriptive analysis).[16,17] Patients perceived the usability of the system between moderate and good.[17]

The limitations of both systems are that only the plantar foot surface can be assessed. Future designs of the system should involve dorsal foot imaging since only half of the ulcers are located at the plantar side. Future research should study the validity and reliability of assessing blisters, fissures and erythema as precursor to foot infection, as well as the (cost-) effectiveness of photographic foot imaging.

Video and audio communication

The treatment of foot ulcers may benefit from video and audio communication as a telemedical support tool. Most studies used telemedicine consultations using video interaction and face-to-face treatment, or a mobile phone to link the physician and home visiting nurse to support ulcer treatment. These approaches were found to be feasible with potential to expand the delivery of specialised foot care to rural areas, but mostly only small descriptive studies were conducted.[11–13,43] On effectiveness, one case-control study and one randomised controlled trial showed no significant difference in healing time and number of ulcers healed between treatment with support of real-time interactive video consultation, and standard treatment.[14,43] Well-designed studies on the feasibility and effectiveness of video and audio communication are needed. A potential disadvantage of video or audio consultation, compared, for example, with photographic imaging, is that both patient and physician need to be available at the same time. Future studies should further explore the value of this approach to telemedical healthcare for the diabetic foot.

Development of an intelligent telemedicine system

The previously discussed technologies still require active involvement of the users, for example, in writing down the temperature and calculating the difference between the left and right foot in the infrared temperature randomised controlled trials,[22–24] or in assessment of the photos by trained professionals. This can be overcome with an intelligent telemedicine system, whereby the automated analyses are performed using trained software. Such a system could greatly reduce the burden for patients and professionals in using telemedical healthcare, while it also allows for easy application of the technology to large groups of users.

In view of such an intelligent telemedicine system, Liu *et al* demonstrated the possibility for automated detection of foot complications based on asymmetric analysis of thermal images in combination with colour imaging (sensitivity and specificity >97% in comparison with manual annotation of foot complications).[44] An intelligent telemedicine system would greatly profit from the combination of different technologies. Liu and colleagues, therefore, also investigated application of hyperspectral data, describing a methodology with a sensitivity of 97% and a specificity of 96% compared to live assessment for the detection of diabetic foot complications, based on a discrimination between (pre-) signs of ulceration and healthy skin spots.[45] Future research is still needed before such a system is functional and ready to use, but the promising early results suggest that the future of telemedical healthcare in the diabetic foot lies in an intelligent system where different technologies are combined.

Cost aspects

For all described telemedical approaches, the benefit for the patient and the healthcare system will have to be evaluated in association with the required investment to setup and use the telemedical system. Cost-effectiveness is the key aspect here that will determine potential for acceptance and implementation in diabetic foot care. Some telemedical systems are low in cost, such as infrared thermometers, while other systems that in the future may serve a telemedical purpose are expensive such as hyperspectral imaging. However, the prevention of a foot ulcer or an amputation may save the healthcare system between US$5,000 and US$40,000 per event, and therefore effective telemedical approaches have a good chance of being cost-effective for the management of diabetic patients with a high-risk of developing serious foot complications.

If proven (cost-) effective and if implemented successfully, telemedical support in the screening, monitoring or treatment of diabetic foot disease can improve patient mobility, autonomy, and health-related quality of life, in particular for patients who may be best served with telemedical support such as those that live alone, have cognitive, visual or physical impairments, or lack knowledge about the disease. Due to the further increasing global internet penetration, such telemedical tools may also serve those patients living in remote areas with limited and time-consuming access to healthcare services.

Conclusion

There are several promising technologies available for the development of an intelligent telemedicine system, which may be of additional value in the prevention, assessment, and/or treatment of diabetic foot disease. For some of these approaches, effectiveness, and in some cases even feasibility, is not yet known and these aspects require further investigations, while for all approaches it is important that cost-effectiveness is demonstrated to achieve widespread acceptance and use in diabetic foot care. However, with advancements in technology and the positive early results, an intelligent telemedicine system could well be within reach.

Summary

- An intelligent telemedicine system may be a great asset for diabetic foot management; it would have major positive impact on patient wellbeing and would lead to significant savings on healthcare expenditure.

- Several promising approaches and technologies exist for the development of an intelligent telemedicine system for the management of diabetic foot disease.

- Available technologies are: dermal thermography (infrared and liquid-crystal themography), hyperspectral imaging, photographic imaging, and video/audio communication.

- An intelligent telemedicine system would profit from the combination of different technologies.

References

1. Singh N, Armstrong DG, Lipsky BA. Preventing foot ulcers in patients with diabetes. *JAMA* 2005; **293** (2): 217–28.
2. Armstrong DG, *et al.* Mind the gap: Disparity between research funding and costs of care for diabetic foot ulcers. *Diabetes Care* 2013; **36**: 1815–17.
3. Driver VR, Fabbi M, Lavery LA, Gibbons G. Strategies to prevent and heal diabetic foot ulcers : The costs of diabetic foot the economic case for the limb salvage team. *J Am Podiatr Med Assoc* 2010; **100**: 335–41.

4. Matricali GA, Dereymaeker G, Muls E, Flour M, *et al.* Economic aspects of diabetic foot care in a multidisciplinary setting: a review. *Diabetes Metab Res Rev* 2007; **23**: 339–47.

5. Bakker K, Schaper NC, Apelqvist J. Practical guidelines on the management and prevention of the diabetic foot 2011. *Diabetes Metab Res Rev* 2012; **28** (Suppl 1): 225–31.

6. Boyko EJ, Ahroni JH, Cohen V, Nelson KM *et al.* Prediction of diabetic foot ulcer occurrence using commonly available clinical information: the Seattle Diabetic Foot Study. *Diabetes Care* 2006; **29**: 1202–07.

7. Fontbonne A, Berr C, Ducimetiere P, Alperovitch A. Changes in cognitive abilities over a 4-year period are unfavorably affected in elderly diabetic subjects: Results of the epidemiology of vascular aging study. *Diabetes Care* 2001; **24**; 366–70.

8. Lavery, LA, Armstrong, DG, Vela, SA, Quebedeaux, TL *et al.* Practical criteria for screening patients at high risk for diabetic foot ulceration. *Arch Intern Med* 1998; **158**: 157–62.

9. Wootton, R. Twenty years of telemedicine in chronic disease management – an evidence synthesis. *J Telemed Telecare* 2012; **18**; 211–20.

10. Jennett, PA, *et al.* The socio-economic impact of telehealth: a systematic review. *J Telemed Telecare* 2003; **9**: 311–20.

11. Clemensen, J, Larsen, SB, Ejskjaer, N. Telemedical treatment at home of diabetic foot ulcers. *J Telemed Telecare* 2005; **11** (Suppl 2): S14–16.

12. Clemensen J, Larsen SB, Kirkevold M, Ejskjaer N. Treatment of diabetic foot ulcers in the home: video consultations as an alternative to outpatient hospital care. *Int J Telemed Appl* 2008: 1–6.

13. Larsen SB, Clemensen J, Ejskjaer N. A feasibility study of UMTS mobile phones for supporting nurses doing home visits to patients with diabetic foot ulcers. *J Telemed Telecare* 2006; **12**: 358–62.

14. Rasmussen, BSB, *et al.* A randomized controlled trial comparing telemedical and standard outpatient monitoring of diabetic foot ulcers. *Diabetes Care* 2015; doi:10.2337/dc15-0332.

15. Bus SA, Hazenberg CE, Klein M, Van Baal JG. Assessment of foot disease in the home environment of diabetic patients using a new photographic foot imaging device. *J Med Eng Technol* 2010; **34**: 43–50.

16. Foltynski P, *et al.* A new imaging and data transmitting device for telemonitoring of diabetic foot syndrome patients. *Diabetes Technol Ther* 2011; **13**: 861–67.

17. Foltynski P, *et al.* Monitoring of diabetic foot syndrome treatment: Some new perspectives. *Artif Organs* 2011; **35**: 176–82.

18. Hazenberg CEVB, van Baal JG, Manning E, Bril A, *et al.* The validity and reliability of diagnosing foot ulcers and pre-ulcerative lesions in diabetes using advanced digital photography. *Diabetes Technol Ther* 2010; **12**: 1011–17.

19. Hazenberg CEVB, *et al.* Telemedical home-monitoring of diabetic foot disease using photographic foot imaging--a feasibility study. *J Telemed Telecare* 2012; **18**: 32–36.

20. Ladyzynski P, *et al.* Area of the diabetic ulcers estimated applying a foot scanner-based home telecare system and three reference methods. *Diabetes Technol Ther* 2011; **13**: 1101–07.

21. Foltynski P, Ladyzynski P, Sabalinska, S, Wojcicki JM. Accuracy and precision of selected wound area measurement methods in diabetic foot ulceration. *Diabetes Technol Ther* 2013; **15**: 712–21.

22. Lavery LA, *et al.* Preventing diabetic foot ulcer recurrence in high-risk patients: use of temperature monitoring as a self-assessment tool. *Diabetes Care* 2007; **30**: 14–20.

23. Armstrong, DG, *et al.* Skin temperature monitoring reduces the risk for diabetic foot ulceration in high-risk patients. *Am J Med* 2007; **120**: 1042–46.

24. Lavery LA, *et al.* Home monitoring of foot skin temperatures to prevent ulceration. *Diabetes Care* 2004; **27**: 2642–47.

25. Skafjeld A, *et al.* A pilot study testing the feasibility of skin temperature monitoring to reduce recurrent foot ulcers in patients with diabetes – a randomized controlled trial. *BMC Endocr Disord* 2015; **15**: 55.

26. Houghton VJ, Bower VM, Chant DC. Is an increase in skin temperature predictive of neuropathic foot ulceration in people with diabetes? A systematic review and meta-analysis. *J Foot Ankle Res* 2013; **6**: 31.

27. van Netten JJ, *et al.* Diagnostic values for skin temperature assessment to detect diabetes-related foot complications. *Diabetes Technol Ther* 2014; **16**: 714–21.

28. National Horizon Scanning Unit Horizon scanning prioritising summary Volume 10, Number 1 : Temptouch: Infrared thermometer device for prevention of foot ulcers in people with diabetic foot disease. *Horizon* 2005; **10**: 1–8.

29. Benbow SJ, Chan AW, Bowsher DR, *et al.* The prediction of diabetic neuropathic plantar foot ulceration by liquid-crystal contact thermography. *Diabetes Care* 1994; **17**: 835–39.

30. Roback, K, Johansson, M, Starkhammar, A. Feasibility of a thermographic method for early detection of foot disorders in diabetes. *Diabetes Technol Ther* 2009; **11**: 663–67.

31. Khaodhiar L, *et al.* The use of medical hyperspectral technology to evaluate microcirculatory changes in diabetic foot ulcers and to predict clinical outcomes. *Diabetes Care* 2007; **30**: 903–10.

32. Neidrauer, M, Zubkov, L, Weingarten, MS, Pourrezaei, K, *et al.* Near infrared wound monitor helps clinical assessment of diabetic foot ulcers. *J Diabetes Sci Technol* 2010; **4**: 792–98.

33. Nouvong A, *et al.* Evaluation of diabetic foot ulcer healing with hyperspectral imaging of oxyhemoglobin and deoxyhemoglobin. *Diabetes Care* 2009; **32**: 2056–61.

34. Papazoglou, ES, Neidrauer, M, Zubkov, L, Weingarten, MS, *et al.* Noninvasive assessment of diabetic foot ulcers with diffuse photon density wave methodology: pilot human study. *J Biomed Opt* 2011; **14**: 064032.

35. Weingarten MS, *et al.* Prediction of wound healing in human diabetic foot ulcers by diffuse near-infrared spectroscopy: A pilot study. *Wound Repair Regen* 2010; **18**: 180–85.

36. Weingarten MS, *et al.* Diffuse near-infrared spectroscopy prediction of healing in diabetic foot ulcers: a human study and cost analysis. *Wound Repair Regen* 2012; **20**: 911–17.

37. Calin MA, *et al.* Assessing diabetic foot ulcer development risk with hyperspectral tissue oximetry. *Johns Hopkins APL Tech Dig* 2014; Applied Phys Lab 26, 026009.

38. Bowling FL, *et al.* An assessment of the accuracy and usability of a novel optical wound measurement system. *Diabet Med* 2009; 26, 93–6.

39. Bowling, FL, *et al.* Remote assessment of diabetic foot ulcers using a novel wound imaging system. Wound Repair Regen 2011; **19**: 25–30.

40. Rajbhandari SM, *et al.* Digital imaging: an accurate and easy method of measuring foot ulcers. *Diabet Med* 1999; **16**: 339–42.

41. Wang L, *et al.* An automatic assessment system of diabetic foot ulcers based on wound area determination, color segmentation, and healing score evaluation. *J Diabetes Sci Technol* 2015; doi:10.1177/1932296815599004.

42. Hazenberg CEVB, van Netten JJ, van Baal SG, Bus SA. Assessment of signs of foot infection in diabetes patients using photographic foot imaging and infrared thermography. *Diabetes Technol Ther* 2014; **16**: 1–8.

43. Wilbright WA, Birke JA, Patout CA, Varnado M, *et al.* The use of telemedicine in the management of diabetes-related foot ulceration: a pilot study. *Adv Ski Wound Care* 2004; **17**: 232–38.

44. Liu C, van Netten JJ, van Baal JG, Bus SA, *et al.* Automatic detection of diabetic foot complications with infrared thermography by asymmetric analysis. *J Biomed Opt* 2015; **20**: 026003.

45. Liu C, *et al.* Statistical analysis of spectral data: a methodology for designing an intelligent monitoring system for the diabetic foot. *J Biomed Opt* 2013; **18**: 126004.

Venous challenges

Acute deep vein thrombosis challenges

Conservative management of deep vein thrombosis

V Bhattacharya, T Barakat and G Stansby

Introduction

Deep vein thrombosis management is usually conservative, involving systemic anticoagulants to prevent the propagation of existing thrombi, formation of new deep vein thrombosis or pulmonary embolism. Current evidence only supports the use of thrombolysis for iliofemoral deep vein thrombosis in cases with symptom duration of 14 days or fewer and in those with a good life expectancy.

Duration of treatment

A key initial step is to determine if the deep vein thrombosis was "provoked" or "unprovoked" and if provoked, whether the provoking factor is ongoing. A provoked deep vein thrombosis or pulmonary embolism is defined as one in which a patient has had a previous deep vein thrombosis (within three months), has transient major clinical risk factors—such as surgery, trauma or significant immobility or is on the oral contraceptive pill or on hormone replacement therapy. In contrast, an unprovoked deep vein thrombosis or pulmonary embolism is one in which the patient does not have transient major clinical risk factors, has active cancer, thrombophilia, or a family history because these are underlying risks that remain constant in the patient. A clear understanding of this is required to guide decisions on treatment duration.

For proximal provoked deep vein thrombosis with no ongoing risk factors, treatment involves three months of anticoagulation. For unprovoked deep vein thrombosis, treatment may be given for six months or even permanently.[1] Venous thromboembolism that is associated with active cancer, or with a second unprovoked venous thromboembolism, is associated with a high risk of recurrence and is usually treated indefinitely. Anticoagulation is often given indefinitely if there is a low risk of bleeding, but is usually stopped at three months if there is a high risk of bleeding. Unfortunately, there is no agreed score for bleeding risk in this context to aid this decision; however, the HAS-BLED score, which was developed for atrial fibrillation, has been used (one point each for hypertension history, renal disease, liver disease, stroke history, prior major bleeding or predisposition to bleeding, labile international normalised ratio [INR], age >65, medication predisposing to bleeding, and alcohol or drug usage history).[2]

When deciding whether or not to prescribe permanent anticoagulation, there needs to be consideration of the risk of long-term anticoagulants *versus* the ongoing risk of venous thromboembolism. The recurrence risk of venous thromboembolism is 50% for an unprovoked event after 10 years and 20–30% after five years, and iliofemoral deep vein thrombosis tend to be associated with a higher recurrence rate than are femoral or popliteal deep vein thromboses. The case for continuing anticoagulation indefinitely after a first unprovoked proximal deep vein thrombosis or pulmonary embolism is further strengthened if the patient is male, the index event was pulmonary embolism rather than a deep vein thrombosis, and/or D-dimer testing is positive one month after stopping anticoagulant therapy.

The PROLONG (D-dimer testing to determine the duration of anticoagulation therapy) trial showed that a normal D Dimer one month after anticoagulation suspension for unprovoked venous thromboembolism was associated with a low risk of late recurrences (4.4% patient years).[3] The DASH (D Dimer, age, sex, hormone therapy) study of 1,800 patients found that abnormal D-Dimer levels after stopping anticoagulation, age <50 years, male sex and venous thromboembolism not associated with hormone replacement therapy were the main predictors of recurrence and these were, therefore, used to derive a prognostic recurrence score.[4] This DASH prediction rule appears to forecast recurrent rate in patients with a first unprovoked venous thromboembolism and maybe a useful tool to decide whether anticoagulation should be continued indefinitely or stopped after an initial treatment of at least three months.

Distal (calf vein) deep vein thrombosis

A deep vein thrombosis that is isolated to the calf veins is termed a "distal" deep vein thrombosis" compared with a "proximal" deep vein thrombosis, which occurs proximal to the knee joint level and popliteal vein. We strongly recommend that the terms "proximal" and "distal" in relation to deep vein thrombosis are used solely to refer to above and below knee deep vein thromboses and should not be used to differentiate between iliofemoral and solely infrainguinal events. Calf vein thrombosis is less likely to embolise to the lungs than a more proximal thrombosis. Many such thromboses are probably asymptomatic and are never identified. The natural history has not been studied well.

A trial of compression stockings with and without anticoagulation for calf vein thrombosis in 107 patients showed that during the follow up of three months, only two patients in each group developed progression of clot proximally and no patient had a pulmonary embolism or died.[5] This study showed that there was no superiority of short-term regiment of low-molecular-weight heparin and compression therapy compared with compression therapy alone in patients with isolated calf vein thrombosis in a low-risk population.

Two management strategies have, therefore, been proposed for symptomatic calf deep vein thrombosis. One is to follow with serial duplex ultrasound examinations and treat only if there is propagation to a proximal deep vein thrombosis. Another is to offer a short course of six weeks to three months of treatment. Further clinical studies are required to investigate the natural history and clinical significance of isolated calf deep vein thrombosis.

Role of aspirin

Aspirin is an inadequate agent for acute treatment of deep vein thrombosis. However, two studies have looked at the efficacy of low-dose aspirin 100mg for prevention of venous thromboembolism following anticoagulation for two years. When results of the two trials were combined in the pre-specified meta-analysis, aspirin was found to significantly reduce the risk of recurrent venous thromboembolism.[6,7]

Therefore, in people who have experienced a first unprovoked deep vein thrombosis or pulmonary embolism and completed initial anticoagulation therapy, low-dose aspirin compared with placebo may reduce the risk of venous thromboembolism and vascular events without increasing the risk of bleeding. Although long-term anticoagulation is the most effective therapy for prevention of venous thromboembolism recurrence, aspirin may be a potential alternative option in patients who have had an unprovoked venous thromboembolism and are unable or unwilling to go on long-term anticoagulation therapy.

Inferior vena cava filters

Evidence for the use of inferior vena cava filters is weak; essentially, just a single study in 400 patients with proximal deep vein thrombosis, who were randomised to treatment with either standard anticoagulation or anticoagulation and insertion of a filter.[8] After 12 days, there were significantly fewer cases of pulmonary embolism in the filter group (1% vs. 5%). At two years, however, there were no overall significant differences the rate of survival or in the rate of symptomatic pulmonary embolism between the two groups. Patients with a filter had a higher incidence of recurrent deep vein thrombosis (21% vs. 12%). Further evaluation at eight years showed a similar overall incidence of thromboembolism between the two groups, but the filter group had a higher incidence of deep vein thrombosis (35% vs. 27%) and a lower incidence of symptomatic pulmonary embolism (6% vs. 15%).

An inferior vena cava filter is thus only indicated for patients with recurrent pulmonary embolism and with contraindications to anticoagulation or for patients with breakthrough pulmonary embolism where they have had recurrent pulmonary embolism despite adequate anticoagulation. Filters are also indicated for prophylaxis in high-risk surgical patients with deep vein thrombosis or pulmonary embolism who are due to have a resection of a malignancy or other major surgery.[1]

Trauma patients are increasingly considered for prophylactic filter placement. Although endorsed by the American College of Radiology and the Society of Interventional Radiology guidelines, both the American College of Clinical Pharmacy and the National Institute for Health and Care Excellence (NICE) guidelines advise against this.[9,1] It remains unclear as to which group of trauma patients will experience enough benefit to outweigh the harms associated with filter placement.[10,11] Additionally, several studies have shown a very high rate of non-retrieval of temporarily placed filters. The focus should, therefore, be on having clear indications for insertion and formalised pathways to ensure removal.

Role of thrombophilia testing

Thrombophilia is an acquired or inherited predisposition to venous thrombosis. Testing for thrombophilia is indicated only in patients who present with thrombosis at a young age or who have a strong family history of thrombosis and are a known thrombophilic variant. Thrombophilia screening should be carried out with appropriate counselling and a clear explanation of the limitations. Widespread thrombophilia testing is not cost-effective and should be largely restricted to cases where the result may alter management.[1]

The normal standard laboratory thrombophilia screen consists of: protein C; protein S; antithrombin; activated protein C resistance and Factor V Leiden; protein gene mutation Lupus anticoagulant; and Anti-Cardiolipin antibodies.

The tests are influenced by the use of anticoagulation and if there is an active thrombosis present. Therefore, thrombophilia screening should not be requested in an acute situation. It would be usual to do it four to six weeks after stopping warfarin. During warfarin therapy, it is not possible to interpret protein C and S results as these are both vitamin K dependant proteins.

Novel oral anticoagulants *versus* warfarin

The standard treatment for thrombosis has been warfarin for many years, which can easily be reversed if necessary by administering oral vitamin K within 24 hours or intravenous vitamin K (which acts within 12 hours). Additionally, vitamin K antagonists are the only anticoagulants that can be used relatively safely in patients with renal function impairment. However, they have a disadvantage in that the therapeutic window is narrow, monitoring is required, and there are many drug and dietary interactions.

Novel oral anticoagulants have now overcome some of these problems. There are three major drugs that have been licensed to be used in treatment of venous thromboembolism: the direct factor Xa inhibitors rivaroxaban (Xarelto, Bayer) and apixaban (Eliquis, Bristol-Myers Squibb/Pfizer), and the direct thrombin inhibitor dabigatran (Pradaxa, Boehringer Ingelheim). The main difference between these drugs and vitamin K antagonists is that they have smaller molecules that act on a single coagulation factor.

All of the current novel anticoagulants have a rapid onset of action to reach plasma levels quickly within four hours compared with a minimum of 60 hours to reach therapeutic levels with vitamin K antagonists. They also have a relatively short half-life, ranging from six to 17 hours compared with four to six days with vitamin K antagonists. As novel oral anticoagulants have a minimal anticoagulant effect 24 hours after the last dose, bridging with parental anticoagulation may not be necessary in patients undergoing surgery or diagnostic procedures. With these drugs, anticoagulant use could be avoided for one or two days depending on the age and renal function. The novel anticoagulants so far investigated are associated with statistically significant reductions in intracranial bleeds compared with vitamin K antagonists.

Currently the novel anticoagulants are indicated for the majority of patients with unstable INR, providing the renal function is adequate, and in whom laboratory testing is difficult. Some centres, however, use these drugs as the first-line anticoagulation in patients who need relatively short-term treatment. The problem with novel oral anticoagulants has been the absence of an antidote and there is no generally accepted protocol on how to manage a patient presenting with a serious haemorrhage shortly after taking one of these medicines. Currently specific antidotes are becoming available and this may reduce this risk in the future of bleeding and emergency surgery in the future.[12]

Testing for undiagnosed cancer in venous thromboembolism

Many studies have suggested that the underlying rate of unsuspected cancer in patients with an unprovoked primary deep vein thrombosis over the age of 40 years is in the order of 10%.[13] The current NICE recommendation is that all patients with unprovoked venous thromboembolism should be offered a chest X-ray, blood tests (which includes full blood count and serum calcium) and liver functions tests along with urinalysis.[1] These guidelines suggest that consideration should be given to patients over the age of 40 for further investigation with a computed tomography (CT) scan of the abdomen and pelvis and a mammogram in women if no evidence of malignancy is identified on initial investigation. This was based on a randomised controlled trial of 200 patients diagnosed with idiopathic venous thromboembolism. One group of patients received extensive investigations, including CT scan, mammography and tumour markers, and a second group received no additional investigation beyond history, examination, full blood count, liver function tests, calcium and chest X-ray. Patients in the extensive investigation group had cancers diagnosed at less advanced stage with 64% of patients diagnosed with stage T1 or T2 compared with 20% in the group receiving no screening.[14] In another study of 630 patients with idiopathic venous thromboembolism, comparing limited and extensive investigation, more patients with cancer were identified at presentation following extensive investigation although there were no significant differences between the two groups.[15]

However in a more recent study of 854 patients with unprovoked venous thromboembolism, there was no significant difference between the two study groups in the mean time to a cancer diagnosis (4.2 months vs. 4 months) or in cancer-related mortality (1.4% and 0.9%). Notably, the overall rate of a new diagnosis of occult cancer between randomisation and the one-year follow-up was low at 3.9%. Routine screening with CT of the abdomen and pelvis did not provide a clinically significant benefit.[16] A recent Cochrane review has also concluded that although testing for cancer in patients with idiopathic venous thromboembolism may lead to an earlier diagnosis of cancer, there is currently insufficient evidence to draw definitive conclusions concerning the effectiveness of testing for undiagnosed cancer in patients with a first episode of unprovoked deep vein thromboembolism or pulmonary embolism. Further good-quality large-scale randomised controlled trials are required.[17]

Treatment strategies in patients with cancer-related venous thromboembolism

There is a 5–10 fold increased risk of venous thromboembolism in malignancy, and cancer associated venous thromboembolism can predate the diagnosis of cancer. Around 15–20% of patients with malignancy develop venous thromboembolism during their illness and venous thromboembolism is the second most common cause of death in cancer patients. In an American cohort controlled study of patients receiving chemotherapy for a known cancer, observed over five years, the incidence of venous thromboembolism was 12.6% compared with 1.4% in the control group without cancer.[18]

A Cochrane review has shown benefit for the use of low molecular weight heparin for the treatment of cancer venous thromboembolism. The duration of treatment has been recommended for six months or indefinitely.[19] However in patients with active metastatic disease, the patients should be kept on low molecular weight heparin lifelong for ongoing venous thromboembolism risk although evidence from trials for this is lacking.

In the CLOT (Clots in legs or stocking) study of patients with cancer-related venous thromboembolism, a strategy of low molecular weight heparin followed by a switch to oral vitamin K antagonist was compared with no vitamin K antagonist and dalteparin treatment for six months.[20] This study showed a significant reduction in venous thromboembolism recurrence in patients treated with low molecular weight heparin compared with an oral vitamin K anticoagulant. However no difference in venous thromboembolism-associated mortality was seen.

The efficacy and safety of novel oral anticoagulants for treatment of cancer-related venous thromboembolism appears at least comparable to those of vitamin K antagonists in existing trials. However, the current novel anticoagulant trials in venous thromboembolism management were not direct comparisons with low molecular weight heparin. As a result, the drugs cannot yet be recommended in preference to heparin as the first-line treatment for venous thromboembolism in cancer patients.

Prevention of post-thrombotic syndrome

Recurrence of deep vein thrombosis is an independent risk factor for the development of post thrombotic syndrome and so effective treatment and prevention after a first episode is key. Patients with two or more episodes of thrombosis have a significantly increased risk of post thrombotic syndrome, which may be due to residual thrombus further aggravating previously damaged veins along with thrombus extension and venous outflow obstruction. It has also been shown that subtherapeutic levels of anticoagulation for significant periods during treatment increases the incidence of post-thrombotic syndrome. It has also been noted to be more frequent in patients who have thrombi in the iliac and femoral veins.

It has been standard practice to recommend graduated compression stockings to patients with post-deep vein thrombosis for a minimum of two years, although compliance with this has always been problematic. This may not now be justified. The SOX (compression stockings to prevent post-thrombotic syndrome) trial was a randomised controlled trial comparing stockings with placebo in preventing post-thrombotic syndrome after the first episode of deep vein thrombosis. It showed that stockings do not prevent the syndrome after a first proximal deep vein thrombosis.[21] However, we would still recommend their use until symptoms such as swelling have fully resolved.

Summary

- Most deep vein thrombosis patients should be managed conservatively (thrombolysis for iliofemoral deep vein thrombosis only).

- Decisions on duration of anticoagulants mostly depend on: the deep vein thrombosis being provoked or unprovoked; the risk of bleeding with anticoagulants; and the ongoing risk of thrombosis.

- Distal (calf vein) deep vein thrombosis natural history is unclear.

- D-Dimer levels may help identify which patients will require ongoing anticoagulants.

- Inferior vena cava filters should be used for those who have further thromboses despite adequate anticoagulants or those who cannot have anticoagulants. Use of prophylactic filters in trauma is not evidence based and temporary filters must be removed.

- Use of novel oral anticoagulants is increasing; they have a rapid onset and a shorter half-life compared with vitamin K antagonists; and specific antidotes are in development.

- Cancer patients should still be treated with low molecular weight heparin and there is weak evidence for extended screening for cancer after unprovoked deep vein thrombosis.

- Thrombophilia testing is not cost-effective, so should be restricted to cases where the result may alter management.

- Aspirin may be a potential long-term alternative option in patients who have had an unprovoked venous thromboembolism and are unable or unwilling to go on long-term anticoagulation therapy after initial treatment.

- Good anticoagulation reduces post-thrombotic syndrome incidence, graduated compression stockings should only be used for symptom management not prevention, and there is poor evidence for extended (two-year) use of graduated compression stockings.

References

1. NICE. The management of venous thromboembolic diseases and the role of thrombophilia testing (CG144). https://www.nice.org.uk/guidance/cg144 (date accessed 29 January 2016).
2. Pisters R, Lane DA, Nieuwlaat R, *et al.* A novel user friendly score (HAS- BLED) to assess one year risk of major bleeding in atrial fibrillation. The European Heart Survey. *Chest* 2010; **138** (5):1093–00.
3. PROLONG Investigators. Usefulness of repeated D-dimer testing after stopping anticoagulation for a first episode of unprovoked venous thromboembolism: The PROLONG II prospective study. *Blood* 2010; **115**: 481–88.
4. Tosetto A, Iorio A, Marcucci M, *et al.* Predicting disease recurrence in patients with previous unprovoked venous thromboembolism: A proposed prediction score (DASH). *J Thromb Haemost* 2012; **366**: 1019–25.
5. Schwarz T, Buschmann L, Beyer J, *et al.* Therapy of isolated calf muscle vein thrombosis: A randomized, controlled study. *J of Vasc Surgery* 2010; **5**: 1246–50.
6. Becattini C, Agnelli, G, Schenone A, *et al* for the WARFASA Investigators. Aspirin for preventing the recurrence of venous thromboembolism. *N Engl J Med* 2012; **366**: 1959–67.
7. Brighton TA, Eikelboom JW, Mann K, *et al* for the ASPIRE Investigators Low-Dose Aspirin for Preventing Recurrent Venous Thromboembolism *N Engl J Med* 2012; **367**: 1979–87.

8. Decousus H, Leizorovicz A, Parent F, *et al.* A clinic al trial of vena caval filters in the prevention of pulmonary embolism in patients with proximal deep-vein thrombosis. Prévention du Risque d'EmboliePulmonaire par Interruption Cave Study Group. *N Engl J Med* 1998; **338**: 409.

9. Molvar C. Inferior vena cava filtration in the management of venous thromboembolism: filtering the data Seminars. *Interventional Radiology* 2012; **29** (3): 204–17.

10. Haut ER, Garcia LJ, Shihab HM, *et al.* The effectiveness of prophylactic inferior vena cava filters in trauma patients: a systematic review and meta-analysis. *JAMA Surg* 2014; **149** (2):194–02.

11. Wang SL, Lloyd AJ. Clinical review: inferior vena cava filters in the age of patient- centered outcomes. *Ann Med* 2013; **45** (7): 474–81.

12. Das A, Liu D. Novel antidotes for target specific oral anticoagulants. Exp Haematol Oncol 2015; 4: 25.

13. Sorensen HT, Mellemkjaer L, Steffensen FH, *et al.* The risk of a diagnosis of cancer after primary deep venous thrombosis or pulmonary embolism. *N Eng J Med* 1998; **23**; 338: 1169–73.

14. Piccioli A, Lensing AW, Prins MH, *et al.* SOMIT Investigators Group. Extensive screening for occult malignant disease in idiopathic venous thromboembolism: A prospective randomized clinical trial. *J ThrombHaemost* 2004; **2**: 884–89.

15. Van Doormaal FF, Terpstra W, Van der Griend R, *et al.* Is extensive screening for cancer in idiopathic venous thromboembolism warranted? *J Throm Haemost* 2011; **9** (1): 79–84.

16. Carrier M, Lazo Langner A, Shivakumar S, *et al.* Screening for occult cancer in unprovoked venous thromboembolism. *N Engl J Med* 2015; **373**: 697–704.

17. Robertson L, Yeoh SE, Stansby G, Agarwal R. effect of testing for cancer on cancer and venous thromboembolism (VTE)- related mortality and morbidity in patients with unprovoked VTE. Cochrane Database Syst Rev. 2015 Mar 6; 3: CD 010837.

18. Khorana AA, Dalal M, Lin J, Connolly GC. Incidence and predictors of venous thromboembolism among ambulatory high risk cancer patients undergoing chemotherapy in the United States. *Cancer* 2013; **119** (3): 648–55.

19. Aki EA, Labedi N, Barba M, *et al.* Anticoagulation for the long-term treatment of venous thromboembolism in patients with cancer. Cochrane Database Syst Rev, 2011; 11:CD009447.

20. Dennis M, Sandercock P, Graham C, *et al.* Effectiveness of intermittent pneumatic compression in reduction of risk of deep vein thrombosis in patients who have had a stroke collaborators (CLOTS 3) clots in legs or stockings after Stroke : a multicentre randomized controlled trial. *Lancet* 2014; **383** (9920): 880–88.

21. Kahn SR, Shapiro S, Wells PS, *et al:* SOX trial investigators Compression stockings to prevent post-thrombotic syndrome: a randomized placebo-controlled trial. *BMC Cardiovasc Disord* 2007; **7**: 21.

Selection of patients for acute deep vein thrombosis treatment

CWKP Arnoldussen and RHW Strijkers

Introduction

Long-term sequelae after deep vein thrombosis may develop in approximately 25–60% of cases; these are designated as post-thrombotic syndrome.[1-6] The incidence of the syndrome shows a strong positive correlation with age, level of the deep vein thrombosis (proximal *versus* distal), ipsilateral recurrence of deep vein thrombosis, residual occlusion after deep vein thrombosis and residual reflux after deep vein thrombosis. Diagnosis of post-thrombotic syndrome is made by confirming presence of both a deep vein thrombosis in the medical history of a patient and by signs and symptoms related to chronic venous disease—as described in the Clinical Etiology Anatomy and Pathophysiology (CEAP) score, the Venous Clinical Severity Score (VCSS), and the Villalta score.[7-9] In severe cases of post-thrombotic syndrome, patients are greatly disabled by venous claudication and venous ulcers, and this leads to both a severe reduction in quality of life for the patient and high socioeconomic costs (by a combination of high medical care costs and decreased productivity of these patients).

Historically, an acute deep vein thrombosis was treated with anticoagulation therapy for three to six months, to prevent occurrence of pulmonary embolism, thrombus propagation and rethrombosis. Oral anticoagulants, however, have no effect on elimination of the thrombus; this is only realised by the innate thrombolytic system of the body. This system shows suboptimal removal of thrombosis, however, especially in iliofemoral deep vein thrombosis, as complete thrombus resolution is observed only in a minority of cases. Moreover, this process is characterised by an inflammation reaction leading to vein wall scarification and venous valve destruction, resulting in residual vein lumen obstruction and deep venous reflux respectively, the two cornerstones of post-thrombotic syndrome aetiology. Since the findings of Brandjes *et al* that treatment with elastic compression stockings and quick mobilisation following deep vein thrombosis reduces the incidence of post-thrombotic syndrome, the gold standard for deep vein thrombosis treatment has been a combination of oral anticoagulants, elastic compression stockings and mobilisation (as described by multiple international guidelines).[10-11]

During the last decade, however, a new treatment modality arose: catheter-directed thrombolysis, in which the thrombus is resolved by direct infusion of thrombolytic agents into the clot through a catheter placed inside the thrombus. Thereby, systemic levels of thrombolytic agents remain low during treatment. In

2012, Enden *et al* reported on the use of catheter-directed thrombolysis in deep vein thrombosis for the prevention of post-thrombotic syndrome in a multicentre randomised controlled trial.[12] Compared with the standard conservative therapy, the group with additional catheter-directed thrombolysis showed an absolute risk reduction of 14.4% in the incidence of post-thrombotic syndrome. Moreover, during the same period, percutaneous transluminal angioplasty and stenting have been described as a technique to treat the residual obstruction after a deep vein thrombosis, improving in particular the common and external iliac vein patency and thereby further reduce the chances of developing post-thrombotic syndrome.[13]

Catheter-directed thrombolysis

Current standard treatment of deep vein thrombosis consists of oral anticoagulation therapy for three to six months, compression therapy for two years and direct mobilisation of the patient. Short-term results of this treatment are good with low mortality of pulmonary embolism and limitation of thrombus propagation. However in the long term, results are not that good. In 30% of all patients, a recurrent deep vein thrombosis episode occurs within five years after cessation of anticoagulation therapy.[5] In 20–50% of all deep vein thrombosis patients, post-thrombotic syndrome occurs within the first two years after the first deep vein thrombosis episode.[14] Patients with an iliofemoral deep vein thrombosis have a two-fold increased risk of developing post-thrombotic syndrome.[15] Post-thrombotic syndrome diminishes quality of life and is a heavy burden on healthcare costs.[16] Post-thrombotic syndrome cannot be cured and current research, therefore, focuses on prevention of post-thrombotic syndrome in patients with iliofemoral deep vein thrombosis. Early clot lysis is associated with a higher patency of the iliofemoral tract and valve preservation.[17] Obstruction and reflux are associated with high incidence of post-thrombotic syndrome. Therefore, early lysis of the clot is hypothesised to prevent post-thrombotic syndrome. The literature has shown good results for catheter-directed thrombolysis and the reduction of post-thrombotic syndrome. Early 2012, the CAVENT (Catheter-directed venous thrombolysis) study showed an absolute risk reduction of 14.4% in patients treated with additional catheter-directed thrombolysis for (ilio)femoral deep vein thrombosis compared with patients with standard anticoagulation therapy. This is the first major randomised trial showing the additional benefit of catheter-directed thrombolysis for the prevention of post-thrombotic syndrome.[12] In addition to the data provided by the CAVENT study, there are multiple studies suggesting specific benefit for patients with (extensive) iliofemoral deep vein thrombosis, which is being investigated by the ongoing CAVA (Catheter *versus* anticoagulation alone) trial and the ATTRACT (Acute venous thrombosis: thrombus removal with adjunctive catheter-directed thrombolysis) trial.[18,19]

Considerations when selecting patients for intervention

Although initially the lytic drugs are given locally, during the treatment period, the drugs will diffuse and become systemic. The lytic drug will also dissolve thrombus elsewhere in the body and can cause bleeding. Patients with enhanced bleeding risks are, therefore, not candidates for catheter-directed thrombolysis. Patients with recent surgery (in the past six weeks), a history of bleeding in the past six

Exclusion criteria for catheter directed thrombolysis
History of Gastro-intestinal bleeding within six months
History of Cerebral Vascular Accident (CVA)/central nervous system disease
Severe hypertension (>180/100mmHg)
Active malignancy
Surgery within two weeks
Previous thrombosis of the affected limb (secondary thrombosis)
Pregnancy
Alanine transaminase (ALAT) >3 times normal range
Glomular Filtration Rate (eGFR) <30ml/min

Table 1: Exclusion criteria for catheter-directed thrombolysis.

months, or gastrointestinal bleeding—as well as patients with a cerebrovascular incident—in the past year have a strict contraindication for catheter-directed thrombolysis. Patients with active malignancies that are treated with surgery, chemo- or radiotherapy or those who have intracranial metastases are excluded from catheter-directed thrombolysis. Patients with decreased kidney function or decreased liver function also have a contraindication for ultrasound-assisted catheter-directed thrombolysis, because of potentially prolonged bleeding time and the use of contrast fluids to monitor treatment progress. Pregnant women and women until two weeks post-partum are also excluded from catheter-directed thrombolysis. The exclusion criteria are listed in Table 1.

Implications for interventional deep vein thrombosis treatment

Even though the reported risks for complications are low, we have to take these potentially serious adverse events into account when selecting patients for catheter-directed thrombolysis. In addition to the mentioned exclusion criteria, it is with the aid of non-invasive imaging that further patient selection can be performed. The aim of pre-interventional imaging should be the identification of acute *versus*

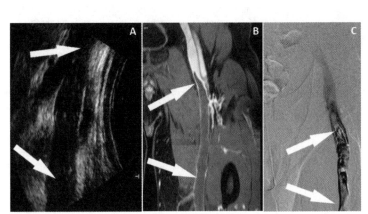

Figure 1: Evaluation of deep vein thrombosis at the level of the femoral and common femoral vein with (A) duplex ultrasound, (B) contrast-enhanced MR venography and (C) phlebography.

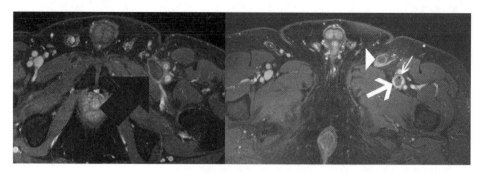

Figure 2: Assessment of thrombus characteristics with MR venograpy. An acute deep vein thrombosis of the left common femoral vein is shown on the left (black arrow). On the right an unknown deep vein thrombosis recurrence was identified in the common femoral vein with chronic remnants shown adhering to the vein wall (small white arrow) and acute clot obstructing the lumen (large white arrow). The greater saphenous vein is also thrombosed (arrowhead).

chronic obstructive components and external compression. Catheter-directed thrombolysis is effective and can be performed within a reasonable time window in the acute stage of deep vein thrombosis. Progression from acute to a more chronic state of deep vein thrombosis (transformation from clot to more "structured"' remnants) implies less effective or ineffective lysis, unnecessary prolonging the treatment time and increasing the risk of bleeding. External compression as a contributing cause to iliofemoral deep vein thrombosis refers to a significant lumen reduction or total occlusion in mainly the iliac deep vein tract requiring additional stenting to restore patency of the outflow to the inferior vena cava. With regard to thrombus location (to select iliofemoral deep vein thrombosis patients) duplex ultrasound, computed tomography (CT) and magnetic resonance (MR) imaging are capable of identifying thrombus in the veins from the calf up to the heart (Figure 1). In particular for duplex ultrasound, operator experience is vital for obtaining a complete overview of the deep vein system. CT venography and MR venography can provide a reliable alternative. Thrombus characteristics have been studied most extensively with MR imaging and there are some recent publications suggesting thrombus age can be measured.[20,21] The concept is to select patients with a high probability of successful catheter-directed thrombolysis and exclude those in which catheter-directed thrombolysis will not be effective based on thrombus characteristics (Figure 2).[20] Identification of external compression can be identified

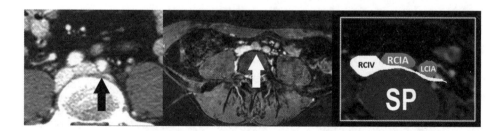

Figure 3: Non-thrombotic common iliac vein obstruction as shown with CT venography (left image, black arrow), MR venography (middle image, white arrow) and schematically (right image). The schematic shows an example of compression of the left common iliac vein proximally by the right common iliac artery and more distally by the left common iliac artery against the spine. Key: RCIV = right common iliac vein; RCIA = right common iliac artery; LCIA = left common iliac artery; and SP = spine.

with all the above mentioned modalities with a lower accuracy of identification of obstruction for duplex ultrasound in comparison to CT and MRI (Figure 3).

Conclusion

The evidence to support early intervention for iliofemoral deep vein thrombosis is clearly increasing. Patient selection is a key element to the primary success, the prevention of complications and (long-term) outcome of catheter-directed thrombolysis. Therefore, when considering catheter-directed thrombolysis, the pre-interventional work-up requires strict adherence to the exclusion criteria and (non-invasive) detailed analysis of the deep vein system.

Summary

- The strength of the evidence to support catheter-directed thrombolysis for deep vein thrombosis is increasing and we expect the ATTRACT trial and CAVA trial to establish catheter-directed thrombolysis as the standard of care for (ilio)femoral deep vein thrombosis.

- The rates of complications of catheter-directed thrombolysis are low in comparison to those of systemic thrombolytic therapy as long as strict exclusion criteria are applied.

- To further increase the success rate and potentially further reduce the risks of catheter-directed thrombolysis, non-invasive imaging should be performed prior to the intervention.

- Prior to the intervention non-invasive imaging should be used for two reasons:

  - Excluding non-acute deep vein thrombosis to ensure no unnecessary (prolonged) thrombolysis is performed that imposes an increased bleeding risk.

  - Non-thrombotic obstruction can (and should) be identified prior to starting catheter-directed thrombolysis and treated with recanalisation and stenting in conjunction with catheter-directed thrombolysis.

References

1. Tick LW, Kramer MHH, Rosendaal FR, et al. Risk factors for post-thrombotic syndrome in patients with a first deep venous thrombosis. *Journal of Thrombosis and Haemostasis* 2008; **6** (12): 2075–81.
2. Schulman S, Lindmarker P, Holmström M, et al. Post-thrombotic syndrome, recurrence, and death 10 years after the first episode of venous thromboembolism treated with warfarin for 6 weeks or 6 months. *Journal of Thrombosis and Haemostasis* 2006; **4** (4): 734–42.
3. Mohr DN, Silverstein MD, Heit JA, et al. The venous stasis syndrome after deep venous thrombosis or pulmonary embolism: a population-based study. *Mayo Clin Proc* 2000; **75** (12): 1249–56.
4. Stain M, Schönauer V, Minar E, et al. The post-thrombotic syndrome: risk factors and impact on the course of thrombotic disease. *Journal of Thrombosis and Haemostasis* 2005; **3** (12): 2671–76.
5. Prandoni P, Lensing AWA, Cogo A, et al. The long-term clinical course of acute deep venous thrombosis. *Ann Intern Med* 1996; **125** (1): 1.
6. Prandoni P, Villalta S, Bagatella P, et al. The clinical course of deep-vein thrombosis. Prospective long-term follow-up of 528 symptomatic patients. *Haematologica* 1997; **82** (4): 423–28.

7. Eklof B, Rutherford RB, Bergan JJ, *et al.* Revision of the CEAP classification for chronic venous disorders: consensus statement 2004. pp. 1248–52.

8. Vasquez MA, Munschauer CE. Revised venous clinical severity score: a facile measurement of outcomes in venous disease. *Phlebology* 2012; **27** Suppl 1: 119–29.

9. Villalta S, Bagatella P, Piccioli A, *et al.* Assessment of validity and reproducibility of a clinical scale for the post-thrombotic syndrome. *Haemostasis* 1994; **24** (158a).

10. Brandjes DP, Büller HR, Heijboer H, *et al.* Randomised trial of effect of compression stockings in patients with symptomatic proximal-vein thrombosis. *The Lancet* 1997; 349 **(9054):** 759–62.

11. Kearon C, Akl EA, Comerota AJ, *et al.* Antithrombotic therapy for VTE disease: Antithrombotic Therapy and Prevention of Thrombosis, 9th ed: American College of Chest Physicians Evidence-Based Clinical Practice Guidelines. *Chest* 2012; **141** (2 Suppl): e419S–94S.

12. Enden T, Haig Y, Kløw N-E, *et al.* Long-term outcome after additional catheter-directed thrombolysis *versus* standard treatment for acute iliofemoral deep vein thrombosis (the CaVenT study): a randomised controlled trial. *Lancet* 2012; **379** (9810): 31–38.

13. Baekgaard N, Broholm R, Just S, *et al.* Long-term results using catheter-directed thrombolysis in 103 lower limbs with acute iliofemoral venous thrombosis. *Eur J Vasc Endovasc Surg* 2010; 39(1): 112–17.

14. Kahn SR, Ginsberg JS. Relationship between deep venous thrombosis and the postthrombotic syndrome. *Arch Intern Med* 2004; **164** (1): 17–26.

15. Kahn SR, Shrier I, Julian JA, *et al.* Determinants and time course of the postthrombotic syndrome after acute deep venous thrombosis. *Ann Intern Med* 2008; **149** (10): 698–707.

16. Kahn SR, Shbaklo H, Lamping DL, *et al.* Determinants of health-related quality of life during the 2 years following deep vein thrombosis. *Journal of Thrombosis and Haemostasis* 2008; **6** (7): 1105–12.

17. Grewal NK, Martinez JT, Andrews L, *et al.* Quantity of clot lysed after catheter-directed thrombolysis for iliofemoral deep venous thrombosis correlates with postthrombotic morbidity. *Journal of Vascular Surgery*; 2010; **51** (5): 1209–14.

18. Strijkers RH, Cate-Hoek AJ, Bukkems SF, *et al.* Management of deep vein thrombosis and prevention of post-thrombotic syndrome. *BMJ* 2011; **343:** d5916.

19. Vedantham S, Goldhaber SZ, Kahn SR, *et al.* Rationale and design of the ATTRACT Study: a multicenter randomized trial to evaluate pharmacomechanical catheter-directed thrombolysis for the prevention of postthrombotic syndrome in patients with proximal deep vein thrombosis. *Am Heart J* 2013; **165** (4): 523–530.e3.

20. Arnoldussen C, Strijkers R, Lambregts D, *et al.* Feasibility of identifying deep vein thrombosis characteristics with contrast enhanced MR-Venography. *Phlebology* 2014; **29** (1 suppl): 119–24.

21. Tan M, Mol GC, van Rooden CJ, Klok FA, *et al.* Magnetic resonance direct thrombus imaging differentiates acute recurrent ipsilateral deep vein thrombosis from residual thrombosis. *Blood* 2014; **124** (4): 623–27

It is not just about patency—scales and quality of life outcomes

TRA Lane and AH Davies

Introduction

Vascular surgeons have spent many years treating patients as "technical conundrums", primarily because of the difficulties of providing them with "working plumbing" (i.e. patent veins). As technology and surgical techniques have advanced, providing this has become less difficult. Also, these advances have allowed assessment of how treatments and their failure can affect patients and their quality of life.[1-3] Indeed, most arterial trials now include a quality of life assessment.[4] Because of the benign nature of venous disease, and the complex haemodynamics and time lag associated with the development of venous ulceration,[5,6] justification for intervention in superficial venous disease has long had to involve the use of quality of life scores and clinical severity scores.[7,8]

Furthermore, recent developments in deep venous disease have radically changed the understanding of interventional options and their sequelae. The advent of cheap reliable non-invasive imaging with duplex ultrasound, and comparison with intravascular ultrasound (IVUS), has revealed new anatomical and haemodynamic information.

Deep venous disease pathology comprises of two main components—obstruction and reflux—and is less common than superficial venous disease. Obstruction and reflux may both be present and can be primary (non-thrombotic iliac vein lesions) or secondary to thrombosis (or less commonly, trauma). The most common finding is obstruction; in primary cases, it often presents as the eponymous May-Thurner or Cockett's Syndrome, but this is present in a significant percentage of the asymptomatic population.[9] Obstruction secondary to thrombosis is often associated with pre-existing non-thrombotic stenoses or occlusions, and so this clinical picture provides evidence that such lesions appear to be a permissive phenomenon rather than necessarily pathogenic.[10] Complete obstruction of the iliac vein is most commonly secondary to thrombosis, with iliac veins demonstrating poor recanalisation and collateralisation behaviours. After a thrombotic event, few veins recanalise fully, with scarring, webbing and incompetent valves a significant feature, leading to reflux in high resistance outflow tracts.

Post-thrombotic syndrome

This syndrome has a wide spectrum and affects 25–50% of those who have suffered a deep vein thrombosis despite post-diagnosis anticoagulation.[11] Symptoms vary from mild limb swelling and moderate aching through to intractable oedema and pain, skin changes and treatment-resistant ulceration. It is thought to be due to poor venous outflow of the affected limb due to obstruction, leading to persistent venous hypertension and, therefore, reduced capillary flow.

Treatment of post-thrombotic syndrome has been largely limited to symptomatic relief; in a recent study, compression hosiery was not found to prevent post-thrombotic syndrome or to improve quality of life or symptom scores.[12] In severe cases, phlebotonics (such as horse chestnut extract) therapy may offer some symptomatic benefit.[11]

Deep venous stenting

Deep venous stenting has become a new weapon in the battle against the debilitating and chronic swollen legs of post-thrombotic syndrome and chronic venous disease. This approach has been popularised by pioneering work by Raju and Neglen,[13] who used IVUS to delineate lesions not previously identified on duplex ultrasound or conventional venography. This early work has been replicated in other centres to provide a firm foundation for intervention.[14,15] However, randomised trials are lacking. Interestingly, though stenting the deep venous system does not produce competent veins, the reduction of outflow obstruction provides sufficient haemodynamic improvement.[16] Stenting provides an attractive intervention—percutaneous access and straightforward procedures.

Clinical scoring systems

The standard clinical scoring systems for venous disease are appropriate for use in deep venous disease, and international guidance recommend use of both clinical scoring scales and quality of life scales.[17] The Clinical Etiological Anatomical Pathological (CEAP) score is a clinician completed score that allows for broad classification of the clinical sequelae of venous disease (and is most commonly used as a "basic" C component only). However, it is insensitive to change and provides only six classes for all of venous disease.[18] The revised Venous Clinical Severity Score (VCSS) and its lesser used additional components (Venous Segmental Disease Score and Venous Disability Score) allow assessment of the complete symptomatic and clinical picture. It is, however, a clinician-completed score and combines both subjective and objective findings (for example pain experienced, use of stockings and degree of haemosiderin deposition), which reduces comparability.[18]

The Villalta scale is a specific scoring system for patients with deep vein thrombosis and is used in the assessment of post-thrombotic syndrome. The Ginsberg measure is a similar scoring system. Both are designed for assessment of post-thrombotic syndrome after deep vein thrombosis rather than unfiltered cases.[19] Other scoring systems used infrequently for post-thrombotic syndrome are Brandjes and Widmer scales, although these have been superseded.[19] International consensus has recommended the use of the Villalta scale for assessment of post-thrombotic syndrome;[11,20] however, the largest study on treatment of post-thrombotic syndrome (SOX—Compression stockings to prevent post-thrombotic syndrome—trial) used the Ginsberg measure as a primary outcome[12] and thus comparison of studies is often difficult.

Quality of life scales

Quality of life scores in deep venous disease are less well investigated than their superficial venous cousins.

Generic scores—such as the EuroQol 5 Domain (EQ-5D) and EuroQol Visual Analogue Scale (EQ-VAS) or the Short Form 36 (SF-36) and its derivations—allow holistic assessment of the person's quality of life. This holistic assessment also allows comparison between diseases and interpretation of the impact of treatment with the culprit disease—patient success rather than technical success.[18]

Disease-specific scores—such as those used in varicose vein disease (Aberdeen Varicose Vein Questionnaire or Chronic Venous Insufficiency quality of life Questionnaire)—provide some ability to assess quality of life in patients superficial venous disease; however, these questionnaires are not designed to assess deep venous disease.[18] The Venous Insufficiency Epidemiological and Economic Study Quality of Life/Symptoms score (VEINES-QOL/Sym) has been shown to be an effective tool for assessing quality of life of patients with both superficial venous disease and deep venous disease,[18] and, therefore, allows comparative assessment. Additionally, it has been shown to correlate with disease severity as assessed by CEAP classification.[21]

Outcomes of stenting

Stent outcomes are extremely difficult to generalise with the majority of the data available coming from small scale studies using differing stent technologies and post-procedural anticoagulation techniques.

A recent systematic review by the Imperial group identified extremely disparate data, with multiple different outcomes quoted (akin to the early days of superficial venous treatment).[22,23]

The review identified six main outcome classes in 17 studies, but was not able to calculate a treatment effect in any of these classes because none of the studies included a control group. Patency rates were 32–99% over a time period of 6–48 months follow-up, with ulcer healing rates of 56–100%. Clinical severity and quality of life scores improved in most studies reporting them (five for clinical severity and four for quality of life), but with disparate tools and systems used, comparison was exceptionally difficult. In the management of a long-term, symptomatic syndrome, quality of life tools must be a key marker of treatment as it is in superficial venous disease.[17]

Significantly, multiple different venous stents exist, with the majority of longer term data available for off-licence use of Wallstent endoprostheses (Boston Scientific). No comparator study has investigated individual stents and, as with endovascular aneurysm repair (EVAR) or endovenous laser ablation, technological advances are far beyond their supportive data. With the advent of bespoke venous stents, it is hoped that the variation in outcomes will be vastly reduced.

Conclusion

It appears that early data support the use of deep venous stents to treat deep venous obstruction, with improved clinical status and quality of life scores. However, the data available are extremely sparse and further work, with randomised clinical trials and long-term, prospective cohort-based studies, is needed to clarify optimal treatment pathways and stent usage. This will allow understanding of how patency and symptom outcomes are related and which patients and lesions will benefit the most from intervention. Additionally, as stent technologies advance, the evidence base must keep pace.

Summary

- Deep venous stenting has been shown to improve clinical status and quality of life at early follow-up.

- The use of IVUS in conjunction with biplanar venography has allowed comprehensive assessment of venous outflow obstructions.

- The use of clinical scores and quality of life scores allow better understanding of the complex nature of deep venous disease beyond basic technical success.

- Venous stent technology is rapidly advancing and new stents are being introduced far in advance of robust long-term data.

- The use of the CEAP classification, Venous Clinical Severity Score (VCSS) and Venous Insufficiency Epidemiological and Economic Study Qulity of Life/Symptoms (VEINES-QOL/Sym) score is recommended as a minimum dataset for studies investigating deep venous disease.

References

1. Bulpitt CJ. Quality of life as an outcome measure. *Postgraduate Medical Journal* 1997; **73** (864): 613–16.
2. Kayssi A, DeBord Smith A, *et al.* Health-related quality-of-life outcomes after open *versus* endovascular abdominal aortic aneurysm repair. *JVS* 2015; **62** (2): 491–98.
3. Donker J, de Vries J, Ho G, *et al.* Review: Quality of life in lower limb peripheral vascular surgery. *Vascular* 2016; **4**(1): 88–95.
4. Werner M, Schmidt A, Scheinert S, *et al.* Evaluation of the Biodegradable Igaki-Tamai Scaffold After Drug-Eluting Balloon Treatment of De Novo Superficial Femoral Artery Lesions: The GAIA-DEB Study. *JEVT* 2016; **23** (1): 92–97.
5. Rabe E, Pannier-Fischer F, Bromen K, *et al.* Bonner Venenstudie der Deutschen Gesellschaft für Phlebologie* Epidemiologische Untersuchung zur Frage der Häufigkeit und Ausprägung von chronischen Venenkrankheiten in der städtischen und ländlichen Wohnbevölkerung. *Phlebologie* 2003; **32** (1): 1–14.
6. Pannier F, Rabe E. Progression in venous pathology. *Phlebology* 2015; **30** (1 Suppl): 95–97.
7. Andreozzi GM, Cordova RM, Scomparin A, *et al.* Quality of life in chronic venous insufficiency. An Italian pilot study of the Triveneto Region. *Int Angio* 2005; **24** (3): 272–77.
8. Çeviker K, Şahinalp Ş, Çiçek E, *et al.* Quality of life in patients with chronic venous disease in Turkey: influence of different treatment modalities at 6-month follow-up. *Quality of Life Research* 2015. Epub
9. Kibbe MR, Ujiki M, Goodwin AL, *et al* J. Iliac vein compression in an asymptomatic patient population. *JVS* 2004; **39** (5): 937–43.
10. Raju S, Neglén P. High prevalence of nonthrombotic iliac vein lesions in chronic venous disease: a permissive role in pathogenicity. *JVS* 2006; **44** (1): 136–43.
11. Kahn SR. The post thrombotic syndrome. *Thromb Res* 2011; **127** (Suppl 3): S89–92.
12. Kahn S, Shapiro S, Wells PS, *et al.* Compression stockings to prevent post-thrombotic syndrome: a randomised placebo-controlled trial. *Lancet* 2014; **383** (9920): 880–88.
13. Neglén P, Raju S. Balloon dilation and stenting of chronic iliac vein obstruction: technical aspects and early clinical outcome. *J Endovasc Ther* 2000; **7** (2): 79–91.
14. Alhalbouni S, Hingorani A, Shiferson A, *et al.* Iliac-femoral venous stenting for lower extremity venous stasis symptoms. *Ann Vasc Surg* 2012; **26** (2): 185–89.
15. Gaweesh AS, Kayed MH, Gaweesh TY, *et al.* Underlying deep venous abnormalities in patients with unilateral chronic venous disease. *Phlebology* 2013; **28** (8): 426–31.

16. Raju S, Darcey R, Neglén P. Unexpected major role for venous stenting in deep reflux disease. *JVS* 2010; **51** (2): 401–8

17. Gloviczki P, Comerota AJ, Dalsing MC, *et al.* The care of patients with varicose veins and associated chronic venous diseases: clinical practice guidelines of the Society for Vascular Surgery and the American Venous Forum. *Journal of Vascular Surgery* 2011: 2S–48S.

18. Catarinella FS, Nieman FHM, Wittens CHA. An overview of the most commonly used venous quality of life and clinical outcome measurements. *JVS:VLD* 2015; **3** (3): 333–40.

19. Soosainathan A, Moore HM, Gohel MS, Davies AH. Scoring systems for the post-thrombotic syndrome. JVS. *Society for Vascular Surgery;* 2013; **57** (1): 254–61.

20. Saedon M, Stansby G. Post-thrombotic syndrome: prevention is better than cure. *Phlebology* 2010; **25** Suppl 1:14–9.

21. Kahn SR, M'lan CE, Lamping DL, *et al.* Relationship between clinical classification of chronic venous disease and patient-reported quality of life: results from an international cohort study. *JVS* 2004; **39** (4): 823–28.

22. Seager MJ, Busuttil A, Dharmarajah B, Davies AH. A Systematic Review of Endovenous Stenting in Chronic Venous Disease Secondary to Iliac Vein Obstruction *EJVES* 2016; **51** (1): 100–20.

23. Vedantham S, Grassi CJ, Ferral H, *et al.* Reporting standards for endovascular treatment of lower extremity deep vein thrombosis. *JVIR* 2006; **17** (3): 417–34.

Molecular and cellular basis of lymphoedema and venous disease

O Lyons and S Black

Introduction

The most frequent lymphatic vascular anomaly is lymphoedema, which is characterised by an abnormal accumulation of interstitial fluid due to insufficient lymphatic function, and affects approximately 1.3/1000 population in the UK.[1,2] Lymphoedema may be primary (genetic) or secondary (due to some other insult, most commonly treatment of malignancy, or infection). In the past, primary lymphoedemas have been seen as a relatively homogeneous group of diseases. On the basis of age at onset and variable lymphangiographic appearances, they were classified as congenital, praecox and tarda.[3] This system is now outmoded and has been replaced by an approach focusing on accurate phenotyping and identification of the underlying genetic aetiology.[4,5] Treatment is usually limited to conservative measures—compression and manual lymphatic drainage, but can include physiological operations to improve flow, or liposuction to reduce limb volume. Debulking procedures are reserved for advanced disease.[6] Understanding of the molecular and cellular basis of primary (and secondary) lymphoedema has revealed a range of disorders with variable effects on fluid uptake, transport and reflux. Treatment of secondary lymphoedema by stimulation of lymphangiogenesis with adenovirally transfected vascular endothelial growth factor C has shown success in small and large animal models and is now being evaluated in first-in-man clinical studies. There has been progress in understanding the relationship of primary lymphoedema to venous reflux, but the causes of primary venous reflux remain unclear, and understanding of the molecular regulation of veins and valves is lacking.[7] In this chapter, recent progress is summarised and a route to replicating in venous disease the progress seen in lymphoedema is discussed.

Improved classification of primary lymphoedema

The primary lymphoedemas vary widely in their phenotype and associated features.[4,5,8] Alongside improvements in DNA sequencing technology and analysis pipelines, progress has been enabled by accurate and detailed phenotyping of the lymphatic anatomical defects, functional disorders, and associated features (e.g. distichiasis). The classification pathway of primary lymphoedema now includes increasingly well-described single gene disorders.[4,5] Five sections of the classification pathway are outlined as follows:

- Syndromic. Lymphoedema is recognised as part of several syndromes, and these patients display a number of abnormal features alongside their oedema. Examples of such syndromes include Turner's (*45XO*), Noonan's (mutations in *PTPN11* and others), Prader Willi (mainly *15q11* microdeletion) and Oculo-dento-digital dysplasia (mutation in *GJA1*).
- Systemic/visceral involvement. These individuals show a widespread developmental abnormality of the lymphatic system, not confined to the peripheries. Disease may be segmental/multisegmental, or show a uniform and widespread pattern of oedema in all body segments (e.g. Hennekam Syndrome, caused by mutations in *CCBE1* and *FAT4*).
- Disturbed growth and/or cutaneous/vascular anomalies. This group includes individuals with CLOVE syndrome due to increased signalling via the *PIK3/AKT/mTOR* signalling pathway, giving rise to the potential utility of mTOR inhibitors (e.g. rapamycin) in treating these patients. Klippel Trenauney, Parkes-Weber and Lymphangiomatosis are also grouped here.
- Congenital (<1 year of age) onset lymphoedema. This group includes patients with Milroy disease, of which approximately 70% of cases are due to mutations in vascular endothelial growth factor receptor 3. In Milroy's, the lymphoedema is typically present at birth and is bilateral, and associated with upturned toenails.
- Late onset (>one year) primary lymphoedema. This group includes patients with lymphoedema distichiasis (which is caused by mutations in *FOXC2*) and Meige's disease (genetic cause unknown).

The molecular and cellular basis for lymphoedema

Identification of markers for identifying lymphatic endothelial cells has led to enormous progress in understanding how the lymphatic system develops, is maintained in adult life, and responds to disease.[8] Populations of lymphatic cells arise via sprouting from veins and also non-venous sources, and subsequently develop into the network of vessels required to function as a critical component of the circulatory system.[9,10] Studies of lymphatic cells *in vitro* and in animal models are leading to great progress in understanding at a molecular level the broad range of mechanisms by which lymphatic diseases occur.[8,11]

The first gene identified in which mutations are responsible for lymphoedema was *FLT-4*, which encodes vascular endothelial growth factor receptor 3 (VEGFR3), a tyrosine kinase receptor initially required for normal development of the blood vascular system, and then at later stages critically required for lymphatic development.[11] Missense mutations in the tyrosine kinase domain of VEGFR3 result in Milroy's disease, which is usually inherited in an autosomal dominant manner and presents at birth with bilateral oedema, eventually extending up to the knees. Patients can present with prenatal pleural effusion or in utero hydrops.[11-13] In patients, initial lymphatics are present but are unable to properly absorb interstitial fluid, which is seen on lymphoscintigraphy as a failure of uptake.[14] A similar pattern of oedema is seen with haploinsufficiency of vascular endothelial growth factor C (*VEGFC*), the major ligand for *VEGFR3*.[5]

Discovery of the role of *FLT-4* was followed by identification of mutations in the transcription factor *FOXC2* as being causative of lymphoedema distichiasis, in which lymphoedema is accompanied by abnormal growth of additional eyelashes from the meibomian glands.[15] In both Milroy's and lymphoedema distichiasis there is an increased incidence of venous reflux, for unknown reasons.[14] In mice, Foxc2 is required for maturation of lymphatic collecting vessels and lymphatic valve formation, and in patients lymphoscintigraphy, typically shows dermal reflux of tracer that is presumably due to refluxing hyperplastic lymphatics.[5,16]

These early discoveries have been followed by more rapid recent developments, including the finding that mutations in *SOX18* cause the very rare syndrome Hypotrichosis-lymphoedema-telangiectasia. Mutations in *CCBE1* cause the generalised lymphatic dysplasia seen in children with Hennekam Syndrome. Mutations in two genes, *GJC2* and *GJA1*, which encode connexins (the components of gap junctions), have also been shown to cause lymphoedema. *GJC2* mutations are causative of a typically (but variable) four limb oedema. Lymphoscintigraphy in these patients shows a normal appearance of lymphatic tracts, but upon quantification the transport of tracer is reduced.[5] *GJA1* mutations form part of oculo-dento-digital dysplasia, causing typically lower limb oedema. Mutations in *PIEZO1* can cause lymphoedema with mild spherocytosis.[17] *KIF11* encodes a protein (EG5) involved in spindle formation.[18] The mechanisms by which mutations in *PIEZO1* and *KIF11* cause lymphoedema remain unknown.[5] Mutations in *GATA2* cause lymphoedema as part of Emberger syndrome, with a predisposition towards acute myeloid leukaemia, and a lower limb functional lymphatic hypoplasia on lymphoscintigraphy.[5]

Progress towards curative therapies for lymphoedema

Understanding of the genetic basis of human lymphoedema, and of mechanisms of disease in animal models, is leading towards novel therapies for lymphoedema in man.[19,20] In mice, lymphatics have been stimulated with VEGFC—the major ligand for VEGFR3—to regrow following axillary dissection.[21] In large animal models (sheep, pigs), lymphatics can be stimulated to re-grow following a disruption of lymphatics similar to that commonly seen after surgery in patients. Postoperative oedema was reduced following intervention.[22,23] Following on from these key advances, clinical studies of adenoviral transfection of VEGFC in combination with lymph node transfer, initially for the treatment of breast cancer-associated lymphoedema, are due to begin recruiting in Europe in 2016.

Treating genetic vascular disease with drugs is becoming feasible

Understanding the molecular basis of venous malformations has led to the development of cell and mouse models, and an understanding that these malformations frequently result from increased signalling through an intracellular signalling pathway (*PI3K*/AKT/mTOR), often due to mutations in the gene encoding the surface receptor Tie2 that increase its signalling activity. The drug rapamycin inhibits AKT signalling downstream of Tie2, and so is able to bypass the effects of the abnormal Tie2 protein. Recent studies in patients have shown benefit from treatment with rapamycin.[24] In a clinical pilot study of the treatment of vascular malformations refractory to standard care, systemic treatment with rapamycin resulted in reduced lesion size and pain, and improved quality of life and function in affected limbs. Patients who were previously affected by episodes of bleeding or infections noted reductions in these events. The side effects of treatment were primarily mucositis and headaches.[24] The use of rapamycin to treat these lesions is particularly notable since it was already in use for another indication, so developing drug therapies does not necessarily require development of novel molecules, providing hope for patients with other relatively rare vascular disorders and proving the merits of delineating the mechanisms of other rare diseases in the laboratory. In a further study, a low dose of rapamycin resulted in successful treatment of blue rubber bleb nevus syndrome.[25] Independently, treatment was associated with clinical improvement in children with complex vascular anomalies.[26] It is also currently undergoing phase 2 testing in a multicentre clinical trial of treatment for lymphatico-vascular malformations in young patients.[27]

Progress in venous disease is lacking

In contrast to the developments in understanding and the development of novel therapies for lymphoedema, progress in venous disease has been painfully slow.[7,28,29] Primary venous disease probably encompasses a broad range of genetic defects and molecular aetiologies that may require different treatments. These subgroups are not identified, and there has been little or no progress in understanding their underlying mechanisms. It has long been known that patients with primary lymphoedema have an increased incidence of venous reflux.[29,30] Whilst this has previously been thought to reflect the venous origin of the lymphatic system, this has not made sense on a molecular level, and does not sit well with recent findings of additional non-venous origins of lymphatics.[9,10] Recently, it has become clear that venous valves show a high degree of molecular similarity to lymphatics; they express and are regulated by genes that regulate lymphangiogenesis.[31] This finding can explain the increased incidence of venous reflux in patients with lymphoedema. Venous insufficiency may contribute to the oedema and skin disease in these patients.

Identification of genetic causes of venous failure has lagged behind progress in the lymphatic system; although venous disease is far more common, a lack of accurate methods with which to visualise valves, and phenotype valve failure, has precluded identification of groups of patients with similar defects. It is now possible to systematically visualise and quantify venous valves in patients, enabling a more detailed characterisation of venous valve disease. This can now be utilised to identify patients with primary venous valve failure, and phenotype distribution and characteristics of their disease enabling modern approaches to identification of causative genes. Progress is most likely to be made with extreme phenotypes, such as early onset widespread venous reflux. Understanding the mechanisms of these rarer conditions is directly applicable to understanding the molecular regulation of veins and valves in the general population. Furthermore, as with lymphatic disease and venous malformations, this understanding will be applicable to secondary venous disease requiring restoration of normal venous function, including the setting of

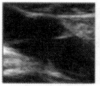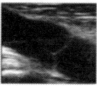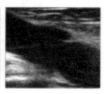

Figure 1: Venous valves can now be visualised on a systematic basis, allowing quantification of valve phenotypes in primary valve disease.

post thrombotic reflux. Developing pharmacological therapy for a failing venous system may not necessarily require development of new molecules (as has been seen with re-purposing of Rapamycin to treating vascular malformations).

Summary

- In the lymphatic system, understanding of the broad range of the genetic causes of primary (and secondary) lymphoedema and understanding of the mechanisms of disease at the molecular and cellular level is leading to the development of novel therapies.

- Adenoviral transfection of *VEGFC* in combination with lymph node transfer is entering first in man studies for treatment of breast cancer associated lymphoedema in 2016.

- Drug therapies (e.g. rapamycin) for vascular malformations are undergoing pilot studies and reported results indicate improvements in lesion size, function and haematological function.

- Our understanding of the basis of venous disease is lagging but molecular markers for venous valves have been identified, and the first genes required for the development and subsequent maintenance of venous valves described.

- Venous valves can now be visualised and quantified in patients. Accurate disease phenotyping may lead to identification of underlying genetic aetiologies and allow development of novel therapies. Initial progress may be made with extreme phenotypes, such as early onset widespread venous reflux.

References

1. Moffatt CJ, Franks PJ, Doherty DC, Williams AF, *et al.* Lymphoedema: an underestimated health problem. *QJM* 2003; **96** (10): 731–8.
2. Mortimer PS, and Rockson SG. New developments in clinical aspects of lymphatic disease. *J Clin Invest* 2014; **124** (3): 915–21.
3. Kinmonth JB, Taylor GW, Tracy GD, and Marsh JD. Primary lymphoedema; clinical and lymphangiographic studies of a series of 107 patients in which the lower limbs were affected. *Br J Surg* 1957; **45** (189): 1–9.
4. Connell F, Brice G, Jeffery S, Keeley V, *et al.* A new classification system for primary lymphatic dysplasias based on phenotype. *Clinical Genetics* 2010; **77** (5): 438–52.
5. Connell FC, Gordon K, Brice G, Keeley V, *et al.* The classification and diagnostic algorithm for primary lymphatic dysplasia: an update from 2010 to include molecular findings. *Clin Genet* 2013; **84** (4): 303–14.
6. Cormier JN, Rourke L, Crosby M, Chang D, *et al.* The surgical treatment of lymphedema: a systematic review of the contemporary literature (2004-2010). *Annals of Surgical Oncology* 2012; **19** (2): 642–51.
7. Ng MYM. Linkage to the FOXC2 region of chromosome 16 for varicose veins in otherwise healthy, unselected sibling pairs. *Journal of Medical Genetics* 2005; **42** (3): 235–39.
8. Alitalo K. The lymphatic vasculature in disease. *Nat Med* 2011; **17** (11): 1371–80.
9. Stanczuk L, Martinez-Corral I, Ulvmar MH, Zhang Y, *et al.* cKit lineage hemogenic endothelium-derived cells contribute to mesenteric lymphatic vessels. *Cell reports* 2015.
10. Martinez-Corral I, Ulvmar MH, Stanczuk L, Tatin F, *et al.* Nonvenous origin of dermal lymphatic vasculature. *Circ Res* 2015; **116** (10): 1649–54.
11. Brouillard P, Boon L, and Vikkula M. Genetics of lymphatic anomalies. *J Clin Invest* 2014; **124** (3): 898–904.

12. Ferrell RE, Levinson KL, Esman JH, Kimak MA, *et al.* Hereditary lymphedema: evidence for linkage and genetic heterogeneity. *Hum Mol Genet* 1998; **7** (13): 2073–78.

13. Karkkainen MJ, Ferrell RE, Lawrence EC, Kimak MA, *et al.* Missense mutations interfere with VEGFR-3 signalling in primary lymphoedema. *Nat Genet* 2000; **25** (2): 153–59.

14. Mellor RH, Hubert CE, Stanton AWB, Tate N, *et al.* Lymphatic dysfunction, not aplasia, underlies Milroy disease. *Microcirculation* 2010; **17** (4): 281–96.

15. Fang J, Dagenais SL, Erickson RP, Arlt MF, *et al.* Mutations in FOXC2 (MFH-1), a forkhead family transcription factor, are responsible for the hereditary lymphedema-distichiasis syndrome. *Am J Hum Genet* 2000; **67** (6): 1382–88.

16. Petrova TV, Karpanen T, Norrmén C, Mellor R, *et al.* Defective valves and abnormal mural cell recruitment underlie lymphatic vascular failure in lymphedema distichiasis. *Nature Medicine* 2004; **10** (9): 974–81.

17. Fotiou E, Martin-Almedina S, Simpson MA, Lin S, *et al.* Novel mutations in PIEZO1 cause an autosomal recessive generalized lymphatic dysplasia with non-immune hydrops fetalis. *Nature communications* 2015; **6:** 8085.

18. Ostergaard P, Simpson MA, Mendola A, *et al.* Mutations in KIF11 cause autosomal-dominant microcephaly variably associated with congenital lymphedema and chorioretinopathy. *Am J Hum Genet* 2012; **90** (2): 356–62.

19. Yoon YS, Murayama T, Gravereaux E, Tkebuchava T, *et al.* VEGF-C gene therapy augments postnatal lymphangiogenesis and ameliorates secondary lymphedema. *J Clin Invest* 2003; **111** (5): 717–25.

20. Baker A, Kim H, Semple JL, Dumont D, *et al.* Experimental assessment of pro-lymphangiogenic growth factors in the treatment of post-surgical lymphedema following lymphadenectomy. Breast cancer research: *BCR* 2010; **12** (5): R70.

21. Tammela T, Saaristo A, Holopainen T, Lyytikkä J, *et al.* Therapeutic differentiation and maturation of lymphatic vessels after lymph node dissection and transplantation. *Nature Medicine* 2007; **13** (12): 1458–66.

22. Szuba A, Skobe M, Karkkainen MJ, Shin WS, *et al.* Therapeutic lymphangiogenesis with human recombinant VEGF-C. FASEB J 2002; **16** (14): 1985–87.

23. Lahteenvuo M, Honkonen K, Tervala T, Tammela T, *et al.* Growth factor therapy and autologous lymph node transfer in lymphedema. *Circulation* 2011; **123** (6): 613–20.

24. Boscolo E, Limaye N, Huang L, Kang KT, *et al.* Rapamycin improves TIE2-mutated venous malformation in murine model and human subjects. *J Clin Invest* 2015; **125** (9): 3491–504.

25. Yuksekkaya H, Ozbek O, Keser M, and Toy H. Blue rubber bleb nevus syndrome: successful treatment with sirolimus. *Pediatrics* 2012; **129** (4): e1080–4.

26. Lackner H, Karastaneva A, Schwinger W, Benesch M, *et al.* Sirolimus for the treatment of children with various complicated vascular anomalies. European Journal of Pediatrics 2015; **174 (12):** 1579–84.

27. Hammill AM, Wentzel M, Gupta A, Nelson S, *et al.* Sirolimus for the treatment of complicated vascular anomalies in children. *Pediatric Blood & Cancer* 2011; **57** (6): 1018–24.

28. Anwar MA, Georgiadis KA, Shalhoub J, Lim CS, *et al.* A review of familial, genetic, and congenital aspects of primary varicose vein disease. *Circulation Cardiovascular Genetics* 2012; **5** (4): 460–6.

29. Mellor RH, Brice G, Stanton AWB, French J, *et al.* Mutations in FOXC2 are strongly associated with primary valve failure in veins of the lower limb. *Circulation* 2007; **115** (14): 1912–20.

30. Rosbotham JL, Brice GW, Child AH, Nunan TO, *et al.* Distichiasis-lymphoedema: clinical features, venous function and lymphoscintigraphy. The British Journal of Dermatology 2000; **142** (1): 148–52.

31. Bazigou E, Lyons OT, Smith A, Venn GE, *et al.* Genes regulating lymphangiogenesis control venous valve formation and maintenance in mice. *J Clin Invest* 2011; **121** (8): 2984–92.

Superficial venous challenges

Ultrasound-placed percutaneous clips will make CHIVA more widely applicable

L Kabnick and A Miller

Introduction

Varicose veins, which are estimated to affect approximately 23% of adults in the USA, are part of a spectrum of chronic venous disease and are generally more common in women than men (between the ages of 40 years and 80 years).[1,2] Untreated, varicose veins may eventually progress to severe chronic venous insufficiency with symptoms and other manifestations including lower extremity venous ulceration. Until the turn of the century, the standard of care in the USA for the treatment of varicose veins was surgery with high ligation, stripping of the saphenous vein, and phlebectomy of the presenting varicosities. More recently, alternative treatments for varicose veins—including endothermal ablation with laser or radiofrequency, together with chemical treatments and chemical adhesives—have replaced surgery as the standard of care.[3] These procedures have brought the treatment of varicose veins out of the hospital surgical operating rooms and into the outpatient surgical clinics and offices, reducing hospital costs for patient management and minimising patient morbidity; however, the underlying pathophysiological approach to the treatment of these patients has not changed. The treatment remains aimed at preventing reflux in the lower extremity veins with occlusion of the incompetent saphenous vein(s) and phlebectomy of the superficial varicosities.

In the early 1990s, Claude Franceschi described an alternative approach, saphenous sparing, to treat venous insufficiency associated with varicose veins.[4] Unlike other surgical and endovascular approaches, the "CHIVA" (Cure conservatrice et Hemodynamique de L'Issufsance veineuse en Ambulatoire or conservative hemodynamic cure for varicose veins) approach does not aim to eliminate all of the reflux in the lower extremity veins but rather aims to direct the flow of the "refluxing" blood into the deep veins of the lower extremity. Ultimately, the CHIVA method attempts to relieve the pressure in the superficial veins, thus eliminating the problem of superficial venous hypertension and the clinical consequences of varicose veins.

This method of treatment has two main requirements: an accurate ultrasonic assessment of the flow patterns in the extremity veins to select the optimal flow diversions that need to be performed; and accurate open surgical ligation.[5] These minimally invasive surgical procedures require some surgical expertise. Additionally, because multiple occlusions may be required, they are also time

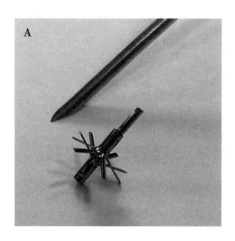

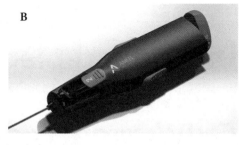

Figure 1: (A) The deployed Amsel vessel occluder, with the two occluding elements locked together. (B) The unoccluded occlusion elements are provided preloaded into the 18G needle of the delivery device.

consuming and disfiguring. Because of the combination of demanding ultrasonic expertise and the associated surgical skills required to execute the plan, CHIVA has not been adopted by the majority of venous interventionalists. However, as a result of the expense of the endothermal or chemical ablation devices, there may be a developing interest in the CHIVA technique if it is simplified.

In this chapter, we describe an alternative simple, percutaneous, mechanical method of vessel occlusion with a device that eliminates the need for these time-consuming and skilled surgical procedures. This technique will simplify and expedite the CHIVA procedure for the doctor and minimise the patient's discomfort and recovery. Currently, the device and the delivery system (Amsel Vessel Occluder, Amsel Medical) is pending Food and Drug Administration (FDA) clearance for percutaneous use. The FDA has approved the occlusion device for "open" surgical vessel and tubular structure occlusion ranging from 2mm to 7mm in diameter.[6–8]

Device description

The device is preloaded into an 18G needle of the delivery system (Figure 1) and, when deployed, transfixes and occludes the target vessel. It consists of two "star" shaped compression elements and a titanium fine strut, which connects and locks the compression elements together. The proximal element (which compresses the near wall of the vessel) and the distal element (which compresses the far wall of the vessel) are made of nitinol, which, once deployed, assumes its designated configuration closing off the vessel (Figure 2); the individual "arms" of the proximal occlusion component alternate with and interdigitate with the individual "arms' of the distal occlusion components. This interdigitation is important as it obviates the problem with different vessel wall thicknesses and creates a zone of occlusion that surrounds the site of penetration, preventing leaks at the needle entry site (Figure 3).

Technique and results of the occluder device

The ultrasound is held in the one hand and the occluder device held in the other hand. Clear identification of the vessel is essential in order to transfix the vessel by passing the needle through both walls of the vessel. A small opening in the transfixing needle allows the escape of blood as the needle enters into the lumen

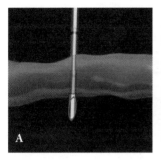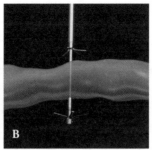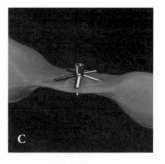

Figure 2: The illustration of steps in deployment of the Amsel Vessel Occluder (A) through needle penetration of targeted vessel. (B) Deployment of two separate occluding elements. (C) Locking together of the two occluding elements thus securely occluding the vessel and finally, detachment and removal of the introducer elements.[7]

of the vessel to confirm accuracy of needle placement within the targeted vessel, as well as confirm the identity of the vessel and determine whether it is an artery *versus* a vein. Once the vessel is transfixed, further ultrasound guidance is not required. The two occluding elements are released, locked together, and the vessel is occluded. The delivery device is then detached and withdrawn.

In a porcine model, we successfully performed 30 ultrasound guided percutaneous occlusions, in vessels ranging from 2mm to 12mm. These vessels include the proximal femoral vessels, distal (superficial) femoral arteries and veins, carotid arteries, and jugular veins.[8] For the larger vessel size (>7mm), a second clip was necessary to completely occlude the targeted vessel. In the future, for clinical patient use, the size of the clip will be determined by need; thus, for the larger vessel, a larger clip will be made available.

All targeted vessels in this study were successfully occluded and occlusion was confirmed by Duplex ultrasound as well as open surgical exposure. Additionally, no injury to any of the adjacent structures was identified.

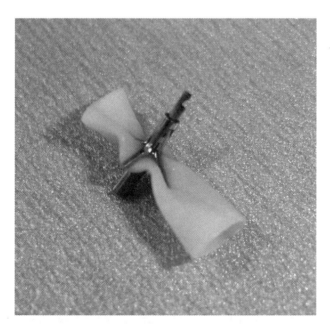

Figure 3: The "arms" of the proximal and distal occlusion components alternate and interdigitate with one another while transfixing the vessel. In the figure, the vessel is a synthetic saphenous vein (Lifelike Biotissues).

Conclusion

This vessel occluder, with its ability to accurately occlude vessels percutaneously under ultrasound guidance, simplifies the technique of the CHIVA procedure. Additionally, the instrument will allow a wider spectrum of healthcare professionals to adopt this more conservative approach with saphenous vein preservation for the treatment of symptomatic varicose veins and chronic venous insufficiency. Finally, the percutaneous vessel occluder will improve patient comfort and acceptance of the procedure, speed recovery, decrease the procedural morbidity, and reduce the associated healthcare costs.

Summary

- Varicose veins are estimated to affect approximately 23% of US adults.

- With regard to the descending theory for the aetiology for varicose veins, endothermal ablation with laser or radiofrequency has replaced surgery as the standard of care together with chemical treatments and chemical adhesives.

- These procedures have brought the treatment of varicose veins out of the hospital surgical operating rooms and into the outpatient surgical clinics or offices.

- In the early 1990s, an alternative approach, saphenous sparing, to treat the venous insufficiency associated with varicose veins was described.

- The saphenous sparing approach CHIVA does not aim to eliminate all of the reflux in the lower extremity veins, but to direct the flow of the "refluxing" blood into the deep veins of the lower extremity.

- Because of the combination of demanding ultrasonic expertise, and the associated surgical skills required to execute the plan, CHIVA has not been adopted by the majority of venous interventionalists.

- An alternative simple, percutaneous, mechanical method of vessel occlusion with a device should eliminate the need for these time-consuming and skilled-surgical procedures. This technique will simplify, expedite, minimise recovery, and reduce the costs the CHIVA procedure for the interventionalists.

References

1. Bergan JJ, Schmid-Schönbein GW, Coleridge Smith DM, *et al.* Chronic Venous Disease. *N Engl J Med* 2006; **355**: 488–98.
2. Hamdan A. Management of varicose veins and venous insufficiency. *JAMA* 2012; **308**: 2612–21.
3. Gloviczki P, Comerota AJ, Dalsing MC, *et al:* The care of patients with varicose veins and associated chronic venous diseases: Clinical practice guidelines of the Society for Vascular Surgery and the American Venous Forum. *J Vasc Surg* 2011; **53**: 2S–48S.
4. Franceschi C. Theory and Practice of the Conservative Haemodynamic Cure of Incompetent and Varicose Veins in Ambulatory Patients, translated by Evans J. Precy-sous-Thil 1988
5. Zamboni P, Escribano JM. Regarding reflux elimination without any ablation or disconnection of the saphenous vein. A haemodynamic model for surgery and 'durability of reflux-elimination by a minimal invasive CHIVA procedure on patients with varicose veins. a 3-year prospective case study. *Eur J Vasc Endovasc Surg* 2004; **28**: 567–68.

6. Miller A, Lilach N, Miller R. A novel secure vessel occluder for minimally invasive and percutaneous rreatments. *J Vasc Surg* 2014; **59** (suppl6S): PS234–89S.
7. Miller A, Lilach N, Botero-Anug A, *et al*. Comparison of a Novel Secure Transfixing Blood Vessel Occluder with the Hemoclip in the Porcine Model. J Laparoendoscopic Surgery. Submitted for publication.
8. Miller A, Lilach N, Miller R, Kabnick L. A novel, simple, and secure, percutaneous vessel occluder for the treatment of varicose veins. American Venous Forum, Orlando, FL February 2016.

Management of anatomically difficult revascularisation— the "hedgehog" technique

BA Price

Introduction

Recurrent varicose veins present a considerable challenge. In recent times other methods other than traditional saphenous ligation combined with avulsion by stripping of the great and/or small saphenous vein(s) have become popular alternatives. However, there remains a large cohort of patients who have undergone traditional treatment in the past and they make up a significant percentage of the presenting case load in most practices. In our unit, the ratio of recurrent patterns presenting to us is consistently in the order of 30% of affected limbs. Further traditional treatment methods continue to be applied to these patients despite the increased difficulty especially if groin re-exploration is contemplated. In a consensus debate held at the Charing Cross Symposium in 2014,[1] delegates found in favour of the argument for re-exploration of the groin even considering its morbidity risks.[2] Endovenous laser ablation can be used to treat recurrent patterns,[3] especially if there are segmental lengths of recurrent vein or accessory veins that can be accessed to allow insertion of the device of choice.

It has been suggested that incomplete removal of the original truncal vein is the major cause of recurrent varicose veins;[4] although, our group has demonstrated that neovascularisation occurs after ultrasound-guided complete stripping of the great saphenous vein and that neovascular process was complete in 6% and partial in a further 17% followed ultrasonically to one year.[5] This type of neovascularisation does not appear to occur after thermoablation and if recurrence is observed, it appears to be the result of recannalisation of the treated vein. This distinction has been made previously.[6] Ultrasound-guided foam sclerotherapy has been proposed as a method of tackling complicated varicose veins but care has to be taken in defining complexity. O'Hare et al[7] defined complex cases according to their comprehensive classification system for chronic venous disorder (Clinical, Etiological, Anatomical, and Pathophysiological or "CEAP"), clinical scoring between four and six as opposed to uncomplicated cases which fell into the category one to three. The problem with considering case complexity in this way is that the patient with recurrence who has extensive neovascularisation in the groin and along the truncal vein track who exhibits small vessels only on the surface and may or may not show signs of oedema will fall into the category of "uncomplicated" according to this description. It does not suggest the technical realities of treatment in someone who nevertheless may present significant symptoms. Therefore, for the purposes of this

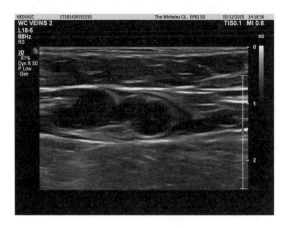

Figure 1: Ultrasound image showing typical neovascularised segment in the groin following truncal ligation and stripping.

discussion, I am referring to the pattern shown on ultrasound appearances rather than the overall clinical view when discussing complexity. In the aforementioned study, there was no difference shown in results following foam sclerotherapy when primary and recurrent cases were compared. High recannalisation rates of 25% and 22%, respectively, were demonstrated after a mere six months post-treatment. This suggests that foam sclerotherapy as a single modality cannot be considered reliable and compares poorly to thermoablation[8] if long-term vein occlusion is considered the primary endpoint.

Neovascular segments, even if they occur in relatively few patients according to some authors,[9] still present a difficult challenge to the clinician when they do and it is easy to see why ultrasound-guided foam sclerotherapy is appealing as a form of treatment.[10] The segments are rarely suitable to the insertion of long introduction cannulas such as the Terumo cannula because they are serpiginous with scarred walls and internal webs. However, with care these challenging vessels can be accessed with shorter cannulae and some of the webs traversed to obtain longer lengths for treatment. They contract under exposure to heat energy delivered by either laser or

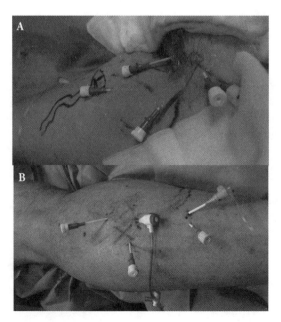

Figure 2: (A) "Hedgehog" multiple cannulae inserted into groin neovascularised segments (upper picture) and (B) into small saphenous vein recurrent segments.

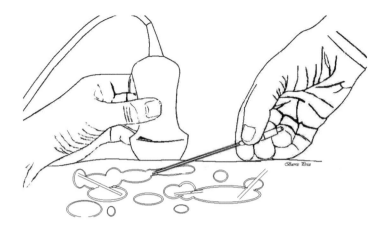

Figure 3: Diagram showing technique of multiple cannulae insertions into recurrent venous segments.

radiofrequency and it obviates the risk of them filling with sclerothrombus at the time of foam injection only for recanalisation to occur later.

A strategy for treatment

The National Institute for Health and Care Excellence (NICE) guidelines formulated in 2013[11] suggest that thermoablation is the treatment of first choice for truncal vein reflux based on the evidence to date with ultrasound-guided foam sclerotherapy as the next alternative. Traditional vein stripping is relegated to third place although it is still considered an acceptable treatment modality. One could argue that this order of march applies equally to recurrent patterns but the difficulty arises when one is dealing with multiple segments as shown in Figure 1. These segments are short, highly tortuous, containing multiple scarred webs and do not lend themselves to Seldinger access[12] via a Terumo-like cannula. It is tempting, therefore, to resort to ultrasound-guided foam sclerotherapy for these segments but these lesions can be very extensive especially in the groin and it is difficult to apply effective, prolonged compression, essential for optimal results, to these areas. However, there is a way based on the Holdstock-Whiteley method[13] developed in our unit for the thermoablation of perforator veins to access these segments effectively. The next problem to overcome is the close proximity of the various vein segments, which means that the act of placing tumescent anaesthetic fluid around an accessed segment will make insertion of an appropriate intravenous cannula into the next segment close by difficult or even impossible. It is important, therefore, to access all the numerous segments prior to submitting the whole area to high-volume tumescent anaesthesia to compress all the cavernous vessels before insertion of a laser fibre to each segment in turn to impart the appropriate linear endovenous energy density. Foam sclerosant can be administered to individual segments immediately prior to laser ablation to theoretically chemically close any areas still not accessible to the laser fibre taking advantage of the collapsed state of the tortuous recurrent tributaries. Catheter-directed foam sclerotherapy under tumescence has been suggested before for treatment of truncal vein reflux in the great saphenous vein but in a small randomised trial, there appeared to be no advantage in volume reduction of the targeted vein.[14]

Method

Careful and thorough ultrasound mapping of the various neovascular segments is essential before proceeding. The segments are carefully marked with an indelible pen and a plan formulated as to the number of cannulae insertions required to cover as much of the neovascular field as possible. Intradermal local anaesthesia is infiltrated into the skin at the pole of the ultrasound probe with the target vessel demonstrated in the parasagittal plane. The author favours a 14G Abbocath cannula (Venisystems; Abbocath; Hospira) for insertion into the vessel, which should be penetrated under guidance for a long a length as possible piercing any webs in the path of the cannula needle. Once in the desired position, the needle is extracted as a plastic Luer-Lok cannula cap applied to stop back bleeding as shown in Figure 2. The process is repeated until as many as possible of the neovascularised segments have been cannulated. Figure 3 is a diagrammatic representation of the appearance and several cannulae are in place as shown. The vessels concerned are very tortuous and so only part of the cannulae previously inserted may be visible. Once all desired cannulae are in place the whole field can then be flooded with Klein's solution. A 4Fr jacketed laser fibre (Angiodynamics VenaCure EVLT NeverTouch Direct; Angiodynamics) is passed individually down each of the Abbocath cannulae in turn. Energy transfers of 70–80J/cm are delivered under ultrasound surveillance to the segment lengths. Ultrasound-guided foam sclerotherapy may be added to theoretically take advantage of the reduced volume of the recurrent vessels prior to endovenous laser ablation if desired but this is in no means obligatory. Figure 4 shows before and after ultrasound pictures of neovascular tissue treated as described without additional ultrasound-guided foam sclerotherapy and the previously cavernous vessels have been obliterated.

Conclusion

Traditional truncal vein ligation and stripping remains a common method of treatment of primary varicose veins and neovascularisation in the groin, popliteal

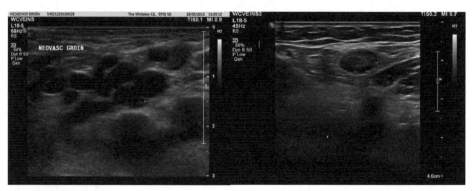

Figure 4: Ultrasound images demonstrating before and after appearances of laser ablations of multiple groin neovascular vein segments.

fossa and strip track are common and well recognised.[15,16] It is to be expected, therefore that in the future clinicians are going to continue to be confronted with cases where significant recurrence secondary to neovascular development is present. Repeated traditional surgery not only carries risks but is time-consuming and costly.[17] It would appear that despite the previous consensus[1] serious questions remain as to the validity of further invasive treatment especially as further neovascular changes are to be expected with time. Therefore, any alternative method that avoids further invasive surgical trauma to the tissues, especially in the groin and popliteal fossa, has to be seriously considered. The argument for ultrasound-guided foam sclerotherapy is compelling and has its supporters[18] but there are areas such as the femoral triangle and proximal parts of the thigh where it is impossible to maintain continuous effective compression postprocedure. Vessels with minimal length such as perforator veins can be effectively ablated using endovenous laser ablation or radiofrequency[13] and these skills can be transferred effectively to the treatment of short lengths of neovascular track which unlike ultrasound-guided foam sclerotherapy is not dependant on sustained compression postprocedure and early results show that it appears effective.

Summary

- Recurrent varicose veins associated with neovascularisation are common and are estimated to represent 30% of the workload in new referrals.

- Repeat traditional surgery is difficult, morbidity-associated, time-consuming and costly especially if re-exploration of the groin or popliteal fossa is contemplated.

- Thermoablation using radiofrequency or endovenous laser ablation is a viable and effective alternative to repeat surgery for groin, popliteal fossa and strip track revascularisation.

- Multiple punctures may be necessary to ablate extensive neovascular fields producing a "hedgehog" technique prior to high-volume tumescent infiltration.

- Ultrasound-guided foam sclerotherapy can be used in conjunction with the hedgehog technique to take advantage of the compression afforded by tumescence.

- A variety of techniques and skills should be employed to treat highly complex venous patterns.

References

1. Chaloner E, Scurr J. Varicose vein treatment consensus update debate; "There is no indication for groin exploration for recurrent varicose veins." Charing Cross International Conference CX 36: 8 April 2014.
2. Hayden A, Holdsworth Complications following re-exploration of the groin for recurrent varicose veins. *J Ann R Coll Surg Engl* 2001; **83**: 272–73.
3. Theivacumar NS, Gough MJ. Endovenous Laser Ablation (EVLA) to treat recurrent varicose veins. *Eur J Vasc Endovasc Surg* 2011: **41** (5): 691–96.
4. Joshi D, Sinclair A, Tsui J, Sarin S. Incomplete removal of great saphenous vein is the most common cause of recurrent varicose veins. *Angiology* 2011: **62**: 198–201.

5. Munasinghe A, Smith C, Kianifard B, Price BA, *et al.* Strip-track revascularization after stripping of the great saphenous vein. *Br J Surg* 2007: **94**: 840–43.

6. Theivacumar NS, Darwood R, Gough MJ. Neovascularisation and recurrence 2 years after varicose vein treatment for saphenofemoral and great saphenous vein reflux; a comparison of surgery and endovenous laser surgery. *Eur J Vasc Endovasc Surg* 2009: **38** (2): 203–07.

7. O'Hare JL, Parkin D, Vandenbroeck CP, Earnshaw JJ. Midterm results of ultrasound-guided foam sclerotherapy for complicated and uncomplicated varicose veins. *Eur J Vasc Endovasc Surg* 2008: **36** (1); 109–13.

8. Rasmussen LH, Lawaetz M, Bjoern L, Vennits B, *et al.* Randomized clinical trial comparing endovenous laser ablation, radiofrequency ablation, foam sclerotherapy and surgical stripping for great saphenous varicose veins. *Br J Surg* 2011; **98**: 1079–87.

9. Egan B, Donnelly M, Bresnihan M, Tierney S, Feeley M. Neovascularization: an "innocent bystander" in recurrent varicose veins. *J Vasc Surg*. 200; **44:** 1279–84.

10. Perrin, Gillet JL. Management of recurrent varices at the popliteal fossa after surgical treatment. Phlebology 2008; **23:** 64–68.

11. NICE. Varicose veins in the legs: The diagnosis and management of varicose veins. National Institute for Health and Care Excellence. https://www.nice.org.uk/guidance/cg168 (date accessed 19 February 2016).

12. Seldinger SI. Catheter replacement of the needle in percutaneous arteriography; a new technique. *Acta Radiologica* 1953: **39** (5): 368–76.

13. Bacon JL, Dineen AJ, Marsh P, Holdstock JM, *et al.* Five-year results of incompetent perforator vein closure using Trans-Luminal Occlusion of Perforator. *Phlebology* 2009; **24:** 74–78.

14. Devereux N, Recke AL, Westermann L, Recke A, *et al.* Catheter-directed foam sclerotherapy of great saphenous veins in combination with pre-treatment reduction of the diameter employing the principals of perivenous tumescent local anesthesia. *Eur J Vasc Endovasc Surg* 2014: **47** (2): 187–95.

15. Klein JA. The tumescent technique for liposuction surgery. *Am J Cosmetic Surg* 1987; **4:** 1124–32.

16. Corbett CRR, Prakash V. Neovascularisation is not an innocent bystander in recurrence after great saphenous vein surgery. *Ann R Coll Surg Engl* 2015; **97:** 102–08.

17. Pittaluga P, Chastanet S, Locret T, Rousset O. Retrospective evaluation of the need of a redo surgery at the groin for the surgical treatment of varicose vein. *J Vasc Surg* 2010: **51;** 1442–50.

Rational anti-DVT prophylaxis for ambulatory varicose vein procedures

SJ Goodyear and IK Nyamekye

Introduction

Postoperative venous thromboembolism is associated with a considerable burden of morbidity and mortality.[1] In addition to acute symptoms, deep vein thrombosis (DVT) may cause recurrent thrombosis, post-thrombotic syndrome and potentially fatal pulmonary embolism even when deep vein thrombosis has been diagnosed and treated. This underscores the need for active deep vein thrombosis prevention. There is a lack of evidence for the requirement for, modalities of, or duration for DVT prophylaxis in patients undergoing local anaesthetic ambulatory varicose vein (LA-AVV) procedures.[2] This deficiency will form the focus of this chapter.

The incidence of DVT following local anaesthetic ambulatory varicose vein procedures is likely to be lower than that for open surgery performed under general anaesthesia.[3] However, its true incidence is unknown and further confounded by heterogenous reporting of often self-resolving non-occlusive junctional thrombus.[4–6]

Lack of evidence and specific guidance for DVT prevention after local anaesthetic ambulatory varicose vein procedures has led to inconsistent provision of pharmacological thromboprophylaxis. Practices of no low-molecular-weight heparin (LMWH) prophylaxis and selective prophylaxis (with variabilies in indication for, and duration of, treatment) are common, with many phlebologists administering "single-dose" LMWH. One text promoting avoidance of vascular complications recommends this "single-dose" LMWH administration, especially for "moderate -risk groups".[7] Haematologists do not support this advice and practice. Available clinical guidance is also equivocal.[8–10] We address the limitations of current anti-DVT prophylaxis in local anaesthetic ambulatory varicose vein treatment and emphasise the futility of "single-dose" LMWH prophylaxis.

Clinical Guidance for DVT risk during ambulatory varicose vein procedures

Guidelines for venous thromboembolism prophylaxis have focussed on in-patient major surgery. Major guidelines—from the UK's National Institute for Health and Care Excellence (NICE), the American College of Chest Physicians (ACCP), and the Society for Vascular Surgery (SVS)—offer no specific advice for local anaesthetic ambulatory varicose vein interventions, despite proliferation of these techniques.[8–10] Generic guidance from NICE (2010) states: "Do not routinely offer pharmacological or mechanical venous thromboembolism prophylaxis to patients undergoing a surgical procedure with local anaesthesia by local infiltration who have no limitation of mobility."[8] Further guidance for vascular procedures advises mechanical prophylaxis (foot impulse devices or intermittent pneumatic compression) as alternatives to antiembolism stockings. Additional LMWH is advised for individuals who are assessed to be at increased risk of DVT.[8] This guidance is not specific for endovenous treatments where patients are immediately mobile.

Varicose veins, by having a female preponderance and increasing with advancing age, are commonly associated with oral contraceptives and hormone replacement therapy and medical comorbidities—all known risk factors for postoperative deep vein thrombosis.[8,11,12] Many of these risk factors are present in patients presenting for local anaesthetic ambulatory varicose vein treatment.

The Scottish Intercollegiate Guideline Network (SIGN) is unique in specifically mentioning endovenous treatment. SIGN advises prophylaxis with stockings alone after varicose veins surgery, unless patients have additional thromboembolic risk factors, when LMWH is added. It notes: "There is no evidence that the incidence of DVT following endovenous treatment is any different from that following open surgery." SIGN, thereby, also implies its strategy should be followed for endovenous procedures. The assignment of its recommendation as grade "D" indicates guidance based on weak evidence or expert opinion.[2]

DVT risk in ambulatory varicose veins procedures

Local anaesthetic ambulatory varicose vein procedures are office-based or day-case interventions, patients are immediately ambulant post-intervention, and low incidence of DVT has been reported. Post-hoc analysis of varicose vein procedures (of Hospital Episode Statistics data) conducted by Sutton in 2012 identified 35,374 treatment episodes.[3] The overall DVT rate was 0.51% but the incidence in the small number of local anaesthetic ambulatory varicose vein procedures was zero. However, other published studies report differing rates after endovenous techniques, especially when the techniques were performed under general anaesthesia. Rates of 0–16% for thermal modalities and 0–5.7% for foam sclerotherapy have been reported over the last 15 years.[5,13–15] These quoted incidences are further complicated by heterogenous reporting of "endothermal heat-induced thrombosis" and "endovenous foam-induced thrombosis", defined as protrusion of non-occlusive thrombus from the treated saphenous junction into the deep venous system (Figure 1) and occlusive DVT.[4,5,13,16] Large contemporary series have reported lower rates (0–2%)[17] whilst recent systematic reviews have failed to identify sufficient events for meta-analysis.[18,19] NICE guideline CG168 identified a DVT incidence of 0.4%.[20] However, few studies were of adequate quality and many were graded as low or very low quality.

Several factors contribute to the inability to report accurate DVT rates after local anaesthetic ambulatory varicose vein techniques in clinical practice. Asymptomatic DVT is missed unless there is a policy of systematic interval duplex imaging for all patients. This is particularly so when there is failure to follow up patients from surgeon choice, lack of funding from providers, or non-attendance. Surgeon-performed duplex scans may lack objectivity and detail and may not identify small calf vein DVTs. With the protracted time-course (discussed later in this chapter)

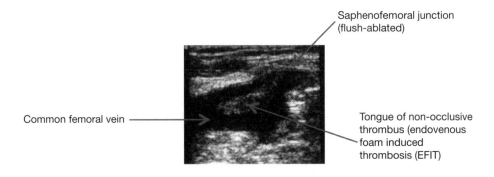

Figure 1: Asymptomatic thrombus seen on routine duplex imaging two weeks after great saphenous vein foam sclerotherapy.

over which DVT develop even detailed scans performed by vascular scientists at a single time-point will miss some postoperative thrombotic events. Finally some events are missed when symptomatic patients present to specialist DVT clinics, especially if this is in a different hospital.

There is relatively robust evidence for the influence of generic surgical interventions on DVT incidence from epidemiological publications such as the Million Women Study.[21] Sweetland *et al* compared women who underwent surgery with those who did not. Despite groups being well matched for factors such as age, body mass index, hormonal therapy and use of oral contraceptives, patients who had surgery had considerably more DVTs compared with controls. This supports an inherent increase in incidence for patients undergoing endovenous (albeit minimally invasive) procedures. However, we must be cautious in directly extrapolating this evidence, derived largely from general anaesthesia operations performed as inpatients, to our local anaesthetic ambulatory varicose vein patients. Day-case surgery also increased DVT risk within six weeks in Sweetland *et al's* paper, with a lesser level of risk persisting beyond six weeks. However, many day-case patients were also treated under general anaesthesia. This inherent period of postoperative immobilisation differentiates them from our local anaesthetic ambulatory varicose vein patients. Data provided for day-case vascular surgery was not specific to patients undergoing endovenous interventions.

Managing DVT risk in ambulatory varicose veins procedures

Patients' DVT risk may be mitigated by established methods of mechanical and pharmacological prophylaxis. Because patients are immediately ambulant, early mobilisation and graduated compression stocking are the mechanical methods of choice. But just how effective are stockings? In a recent Cochrane review, Sachdeva and Lees showed that graduated compression stockings reduced postoperative DVT rates from 21% to 9% for surgical procedures across multiple specialities. They concluded that "stockings should be considered in all surgical patients" unless there are specific contraindications.[22] However, the procedures reviewed comprised major in-patient general anaesthesia operations, which limits the relevance and applicability of the data to the local anaesthetic ambulatory varicose vein cohort. We do not know the extent (if any) to which graduated compression stockings confer additional thromboprophylactic benefit over aggressive mobilisation after local anaesthetic ambulatory varicose vein procedures. Additional limitations of graduated compression stockings include lack of standardisation in compression graduations across different stocking types, difficulties in fitting unusual leg shapes/ sizes and variable patient compliance. A good quality trial is required to address whether graduated compression stockings confer additional thromboprophylaxis benefit for patients undergoing local anaesthetic ambulatory varicose vein procedures.

LMWH, the mainstay of pharmacological prophylaxis for surgical DVT, consistently delivers 60–70% reduction in postoperative DVT.[23] Low-dose unfractionated heparin and fondaparinux are effective alternatives advocated in patients with impaired renal function or when heparin is contraindicated.[8] Currently there is no defined role for the direct oral anticoagulants in DVT prophylaxis for varicose veins interventions. Caprini's chapter of *The Vein Book* provides a balanced comparison and summary of the various methods of pharmacological DVT thromboprophylaxis with placebo for inpatient surgery under general anaesthesia.[23]

Duration of pharmacological thromboprophylaxis

When LMWH is prescribed, NICE recommends LMWH prophylaxis until the patient is mobile, stated as being five to seven days, but without supporting objective data.[8] Data from Sweetland *et al's* study demonstrate sustained DVT risk for several weeks following day-case vascular surgery.[21] Both venous and arterial day-case procedures were grouped for analysis in this study, including treatments under general anaesthesia. Sweetland *et al*, therefore, provides objective data to help guide duration of DVT prophylaxis for day-cases. The extended at-risk period demonstrates the futility of administering DVT prophylaxis in the form of perioperative "single-dose" LMWH as it offers no prophylaxis during the high-risk weeks of the postoperative period. The importance of an adequate duration of thromboprophylaxis might explain the surprising finding of Arcelus *et al* (albeit from general surgical data) that two-thirds of surgical patients who developed postprocedure DVT had received prophylactic LMWH.[24]

In the absence of specific data, the indirect evidence from Sweetland *et al* should inform prescriptions for treatment duration of LMWH for patients undergoing local anaesthetic ambulatory varicose vein procedures who are considered to be at increased risk of thromboembolism. Whilst we accept their DVT rates may be lower than those studied, the prolongation of DVT risk in high-risk patients undergoing local anaesthetic ambulatory varicose vein procedures is likely to follow the overall pattern shown by Sweetland.[21]

Strategies to define increased DVT risk in ambulatory varicose vein procedures

Thromboprophylaxis can be targeted more effectively by stratifying patients for DVT risk. Procedure-based models that stratify risk by surgery type and time are not useful in patients undergoing relatively minor local anaesthetic ambulatory varicose vein treatments that last less than 60 minutes. Assessing individuals' DVT risk is more useful and allows stratification into low, moderate or high-risk groups. However, formal individual patient risk assessment models such as the Rogers' score and the Caprini score are best suited to patients undergoing major surgery, including a period of immobilisation and are not discriminatory for ambulatory endovenous patients.[23,25] For example, only a limited number of the many Caprini factors would apply to most endovenous patients, thus leading to low or very-low Caprini scores.

Until varicose vein specific risk assessment models are available, targeting factors that have established relevance to varicose vein cohorts should provide better risk stratification for patients. Phlebologists have long used factors such as obesity, reduced mobility, hormonal therapy, personal or family history of DVT, active thrombophlebitis and the presence of thrombophilia to guide decisions on pharmacological thromboprophylaxis management. These can also guide thromboprophylaxis in endovenous treatments even though much of their evidence is from open veins surgery performed under general anaesthesia.

A strong case must now be made for focused research concerning the development of specific DVT risk scoring in patients undergoing local anaesthetic ambulatory varicose vein procedures. This much needed tool will facilitate and improved clinician decision-making in this high volume area of vascular practice.

Pragmatic advice on managing DVT risk in ambulatory varicose vein patients

Until specific risk assessment models become available, the authors advocate careful patient selection as previously indicated to place patients into risk groups, whilst being mindful of the limitations of their evidence in local anaesthetic ambulatory varicose vein procedures. Such risk assignment will necessarily involve a degree of subjectivity as a consequence of observer variability and the dearth of our existing knowledge. However, experienced phlebologists are likely to classify patients into broadly appropriate risk groups for DVT. This will allow the use of targeted thromboprophylaxis management based on practical treatment models such as the treatment ladder used by the senior author (Figure 2). Here, in addition to the operator's usual postprocedural compression regime, all patients are encouraged to comply with early, aggressive and frequent mobilisation. Graduated compression stockings are added for low-risk patients and worn for at least one week. Moderate-risk patients are given additional LMWH, again, for at least one week. Patients who

DVT Risk	Thromboprophylaxis
Moderate	And LMWH for one week
Low	And graduated compression stockings for seven days
Very Low	Early (aggressive) mobilisation, standard compression

Figure 2: Example of a thromboprophylaxis ladder.

have been assessed as high-risk, for example those with a personal history of DVT, morbid obesity, immobility or thrombophilia are given extended pharmacological thromboprophylaxis with LMWH for at least six weeks. Alternatively, a case could be made for avoiding varicose veins intervention altogether for high-risk individuals, in favour of conservative treatment.

Conclusions

DVT risk is increased by endovenous varicose veins interventions, but to an as-yet unknown extent. However, phlebologists recognise the risk and variably use graduated compression stockings or LMWH prophylaxis to mitigate outcomes. Existing knowledge (derived mainly from inpatient surgery) suggests that for the provision of rational thromboprophylaxis, all patients should be risk-assessed with a view to instituting personalised thromboprophylaxis treatment. No risk assessment models exist for the cohort of patients undergoing ambulatory local anaesthetic endovenous procedures. There is good evidence that the duration of postprocedure DVT risk is significantly longer than current treatment practices recognise and the duration of any prescribed prophylaxis should be extended accordingly.

There is an urgent need for research aimed at developing specific risk assessment models to inform validated rational thromboprophylaxis guidelines for patients undergoing local anaesthetic endovenous interventions.

Summary

- DVT risk is increased by endovenous varicose veins interventions but to an unknown extent.

- Clinicians recognise and variably use stockings and LMWH prophylaxis to mitigate the risk.

- Use of "single-shot" LMWH is not supported by haematological evidence, which shows duration of DVT risk to be in the order of weeks to months.

- Patients should be risk assessed for provision of rational thromboprophylaxis.

- No specific risk assessment models exist for patients undergoing ambulatory local anaesthetic endovenous procedures.

- Duration of prescribed pharmacological prophylaxis should be extended beyond the perioperative period.

- There is urgent need for research to develop specific risk assessment models for patients undergoing local anaesthetic endovenous interventions.

References

1. House of Commons Health Committee. The prevention of venous thromboembolism in hospitalised patients. London: Stationery Office, 2005.
2. Scottish Intercollegiate Guideline Network. Guideline 122: Prevention and management of venous thromboembolism: A national clinical guideline. http://www.sign.ac.uk/guidelines/fulltext/122/ (date accessed 22 February 2016).

3. Sutton PA, El-Dhuwaib Y, Dyer J, Guy AJ. The incidence of postoperative venous thromboembolism in patients undergoing varicose vein surgery recorded in Hospital Episode Statistics. *Ann R Coll Surg Engl* 2012; **94** (7)**:** 481–83.

4. Jones RT, Kabnick LS. Perioperative duplex ultrasound following endothermal ablation of the saphenous vein: is it worthless? *J Invasive Cardiol* 2014; **26** (10)**:** 548–50.

5. Marsh P, Price BA, Holdstock J, *et al.* Deep vein thrombosis (DVT) after venous thermoablation techniques: rates of endovenous heat-induced thrombosis (EHIT) and classical DVT after radiofrequency and endovenous laser ablation in a single centre. *Eur J Vasc Endovasc Surg* 2010; **40** (4)**:** 521–27.

6. Merchant RF, Pichot O; Closure Group. Long-term outcomes of endovenous radiofrequency obliteration of saphenous reflux as a treatment for superficial venous insufficiency. *J Vasc Surg* 2005; **42:** 502–09.

7. Earnshaw JJ and Wyatt MG. (eds). Complications in *Vascular and Endovascular Surgery*: How to Avoid Them and How to Get Out of Trouble, 1st edition. Tfm Pub Ltd, UK, 2011.

8. National Clinical Guideline Centre – Acute and Chronic Conditions (UK). Venous Thromboembolism: Reducing the Risk of Venous Thromboembolism (Deep Vein Thrombosis and Pulmonary Embolism) in Patients Admitted to Hospital. National Institute for Clinical and Health Excellence: Guidance. http://www.ncbi.nlm.nih.gov/pubmedhealth/PMH0051769/pdf/PubMedHealth_PMH0051769.pdf (date accessed 22 February 2016).

9. Kahn SR, Lim W, Dunn AS, *et al.* Prevention of VTE in Nonsurgical Patients: Antithrombotic Therapy and Prevention of Thrombosis, 9th ed: American College of Chest Physicians Evidence-Based Clinical Practice Guidelines. *Chest* 2012; **141** (2_suppl)**:** e195S–e226S.

10. Gloviczki P, Comerota AJ, Dalsing MC, *et al.* The care of patients with varicose veins and associated chronic venous diseases: Clinical practice guidelines of the Society for Vascular Surgery and the American Venous Forum. *J Vasc Surg* 2011; **53** (Suppl): 2S–48S.

11. Bergan JJ, Schmidt-Schonbein GW, Smith PD, *et al* (2006). Chronic Venous Disease. *N Engl J Med* 2006; 355: 488–98.

12. Lee AJ, Evans C, Allan PL, *et al:* Lifestyle factors and the risk of varicose veins: Edinburgh Vein Study. *J Clin Epidemiol* 2003, **564:** 171–79.

13. Kulkarni S, Messenger DE, Slim FJA, *et al.* The incidence and characterization of deep vein thrombosis following ultrasound-guided foam sclerotherapy in 1000 legs with superficial venous reflux. *Journal of Vascular Surgery: Venous and Lymphatic Disorders* 2013; **1** (3): 231–38.

14. Hingorani AP, Ascher E, Markevich N, *et al.* Deep venous thrombosis after radiofrequency ablation of greater saphenous vein: a word of caution. *J Vasc Surg* 2004; **40** (3): 500–04.

15. Carradice D, Leung C, Chetter I. Laser; best practice techniques and evidence. *Phlebology* 2015; **30** (2 Suppl): 36–41

16. Kabnick LS, Ombrellino M, Agis H, *et al.* Endovenous heat induced thrombus (EHIT) at the superficial-deep venous junction: a new post-treatment clinical entity, classification and potential treatment strategies. 18th Annual Meeting of the American Venous Forum, Miami, Florida; 2006.

17. Puggioni A, Kalra M, Carmo M, *et al.* Endovenous laser therapy and radiofrequency ablation of the great saphenous vein: analysis of early efficacy and complications. *J Vasc Surg* 2005; **42** (3): 488–93.

18. Carroll C, Hummel S, Leaviss J, Ren S, *et al.* Clinical effectiveness and cost-effectiveness of minimally invasive techniques to manage varicose veins: a systematic review and economic evaluation. Health *Technol Assess* 2013; **17** (48): i–xvi.

19. Nesbitt C, Bedenis R, Bhattacharya V, *et al.* Endovenous ablation (radiofrequency and laser) and foam sclerotherapy *versus* open surgery for great saphenous vein varices. Cochrane Database Syst Rev. 2014 Jul 30; 7: CD005624.

20. National Institute for Health and Care Excellence. Varicose veins: Diagnosis and Management, Clinical Guideline 168. https://goo.gl/19As0H (date accessed 22 February 2016).

21. Sweetland S, Green J, Liu B, Berrington de González A, *et al.* Million Women Study collaborators. Duration and magnitude of the postoperative risk of venous thromboembolism in middle aged women: prospective cohort study. *BMJ* 2009; **339:** b4583.

22. Sachdeva A, Dalton M, Amaragiri SV, Lees T. Graduated compression stockings for prevention of deep vein thrombosis. Cochrane Database Syst Rev. 2014 Dec 17.

23. Caprini JJ. Chapter 41: Thrombotic Risk Assessment: A Hybrid Approach. The Vein Book (ed. Bergan JJ). 2007 Elselvier inc.

24. Arcelus JI, Caprini JA, Monreal M, *et al.* The management and outcome of acute venous thromboembolism: a prospective registry including 4011 patients. *J Vasc Surg* 2003; **38** (5)**:** 916–22.

25. Rogers SO Jr, Kilaru RK, Hosokawa P, *et al.* Multivariable predictors of postoperative venous thromboembolic events after general and vascular surgery: results from the patient safety in surgery study. J Am Coll Surg 2007; **204** (6): 1211–21.

Sclerotherapy of the sub-ulcer plexus: Practical tips for success

C Sabbagh and MS Gohel

Introduction

With a rapidly ageing and increasingly overweight population, the incidence of chronic venous ulceration (Clinical, Etiological, Anatomical, and Pathophysiological, CEAP, C5 and C6) is likely to increase dramatically in the next 5–10 years. The enormous impact of chronic venous disorders on patients, carers, healthcare providers and society has been widely acknowledged.[1,2] Significant advances in treatment have been achieved, with widespread acceptance that endovenous interventions have largely replaced open surgery for superficial venous reflux and are an essential component of venous care, in addition to compression, elevation and other non-surgical options.[3,4] Multiple endovenous options are available including thermal ablation (using radiofrequency and laser), non-thermal ablation (such as mechanochemical ablation or cyanoacrylate glue) and ultrasound-guided foam sclerotherapy. These local anaesthetic procedures have revolutionised the management of patients with superficial venous reflux. Moreover, these interventions have been embraced by clinicians and are welcomed by patients, as the treatment strategy can now be tailored to their individual circumstances and preferences.

There are enthusiastic advocates for each of the endovenous treatment modalities, but a prevailing opinion among venous specialists is that a combination of endovenous (or open surgical) interventions may be the best approach for individual patients. Rather than focusing on the endovenous modality, there is a general appreciation that treatment technique and strategy is likely to be as important as the type of catheter, or perhaps even more so. Specific targeting of the leash of veins that almost invariably exists under areas of active or healed venous ulceration (known as the "sub-ulcer venous plexus") is a logical and increasingly popular strategy. The rationale for this approach is discussed in this chapter, as well as practical tips to achieve effective ablation.

The rationale for ablating the sub-ulcer plexus

The underlying rationale for all venous interventions is to reduce venous hypertension in the leg and achieve clinical benefits for the patient. In cases of advanced venous disease with ulceration, interventions are intended to promote ulcer healing and reduce the risk of ulcer recurrence. A number of randomised and non-randomised studies, including the ESCHAR (Effect of surgery and compression on healing and recurrence) study,[5–7] have demonstrated the clinical benefits of open surgical and endovenous treatments. Treatment of superficial venous reflux reduces venous ulcer recurrence in patients with isolated superficial reflux and also in some patients with mixed superficial and deep venous reflux. However, the superficial venous interventions utilised in most published studies generally focused on ablation of the refluxing truncal vein, with little standardisation of adjunctive treatments in the ulcer area. One of the reasons for the increasing popularity of the sub-ulcer sclerotherapy technique is the widespread support for ultrasound-guided foam sclerotherapy as an effective treatment modality in a number of international guidelines and consensus statements.

The "sub-ulcer plexus" refers to a tortuous leash of incompetent veins that is almost invariably present under an area of active or healed venous ulceration. While there are multiple causes of chronic venous hypertension, including superficial/deep venous reflux and deep venous occlusion, the precise pathophysiological pathways leading from chronic venous hypertension to skin inflammation and breakdown are poorly understood. However, there is a growing body of opinion that the sub-ulcer plexus may have an important role in transferring chronic venous hypertension to the skin, resulting in microvascular changes, skin damage and ulceration (Figure 1). The principal aim of ablating the sub-ulcer plexus is to interrupt the terminal component of the pathway transmitting venous disease to the ulcerated skin. Advocates have suggested using this approach in isolation, or in combination with other interventions, to address superficial or deep venous disease.[8] However, in view of the clear, unequivocal evidence supporting treatment of the incompetent superficial truncal veins, a strategy of ablating the sub-ulcer plexus in addition to traditional superficial venous intervention seems the most logical.

Practical tips

The authors would suggest a number of tips and techniques to optimise outcomes following sub-ulcer venous plexus ablation. When considering the optimal treatment modality, there have been reports of endovenous thermal ablation at the ulcer bed (usually performed in a retrograde manner), with good results. While this technique may be effective at ablating the truncal refluxing vein

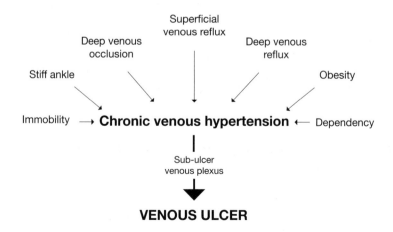

Figure 1: The sub-ulcer venous plexus have an important role in the final pathway between chronic venous hypertension and chronic venous ulceration.

to the level of the ulcer, the sub-ulcer plexus is not ablated and may continue to transmit venous hypertension to the ulcer bed. Ultrasound-guided foam sclerotherapy is the most effective modality for ablating the tortuous and multiple venous channels in the sub-ulcer plexus. Ablating the sub-ulcer veins should be considered for all patients with ulceration or advanced skin changes (C4b, C5 and C6 disease). As with any endovenous intervention, detailed colour duplex mapping should be performed to ascertain the status of deep veins, identify any truncal source of reflux, as well as the location of incompetent perforating veins. Specifically, the location of perforators in the sub-ulcer region should be marked in preparation for treatment.

While some clinicians may treat only the sub-ulcer venous plexus, it is the routine practice of the authors to consider sub-ulcer sclerotherapy as a specific and separate component of the superficial venous intervention, performed in addition to endovenous ablation of any truncal saphenous reflux (usually during the same treatment session). Using colour duplex scanning, feeding veins can usually be identified both proximal and distal to the ulceration area. These vessels are cannulated using 21G butterfly needles, aiming towards the ulcer bed. Where there are multiple tributaries feeding the sub-ulcer region, three to four needles may be necessary, all aiming towards the ulcer from different directions. This "pincer" technique (Figure 2) allows excellent dispersion and coverage on injection of the foam sclerosant. By treating any truncal reflux first, the sub-ulcer veins are depressurised, further improving sclerosant coverage and treatment effectiveness. Sclerosant injections are performed with aggressive leg elevation (with the patient in the Trendelenburg position) in order to maximise venous emptying and optimise sclerosant contact with the venous endothelium. Multiple smaller volume injections may be more effective than single large injections (with "milking" of sclerosant), as the effectiveness of the sclerosant is likely to be diminished by prolonged contact with venous blood.

For ulcers located in the medial gaiter region, the presence of one of more perforators (Cockett's) can add complexity and risk to the sub-ulcer sclerotherapy procedure. As there may be multiple foam injections directly towards these perforators, there are understandable concerns about passage of significant

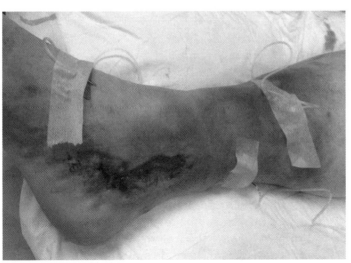

Figure 2: The "pincer" approach to sclerotherapy of the sub-ulcer plexus. Feeding vessels are cannulated using 21G butterfly needles from proximal and distal to the ulcer bed to optimise dispersion of foam sclerosant.

volumes of foam sclerosant into the deep venous system. In general, sclerotherapy of the sub-ulcer plexus is virtually always feasible, even in the presence of multiple perforators. The choice of cannulation sites may need to be adapted to account for the location of perforators. This may involve siting a butterfly needle very close to (or even within) an ulcer to remain distal to a perforator. Slightly aggressive injection of saline solution into the butterfly needles can be seen easily on duplex and may help identify the main "high-risk" perforator that could send foam sclerosant into the deep veins, which can be compressed specifically during foam injection. Where it is impossible to exclude perforators from the sub-ulcer sclerotherapy zone, the authors utilise a compression technique, where the perforator (carefully premarked using duplex) is directly compressed, while foam sclerosant is injected from proximally and distally to ablate the plexus and draining veins around the perforator. Using this "pincer" approach, the passage of foam sclerosant into deep veins can be minimised. It should be noted, however, that passage of some foam sclerosant into the deep system is inevitable and is not usually associated with any adverse events. However, operators should remain vigilant to monitor the passage of foam, as much of the injected volume may pass away from the intended location. In the event of visible passage of sclerosant into deep veins, ankle dorsiflexion/plantar flexion movements are usually very effective at promoting deep venous flow and minimising sclerosant stasis.

Occasionally, foam sclerosant may not dissipate readily throughout the sub-ulcer plexus, despite the usual manoeuvres ("milking" of sclerosant with the ultrasound probe, compression of veins to direct the sclerosant during injection, ankle dorsiflexion repetitions). In such cases, the authors would advocate a further sclerosant injection using a direct puncture technique, through the ulcer bed if necessary. Excellent dispersion throughout the sub-ulcer area is imperative for optimal results. It is the authors' practice to use 3% sodium tetradecyl sulphate agitated with room air in a 1:4 ratio using the Tessera technique. Patients on anticoagulant medications are asked to discontinue these prior to sclerotherapy. Compression therapy is continued for all patients with an active ulcer, as sub-ulcer sclerotherapy is considered an adjunct to the mainstays of management (compression and elevation). Patients without active ulcers wear a class II compression stocking, with additional elastic bandage for five days. It is imperative to maintain a high level of compliance with compression after intervention.

In patients with obvious chronic venous hypertension (as evidenced by skin changes), but no significant superficial reflux, sub-ulcer sclerotherapy may have a role, particularly in patients with intractable ulceration. A significant proportion of patients have predominantly deep venous reflux, and some may present without any venous reflux, but venous hypertension due to other causes (calf muscle pump failure, dependency etc). While the published evidence is limited, the authors have experienced considerable clinical success treating this cohort.

While treatments have progressed, the models of care for patients with chronic venous ulcers remain disjointed in many healthcare systems. Most patients with venous ulcers present to primary care and community nursing services and perhaps the greatest challenges relate to timely investigation and delivery of care, rather than the technique. Perhaps one approach will be to move away from traditional secondary/specialist care based systems, towards more community based venous assessments and treatments. The widespread availability of endovenous interventions, performed using local (or without) anaesthesia certainly makes this aspiration feasible.

Conclusion

The demographic changes seen in western countries in recent decades indicate that significant increases in the incidence and prevalence of chronic venous ulceration are inexorable. There have been enormous advances in the management of patients with chronic venous disorders, including the development of a range of minimally invasive endovenous interventions to ablate superficial incompetent veins. Sub-ulcer sclerotherapy is an evolution of the widely adopted ultrasound-guided foam sclerotherapy procedure, with specific ablation of the leash of incompetent veins in the sub-ulcer region.[8] Outcomes can be improved with detailed preprocedure duplex mapping, with specific emphasis on perforators, primary ablation of superficial reflux and use of a "pincer" injection technique to fill the entire plexus of veins. Further studies are needed to quantify the impact of this specific component of care, but this approach is logical, feasible and offers an excellent therapeutic option for patients with advanced venous skin changes and ulceration.

Summary

- Chronic venous ulcers are common, distressing, expensive to treat and increasing in prevalence due to an ageing and increasingly overweight population.

- The benefits of treating superficial reflux in patients with venous ulcers have been demonstrated unequivocally in a number of studies.

- Minimally invasive, endovenous techniques have superseded traditional venous surgery and are ideally suited for treating the elderly, frail leg ulcer population.

- The sub-ulcer venous plexus is a leash of tortuous, incompetent veins that are almost invariably present under an area of ulceration or severe skin damage. This may have an important role in transmitting venous hypertension to the ulcerated skin and therefore is a logical target for ablation.

- Effective ablation of the sub-ulcer venous plexus can be achieved using ultrasound guided foam sclerotherapy, with multiple injections to target the sub-ulcer area.

- Although there is a growing body of anecdotal evidence, studies are needed to define the additional benefit offered by sub-ulcer plexus sclerotherapy in addition to truncal venous ablation.

References

1. Rabe E, Guex JJ, Puskas A, Scuderi A, *et al*, VCP Coordinators. Epidemiology of chronic venous disorders in geographically diverse populations: results from the Vein Consult Program. *Int Angiol* 2012; **31**: 105–15.
2. Pannier F, Rabe E. The relevance of the natural history of varicose veins and refunded care. *Phlebology* 2012; **27** (Suppl 1): 23–26.

3. Wittens C, Davies AH, Bækgaard N, Broholm R, *et al.* Editor's Choice - Management of Chronic Venous Disease: Clinical Practice Guidelines of the European Society for Vascular Surgery (ESVS). *Eur J Vasc Endovasc Surg* 2015; **49**: 678–737.

4. O'Donnell TF, Passman MA. Clinical practice guidelines of the Society for Vascular Surgery (SVS) and the American Venous Forum (AVF)--Management of venous leg ulcers. Introduction. *J Vasc Surg* 2014; **60:** 1S–2S.

5. Gohel MS, Barwell JR, Taylor M, Chant T, *et al.* Long term results of compression therapy alone *versus* compression plus surgery in chronic venous ulceration (ESCHAR): randomised controlled trial. *BMJ* 2007; **335:** 83.

6. Kulkarni SR, Slim FJA, Emerson LG, *et al.* Effect of foam sclerotherapy on healing and long-term recurrence in chronic venous leg ulcers. *Phlebology* 2013; **28:** 140–46.

7. Pang KH, Bate GR, Darvall KAL, Adam DJ, *et al.* Healing and recurrence rates following ultrasound-guided foam sclerotherapy of superficial venous reflux in patients with chronic venous ulceration. *Eur J Vasc Endovasc Surg* 2010; **40:** 790–95.

8. Bush RG. New technique to heal venous ulcers: terminal interruption of the reflux source (TIRS). *Perspect Vasc Surg Endovasc Ther* 2010; **22:** 194–99.

Laser treatment of reticular and subcuticular veins

K Miyake

Introduction

"Aesthetic phlebology" is a new concept globally, but has been known for about half a century in Brazil. It involves treating veins and spider veins, particularly those in the legs and face—unsightly vessels can affect a patient's self-esteem and, therefore, their quality of life.

Often, in the same patient, lasers (or other techniques) can be an effective treatment for facial veins but not for treating similar veins in the legs. Therefore, this raises the question of why there is such a difference in treatment response with veins of apparently the same type.

The treatment of spider veins in the lower limbs is seen as something palliative and is often done by injection of sclerosing agents without any prior diagnosis. Worldwide, payment for sclerotherapy session is sometimes made through government or healthcare insurance; this limits investment in equipment for aesthetic phlebology and also makes it impossible to dedicate 10–20 minutes for a detailed comparative photo-documentation. There is also the need to separate sclerotherapy for treatment of disease (paid by healthcare insurance or government) and aesthetic treatment (paid by the patient). In this chapter, we discuss how diagnosis, classification and cryo laser and cryo sclerotherapy (CLaCS) treatment of telangiectasias and feeder vein(s)—connected or not to refluxing perforator vein(s) and/or saphenous vein(s)—leads to excellent results and low rate of recurrence.

Augmented reality and duplex scan

The use of augmented reality and duplex scan are substantial advances in aesthetic phlebology. Regardless of the technique of choice for telangiectasias and feeder veins, accurate diagnosis leads to better results and a lower complication rate. Augmented reality devices, such as the VeinViewer (VV, Christie), can help with the diagnostic process.

The VV was designed in 2004 to help venous punctures in the upper limbs. It brightens skin with infrared light, films it with an infrared camera, processes the data, and projects the image onto the skin in a fraction of a second delay. It enables you to see veins that are too shallow (e.g. 2–5mm in depth).

By combining real images with images processed by computer, the VV is classified as augmented reality.[1] Furthermore if the infrared light can reach the veins and go back to the infrared camera, the transdermal laser, and the much more intense and collimated laser, also will.

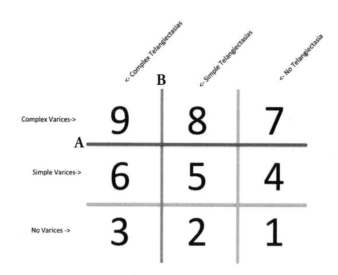

Figure 1: Score 9–1. Line (A) represents the duplex scan and the line (B) represents augmented reality. When there is no duplex scan or augmented reality, tourniquet, palpation, illumination, trans-illumination and treatment failure can be a resource to assist the Score 9–1.

Classification of the superficial venous lesions

The success in aesthetic treatment depends on the careful classification of lesions. Often the aesthetic vein lesions are just the "tip of the iceberg", and the differentiation between complex and simple telangiectasia is the most important concept for lower limbs telangiectasias treatment success. According to Hiroshi Miyake, there are three ways to diagnose complex telangiectasias: presence of at least one feeder vein visible to the naked eye; rapid refill of telangiectasias after the sudden digital decompression; and failure or low response to the treatment of telangiectasia. Therefore, to optimise treatment outcome, two questions should be asked—are there varicosities connected or not to an axial reflux (saphenous and/or perforating)? And, are there telangiectasias with or without feeder veins?[2,3]

From these questions, the 9–1 score was developed (Figure 1). Using this score, we can define the optimal therapeutic approach and monitor the progressive improvement afterwards. The score is not meant to replace the comprehensive classification system for chronic venous disorders (Clinical Etiology Anatomy Pathophysiology, CEAP) or the Validation of Venous Clinical Severity Score (VCSS).[4–13]

Value of photography

A photograph should be made with an at least semi-professional machine—digital single lens reflex (DSLR)—with an external flash. The flash head should be rotated 180 degrees and directed to the ceiling, which should be white. This way, using the automatic mode of the camera, we can obtain high-resolution photos without the need for photographic experience or expensive medical photo-documentation software/hardware. Two tablet devices (e.g. iPad, Apple) can be used to provide before and after comparisons. Patients frequently forget how the lesion looked prior to treatment; therefore, showing the comparison helps them to evaluate outcome. We strongly recommend at least 20 pre-treatment photos; at our clinic, we take about 40 pre-treatment photographs on average. Only the pre and post photo-documentation can give an objective evidence of the outcome. Neither the patient nor the doctor can appreciate the improvement without the use of photography (Figure 2).

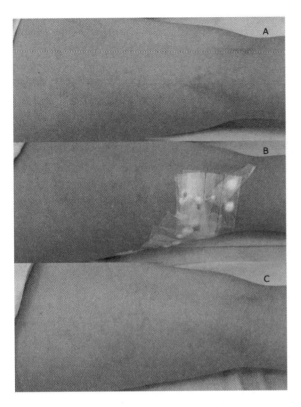

Figure 2: (A) Photograph before treatment; (B) photograph showing which veins received CLaCS; and (C) photograph after the patient returned one month after CLaCS. She was reporting that some veins on the back of her thigh did not respond but the photo (B) shows that only some veins of the back of her thigh were treated.

CLaCS guided by augmented reality

CLaCS is a new technique to treat the combination of telangiectasias and the associated causative reticular veins ("feeder veins") of the leg. It employs the following features: augmented reality viewing of the feeder veins; application of transdermal laser energy to the feeder veins and overlying telangiectasias; injection of the feeder vein and surface telangiectasias with a Dextrose 75%; and skin temperature protection and numbing of the skin with application of a flow of cold air throughout the procedure. A photograph is taken before and after the procedure in all patients at our clinic.

The purpose of CLaCS technique is to achieve efficacy through the synergy between the transdermal laser, injection sclerotherapy and skin cooling. The transdermal laser has the ability to perform selective photo-thermolysis (penetrate the skin, without damage, and injure the vein).[14] The vein contains oxy-haemoglobin and deoxy-haemoglobin, having a higher absorption coefficient compared with the skin.

Importantly, the transdermal laser and sclerotherapy with Dextrose 75% are just "supporting actors" in CLaCS. The main "actor" is the doctor. In 1995, when the pulsed light began to be studied and associated with sclerotherapy, it was proposed to use a synergy to obtain the final result.[15,16]

The ideal laser for CLaCS is the neodymium-doped yttrium aluminium garnet (ND: Yag 1064 (nm), long pulse (>15ms), large spot size (>5mm in diameter) laser. Such lasers typically have more than 1000W of power. Other lasers, such as 980nm wavelengths or small spot size lasers, have generally much less power (10–30W).

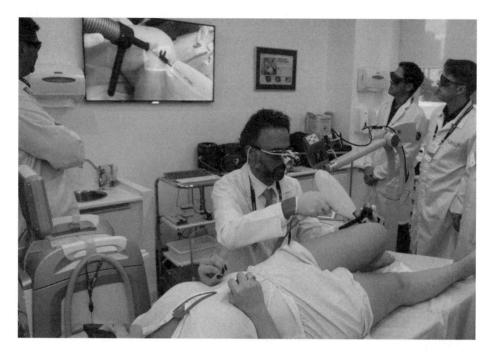

Figure 3: "Flebosuite" is a room prepared for diagnosis and aesthetic vein treatment. Ideally it should include photo equipment, duplex ultrasound, augmented reality, skin cooler, transdermal laser and magnification loupe. A complete flebosuite may also contain endovenous laser/radiofrequency equipment.

In CLaCS, the skin and the sclerosing agent are cooled by a cold air blower; skin cooling decreases pain both during laser and injection sclerotherapy. Low initial temperature also helps to protect the skin.[17–21]

At our clinic, we use the ND:Yag Harmony 1064nm transdermal laser set to a 6mm spot size, (average 70J/cm^2 fluency, and 15ms pulse width). Transdermal laser is directed at the feeder veins identified through augmented reality, overlying and nearby the telangiectasia vessels that are being targeted with transdermal laser (Figure 3). After a few minutes, we see a reduction of the internal diameter caused by tunica media swelling.[22,23] If there is no immediate collapse, each segment 5mm vein or telangiectasia receives at least two laser shots.

Sclerotherapy is made with Dextrose 75%, 3ml syringe and 27G needle (due to high viscosity with Dextrose 75%, it is difficult to inject with 30G needles). The use of 2.5x magnifying loupe is advised as with magnification, you are able to visualise the needle bevel filling with blood indicating the ideal injection point. After injection, a cotton ball is placed about 2–3mm and taped.

The effectiveness and safety of CLaCS

CLaCS results in partial or total injury in the tunica media and endothelium caused by transdermal laser and osmolar injury caused by Dextrose 75%. And with the synergy, laser injury, Dextrose 75% injury and oedema are caused by laser generating a trapping effect for the Dextrose 75%. This trapping causes longer Dextrose 75% contact time within the vein, increasing sclerotherapy effectiveness. The reduction of the internal diameter that may appear right after or minutes after transdermal laser and it also helps to lower pigmentation rates.

CLaCS complication rate is very low. According to a survey we conducted (November 2007 to March 2009 in 1,909 sessions), the rate of pigmentation was 0.67%; the rate of skin burn was 0.11%, and there were no reported skin ulcers, deep vein thromboses, embolism, neuro-functional disorders, anaphylaxis or deaths.

However, anecdotal reports suggest that there have been three deaths related to aesthetic treatment with foam sclerotherapy in Brazil. Unfortunately, such complications are not published in medical literature.

One of the biggest concerns with transdermal laser is the risk of burning. During the reported period in Clínica Miyake, we had just two minor cases of burnings caused by laser. One of them was a patient with Fitzpatrick 5 skin type where we started treatment with 60J/cm². In the popliteal fossa region, fine dermal "crustings" were observed after laser stacking. Those lesions disappeared after three months. The other case was a patient who was undergoing CLaCS and the air cooling device was not cold enough because of mechanical problems. One foot was treated without proper cooling and blisters were observed after some minutes. Such blisters generated light pigmentation that disappeared completely after six months. In both cases, the patients were happy with the result in other areas and did not complain about the temporary complication.

Discussion

Even if the patient is CEAP 1, duplex scanning, detailed photo-documentation and examination with augmented reality are mandatory. We have never used detergents or foam as we aim to have a zero risk of anaphylaxis or post-sclerotherapy skin ulcer.[24,25] CLaCS has been the method of choice for more than 10 years in our clinic (Figures 4 and 5).

The Score 9-1 system may be also used to determine if the case is functional, aesthetic or both. The scores "9, 8 and 7" are, in general, functional problems. Scores "6, 5, 4, 3 and 2" are "aesthetic". We use the word aesthetic because it helps both the physician and the patient to understand that treatment for these lesions should not be paid by government healthcare insurance. It is a cosmetic treatment, and should be paid for with the patient's own funds rather than insurance, just as breast augmentation or dermatologic rejuvenation treatments are. Therefore, the scores 9, 8 and 7 indicate the treatment of saphenous and/or perforating veins. Our treatment option is 1470nm double ring radial fibre endovenous laser. For scores 6, 5, 4, 3 and 2, we indicate CLaCS. The chance of obtaining success with CLaCS in this situation is about 90%. Average rate of clearance is over 75% after two

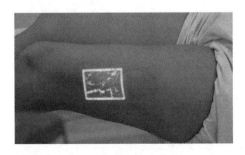

Figure 4: Augmented reality showing feeder veins in a Score 6 patient.

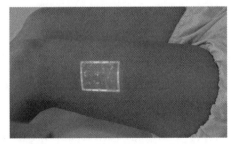

Figure 5: Same patient from figure 4 after three years (almost no recurrence).

sessions. Failure of the treatment occurs if the initial diagnosis was incorrect (e.g. undetected feeder veins and/or varicose veins with more than 2mm in diameter). In this situation, phlebectomy is indicated. Skin burning is easy to avoid because we have been using less energy at our clinic (50–70J/cm²) with multiple passes. By doing this, the treatment is also less painful.

We believe that the healthcare insurance companies and the government should only pay for surgery, endovenous laser, radiofrequency or sclerotherapy in Score 9, 8 and 7 cases—i.e. symptomatic cases. All of the rest of the cases should be considered private and thus aesthetic treatment; such an approach would help healthcare economics. The score 9-1 can be printed and shown to patients in order to help them understand what is functional and what is aesthetic.

Other forms of aesthetic treatment of varicose veins and sclerotherapy with detergents (foamed) are certainly not effective. CLaCS technique follows the principle of "*primum non nocere*" or "first, do no harm". While the cost of CLaCS equipment is high, the cost of a serious complication when it is the result of an aesthetic procedure is much higher.[26–33] For this reason, it is recommended to do CLaCS only with Dextrose 75%. If detergents (or just blending a small percentage of detergents or anaesthetics) are used, there is associated risk of anaphylaxis. It is important to remember that anaphylaxis is idiosyncratic. Thus, to have zero risk of anaphylaxis, Dextrose 75% should be the chosen sclerosing agent.[34]

Since 1984, at our clinic, we have not used detergents to do sclerotherapy; only Dextrose 75%. Prior to the creation of CLaCS (circa 2001), resilient telangiectasias were treated by phlebectomy of the feeder veins. Tedious palpation, illumination and treatment failure were the indicators of the presence of a feeder vein. Since 2005, CLaCS guided by augmented reality is our method of choice for 100% of our patients with score 6 or less.

The CLaCS can be used throughout the body. In the abdomen, lumbar area, reticular veins in breasts after breast implant and even some tortuous veins on hands. However, in the face, we just do cryo laser without cryo-sclerotherapy. The injection of sclerosing agents in facial veins can lead to cavernous sinus thrombosis, blindness and death.[35] Facial veins have no valves and respond better

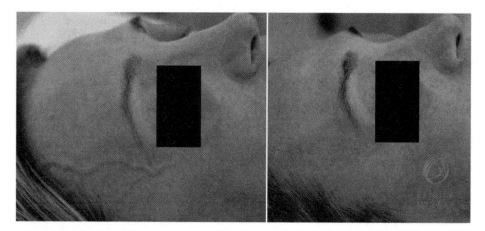

Figure 6: Facial vein treated with cryo laser after five sessions.

to transdermal laser due to the lower pressure regimen. Complete result may appear in one to five sessions (Figure 6).

Conclusion

Score 9-1 helps to increase diagnostic accuracy thus improving the result. Visualisation and treatment of feeder veins is key to produce optimal resolution on telangiectasia treatment and to prevent recurrences. Detailed photo-documentation should be mandatory in aesthetic phlebology. CLaCS technique is efficient and safe.

Summary

- Augmented reality helps diagnose feeder veins that may cause telangiectasia treatment failure.

- CLaCS is a synergy of a "medium power" thermal sclerosing method with a "medium power" injection sclerosing agent (Dextrose75%).

- One of CLaCS highlights is effectiveness due to vein edema and contraction caused by transdermal laser.

- The synergy between methods causes less trapped blood and thus very low hyperpigmentation rate.

- Photo-documentation should be mandatory in aesthetic phlebolgy (private practice).

- CLaCS is a combination of light, sugar and cold air.

References

1. Miyake RK, Zeman HD, Lovhoiden G, et al. Vein Imaging: A new method of Near infrared imaging, where a processed image is projected onto the skin for the enhancement of vein treatment. *Dermatol Surg* 2006; **32**: 1031–38.
2. Miyake RK, Duarte FH, Kikuchi R, Fidelis RJR. Escleroterapia intra-operatória no tratamento das telangiectasias combinadas. Há forma de prever o desaparecimento da lesão? Pan American Congress of Angiology e Vascular Surgery, Rio de Janeiro, 2002.
3. Miyake K. Prevalence of small varicosities among patients with or without telangiectasias on the lower limbs estimated by augmented reality examination. *Int Angiology* 2013; **32** (5) (Suppl 1): S124.
4. Eklöf B, Rutherford RB, Bergan JJ, et al. American Venous Forum International Ad Hoc Committee for Revision of the CEAP Classification. Revision of the CEAP classification for chronic venous disorders: consensus statement. *J Vasc Surg* 2004; **40** (6): 1248–52.
5. Allegra C, Antignani PL, Bergan JJ, et al. International Union of Phlebology Working Group. The "C" of CEAP: suggested definitions and refinements: an International Union of Phlebology conference of experts. *J Vasc Surg* 2003; **37** (1): 129–31.
6. Moneta GL. Regarding "The 'C' of CEAP: suggested definitions and refinements: an International Union of Phlebology conference of experts". *J Vasc Surg* 2003; 37 (1): 224–25.
7. Kistner RL. Definitive diagnosis and definitive treatment in chronic venous disease: a concept whose time has come. *J Vasc Surg* 1996; **24** (5): 703–10.
8. Kistner RL, Eklof B, Masuda EM. Diagnosis of chronic venous disease of the lower extremities: the "CEAP" classification. *Mayo Clin Proc* 1996; **71** (4): 338–45.
9. Rutherford RB, Padberg FT Jr, Comerota AJ, et al. Venous severity scoring: An adjunct to venous outcome assessment. *J Vasc Surg* 2000; **31** (6): 1307–12.
10. Kakkos SK, Rivera MA, Matsagas MI, Lazarides MK, Robless P, Belcaro G, Geroulakos G. Validation of the new venous severity scoring system in varicose vein surgery. *J Vasc Surg*; 2003; **38** (2): 224–28.

11. Perrin M, Dedieu F, Jessent V, Blank MP. Evaluation of the new severity scoring in chronic venous disease of the lower limbs: an observational survey conducted by French angiologists. *Phlebologie* 2003; **56:** 127–36.

12. Perrin MR, Guex JJ, Ruckley CV, *et al.* Recurrent varices after surgery (REVAS), a consensus document. REVAS group. *Cardiovasc Surg* 2000; **8** (4): 233–45.

13. Beebe HG, Bergan JJ, Bergqvist D, *et al.* Classification and grading of chronic venous disease in the lower limbs. A consensus statement. *Eur J Vasc Endovasc Surg* 1996; **12** (4): 487–91.

14. Anderson RR, Parrish JA. Selective photothermolisis: precise microsurgery by selective absorption of pulsed radiation. *Science* 1983; **220:** 524–27.

15. Miyake RK. Fatores preditivos da lesão cutânea por luz intensa pulsada. (Tese de Doutorado). São Paulo: Faculdade de Medicina da Universidade de São Paulo, 1999. p47.

16. Miyake RK, Kauffman P, Miyake H. Skin temperature measurements during intense pulsed light emission. *Dermatol Surg* 2001; **27:** 549–54.

17. Miyake RK, Duarte FH, Fidelis RJ, *et al.* Pain reduction using cooled forced air at -20°C during laser and injection sclerotherapy. *Lasers Surg Med* 2006; **16** (suppl): 69.

18. Miyake RK, Duarte FH, Fidelis RJ, Miyake H. New leg veins air cooled treatment using 1064nm laser combined with sclerotherapy. Technique description and one year follow-up. *Las Med Sci* 2003; **18:** S22.

19. Rivello T. A crioterapia no tratamento das varizes de membros inferiores. In: VI Jornada Brasileira de Angiologia e Cirurgia Vascular. Hospital Naval Marcílio Dias. Rio de Janeiro, 1986.

20. Francischeli M. Tese defendida na Faculdade de Medicina da Universidade de São Paulo para a obtenção do título de doutor.

21. Miyake RK, Duarte FH, Kikuchi R, Fidelis RJR. Pain reduction using cooled forced air at -20°C during laser and sclerotherapy. In anais of American Society of Laser in Medicine Surgery, Dallas, 2002.

22. Miyake RK, Miyake H, Telles MA, *et al.* Avaliação anatomopatológica do efeito do laser "Vasculight" (1.064 nm) sobre microvarizes. In: Resumos. XXXIII Congresso Brasileiro de Angiologia e Cirurgia Vascular. Belo Horizonte, 1999; **60**.

23. Miyake RK. Cryo-Laser and Cryo-Sclerotherapy guided by augmented reality. Report of 140 Cases. *Phlebologie* 2014; **5;** 257–61.

24. Miyake H. Necroses cutâneas provocadas por injeções de substâncias esclerosantes utilizadas no tratamento de microvarizes e telangiectasias: estudo experimental (Tese de Doutorado). São Paulo: Faculdade de Medicina da Universidade de São Paulo, 1972;.

25. Miyake RK, King JT, Kikuchi R, Duarte FH, Davidson JRP, Oba C. Role of injection pressure, flow and sclerosant viscosity in causing cutaneous ulceration during sclerotherapy. *Phlebology* 2012; **27:** 383–89.

26. Hagen PT, Scholz DG, Edward WD. Incidence and size of patent foramen ovale during the first 10 decades of life: an autopsy study of 965 normal hearts. *Mayo Clin Proc* 1984; **59:** 17.

27. Forlee MV, Grouden M, Moore DJ, Shanik G. Stroke after varicose vein foam injection sclerotherapy. *J Vasc Surg* 2006; **43** (1): 162–64.

28. Morrison N, Cavezzi A, Bergan J, Partsch H. Regarding "Stroke after varicose vein foam injection sclerotherapy". *J Vasc Surg* 2006; **44** (1): 224–26.

29. Asbjornsen CB, Rogers CD, Russel BL. Middle cerebral air embolism after foam sclerotherapy. *Phlebology* 2012; **8:** 430–33.

30. Parsi K. Paradoxical embolism, stroke and sclerotherapy. *Phlebology* 2012; **27** (4): 147-67.

31. Bergan J, Pascarella L, Mekenas L. In Venous disorders: treatment with sclerosant foam. *J Cardiovasc Surg* 2006; **47** (1): 9–18.

32. Paysant F, Baert A, Morel I, *et al.* Case of death occurred after an injection of aetoxisclerol. The responsibility of the product should be discussed. *Acta Clin Belg Suppl* 2006; **1:** 51–53.

33. Lewis KM. Anaphylaxis due to sodium morrhuate. *JAMA* 1936; **107** (1): 298.

34. Miyake K. Case Report of 195 Patients Classified by Duplex Scanning and Augmented Reality, and Treated by Cryo-Laser & Cryo-Sclerotherapy: Results and Complications. *Int Angiol* 2013; **32** (5) (Suppl 1): S153.

35. Hoffman K. An unusual complication of facial sclerotherapy. *Dermatol Surg* 2003; **29** (4): 423–24.

Evidence of choice of sclerosant for treatment of telangiectasia

G Dovell and S Ashley

Introduction

Telangiectasias are a confluence of unsightly dilated intradermal venules that are less than 1mm in diameter. Commonly found on the lower extremities, they are synonymous with spider veins, hyphen webs and thread veins. The word telangiectasia is derived from the greek for "end" (telos), "vessel" (angeion) and "dilation" (ektasis).[1] Telangiectasias are, for the most part, asymptomatic, but may present with throbbing or aching pain, itching and inflammation, or with cosmetic concerns. They may be associated with concurrent superficial venous reflux and varicose veins.[2,3]

It has been hypothesised that the underlying pathophysiology of telangiectasias is similar to that of varicose veins, in that venous hypertension leads to valvular damage, reflux and venous dilatation. It has also been suggested that local cellular inflammatory processes in the endothelium, and vascular neogenesis in response to hypoxia, may have a role. Despite these hypotheses the exact pathophysiology remains unknown.[4] Studies suggest that between 50% and 77% of patients with telangiectasias have no significant underlying chronic venous disease, suggesting that venous hypertension and reflux alone cannot account for the aetiology.[3,5,6]

Telangiectasias are extremely common. Epidemiological studies suggest that the majority of adults will develop them throughout their life, and that women are more likely to develop telangiectasias than men.[3,5] Risk factors identified for telangiectasias include increasing age, family history, lax connective tissue, prolonged standing, high body mass index (BMI), smoking, sedentary lifestyle, topical steroids, trauma in the affected area, previous venous thrombosis (superficial or deep), arterio-venous shunting, hereditary conditions (hereditary haemorrhagic telangiectasia, Osler Webber Rendu), exposure to female hormones and pregnancy.[4, 5,7,8]

Telangiectasias are classified by the "CEAP" (Cinical, Etiology, Anatomy, Pathophysiology) classification for chronic venous disease, which was developed in 1994 and updated in 2004 by Eklof et al.[9] It consists of seven major categories (0–6) classifying venous disease based upon clinical examination. Telangiectasias are classified as category one, alongside the larger subdermal reticular veins.[10]

Sclerotherapy has been used for centuries, but there remains no overwhelming consensus as to the ideal sclerosant for the treatment of telangiectasias.[1,4]

Sclerotherapy

Sclerotherapy is still considered the "gold standard" first-line technique in the treatment of telangiectasias.[11] It involves injection of a "sclerosing agent" into the target vessel. Often referred to as "microsclerotherapy" or "micro-injection sclerotherapy", this is usually performed under direct vision with the aid of magnification. The sclerosing agent causes endothelial damage to the vessels leading to inflammation, thrombus formation, collapse and fibrosis of the vein.[1] The majority of patients seek treatment for cosmetic reasons. Therefore, the ideal sclerosing agent would cause complete vessel destruction and resolution of symptoms with minimal side effects as well as being a cost effective solution.

There are three main categories of sclerosant; detergents, osmotic agents and chemical irritants/corrosives. Detergents (for example, polidocanol or sodium tetradecyl sulphate) form micelles due to their hydrophobic and hydrophilic poles. These micelles cause endothelial injury by altering the surface tension around cells. Osmotic agents (hypertonic saline or dextrose saline) cause endothelial injury by dehydration and chemical irritants (chromated glycerine and glycerine) have a corrosive effect directly on the endothelium by cauterisation.[1,12]

There are four main sclerosing agents commonly used in the treatment of telangiectasias. These are hypertonic saline, sodium tetradecyl sulphate, polidocanol and glycerine. Sodium tetradecyl sulphate is US Food and Drug Administration (FDA) approved, and the only drug discussed here which is licensed for use in the UK. Polidocanol has recently gained FDA approval. However, these sclerosants are used widely "off-licence" in North America, the UK and across Europe.[12]

Choice of sclerosant—efficacy

There is clear evidence within the literature that the use of sclerotherapy is superior to placebo in the treatment of telangiectasias. This is demonstrated both in physician assessed trials (blinded and un-blinded) and in those assessed by patient satisfaction.[1,13–15] Polidocanol and sodium tetradecyl sulphate have been most extensively compared in the literature.

A 1987 study by Carlin compared heparsal (hypertonic saline), sodium tetradecyl sulphate, polidocanol and normal saline as sclerosants for telangiectasias.[13] This was a prospective, split body (four quadrant) 20-patient trial. Outcome was measured by improvement scores by the treating physician, and a statistically significant difference was demonstrated between treatment with sclerotherapy compared with normal saline (p=0.0001).

This is supported by two further studies. Firstly, Kahle in 2006 compared polidocanol and normal saline; this single blinded trial compared 48 patients randomised to either polidocanol or normal saline.[14] Outcomes were measured by two blinded consultants. They scored the results based upon photographs, and demonstrated there was a statistically significant difference in the treatment of telangiectasias with polidocanol (p=0.0013). Patients were also more satisfied following treatment with polidocanol, but a statistical analysis was not carried out on these scores. Secondly, Rabe in 2010—in a study commissioned by Kreussler pharmaceuticals—conducted a double blind, randomised, prospective, multicentre trial which recruited 157 patients. Results demonstrated a significant difference between polidocanol and sodium tetradecyl sulphate *versus* placebo (p≤0.0001).[15]

Polidocanol has been compared in foam *versus* liquid form by Benigni in 1999, this was a small (24 patients) pilot study, and no significant statistical workings were carried out.[16] This left insufficient information to conclude about the differences in foam or liquid microsclerotherapy from that study alone.

Different polidocanol concentrations have been compared by a 20-patient, randomised, split body, non-blinded trial conducted by Norris in 1989.[17] Reported outcomes included visual assessments of physicians, as well as patient satisfaction. There was no significant statistical difference found between the efficacies of the concentrations of polidocanol. A significant difference was found in the degree of hyperpigmentation caused by a 1% *versus* a 0.25% solution. Eighty per cent of patients were satisfied or very satisfied with their treatment, suggesting efficacy at the 0.25% concentration.

There is no sound evidence to support the use of one sclerosant over another. Furthermore, the patient numbers used in the studies to date are small and do not have the power to demonstrate significant differences between the sclerosants.[1]

As previously discussed, Carlin in 1987 demonstrated no significant difference in polidocanol, sodium tetradecyl sulphate or heparsal (hypertonic saline) as sclerosant agents.[13] McCoy in 1999 compared polidocanol and hypertonic saline in a randomised, split body trial, which included 81 patients.[18] The treating physician was un-blinded, and efficacy was measured by the un-blinded and by a blinded doctor. In the un-blinded assessment there was no significant difference in improvement scores (p=0.05) but in the blinded assessment there was a statistically significant difference (p=0.04). This trial presents conflicting evidence and suggests an element of bias in the study.[1] Patient satisfaction was also measured in this trial, and there was no statistically significant difference in patient satisfaction between the two agents.

In 2002 Goldman conducted a double blind, prospective, comparative trial of 42 patients. They were treated with polidocanol and sodium tetradecyl sulphate on either leg.[19] Confusingly, there is discrepancy in the data presented, and the number of patients included *versus* the outcomes did not add up.[1] This inconsistency could not be tracked in the methodology. Regardless, no significant difference was found between polidocanol (0.25%) and sodium tetradecyl sulphate (0.5%). Satisfaction was presented as 70% and 72% respectively suggesting no difference between these two agents.[19]

In a very small study in 2003 by Leach, sodium tetradecyl sulphate was compared with glycerine.[20] Thirteen patients were included in this split-body trial. Seven out of 13 patients achieved clearance of vessels with glycerine, but only one out of 13 achieved vessel clearance with sodium tetradecyl sulphate. The study size was too small to make meaningful conclusions, and no statistical analysis was undertaken.

Prescott compared sodium tetradecyl sulphate and hypertonic dextrose in 1992 in a 60-patient comparative study.[21] The authors reported the average clearance of telangiectasias as 70% for each sclerosant, but also noted that it took 61% more treatments for hypertonic dextrose to achieve the same clearance as sodium tetradecyl sulphate.

Further difficulties are encountered when trying to make sense of the literature. The assessment of the efficacy of sclerosants is not standardised throughout the literature and often un-blinded clinicians are used to assess outcome. Also, despite treatment being sought primarily for cosmetic reasons within a private practice setting, assessment of patient satisfaction is often lacking. Treatment length and numbers of sclerotherapy sessions were only compared in one trial, and injection technique, although well documented to lead to adverse effects and poor outcome in the sclerosant treatment of varicose veins, is not cited as a potentially confounding factor in the outcome of microsclerotherapy treatment for telangiectasias.

In summary, a Cochrane review of the literature in 2011 concluded "the evidence did not suggest superior efficacy or patient satisfaction for any one sclerosing agent".[1]

Choice of sclerosant—adverse effects

Data for the adverse effects of sclerosants is well documented for each individual sclerosant in the treatment of varicose veins. However, the literature poorly records the complications that are specifically associated with sclerotherapy for telangiectasias.[1]

Some of the most commonly observed side effects of microsclerotherapy treatment are pain at the injection site, telangiectatic matting and hyperpigmentation.

Pain at the sclerotherapy injection site is a common side effect of treatment, and many patients report minor pain. Severe pain is most often associated with extravasation or extra-vascular injection of the sclerosant agent. The literature suggests that polidocanol is the least painful in treatment of telangiectasias; both Carlin in 1987 and McCoy in 1999 demonstrated a statistically significant difference in the degree of pain experienced by patients when polidocanol was used, compared with sodium tetradecyl sulphate and hypertonic saline respectively (p=0.007, p=0.00001).[13,18]

Telangiectatic matting is a phenomenon whereby multiple fine dilated vessels occur in the region of the injection site. It is common and has been seen to occur at up to 24% of injection sites.[22] It usually resolves over the coming months, and in a large retrospective study in 1990 containing 2,120 patients it was observed that there were significantly more overweight patients, on female hormones, with positive family history, and a long disease course in the group that developed telangiectatic matting. The results were not separated for telangiectasias and sclerotherapy for larger veins, however, it suggests multiple confounding variables other than sclerosant choice in the development of telangiectatic matting. It has been suggested that sodium tetradecyl sulphate has been associated with a lower incidence of telangiectatic matting in the treatment of varicose veins but this has not been demonstrated for telangiectasias.[22] McCoy in 1999 reported a statistically significant difference (p=0.04) in telangiectatic matting with use of hypertonic saline when compared to polidocanol.[18] However, the dose of polidocanol used in this study was 1%, a dose not commonly used in clinical practice and, as Norris demonstrated in 1989, side effects increased with increasing doses of polidocanol.[17] Therefore, there is currently no sound evidence on which to conclude that any one sclerosant causes more telangiectatic matting than another.

Hyperpigmentation is the brownish discolouration of skin, surrounding injected areas following microsclerotherapy. It occurs due to extravasation of red blood cells leading to haemosiderin deposition. It usually arises a month or so following sclerotherapy. Again, limited evidence is available to suggest which sclerosant causes the least amount of hyperpigmentation in the treatment of telangiectasias. However, in the treatment of varicose veins it has been suggested that sodium tetradecyl sulphate is associated with less hyperpigmentation.[23] There is some evidence to show that there is statistically more hyperpigmentation when concentrations of 1% polidocanol are used compared with 0.25%, with no difference to patient satisfaction suggesting that the lower concentration is more favourable.[17] McCoy's paper suggested that there was statistically more hyperpigmentation with polidocanol than hypertonic saline, but this paper used 1% polidocanol for comparison, which, as previously discussed, is associated with increased hyperpigmentation.[18]

Injection site skin ulceration is another potential, albeit rare, complication that can arise when sclerosant extravasates into the surrounding tissue and/or an arteriolar vessel is inadvertently injected. Operator technique has a large part to play in its occurrence. Both hypertonic saline and sodium tetradecyl sulphate can cause skin ulceration but polidocanol is rarely associated with this due to its non-toxic properties.[19] However, there is insufficient evidence to determine the frequency of occurrence of ulceration between different sclerosants.

Sclerotherapy for varicose veins is associated with other systemic complications, for example anaphylaxis (which all sclerosants apart from hypertonic saline may cause), deep vein thrombosis, and neurological sequelae. The latter are largely theoretical as telangiectasias can communicate with the deep venous system, but there was no evidence of these complications in the literature.[1,13–19]

Conclusion

There is clear evidence that sclerotherapy is superior to placebo in the treatment of telangiectasia; however, there is no data to support the use of one particular sclerosant over another. There is some data to suggest that polidocanol is less painful on injection than sodium tetradecyl sulphate or hypertonic saline, but no other significant difference in side effect profile other than those deduced from the treatment of varicose veins. No allowance is made in the literature for operator skill, and there is no way of identifying the extent to which the results might have been influenced by poor technique. More studies need to be conducted in the field of sclerotherapy and specifically microsclerotherapy for telangiectasias. Ideally, in order to compare the preferred sclerosant for treatment of telangiectasias, a double-blind randomised controlled trial should be performed. This will be a challenge to undertake as within the UK, and many other countries, telangiectasias are primarily treated within a private practice setting to improve cosmesis.

Summary

- There is good evidence for use of sclerosant over placebo in the treatment of telangiectasias.

- Currently there is no evidence to favour the use of one particular sclerosant over another in the treatment of telangiectasias.

- Further high-quality trials are needed to determine the preferred choice of sclerosant for the treatment of telangiectasias.

References

1. Schwartz L, Maxwell H. Sclerotherapy for lower limb telangiectasias. The Cochrane Collaboration 2011; doi:10.1002/14651858.CD008826.pub2
2. Langer RD, Ho E, Denenberg JO, et al. Relationships between symptoms and venous disease: the San Diego population study. Arch Intern Med 2005; **165**: 1420.

3. Criqui MH, Jamosmos M, Fronek A, *et al.* Chronic venous disease in an ethnically diverse population: the San Diego Population Study. *Am J Epidemiol* 2003; **158**: 448.

4. Goldman MP, Bergan JJ, Guex JJ. Sclerotherapy Treatment of Varicose and Telangiectatic Leg Veins. Fourth Edition. Mosby Elsevier Inc 2007.

5. Chiesa R, Marone EM, Limoni C, *et al.* Chronic venous disorders: correlation between visible signs, symptoms, and presence of functional disease. *J Vasc Surg* 2007; **46**: 322.

6. Thibault PK, Lewis WA. Recurrent varicose veins part 1: evaluation utilizing duplex venous imaging. *The Journal of Dermatologic Surgery and Oncology* 1992; **18** (7): 618–24.

7. Brand FN, Dannenberg AL, Abbott RD, *et al.* The epidemiology of varicose veins: the Framingham Study. *Am J Prev Med* 1988; **4**: 96.

8. Callam MJ. Epidemiology of varicose veins. *Br J Surg* 1994; 81: 167.

9. Eklöf B, Rutherford RB, Bergan JJ, *et al.* Revision of the CEAP classification for chronic venous disorders: consensus statement. *J Vasc Surg* 2004; **40**: 1248.

10. Eklof B, Perrin M, Delis KT, *et al.* Updated terminology of chronic venous disorders: the VEIN-TERM transatlantic interdisciplinary consensus document. *J Vasc Surg* 2009; **49**: 498.

11. Sadick N, Sorhaindo L. "15. Laser Treatment of Telangiectatic and Reticular Veins". The Vein Book. Amsterdam: Elsevier Academic Press 2014.

12. Worthington-Kirsch R L. Injection Sclerotherapy. Semin Intervent Radiol 2005; **22**: 209–17. doi:10.1055/s-2005-921954

13. Carlin MC, Ratz JL. Treatment of telangiectasia: comparison of sclerosing agents. *Journal of Dermatologic Surgery and Oncology* 1987; **13**: 1181–84.

14. Kahle B, Leng K. Efficiency of sclerotherapy of spider leg veins: A prospective, randomized, double-blind, placebocontrolled study. *Vasomed* 2006; **18**: 146.

15. Rabe E, Schliephake D, Otto J, *et al.* Sclerotherapy of telangiectases and reticular veins: a doubleblind, randomized, comparative clinical trial of polidocanol, sodium tetradecyl sulphate and isotonic saline (EASI study). *Phlebology* 2010; **25**: 124–31.

16. Benigni JP, Sadoun S, Thirion V, *et al.* Telangiectases and reticular veins treatment with a 0.25% aetoxisclerol foam. Presentation of a pilot study. *Phlébologie* 1999; **52**: 283–90.

17. Norris MJ, Carlin MC, Ratz JL. Treatment of essential telangiectasia: effects of increasing concentrations of polidocanol. *Journal of the American Academy of Dermatology* 1989; **20**: 643–49.

18. McCoy S, Evans A, Spurrier N. Sclerotherapy for leg telangiectasia - A blinded comparative trial of polidocanol and hypertonic saline. *Dermatologic Surgery* 1999; **25**: 381–86.

19. Goldman MP. Treatment of varicose and telangiectatic leg veins: double-blind prospective comparative trial between aethoxyskerol and sotradecol. *Dermatologic Surgery* 2002; **28**: 52–55

20. Leach BC, Goldman MP. Comparative trial between sodium tetradecyl sulfate and glycerin in the treatment of telangiectatic leg veins. *Dermatologic Surgery* 2003; **29**: 612–14.

21. Prescott RJ. A comparative study of two sclerosing agents in the treatment of telangiectasias. Phlebology '92. Paris: John Libbey Eurotext 1992; **2**: 803–4.

22. Davis LT, Duffy DM. Determination of incidence and risk factors for postsclerotherapy telangiectatic matting of the lower extremity: a retrospective analysis. *J Dermatol Surg Oncol* 1990; **16**: 327.

23. Tisi PV, Beverley C, Rees A. Injection sclerotherapy for varicose veins. Cochrane Database Syst Rev 2006; CD001732.